Infection Control in the Intensive Care Unit

H. K. F. van Saene · L. Silvestri
M. A. de la Cal · A. Gullo
Editors

Infection Control in the Intensive Care Unit

Third Edition

Foreword by Julian Bion

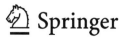
Springer

H. K. F. van Saene
Institute of Aging and Chronic Diseases
University of Liverpool
Liverpool
UK

L. Silvestri
Department of Emergency and Unit of
  Anesthesia and Intensive Care
Presidio Ospedaliero di Gorizia
Gorizia
Italy

M. A. de la Cal
Department of Intensive Care Medicine
Hospital Universitario de Getafe
Getafe, Madrid
Spain

A. Gullo
Department of Anesthesia
  and Intensive Care
School of Medicine
University Hospital Catania
Catania
Italy

ISBN 978-88-470-1600-2   e-ISBN 978-88-470-1601-9
DOI 10.1007/978-88-470-1601-9
Springer Milan Heidelberg Dordrecht London New York

Library of Congress Control Number: 2011929635

© Springer-Verlag Italia 1998, 2005, 2012

This work is subject to copyright. All rights are reserved, whether the whole or part of the material is concerned, specifically the rights of translation, reprinting, reuse of illustrations, recitation, broadcasting, reproduction on microfilm or in any other way, and storage in data banks. Duplication of this publication or parts thereof is permitted only under the provisions of the Italian Copyright Law in its current version, and permission for use must always be obtained from Springer. Violations are liable to prosecution under the Italian Copyright Law.

The use of general descriptive names, registered names, trademarks, etc. in this publication does not imply, even in the absence of a specific statement, that such names are exempt from the relevant protective laws and regulations and therefore free for general use.

Product liability: The publishers cannot guarantee the accuracy of any information about dosage and application contained in this book. In every individual case the user must check such information by consulting the relevant literature.

Printed on acid-free paper

Springer is part of Springer Science+Business Media (www.springer.com)

*The essential of intensive care is the
prevention of complications*
　　　　　C. P. Stoutenbeek 1947–1998

Foreword

In 1847, Ignatius Semmelweis's friend and colleague Jakob Kolletschka died of sepsis after his finger had been cut during a post-mortem examination at the Allgemeine Krankenhaus in Vienna. Semmelweis made the connection between the process which caused the death of his friend, and that which caused the postpartum deaths of so many of the mothers in his obstetric clinic at the hospital. His study of the prevention of puerperal sepsis through effective hand hygiene, and his subsequent career, are classical examples of how inspired insight may fail to be translated into effective action because of defective communication, professional resistance to change, cultural incomprehension that beneficent individuals could also be agents of harm, and lack of an underpinning scientific mechanism.

No such criticisms can be made of the editors and contributors for this valuable and successful book, now in its third edition, which brings together international experts in infection and infection control to review the most recent scientific evidence in preventing critically ill patients from suffering additional harm through the acquisition of autogenous and exogenous infections during their hospital stay. Wider attitudes to one of the components discussed, selective digestive decontamination, do bear some comparison with the Semmelweis story in terms of the gap between the scientific evidence and implementation in practice. Future editions of this book will no doubt contain additional reflections from the behavioural sciences. In the meantime, intensive care and infection control practitioners will find both fact and wisdom in this compendium to guide their practice and improve patient care.

November 2011

Julian Bion
Professor of Intensive Care Medicine
University Department of Anaesthesia and ICM
Queen Elizabeth Hospital
Edgbaston, Birmingham, UK

Preface

A week-long postgraduate course was organised in Trieste, Italy, in 1994. This course was extremely popular Europe wide. Participants were so impressed that they asked for copies of the lectures, and as a result of the many requests, lecturers were asked to provide a manuscript of their lecture(s). These manuscripts resulted in the first edition of this book, published in 1998.

This first edition contained five sections, each based on a day of the course, which comprised six lectures. The five sections Essentials in Clinical Microbiology, Antimicrobials, Infection Control, Infections on ICU, and Special Topics. The format remains the same today.

There are two previous editions to this 2011 edition: 1998 and 2005. The differences between the first edition and this latest one are in the first and last sections. Two chapters from the first edition are merged in the first section: Carriage, and Colonisation and Infection. This occurred because 85% of all infections are endogenous and characterised by these three stages. The other difference is a chapter on microcirculation and infection in Section 5. Perhaps the most important difference between the previous editions and this most recent edition is pictured on the front cover: 15% of all infections are exogenous, and research over the 6 years since the last edition has shown that topically applied antimicrobials are able to control exogenous infections. However, topically applied antimicrobials should only be part of the prophylactic protocol when exogenous infections are endemic.

This third edition is current, with references to publications from 2011. We regard it as important that all statements are justified by the best available evidence. All authors have made efforts to avoid unsubstantiated expert opinion. Although prevention is not entirely separate from therapy, prevention rather than cure is pivotal in this publication.

We are grateful to Donatella Rizza, Catherine Mazars and Hilde Haala for the their superb assistance. We hope that this third edition is instructive, and helpful in your daily practice and that you enjoy it.

November 2011

H. K. F. van Saene
L. Silvestri
M. A. de la Cal
A. Gullo

Contents

Part I Essentials in Clinical Microbiology

1 **Glossary of Terms and Definitions** 3
   R. E. Sarginson, N. Taylor, M. A. de la Cal
   and H. K. F. van Saene

2 **Carriage, Colonization and Infection** 17
   L. Silvestri, H. K. F. van Saene and J. J. M. van Saene

3 **Classification of Microorganisms According
   to Their Pathogenicity** 29
   M. A. de la Cal, E. Cerdà, A. Abella and P. Garcia-Hierro

4 **Classification of ICU Infections** 41
   L. Silvestri, H. K. F. van Saene and A. J. Petros

5 **Gut Microbiology: Surveillance Samples for Detecting
   the Abnormal Carrier State in Overgrowth** 53
   H. K. F. van Saene, G. Riepi, P. Garcia-Hierro,
   B. Ramos and A. Budimir

Part II Antimicrobials

6 **Systemic Antibiotics** 67
   A. R. De Gaudio, S. Rinaldi and C. Adembri

7 **Systemic Antifungals** 99
   C. J. Collins and Th. R. Rogers

8	**Enteral Antimicrobials**	123

M. Sánchez García, M. Nieto Cabrera, M. A. González Gallego and F. Martínez Sagasti

Part III Infection Control

9	**Evidence-Based Infection Control in the Intensive Care Unit**	145

J. Hughes and R. P. Cooke

10	**Device Policies**	159

A. R. De Gaudio, A. Casini and A. Di Filippo

11	**Antibiotic Policies in the Intensive Care Unit**	173

H. K. F. van Saene, N. J. Reilly, A. de Silvestre and F. Rios

12	**Outbreaks of Infection in the ICU: What's up at the Beginning of the Twenty-First Century?**	189

V. Damjanovic, N. Taylor, T. Williets and H. K. F. van Saene

13	**Preventing Infection Using Selective Decontamination of the Digestive Tract**	203

L. Silvestri, H. K. F. van Saene and D. F. Zandstra

Part IV Infections on ICU

14	**Lower Airway Infection**	219

J. Almirall, A. Liapikou, M. Ferrer and A. Torres

15	**Bloodstream Infection in the ICU Patient**	233

J. Vallés and R. Ferrer

16	**Infections of Peritoneum, Mediastinum, Pleura, Wounds, and Urinary Tract**	251

G. Sganga, G. Brisinda, V. Cozza and M. Castagneto

17	**Infection in the NICU and PICU**	289

A. J. Petros, V. Damjanovic, A. Pigna and J. Farias

18	**Early Adequate Antibiotic Therapy**	305

R. Reina and M. A. de la Cal

19	**ICU Patients Following Transplantation**	315
	A. Martinez-Pellus and I. Cortés Puch	
20	**Clinical Virology in NICU, PICU and AICU**	333
	C. Y. W. Tong and S. Schelenz	
21	**AIDS Patients in the ICU**	353
	F. E. Arancibia and M. A. Aguayo	
22	**Therapy of Infection in the ICU**	373
	J. H. Rommes, N. Taylor and L. Silvestri	

Part V Special Topics

23	**The Gut in the Critically Ill: Central Organ in Abnormal Microbiological Carriage, Infections, Systemic Inflammation, Microcirculatory Failure, and MODS**	391
	D. F. Zandstra, H. K. F. van Saene and R. E. Sarginson	
24	**Nonantibiotic Measures to Control Ventilator-Associated Pneumonia**	401
	A. Gullo, A. Paratore and C. M. Celestre	
25	**Impact of Nutritional Route on Infections: Parenteral Versus Enteral**	411
	A. Gullo, C. M. Celestre and A. Paratore	
26	**Gut Mucosal Protection in the Critically Ill Patient: Toward an Integrated Clinical Strategy.**	423
	D. F. Zandstra, P. H. J. van der Voort, K. Thorburn and H. K. F. van Saene	
27	**Selective Decontamination of the Digestive Tract: Role of the Pharmacist**	433
	N. J. Reilly, A. J. Nunn and K. Pollock	
28	**Antimicrobial Resistance**	451
	N. Taylor, I. Cortés Puch, L. Silvestri, D. F. Zandstra and H. K. F. van Saene	

29 ICU-Acquired Infection: Mortality, Morbidity, and Costs 469
J. C. Marshall and K. A. M. Marshall

30 Evidence-Based Medicine in ICU 485
A. J. Petros, K. G. Lowry, H. K. F. van Saene and J. C. Marshall

Index 507

Contributors

A. Abella Department of Intensive Care Medicine, Hospital Universitario de Getafe, Madrid, Spain

C. Adembri Section of Anesthesiology and Intensive Care, Department of Medical and Surgical Critical Care, University of Florence, Azienda Ospedaliero-Universitaria Careggi, Florence, Italy

M. A. Aguayo Unidad de Cuidados Intensivos, Instituto Nacional Tórax, Santiago, Chile

J. Almirall PhD, MD Pneumology, Consorci Sanitari del Maresme, Barcelona, Spain

F. E. Arancibia Unidad de Cuidados Intensivos, Instituto Nacional Tórax, Santiago, Chile

G. Brisinda Istituto di Clinica Chirurgica, Università Cattolica del Sacro Cuore, Rome, Italy

A. Budimir Department for Clinical and Molecular Microbiology, University of Zagreb School of Medicine, University Hospital Centre Zagreb, Zagreb, Croatia

A. Casini MD Careggi Teaching Hospital, Section of Anaesthesia, Department of Critical Care, University of Florence, Florence, Italy

M. Castagneto Istituto di Clinica Chirurgica, Università Cattolica del Sacro Cuore, Rome, Italy

C. M. Celestre MD Department of Anesthesia and Intensive Care, School of Medicine, University Hospital Catania, Catania, Italy

E. Cerdà Department of Intensive Care Medicine, Hospital Universitario de Parla, Madrid, Spain

C. J. Collins Clinical Microbiology, Trinity College Dublin, Dublin, Leinster, Ireland

R. P. Cooke Department of Microbiology, University Hospital Aintree NHS Foundation Trust, Liverpool, Merseyside, UK

I. Cortés Puch Intensive Care Unit, Hospital Universitario de Getafe, Getafe, Madrid, Spain

V. Cozza Dipartimento di Chirurgia "F. Durante", "Sapienza" Università di Roma, Rome, Italy

V. Damjanovic School of Clinical Sciences, University of Liverpool, Liverpool, UK

A. R. De Gaudio MD Careggi Teaching Hospital, Section of Anaesthesia, Department of Critical Care, University of Florence, Florence, Italy

M. A. de la Cal Department of Intensive Care Medicine, Hospital Universitario de Getafe, Getafe, Spain

A. de Silvestre Department of Anesthesiology and Intensive care, University Hospital of S. Maria della Misericordia, Udine, Italy

A. Di Filippo MD Careggi Teaching Hospital, Section of Anaesthesia, Department of Critical Care, University of Florence, Florence, Italy

J. Farias Paediatric Intensive Care Unit, Children's Hospital Ricardo Gutierrez, Buenos Aires, Argentina

M. Ferrer PhD, MD Servei de Pneumologia i Allèrgia Respiratòria, Hospital Clínic, IDIBAPS, CibeRes (CB06/06/0028), Barcelona, Spain

R. Ferrer Critical Care Center, Hospital Sabadell, Sabadell, Barcelona, Spain

P. Garcia-Hierro Department of Medical Microbiology, Hospital Universitario de Getafe, Madrid, Spain

M. A. González Gallego Servicio de Medicina Intensiva, Hospital Clínico San Carlos Universidad Complutense, Madrid, Spain

A. Gullo Department of Anesthesia and Intensive Care, School of Medicine, University Hospital Catania, Catania, Italy

J. Hughes Infection Prevention and Control, 5 Boroughs Partnership NHS Foundation Trust/University of Chester Warrington, Winwick, Warrington, Cheshire, UK

A. Liapikou MD 1st Department of Respiratory Medicine, SOTIRIA Regional Chest Disease Hospital of Athens, Athens, Greece

K. Lowry Intensive Care Unit, Royal Victoria Hospital, Belfast, Northern Ireland, UK

J. C. Marshall Department of Surgery and Intensive Care, St Michael's Hospital, Ontario, Canada

Department of Surgery and Interdepartmental Division of Critical Care, General Hospital and University of Toronto, Toronto, Canada

K. A. M. Marshall Department of Surgery and Interdepartmental Division of Critical Care, General Hospital and University of Toronto, Toronto, Canada

A. Martinez-Pellus Intensive Care Unit, University Hospital "Virgen de la Arrixaca", Murcia, Spain

F. Martínez Sagasti Servicio de Medicina Intensiva, Hospital Clínico San Carlos Universidad Complutense, Madrid, Spain

M. Nieto Cabrera Servicio de Medicina Intensiva, Hospital Clínico San Carlos Universidad Complutense, Madrid, Spain

A. J. Nunn Pharmacy Department, Alder Hey Children's NHS Foundation Trust, Liverpool, Merseyside, UK

A. Paratore MD Department of Anesthesia and Intensive Care, School of Medicine, University Hospital Catania, Catania, Italy

A. J. Petros Pediatric Intensive Care Unit, Great Ormond Street Children's Hospital, London, UK

A. Pigna Neonatal Intensive Care Unit, San Orsola Ospedale, Bologna, Italy

K. Pollock Department of Pharmacy, Western Infirmary, K Pollock, Senior Pharmacist, Glasgow, UK

B. Ramos Department of Medical Microbiology, University Hospital Getafe, Madrid, Spain

N. J. Reilly Pharmacy Department, Royal Liverpool Children's NHS Trust, Alder Hey, Liverpool, UK

R. Reina Intensive Care Unit, Hospital Interzonal de Agudos "General San Martín", La Plata, Buenos Aires, Argentina

G. Riepi Faculty of Medicine, University of Montevideo, Montevideo, Uruguay

S. Rinaldi Section of Anesthesiology, Villa Fiorita Hospital, Prato, Italy

F. Rios Pharmacy, Hospital Nacional Alejandro Posadas, Buenos Aires, Argentina

Th. R. Rogers Clinical Microbiology, St. James's Hospital and Trinity College Dublin, Dublin, Leinster, Ireland

J. H. Rommes PhD, MD Gelre Ziekenhuizen Apeldoorn, Intensive Care, Apeldoorn, The Netherlands

M. Sánchez Garcia PhD, MD Servicio de Medicina Intensiva, Hospital Clínico San Carlos Universidad Complutense, Madrid, Spain

R. E. Sarginson Paediatric Anaesthesia, Royal Liverpool Children's NHS Trust, Liverpool, Merseyside, UK

S. Schelenz Institute of Biomedical and Clinical Sciences, School of Medicine, Health Policy and Practice Faculty of Health University of East Anglia, Norwich, UK

G. Sganga Istituto di Clinica Chirurgica, Università Cattolica del Sacro Cuore, Rome, Italy

L. Silvestri Department of Emergency and Unit of Anesthesia and Intensive Care, Presidio Ospedaliero di Gorizia, Gorizia, Italy

N. Taylor School of Clinical Sciences, University of Liverpool, Liverpool, Merseyside, UK

K. Thorburn Paediatric Intensive Care Unit, Royal Liverpool Children's NHS Trust Alder Hey, Liverpool, UK

C. Y. William Tong Infection, Guy's and St Thomas' NHS Foundation Trust and King's College London School of Medicine, London, UK

A. Torres MD Servei de Pneumologia i Al·lèrgia Respiratòria, Hospital Clínic, Barcelona, Spain

J. Vallés Critical Care Center, Hospital Sabadell, Sabadell, Barcelona, Spain

H. K. F. van Saene Institute of Ageing and Chronic Diseases, University of Liverpool, Duncan Building, Liverpool, UK

School of Clinical Sciences, University of Liverpool, Liverpool, UK

J. J. M. van Saene School of Clinical Sciences, University of Liverpool, Liverpool, Merseyside, UK

P. H. J. van der Voort Department of Intensive Care Medicine, Onze Lieve Vrouwe Gasthuis, Amsterdam, The Netherlands

T. Williets School of Clinical Sciences, University of Liverpool, Liverpool, UK

D. F. Zandstra Department of Intensive Care Unit, Onze Lieve Vrouwe Gasthuis, Amsterdam, The Netherlands

Part I
Essentials in Clinical Microbiology

Glossary of Terms and Definitions

R. E. Sarginson, N. Taylor, M. A. de la Cal
and H. K. F. van Saene

1.1 Introduction

Defining terms is important to avoid ambiguity, particularly in the era of global communication. Words, such as sepsis, nosocomial, colonization, and infection, are often used in an imprecise fashion. Although standardization in terminology is useful, revisions will be needed in the light of progress in biomedical knowledge. Definitions can be based on a variety of concepts, varying from abnormalities in patients' physiology and clinical features to sophisticated laboratory methods. A thoughtful introduction to clinical terminology can be found in the extensive writings of Feinstein [1, 2], who made use of set theory and Venn diagrams to categorize clinical conditions. The choice of boundaries between sets or values on measurement scales can be difficult. In practice, such boundaries are often somewhat fuzzy, for example in the diagnosis of ventilator-associated pneumonia [3].

The situation is further complicated by considering problems in measurement. An apparently simple temperature measurement is subject to variation in time, site, and technique, as well as to errors from device malfunction, displacement, or misuse. Most definitions of infection at various sites include fever as a necessary criterion, typically a temperature of $\geq 38.3°C$. Do we have good evidence that this measurement is a reliable discriminator, in conjunction with other "necessary" criteria, in distinguishing the presence or absence of a particular type of infection [4]?

R. E. Sarginson (✉)
Paediatric Anaesthesia, Royal Liverpool Children's NHS Trust,
Liverpool, Merseyside, UK
e-mail: richard.sarginson@alderhey.nhs.uk

Bone raised some important issues [5–8] for the terms sepsis and inflammation, a debate that continues. Other interesting approaches in the fields of sepsis, systemic inflammatory response, and multiple organ dysfunction are the use of "physiological state space" concepts by Rixen et al. [9] and ideas from "complex adaptive system" and network theory [10–13]. A number of consensus conferences have been held in recent years to seek agreement on definitions of infections as they apply to patients in the intensive care unit (ICU) [14].

The glossary outlined here forms a basis for our clinical practice in various aspects of intensive care infection and microbiology. We advocate definitions that are usable in routine clinical practice and that emphasize the role of surveillance samples in classifying the origins of infection.

1.2 Terms and Definitions

1.2.1 Acquisition

A patient is considered to have acquired a microorganism when a single surveillance sample is positive for a strain that differs from previous and subsequent isolates. This is a transient phenomenon, in contrast to the more persistent state of carriage.

1.2.2 Bloodstream Infection

Bloodstream infections (BSI) were classified into primary, secondary, and catheter related by the International Consensus Forum on ICU infections in 2005 [14]. Debate continues over the number and type of cultures required to detect pathogens in the blood [15]. The clinical impact of BSI depends on the pathogenicity of the invading microorganism, together with the nature and severity of the host response (see "Microorganisms," and "Systemic inflammatory response syndrome (SIRS), sepsis, and septic shock" definitions).

1.2.2.1 Primary Bloodstream Infection
A recognized pathogen, which is not regarded as a common skin contaminant, is cultured from one or more blood cultures and the cultured organism is not related to an infection at another site, including intravenous-access devices. A primary BSI may also be present when a common skin organism, such as coagulase-negative staphylococci, is cultured repeatedly from peripheral cultures.

1.2.2.2 Secondary Bloodstream Infection
A recognized pathogen is cultured from one or more blood cultures and is identical to an organism responsible for an infection at another site.

1.2.2.3 Catheter-Related Bloodstream Infection
A pathogen is isolated from one or more blood cultures and is shown to be simultaneously present in an intravascular device, together with clinical signs of infection. No other source of the pathogen is identified in the patient. In practice, it may be difficult to distinguish between an endogenous and exogenous source unless surveillance cultures are available. If the patient has overgrowth of the relevant pathogen in the gastrointestinal tract, translocation is another possible mechanism for bacteremia.

1.2.3 Carriage/Carrier State

The same strain of microorganism is isolated from two or more surveillance samples in a particular patient. In practice, consecutive throat and/or rectal surveillance samples, taken twice a week (Monday and Thursday), yield identical strains.

1.2.3.1 Normal Carrier State
Surveillance samples yield only the indigenous aerobic and anaerobic flora, including *Escherichia coli* in the rectum. Varying percentages of people carry "normal" potential pathogens in the throat and/or gut. *Streptococcus pneumoniae* and *Haemophilus influenzae* are carried in the oropharynx by more than half of the healthy population. *Staphylococcus aureus* and yeasts are carried in the throat and gut by up to a third of healthy people.

1.2.3.2 Abnormal Carrier State
Opportunistic "abnormal" aerobic Gram-negative bacilli (AGNB) or methicillin-resistant *S. aureus* (MRSA) are persistently present in the oropharynx and/or rectum. MRSA and AGNB are listed under abnormal microorganisms. *E. coli*, isolated from the oropharynx in overgrowth concentrations [$>2+$ or $>10^5$ colony-forming units (CFU)/ml], also represents an abnormal carrier state.

1.2.3.3 Primary Carriage
Primary carriage is the persistent presence of both normal and abnormal potential pathogens in the admission flora surveillance (throat and rectum) samples.

1.2.3.4 Secondary Carriage
Secondary carriage is the persistent presence of abnormal bacteria in throat and/or rectum acquired during treatment in the ICU and which were not present in the admission flora. Commonly used antibiotics eliminate normal bacteria, such as *S. pneumoniae* or *H. influenzae*, but promote the acquisition and subsequent carriage of abnormal AGNB and MRSA. This phenomenon is sometimes referred to as "super" or "secondary" carriage. Overgrowth with microorganisms of low pathogenicity, such as coagulase-negative staphylococci and enterococci, can also occur during selective decontamination of the digestive tract (SDD).

1.2.4 Central Nervous System Infections

This important group of infections includes meningitis, meningoencephalitis, encephalitis, ventriculitis, and shunt infection. These conditions have some overlap and may also coexist with sinus or mastoid infections and septicemia. Microbiological diagnosis usually rests on culture of cerebrospinal fluid (CSF). Frequently, lumbar puncture is contraindicated in suspected meningitis [16]. For example, in meningococcal infection, contraindications include coagulopathy or when computed tomography (CT) scan features suggest a risk of tentorial pressure coning if lumbar puncture were to be done. Also, empirical antibiotics have frequently been started prior to hospital admission. These issues are particularly important in pediatric practice, where meningococcal DNA detection in blood and/or CSF by polymerase chain reaction (PCR) assays, together with bacterial antigen tests, improves diagnostic yield [17]. The use of molecular techniques, including PCR, in detecting septicemia in critically ill patients is still in the developmental stage but shows great promise [18]. In CNS infections, the usual nonspecific criteria of fever or hypothermia, leukocytosis or leukopenia, and tachycardia are present, with specific symptoms that may include headache, lethargy, neck stiffness, irritability, fits, and coma. Cutoff values depend on age and should be defined at age-specific percentile thresholds for physiological variables, e.g., >90th percentile for heart rate. Detailed definitions are not given here, as they would require a separate chapter.

1.2.5 Colonization

Microorganisms are present in body sites that are normally sterile, such as the lower airways or bladder. Clinical features of infection are absent. Diagnostic samples yield $\leq 1+$ leukocytes per high power field (HPF) [19], and microbial growth is $<2+$ or $<10^5$ CFU/ml.

1.2.6 Defense

1.2.6.1 Against Carriage
The defense mechanisms of the oropharynx and gastrointestinal tract, e.g., fibronectin, saliva, and gastric secretions, help prevent abnormal carrier states.

1.2.6.2 Against Colonization
Defense mechanisms of internal organs against microbial invasion, e.g., the mucociliary elevator in the airways and secreted immunoglobulins.

1.2.6.3 Against Infection
Defense mechanisms of the internal organs, beyond skin and mucosa, which include antibodies, lymphocytes, and neutrophils.

1.2.7 Endemicity

Endemicity is defined as at least one new case per month having a diagnostic sample positive for the outbreak strain. Endemicity can be interpreted as an uncontrolled, ongoing outbreak.

1.2.8 Infection

Infection can be remarkably difficult to define in clinical circumstances. Patients have often received empirical antibiotics. In principle, infection is a microbiologically proven clinical diagnosis of local and/or generalized inflammation. The microbiological criteria conventionally include $\geq 10^5$ CFU/ml of diagnostic sample from the infected organ and $\geq 2+$ leukocytes present per HPF in the sample. The thresholds chosen for clinical features and laboratory measurements depend on patient age and assessment timing. Assessment may include temperature changes, heart rate, changes in heart rate variability [10], white blood cell (WBC) counts, C-reactive protein [20], and procalcitonin [21, 22]. Infections can be classified according to the concept of the carrier state [23]:
- primary endogenous infection is caused by microorganisms carried by the patient at the time of admission to the ICU and include both normal and abnormal microorganisms;
- secondary endogenous infection is caused by microorganisms acquired on the ICU and not present in the admission flora. These microorganisms usually belong to the abnormal group. Potentially pathogenic microorganisms are acquired in the oropharynx and followed by carriage and overgrowth in the digestive tract. Subsequently, colonization and then infection of internal organs may occur following migration from the oropharynx into the lower airways or translocation across the gut mucosa into the lymphatics or bloodstream;
- exogenous infection is caused by microorganisms introduced into the patient from the ICU environment. Organisms are transferred directly, omitting the carriage stage, to a site where colonization and then infection occur.

1.2.9 Inflammatory Markers

Inflammatory markers are cells and proteins associated with the proinflammatory process. These include C-reactive protein [20], procalcitonin [21, 22], tumor necrosis factor alpha (TNF)-α, interleukin (IL)-1 and IL-6 [24], lymphocytes, and neutrophils. The onset, magnitude, and duration of changes in these factors vary with infection site and severity.

1.2.10 ICU infection

ICU infection refers to secondary endogenous and exogenous infections, which are infections due to organisms not carried by the patient at the time of ICU admission and transmitted via hands of carers [25]. The term nosocomial (literally, related to the hospital) is widely used but lacks a precise definition.

1.2.11 Intra-Abdominal Infection

Intra-abdominal infection occurs in an abdominal organ and the peritoneal cavity (peritonitis). Peritonitis can be a local or general inflammation of the peritoneal cavity. Local signs such as tenderness and guarding may be difficult to elicit in sedated ICU patients. Generalized, nonspecific features are fever (temperature $\geq$ 38.3°C), leukocytosis (WBC > 12,000/mm^3), or leukopenia (WBC < 4,000/mm^3). Ultrasonography and/or CT evaluation may contribute to the diagnosis. Isolation of microorganisms from diagnostic samples at a concentration of $\geq$2+ or $\geq 10^5$ CFU/ml, with $\geq$2+ leukocytes, confirms the diagnosis. Specific examples include fecal peritonitis due to colon perforation and peritonitis associated with peritoneal dialysis.

1.2.12 Isolation

Patients are nursed in separate cubicles or rooms, with strict hygiene measures, including protective clothing and hand washing by the staff, to control transmission of microorganisms. These measures particularly apply to patients infected with high-level pathogens or resistant microorganisms and those with impaired immunity.

1.2.13 Microorganisms

1.2.13.1 Normal Microorganisms
Normal microorganisms are carried by varying percentages of healthy people and include *S. aureus*, *S. pneumoniae*, *H. influenzae*, *Moraxella catarrhalis*, *E. coli*, and *Candida albicans* [26].

1.2.13.2 Abnormal Microorganisms
Abnormal microorganisms are carried by people with chronic disease or those admitted to the ICU from inpatient wards or other hospitals. These are typically AGNB or MRSA. AGNB include *Pseudomonas, Acinetobacter, Klebsiella, Citrobacter, Enterobacter, Serratia, Proteus,* and *Morganella* spp. These organisms are rarely carried by healthy people [27, 28]. Microorganisms can be ranked by pathogenicity into three types:

- highly pathogenic microorganisms, e.g., *Salmonella* spp, may cause infection in an individual with a normal defense capacity;
- potentially pathogenic microorganisms, e.g., *S. pneumoniae* in community practice and *P. aeruginosa* in hospital practice, can cause infection in a patient with impaired defense mechanisms. These two types of microbes cause both morbidity and mortality;
- microbes of low pathogenicity cause infection under special circumstances only, e.g., anaerobes can cause abscesses when tissue necrosis is present. Low-level pathogens in general cause morbidity and little mortality.

Intrinsic pathogenicity refers to the capacity to cause infection. The intrinsic pathogenicity index (IPI) is defined as the ratio of the number of patients who develop an infection due to a particular microorganism and the number of patients who carry the organism in the throat and/or rectum. Indigenous flora, including anaerobes and *S. viridans*, rarely cause infections despite being carried in high concentrations. The IPI is typically in the range of 0.01–0.03. Coagulase-negative staphylococci and enterococci are also carried in the oropharynx in high concentrations but are unable to cause lower airway infections. High-level pathogens, such as *Salmonella* spp, have an IPI approaching 1 in the gut. Potentially pathogenic microorganisms have an IPI in the range of 0.1–0.3, and include the normal and abnormal potential pathogens, which are the targets of SDD.

1.2.14 Migration

Migration is the process whereby microorganisms carried in the throat and gut move to colonize and possibly infect internal organs. Migration is promoted by underlying chronic disease, some drugs, and invasive devices.

1.2.15 Outbreak

An outbreak is defined as an event in which two or more patients in a defined location are infected by identical, often multidrug-resistant, microorganisms transmitted via the hands of health care workers, usually within an arbitrary time period of 2 weeks. There are two different types of infection involved in outbreaks: secondary endogenous and exogenous. Outbreaks of secondary endogenous infection are preceded by outbreaks of carriage of abnormal flora, whereas outbreaks of exogenous infection are not. Outbreaks of carriage of microbes may therefore have considerable significance for infection control. These two types of outbreaks require different management approaches: SDD is designed to prevent secondary endogenous types of outbreaks, whereas emphasis on hygiene procedures, such as handwashing and cohort nursing, is needed to prevent exogenous outbreaks. SDD paste, applied to tracheostomy wounds, can reduce the risk of exogenous transmission during an outbreak. Such outbreak episodes often occur with multidrug-resistant microorganisms, such as *Pseudomonas*, MRSA, or vancomycin-resistant enterococci (VRE). In the pediatric ICU, viruses such as respiratory syncytial virus or rotavirus can also be a major problem.

1.2.16 Overgrowth

Overgrowth is defined as the presence of a high concentration of potentially pathogenic microorganisms, $\geq 2+$ or $\geq 10^5$ CFU/ml, in surveillance samples from the digestive tract [29]. Gut overgrowth can harm the critically ill patient, as it can cause immunosuppression [30], inflammation [31], infection [32], and antimicrobial resistance [33]. Overgrowth control is the main mechanism of action of SDD. SDD restores immune function [34] and reduces inflammation [35], infection rates [36], and antimicrobial resistance [37].

1.2.17 Pneumonia

1.2.17.1 Microbiologically Confirmed Pneumonia
- presence of new or progressive infiltrates on a chest X-ray for ≥ 48 h, and
- fever $\geq 38.3°C$, and
- leukocytosis (WBC $>$ 12,000/ml) or leukopenia (WBC $<$ 4,000/ml), and
- purulent tracheal aspirate containing $\geq 2+$ WBC/HPF, and
- tracheal aspirate specimen yielding $\geq 10^5$ CFU/ml, or
- protected brush specimen (PBS) yielding $> 10^3$ CFU/ml, or
- bronchoalveolar lavage (BAL) specimen yielding $> 10^4$ CFU/ml.

1.2.17.2 Clinical Diagnosis Only
The first four microbiological criteria are fulfilled, but tracheal aspirates, PBS, or BAL are sterile. Criteria for the diagnosis of pneumonias remain controversial [3]. The situation is sometimes complicated by viral etiologies and/or prior antibiotic treatment, particularly in infants and children. There is also overlap with other pathophysiological terms, such as pneumonitis and bronchiolitis.

1.2.18 Resistance

A microorganism is considered to be resistant to a particular antimicrobial agent if:
- the minimal inhibitory concentration of the antimicrobial agent against a colonizing or infecting microbial species is higher than the nontoxic blood concentration after systemic administration;
- the minimum bactericidal concentration of the antimicrobial agent against microbes carried in throat and gut is higher than the nontoxic concentration achieved by enteral administration.

1.2.19 Samples

1.2.19.1 Diagnostic
Diagnostic or clinical samples are taken from sites that are normally sterile in order to diagnose infection or evaluate response to therapy. Samples are taken on clinical indication only from blood, lower airways, CSF, urinary tract, wounds, peritoneum, joints, sinuses, or conjunctiva.

1.2.19.2 Surveillance
Surveillance samples are taken from the oropharynx and rectum on admission and subsequently at regular intervals (usually twice weekly). These specimens are needed to:
- evaluate the abnormal carriage level of potentially pathogenic microorganisms, in particular, overgrowth;
- assess the eradication of potential pathogens by enteral nonabsorbable antimicrobial regimens used in SDD protocols;
- detect the carriage of resistant strains.

1.2.20 Selective Decontamination of the Digestive Tract

SDD is an antimicrobial prophylaxis method consisting of parenteral cefotaxime and enteral and topical polymyxin E/tobramycin/amphotericin B (PTA) to prevent severe endogenous and exogenous infections of lower airways and blood in the critically ill patient requiring treatment in the ICU. The full SDD protocol has four components [25, 38, 39]:
- parenteral antibiotic (e.g., cefotaxime), is administered for the first few days to prevent or control primary endogenous infection;
- nonabsorbable antimicrobials are administered into the oropharynx and gastrointestinal tract when surveillance cultures show abnormal carriage; the usual combination is PTA;
- a high standard of hygiene is required to prevent exogenous infection episodes;
- regular surveillance samples of throat and rectum are obtained to diagnose carrier states and monitor SDD efficacy.

The policy at Alder Hey, Liverpool, UK is to use SDD "a la carte", guided by the abnormal carrier state detected by surveillance samples. However, most ICUs that use SDD start the regimen on admission, irrespective of surveillance swab results.

1.2.21 Systemic Inflammatory Response Syndrome, Sepsis, and Septic Shock

Definitions for SIRS, sepsis, severe sepsis, and septic shock have been extensively reviewed in recent years, particularly in relation to the inclusion criteria for clinical trials [8, 40, 41]. Consensus definitions form categories based on cutoff points in the value distributions of a number of variables. Cutoff points based perfusion indices can be difficult to evaluate in practice. Furthermore, a patient's clinical state can change rapidly [42]. Microbiological confirmation of infection may occur a considerable time after the clinical diagnosis of septic states. Cutoffs and thresholds must be adjusted in the pediatric population [43].

1.2.21.1 Systemic Inflammatory Response Syndrome

SIRS can be caused by a wide variety of clinical insults [8, 44, 45] and is manifested by two or more of the following:
- temperature >38 or <36°C;
- heart rate >90 bpm;
- respiratory rate >20 breaths/min;
- WBC count >12,000/mm^3 or <4,000/mm^3, or >10% immature forms.

These variables must be adjusted in infants and children [46].

1.2.21.2 Sepsis

Sepsis is defined as SIRS with a clear infectious etiology.

1.2.21.3 Septicemia

Septicemia is sepsis with a positive blood culture. In contrast, bacteremia is defined as a positive blood culture in a patient exhibiting no clinical symptoms.

1.2.21.4 Severe Sepsis

Severe sepsis is defined as sepsis with organ dysfunction, hypoperfusion, or hypotension. Manifestations of hypoperfusion may include, but are not limited to, lactic acidosis, oliguria, and acute alterations in mental state.

1.2.21.5 Septic Shock

Septic shock is sepsis-induced hypotension, persisting despite adequate fluid resuscitation, together with manifestations of hypoperfusion. Hypotension is defined as a systolic blood pressure <90 mmHg or a reduction of >40 mmHg from baseline in the absence of other causes of hypotension.

1.2.22 Sinusitis

Sinusitis is infection of the paranasal sinuses—maxillary, ethmoidal, frontal, or sphenoidal. Symptoms and signs such as localized tenderness and purulent discharge may be absent in the sedated ICU patient. Fever (temperature $\geq 38.3°C$)

and leukocytosis (WBC > 12,000/mm^3) or leukopenia (WBC < 4,000/mm^3) are the main clinical features. Plain radiographs or CT imaging may show fluid levels of obliteration in the sinus air spaces. Surgical drainage is performed to obtain microbiological confirmation ($\geq 2+$ or $\geq 10^5$ CFU/ml of pus, together with $\geq 2+$ leukocytes).

1.2.23 Tracheitis/Bronchitis

In the absence of pulmonary infiltrates on chest X-ray, tracheitis/bronchitis is defined as:
- purulent tracheal aspirate, and
- fever >38.3°C, and
- leukocytosis (WBC > 12,000/mm^3) or leukopenia (WBC < 4,000/mm^3);
- $\geq 2+$ or $\geq 10^5$ CFU/ml of tracheal aspirate.

1.2.24 Translocation (Transmural Migration)

Translocation is defined as the passage of viable microorganisms from the throat and gut through mucosal barriers to regional lymph nodes and internal organs, including the blood.

1.2.25 Transmission

Transmission is defined as the spread of microorganisms between patients by means of "vectors" such as a carer's hands. Transmission of potential pathogens is the crucial stage in the pathogenesis of secondary endogenous and exogenous infections. Measures to control transmission include isolation, hand washing, protective clothing, and care of equipment.

1.2.26 Urinary Tract Infection

Urinary tract infection is defined as infection of the urinary tract, most frequently the bladder. The common clinical features of dysuria, suprapubic pain, frequency, and urgency are often absent in the sedated ICU patient. The diagnosis rests on a freshly voided catheter urine specimen or suprapubic sample containing $\geq 10^5$ bacteria or yeasts per milliliter of urine and ≥ 5 WBC/HPF.

1.2.27 Wound Infection

Wound infection is defined as purulent discharge from wounds, signs of local inflammation, and a culture yielding $\geq 2+$ or $\geq 10^5$ CFU/ml. The isolation of skin flora in the absence of these features is considered contamination.

References

1. Feinstein AR (1967) Clinical judgment. Williams and Wilkins, Baltimore
2. Feinstein AR (1994) Clinical judgment revisited: the distraction of quantitative models. Ann Intern Med 120:799–805
3. Bonten M (1999) Controversies on diagnosis and prevention of ventilator-associated pneumonia. Diagn Microbiol Infect Dis 34:199–204
4. Toltzis P, Rosolowski B, Salvator A (2001) Etiology of fever and opportunities for reduction of antibiotic use in a pediatric intensive care unit. Infect Control Hosp Epidemiol 22:499–504
5. Bone RC (1991) Let's agree on terminology: definitions of sepsis. Crit Care Med 19:973–976
6. Canadian Multiple Organ Failure Study Group (1991) "Sepsis"—clarity of existing terminology…or more confusion? Crit Care Med 19:996–998
7. Bone RC, Grodzin CJ, Balk RA (1997) Sepsis: a new hypothesis for pathogenesis of the disease process. Chest 112:235–243
8. Levy MM, Fink MP, Marshall JC et al (2003) 2001 SCCM/ESICM/ACCP/ATS/SIS international sepsis definitions conference. Crit Care Med 31:1250–1256
9. Rixen D, Siegel JH, Friedman HP (1996) "Sepsis/SIRS", physiologic classification, severity stratification, relation to cytokine elaboration and outcome prediction in post trauma critical illness. J Trauma 41:581–598
10. Seeley AJE, Christou NV (2000) Multiple organ dysfunction syndrome: exploring the paradigm of complex non-linear systems. Crit Care Med 28:2193–2200
11. Toweill DL, Goldstein B (1998) Linear and nonlinear dynamics and the pathophysiology of shock. New Horiz 6:155–168
12. Aird WC (2002) Endothelial cell dynamics and complexity theory. Crit Care Med 30(suppl):S180–S185
13. Strogatz SH (2001) Exploring complex networks. Nature 410:268–276
14. Calandra T, Cohen J (2005) The international sepsis forum consensus conference on definitions of infection in the intensive care unit. Crit Care Med 33(7):1538–1548
15. Lee A, Mirrett S, Reller LB et al (2007) Detection of bloodstream infections in adults: how many blood cultures are needed? J Clin Microbiol 46(3):3546–3548
16. Smith TL, Nathan BR (2002) Central nervous system infections in the immune-competent adult. Curr Treat Options Neurol 4:323–332
17. Carrol ED, Thomson AP, Shears P et al (2000) Performance characteristics of the polymerase chain reaction assay to confirm clinical meningococcal disease. Arch Dis Child 83:271–273
18. Cursons RTM, Jeyerajah E, Sleigh JW (1999) The use of the polymerase chain reaction to detect septicemia in critically ill patients. Crit Care Med 27:937–940
19. A'Court CHD, Garrard CS, Crook D et al (1993) Microbiological lung surveillance in mechanically ventilated patients, using non-directed bronchial lavage and quantitative culture. Q J Med 86:635–648
20. Reny JL, Vuagnat A, Ract C et al (2002) Diagnosis and follow up of infections in intensive care patients: value of C-reactive protein compared with other clinical and biological variables. Crit Care Med 30:529–535
21. Claeys R, Vinken S, Spapen H et al (2002) Plasma procalcitonin and C-reactive protein in acute septic shock: clinical and biological correlates. Crit Care Med 30:757–762

22. Christ-Crain M, Jaccard-Stolz D, Bingisser R et al (2004) Effect of procalcitonin-guided treatment on antibiotic use and outcome in lower respiratory tract infections: cluster-randomised, single-blinded intervention trial. Lancet 363:600–607
23. van Saene HKF, Damjanovic V, Murray AE, de la Cal MA (1996) How to classify infections in intensive care units—the carrier state, a criterion whose time has come? J Hosp Infect 33:1–12
24. Dinarello CA (2000) Pro-inflammatory cytokines. Chest 118:503–508
25. Sarginson RE, Taylor N, Reilly N et al (2004) Infection in prolonged pediatric critical illness: a prospective four-year study based on knowledge of the carrier state. Crit Care Med 32:839–847
26. van Saene HKF, Damjanovic V, Alcock SR (2001) Basics in microbiology for the patient requiring intensive care. Curr Anaesth Crit Care 12:6–17
27. Johanson WG, Pierce AK, Sanford JP (1969) Changing pharyngeal bacterial flora of hospitalized patients. Emergence of gram-negative bacilli. N Engl J Med 281:1137–1140
28. Chang FY, Singh N, Gayowski T et al (1998) *Staphylococcus aureus* nasal colonization in patients with cirrhosis: prospective assessment of association with infection. Infect Control Hosp Epidemiol 19:328–332
29. Husebye E (1995) Gastrointestinal motility disorders and bacterial overgrowth. J Intern Med 237:419–427
30. Deitch EA, Xu DZ, Qi L, Berg RD (1991) Bacterial translocation from the gut impairs systemic immunity. Surgery 104:269–276
31. Silvestri L, van Saene HKF, Zandstra DF et al (2010) Selective decontamination of the digestive tract reduces multiple organ failure and mortality in critically ill patients: systematic review of randomized controlled trials. Crit Care Med 38:1370–1376
32. van Uffelen R, van Saene HK, Fidler V, Löwenberg A (1984) Oropharyngeal flora as a source of bacteria colonizing the lower airways in patients on artificial ventilation. Intensive Care Med 10:233–237
33. van Saene HKF, Taylor N, Damjanovic V et al (2008) Microbial gut overgrowth guarantees increased spontaneous mutation leading to polyclonality and antibiotic resistance in the critically ill. Curr Drug Targ 9:419–421
34. Horton JW, Maass DL, White J, Minei JP (2007) Reducing susceptibility to bacteremia after experimental burn injury: a role for selective decontamination of the digestive tract. J Appl Physiol 102:2207–2216
35. Conraads VM, Jorens PG, De Clerck LS (2004) Selective intestinal decontamination in advanced chronic heart failure: a pilot trial. Eur J Heart Fail 6:483–491
36. de la Cal MA, Cerdá E, van Saene HKF et al (2004) Effectiveness and safety of enteral vancomycin to control endemicity of methicillin-resistant *Staphylococcus aureus* in a medical/surgical intensive care unit. J Hosp Infect 56:175–183
37. de Smet AM, Kluytmans JA, Cooper BS et al (2009) Decontamination of the digestive tract and oropharynx in ICU patients. N Engl J Med 360:20–31
38. Baxby D, van Saene HKF, Stoutenbeek CP, Zandstra DF (1996) Selective decontamination of the digestive tract: 13 years on, what it is, what it is not. Intensive Care Med 22:699–706
39. Silvestri L, de la Cal MA, van Saene HKF (2009) Selective decontamination of the digestive tract (SDD)—twenty-five years of European experience. In: Gullo A, Besso J, Lumb PD, Williams GF (eds) Intensive and critical care medicine. Springer, Milano, pp 273–284
40. Brun-Buisson C (2000) The epidemiology of the systemic inflammatory response. Intensive Care Med 26(suppl):S64–S74
41. Cohen J, Guyatt G, Bernard GR et al (2001) New strategies for clinical trials in patients with sepsis and septic shock. Crit Care Med 29:880–886
42. Rangel-Frausto MS, Pittet D, Costigan M et al (1995) The natural history of the systemic inflammatory response syndrome (SIRS). A prospective study. JAMA 273:117–123
43. Watson RS, Carcillo JA, Linde-Zwirble WT et al (2003) The epidemiology of severe sepsis in children in the United States. Am J Respir Crit Care Med 167:695–701

44. Marik PE (2002) Definition of sepsis: not quite time to dump SIRS. Crit Care Med 30:706–708
45. Zahorec R (2000) Definitions for the septic syndrome should be re-evaluated. Intensive Care Med 26:1870
46. Lucy Lum Chai S (2005) Bloodstream infection in children. Pediatr Crit Care Med 6(Suppl):S42–S44

Carriage, Colonization and Infection

L. Silvestri, H. K. F. van Saene
and J. J. M. van Saene

2.1 Introduction

Physiologically, internal organs such as lower airways and bladder, are sterile. However, colonization of lower airways and bladder by potentially pathogenic microorganisms (PPMs) is common in critically ill patients [1]. Colonization of the internal organs generally follows impaired carriage defense of the digestive tract, which promotes PPM carriage and overgrowth, and impaired defenses of the host against colonization due to illness severity. Failure to clear colonizing microorganisms from the internal organs invariably leads to high concentrations of PPMs, predisposing to infection. The host mobilizes both humoral and cellular defense systems to hinder the invading microorganisms. However, infection requires not only invasion but severity of the underlying disease, which jeopardizes immunocompetence. This chapter defines the concepts of carriage, colonization, and infection and describes the host defense mechanisms against carriage, colonization, and infection.

2.2 Definitions

Carriage is defined as the patient's state in which the same strain is isolated from at least two surveillance samples (saliva, gastric fluid, feces, throat, rectum) in any concentration over a period of at least 1 week (Fig. 2.1). Overgrowth is defined as the presence of $\geq 2+$ or $\geq 10^5$ colony forming units (CFU) per

---

L. Silvestri (✉)
Department of Emergency, Unit of Anesthesia and Intensive Care,
Presidio Ospedaliero di Gorizia, Gorizia, Italy
e-mail: lucianosilvestri@yahoo.it

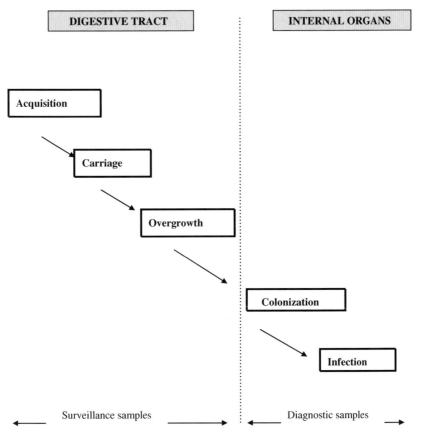

Fig. 2.1 The slippery slope of the pathogenesis of infection in critically ill patients. *Acquisition* develops if only one surveillance sample is positive for a potentially pathogenic microorganism (PPM) that differs from the previous and following isolates. Acquisition refers to the transient presence of a microorganism (usually in the oropharynx and gut), whereas carriage is a persistent phenomenon. *Carriage or carrier state* is the patient's state in which the same bacterial strain is isolated from at least two surveillance samples (saliva, gastric fluid, feces, throat, rectum) in any concentration over a period of at least 1 week. *Overgrowth* is defined as $\geq 10^5$ colony-forming units (CFU)/ml of saliva or gastric fluid or gram of feces and is nearly always present in the critically ill intensive care unit (ICU) patient with impaired gut motility. *Colonization* is the presence of a PPM in an internal organ that is normally sterile (e.g., lower airways, bladder) without inflammatory host response. The diagnostic sample yields $<10^5$ CFU/ml of diagnostic sample. *Infection* is a microbiologically proven clinical diagnosis of inflammation. Apart from the clinical signs of infection, the diagnostic sample obtained from the internal organ contains $\geq 10^5$ CFU/ml or is positive in blood, cerebrospinal fluid, and pleural fluid. *Surveillance samples* are samples from body sites where potentially pathogenic microorganisms are carried, such as digestive tract and skin lesions (tracheotomy, wounds, pressure sores). A surveillance set comprises throat and rectal swabs taken on admission and twice weekly thereafter, e.g., on Monday and Thursday. The purpose of surveillance samples is to determine the microbiological endpoint of the level of PPM carriage. *Diagnostic samples* are samples from internal organs that are normally sterile, such as lower airways, blood, and bladder. The aim of diagnostic samples is clinical, i.e., to microbiologically prove a diagnosis of inflammation, either generalized or local

milliliter of saliva and/or per gram of feces. Colonization must be distinguished from carriage and is defined as the presence of a microorganism in an internal organ that is normally sterile (e.g., lower airways, bladder), without any host inflammatory response (Fig. 2.1). Diagnostic samples such as lower airway secretions, wound fluid, and urine generally yield $<10^5$ CFU of PPMs per milliliter of diagnostic sample. In general, few leukocytes are present in colonized internal organs on a semiquantitative scale of $+$ = few, $++$ = moderate, and $+++$ = many [2]. Carriage and colonization are two different stages in the pathogenesis of endogenous infection in intensive care unit (ICU) patients. The first stage is practically always the oropharyngeal and gastrointestinal carrier state, which is followed by overgrowth. Once the PPMs are present in high concentrations, in general $\geq 10^5$ of potential pathogens per milliliter of saliva and/or gram of feces, they migrate into the sterile internal organs and colonize the lower airways and bladder. Unfortunately, the term colonization is often used to cover both stages of carriage and colonization [3].

Infection is a microbiologically proven clinical diagnosis of inflammation either local and/or generalized. This includes not only clinical signs but also the presence of a moderate $(++)$ number of leukocytes and of $\geq 10^5$ CFU/ml of diagnostic samples obtained from an internal organ, or the isolation of a microorganism from blood, cerebrospinal fluid, or pleural fluid [2]. Diagnostic samples are collected from internal organs that are normally sterile, such as the lower airways, bladder, and blood. They are obtained when clinically indicated and allow the diagnosis of colonization and infection [2].

Surveillance samples are taken from body sites where the potential pathogens are carried, that is, the digestive tract and skin lesions (e.g., tracheostomy, pressure sores). Generally, a set of surveillance samples consists of throat and rectal swabs taken on patient admission to the ICU and twice weekly thereafter. The purpose of surveillance samples is to determine the microbiological endpoint of the level of PPM carriage. They are not useful for diagnosing infection of internal organs, as diagnostic samples are required for this purpose [2].

2.3 Throat/Gut Flora and Internal Organs in Health and Disease

2.3.1 Carriage

Microorganisms are carried in the oropharynx, gut, and vagina. Microorganisms present in healthy people are usually normal flora. They are mainly anaerobes and aerobes of the indigenous flora, together with community microorganisms such as *Streptococcus pneumoniae*, methicillin-sensitive *Staphylococcus aureus*, *Haemophilus influenzae*, *Moraxella catarrhalis*, *Escherichia coli*, and *Candida albicans*. Abnormal flora is uncommon in healthy people and may be only transiently present [4], whereas disease promotes oropharyngeal and gastrointestinal carriage of these abnormal microorganisms. Abnormal microorganisms include the eight aerobic Gram-negative bacilli (AGNB), *Klebsiella, Proteus, Morganella, Enterobacter, Citrobacter, Serratia, Acinetobacter, and Pseudomonas* spp., as well as methicillin-resistant *S. aureus* (MRSA). Approximately one-third of patients with an underlying chronic condition—such as diabetes, alcoholism, chronic obstructive pulmonary disease (COPD)—or neonates receiving total parenteral nutrition, are likely to demonstrate abnormal flora in their oropharynx and gut [4]. Moreover, previously healthy patients admitted to the ICU and requiring long-term ventilatory support due to an acute insult, such as (surgical) trauma, pancreatitis, or acute liver failure, may become carriers of abnormal hospital flora in their digestive tract. Critical illness is the most important factor in conversion from normal to abnormal carrier state [5].

2.3.2 Colonization and Infection

Secretions from internal organs, such as the lower airways, sinuses, middle ear, lachrymal gland, and urinary tract, of healthy individuals are normally sterile. Colonization of internal organs can occur with the two types of PPMs: normal, including *S. pneumoniae* and *H. influenzae*; and abnormal, such as *Klebsiella* and *Pseudomonas* spp. Three examples illustrate the concept of colonization followed by infection:
1. Elderly people cared for in a nursing home carry *S. pneumoniae* and *H. influenzae* in their oropharynx. During winter months, elderly people are at high risk of developing the flu. The flu virus destroys the cilia and causes systemic immunosuppression. Colonization of the lower airways with *S. pneumoniae* and *H. influenzae* invariably occurs in this population during a flu epidemic. If these patients do not receive a short course of commonly used antibiotics, colonization of the lower airways often progresses to pneumonia associated with high mortality rates. A similar pattern has been described for previously healthy trauma patients admitted to the ICU [6–8].
2. COPD patients with a forced expiratory volume in 1 s (FEV_1) <50% are oropharyngeal carriers of both types of flora, including *H. influenzae* and AGNB [9]. The severity of their underlying lung disease promotes colonization of the lower airways with oral flora, including normal and abnormal bacteria. The presence of bacteria in the lower airways, or colonization, is proinflammatory and may result in a range of important effects on the lung, including activation of host defenses with release of inflammatory cytokines and subsequent neutrophil recruitment, mucus hypersecretion, impaired mucociliary clearance, and respiratory cell damage [10, 11, 12]. Bacterial colonization of lower airways in COPD patients modulates the character and frequency of exacerbations and is associated with greater airway inflammation and accelerated decline in FEV_1 [13]. An acute exacerbation of their underlying condition may require intubation and ventilation in the ICU. The immediate administration of an adequate antimicrobial that is active against *H. influenzae*

and AGNB such as *Klebsiella* spp. is required in order to prevent infection of the lower airways.
3. Patients who are transferred from another hospital or ward into the ICU and require ventilatory support often carry abnormal flora, including MRSA or *Pseudomonas* spp., due to the underlying disease. The acute deterioration of their underlying disease requires intubation, leading to colonization of the lower airways with abnormal flora. Colonization may develop into infection depending on the patient's level of immunosuppression.

2.4 Defenses Against Carriage, Colonization, and Infection

2.4.1 Defenses Against Carriage

Healthy individuals efficiently clear abnormal AGNB from the oropharyngeal cavity and digestive tract. This clearing property is called carriage defense [5]. Individuals are continuously exposed to AGNB. Healthy people acquire AGNB in the oropharynx via food intake, whereas unconscious patients acquire bacteria in the oropharynx form the environment, e.g., the ICU. The source of AGNB may be the inanimate or the animate environment, but in general, the other long-term ICU patients are the main sources. AGNB acquisition from such patients commonly results in carriage, as the critically ill patient is unable to clear these abnormal bacteria due to the underlying disease. Seven-mechanisms represent the first line of defense against carriage of PPMs in the digestive tract (Fig. 2.2) [14]:

1. *Intact anatomy of throat and gut.* Chewing, swallowing, and intestinal motility are frequently impaired in critically ill patients [5].
2. *Physiology.* Any severe underlying disease may reduce the exocrine function of the stomach and the gastric acid barrier. Moreover, critically ill patients frequently receive proton pump inhibitors or anti-H_2 receptor antagonists, which impair the gastric-acid barrier [12]. Fibronectin is also reduced during critical illness, resulting in increased AGNB adherence following the increased availability of AGNB receptor sites on the digestive tract mucosa [15]. Macrophages are thought to release elastase, which denudes the fibronectin layer from the mucosa, making AGNB receptor sites available [16].
3. *Secretions.* Bile and mucus secretion is reduced in critically ill patients, particularly in those who receive parenteral nutrition.
4. *Motility.* The regular, cyclical, and contractile activity of the gastrointestinal tract, which flushes out of food remnants, cell debris, and bacteria, is impaired in critically ill patients, leading to bacterial overgrowth. Depending on the severity of the underlying disease, gut paralysis is associated with overgrowth of both normal and abnormal flora [5].
5. *Epithelial renewal.* Intestinal epithelial cells have a rapid turnover, which explains why these cells are highly dependent on adequate nutrient and oxygen supply, which is frequently reduced in ICU patients.

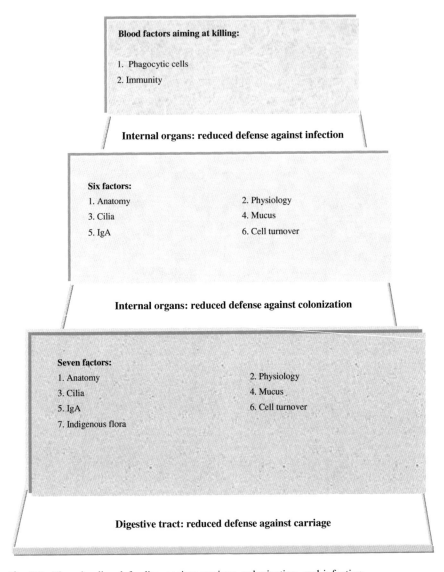

Fig. 2.2 Three hurdles defending against carriage, colonization, and infection

6. *Gut-associated lymphoid tissue (GALT) and IgA.* These are important in eliciting the immune response both locally in the gut and subsequently at a systemic level. Secretory immunoglobulin A (IgA), released by GALT, is the most common immunoglobulin in saliva, bile, and mucus, and the protective effect is due to its ability to inhibit AGNB adherence to the epithelium by coating the microorganisms [17].

7. *Indigenous flora*. These flora are primarily anaerobes and the indigenous *E. coli*. Indigenous flora helps control carriage of acquired AGNB—the so-called colonization resistance. In most cases, the beneficial functions of the indigenous flora outweigh potentially harmful side effects. The microbiota provides digestive functions, modulates host metabolism, and stimulates development of lymphatic tissue and the mucosal immune system [5, 18]. Moreover, it can efficiently limit gut infection by pathogenic bacteria. In fact [5, 18]:
- normal flora acts as living wallpaper covering the mucosal receptor sites, thus preventing AGNB adherence to those receptors;
- anaerobes in high concentration require a huge quantities of nutrients, resulting in AGNB starvation;
- normal flora produces bacteriocidins that are bactericidal for AGNB, release volatile fatty acids that create a growth-inhibiting environment, and are an important source of energy for the gut epithelium (e.g., butyrate produced by *Faecalibacterium prausnitzii* [19]);
- presence of normal flora stimulates peristalsis;
- indigenous flora stimulates host defenses; moreover,
- deconjugation of bile salts by the indigenous flora is crucial for enterohepatic circulation;
- anaerobes produce β-lactamases that neutralize β-lactam antibiotics;
- indigenous flora releases biopeptides, which play a role in gastroendocrine metabolism, maintains water balance, promotes digestive tract motility, and produces vitamins, including vitamin K, biotin, riboflavin, and folate [5].

2.4.2 Defenses Against Colonization of the Internal Organs

Abnormal carriage of AGNB and MRSA inevitably leads to overgrowth of these bacteria in critically ill patients following deterioration of the underlying disease [20]. Intestinal overgrowth of abnormal flora has been shown to promote and maintain systemic immunoparalysis via liver macrophage activation [21] and is considered an independent risk factor for colonization and infection of internal organs [22–24]. PPMs may migrate from the digestive tract toward lower airways or bladder (endogenous colonization) or may be introduced directly into the internal organ from an external source, either animate or inanimate (exogenous colonization). Six clearing factors are present in these internal organs. In the lower airways these are [25] (Fig. 2.2):
1. *Anatomy integrity*. The endotracheal tube damages the mucosa and promotes microorganism adherence;
2. *Physiology integrity*. Inhaled particles or microorganisms must survive and penetrate the aerodynamic filtration system of the tracheobronchial tree. Airflow is turbulent, causing microorganisms to affect mucosal surfaces. Humidification also causes hygroscopic organisms to increase in size, thereby aiding trapping. Mucosal surface adhesins are known to mediate bacterial adherence to host extracellular matrix components, such as collagen, fibrinogen, and fibronectin

[26, 27]. Fibronectin covers surface-cell receptors and thereby blocks attachment of many microorganisms. The mucociliary blanket transports the invading microorganisms out of the lung, and coughing aids this expulsion. In addition, bronchial secretions contain various antimicrobial substances, such as lysozyme, and defensins. Once the microorganism reaches the alveoli, the alveolar macrophages and tissue histiocytes play an important role in protecting the host.
3. *Cilia motility*. In conjunction with mucus, cilia mechanically remove microorganisms reaching its surface. Airway hygiene depends largely on mucociliary clearance, which in turn depends upon movement of viscoelastic mucus along the airway [28]. Aspirated or breathed material sticks to the mucus and is thus cleared from the respiratory tract. Mucociliary clearance can be impaired by (a) genetic defects, e.g., primary ciliary dyskinesia, cystic fibrosis; (b) secondary ciliary dyskinesia due to artificial ventilation or toxins released by microorganisms producing cytotoxic damage of epithelial cells (in this situation, microorganisms may remain longer in the airways, causing colonization and infection); (c) abnormal physicochemical properties of mucus, making it difficult to move it along the airway. A persistent host inflammatory response driven by cytokines fails to eliminate microorganisms and maintains the inflammatory process.
4. *Secretory IgA*. IgA in bronchial secretions coats microorganisms to prevent adherence to mucosal cell receptors. Secretory IgA is the predominant immunoglobulin present in the respiratory tract, nasal secretions, saliva, tears, gastrointestinal fluids, and other mucous secretions. In addition, IgA can neutralize toxin activity [29].
5. *Mucosal cell turnover and desquamation*. This process eliminates adherent bacteria.

Similarly, six mechanisms are present to help prevent fecal PPMs from colonizing the urinary tract [30] (Fig. 2.2):
1. *Anatomical integrity*. The bladder mucosa acts as a barrier to invading microorganisms.
2. *Intact physiology*. Assists with clearing PPMs migrating from the rectal cavity into the urethra and finally into the bladder [31]; extreme levels of osmolality, high urea concentration, and low pH inhibit growth of some bacteria that cause urinary tract infections;
3. *Urinary flow*. Mechanically removes PPMs unless they are capable of adhering to epithelial cells in the urinary tract;
4. *Mucus*. covers the bladder mucosa.
5. *Secretory IgA*. Presence in mucus prevents adherence of fecal bacteria;
6. *Mucosal cell turnover*. Promotes elimination of PPMs already adhering to bladder mucosal cells.

2.4.3 Defenses Against Infection

Colonizing microorganisms that are not eliminated from internal organs invariably lead to a high concentration ($\geq 10^5$) of PPMs, predisposing to invasion. The host mobilizes both humoral and cellular defense systems to hinder the invading microorganisms. However, infection requires both invasion and critical illness, which jeopardize immunocompetence (Fig. 2.2).

2.5 Mechanisms of Colonization and Infection in ICU Patients

There are two basic mechanisms of colonization and infection in ICU patients: migration and translocation. Migration is the movement of live PPMs from one place, e.g., throat and gut, where they are present in overgrowth, to another site, in particular, normally sterile internal organs. Migration is the main mechanism by which microorganisms may cause colonization/infection in ICU patients. Migration of microorganisms in contaminated secretions from the oropharynx into the lower airways within a few days of mechanical ventilation is considered to be the most common route by which PPMs may enter the lung and cause colonization and infection [22, 32, 33]. The severity of the underlying disease, which impairs PPM clearance, is the main factor promoting colonization of the lower airways. The presence of the plastic endotracheal tube is invariably associated with mucosal lesions, which further enhances colonization. Finally, progression toward infection depends on the patient's immune status or defense capacity.

Potential pathogens may also cause colonization and subsequent infection, bypassing the stage of carriage and overgrowth, i.e., exogenous colonization/infection. An example is a lower respiratory tract colonization/infection in a tracheotomized patient due to microorganisms not previously carried in throat and/or gut but directly introduced following breaches of hygiene [34].

Translocation (or transmural migration) was originally defined by Berg and Owens [35] as the passage of viable bacteria from the gut through the epithelium to the lamina propria and hence to mesenteric lymph nodes and possibly other organs. This was subsequently modified by Alexander et al. [36] to refer to the movement of viable and nonviable microorganisms or their toxic products across an intact intestinal barrier. Tsujimoto et al. [37] recently proposed a radical revision of the definition, which includes translocation of pathogen-associated molecular patterns. In normally healthy people, GALT macrophages are generally effective in killing intestinal microorganisms translocating from the gut. When gut function is impaired—as in the critically ill patient—either in the anatomically intact gastrointestinal tract or in altered intestinal mucosa, bacterial translocation can spread into the systemic bloodstream, leading to sepsis and multiple organ failure [38]. Gut overgrowth of PPMs, in particular, in the terminal ileum, is required for translocation [39]. The phenomenon of translocation has been described in surgical patients [40], patients with pancreatitis [23] and neutropenia [41], in surgical neonates and infants receiving parenteral nutrition [42], and in patients requiring intensive care, including mechanical ventilation [43]. Critical illness impacts three elements of the gut: (1) it alters cellular proliferation and death in the epithelium [44, 45]; it has a profound effect on the number of cells in the mucosal immune system [46, 47]; (3) it changes the normal carrier state into abnormal carriage, defined as the persistent presence of abnormal potential pathogens in the oropharynx and/or gut [22, 32, 33].

2.6 Conclusions

Only a general well-being guarantees the efficacy of carriage defenses, which are based on seven innate host factors that facilitate clearing abnormal AGNB from the gut, maintain normal flora, and subsequently prevent colonization and infection of internal organs. Most importantly, the shift from normal to abnormal flora in individuals with an underlying disease is thought to depend on the severity of the illness. The use of antimicrobials, which impair the microbial factor of the carriage defense system, further promotes gut carriage and overgrowth of abnormal flora. Oropharyngeal and gastrointestinal eradication of abnormal flora using enteral, nonabsorbable antimicrobials polymyxin B/tobramycin and amphotericin B is the most logical approach by which to control or minimize the risk of PPM overgrowth in the digestive and control colonization and infection of internal organs [48].

References

1. Kerver AJH, Rommes JH, Mevissen-Verhage EAE et al (1987) Colonization and infection in surgical intensive care patients: a prospective study. Intensive Care Med 13:347–351
2. Sarginson RE, Taylor N, van Saene HKF (2001) Glossary of terms and definitions. Curr Anaesth Crit Care 12:2–5
3. Pittet D, Monod M, Suter PM et al (1994) Candida colonization and subsequent infections in critically ill surgical patients. Ann Surg 220:751–758
4. Mobbs KJ, van Saene HKF, Sunderland D, Davies PDO (1999) Oropharyngeal Gram-negative bacillary carriage. A survey of 120 healthy individuals. Chest 115:1570–1575
5. Rosseneu S, Rios G, Spronk PE, van Saene JJM (2005) Carriage. In: van Saene HKF, Silvestri L, de la Cal MA (eds) Infection control in the intensive care unit, 2nd edn. Springer, Milan, pp 15–36
6. Sirvent JM, Torres A, Vidaur L et al (2000) Tracheal colonisation within 24 h of intubation in patients with head trauma: risk factor for developing early-onset ventilator-associated pneumonia. Intensive Care Med 26:1369–1372
7. Ewig S, Torres A, El-Ebiary M et al (1999) Bacterial colonization patterns in mechanically ventilated patients with traumatic and medical injury. Incidence, risk factors and association with ventilator-associated pneumonia. Am J Respir Crit Care Med 159:188–198
8. Acquarolo A, Urli T, Perone G et al (2005) Antibiotic prophylaxis of early onset pneumonia in critically ill comatose patients. A randomized study. Intensive Care Med 31:510–516
9. Mobbs KJ, van Saene HKF, Sunderland D, Davies PDO (1999) Oropharyngeal Gram-negative bacillary carriage in chronic obstructive pulmonary disease: relation to severity of disease. Respir Med 93:540–545
10. Yamamoto C, Yoneda T, Yoshikawa M et al (1997) Airway inflammation in COPD patients assessed by sputum levels of interleukin-8. Chest 112:505–510
11. Sethi S, Murphy TF (2001) Bacterial infection in chronic obstructive pulmonary disease in 2000: state of the art. Clin Microbiol Rev 14:336–363
12. Hillman KM, Riordan T, O'Farrel SM, Tabacqchali S (1982) Colonization of the gastric content in critically ill patients. Crit Care Med 10:444–447

13. Patel IS, Seemungal TA, Wilks M et al (2002) Relationship between bacterial colonisation and the frequency, character, and severity of COPD exacerbations. Thorax 57:753–754
14. Silvestri L, Lenhart FP, Fox MA (2001) Prevention of intensive care unit infections. Curr Anaesth Crit Care 12:34–40
15. Proctor RA (1987) Fibronectin: a brief overview of its structure function and physiology. Rev Infect Dis 9:S317–S312
16. Dal Nogare AR, Toews GB, Pierce AK (1987) Increased salivary elastase precedes Gram-negative bacillary colonization in post-operative patients. Am Rev Respir Dis 135:671–675
17. Mestesky J, Russel M, Elson CO (1999) Intestinal IgA, novel views on its function in the defence of the largest mucosal surface. Gut 44:2–5
18. Barber S, Wolf-Dietrich H (2011) Mechanisms controlling pathogen colonization of the gut. Curr Opin Microbiol 14:82–91
19. Sokol H, Pigneur B, Watterlot L et al (2008) Faecalibacterium prausnitzii is an anti-inflammatory commensal bacterium identified by gut microbiota analysis of Crohn disease patients. Proc Natl Acad Sci U S A 105:16731–16736
20. van Saene HKF, Damjanovic V, Alcock SR (2001) Basics in microbiology for the patient requiring intensive care. Curr Anaesth Crit Care 12:6–17
21. Marshall JC, Christou NV, Meakins JL (1988) Small-bowel bacterial overgrowth and systemic immuno-suppression in experimental peritonitis. Surgery 104:404–411
22. van Uffelen R, van Saene HKF, Fidler V et al (1984) Oropharyngeal flora as a source of colonizing the lower airways in patients on artificial ventilation. Intensive Care Med 10: 233–237
23. Luiten EJT, Hop WCJ, Endtz HP et al (1988) Prognostic importance of Gram-negative intestinal colonization preceding pancreatic infection in severe acute pancreatitis. Intensive Care Med 24:438–445
24. Oostijk EAN, de Smet AMGA, Kesecioglu J, Bonten MJM, on behalf of the Dutch SOD-SDD trialists group (2011) The role of intestinal colonization with Gram-negative bacteria as a source for intensive care unit-acquired bacteremia. Crit Care Med 39:961–966
25. Manson CM, Summer WR, Nelson S (1992) Pathophysiology of pulmonary defence mechanisms. J Crit Care 7:42–56
26. Peacock SJ, Foster TJ, Cameron BJ, Berend R (1999) Bacterial fibronectin-binding proteins and endothelial cell surface fibronectin mediate adherence of *Staphylococcus aureus* to resting human endothelial cells. Microbiology 145:3477–3486
27. Mongodin E, Bajolet O, Cutrona J et al (2002) Fibronectin-binding proteins of *Staphylococcus aureus* are involved in adherence to human airway epithelium. Infect Immun 70:620–630
28. Cole P (2001) Pathophysiology and treatment of airway mucociliary clearance. Minerva Anestesiol 67:206–209
29. Hienzel FP (2000) Antibodies. In: Mandell GL, Bennett JE, Dolin R (eds) Mandell, Douglas and Bennett's principles and practice of infectious diseases. Churchill Livingstone, Philadelphia, pp 45–67
30. Kass EH, Schneiderman LJ (1957) Entry of bacteria into the urinary tract of patients with implying catheters. N Engl J Med 256:556–557
31. Kunin CM, Evans C, Bartholomew D, Bates DG (2002) The antimicrobial defense mechanism of the female urethra: a reassessment. J Urol 168:413–419
32. Johanson WG Jr, Pierce AK, Sandford JP et al (1972) Nosocomial respiratory tract infections with Gram-negative bacilli: the significance of colonization of the respiratory tract. Ann Intern Med 77:701–706
33. Estes RJ, Meduri GU (1995) The pathogenesis of ventilator associated pneumonia: I. Mechanisms of bacterial trans-colonization and airway inoculation. Intensive Care Med 21:365–383
34. Morar P, Makura Z, Jones A et al (2000) Topical antibiotics on tracheostoma prevent exogenous colonization and infection of lower airways in children. Chest 117:513–518

35. Berg RD, Owens WE (1979) Inhibition of translocation of viable *Escherichia coli* from the gastrointestinal tract of mice by bacterial antagonism. Infect Immun 25:820–827
36. Alexander JW, Boyce ST, Babcock GF et al (1990) The process of microbial translocation. Ann Surg 212:496–510
37. Tsujimoto H, Ono S, Mochizuki H (2009) Role of translocation of pathogen-associated molecular patterns in sepsis. Dig Surg 26:100–109
38. Sganga G, van Saene HKF, Brisinda G, Castagneto M (2001) Bacterial translocation. In: van Saene HKF, Sganga G, Silvestri L (eds) Infection in the critically ill: an ongoing challenge. Springer, Milan, pp 35–45
39. Husebye E (1995) Gastro-intestinal motility disorders and bacterial overgrowth. J Intern Med 237:419–427
40. Kane TD, Wesley Alexander J, Johannigman JA (1998) The detection of microbial DNA in the blood. A sensitive method for diagnosing bacteremia and/or bacterial translocation in surgical patients. Ann Surg 227:1–9
41. Tancrede CH, Andremont AO (1985) Bacterial translocation and Gram-negative bacteremia in patients with hematological malignancies. J Infect Dis 152:99–103
42. van Saene HKF, Taylor N, Donnell SC et al (2003) Gut overgrowth with abnormal flora: the missing link in parenteral nutrition-related sepsis in surgical neonates. Eur J Clin Nutr 57:548–553
43. Feltis BA, Wells CL (2000) Does microbial translocation play a role in critical illness? Curr Opin Crit Care 6:117–122
44. Coopersmith CM, Stromberg PE, Davis CG et al (2003) Sepsis from *Pseudomonas aeruginosa* pneumonia decreases intestinal proliferation and reduces gut epithelial cell cycle arrest. Crit Care Med 39:1630–1637
45. Husain KD, Stromberg PE, Woolsey CA et al (2005) Mechanisms of decreased intestinal epithelial proliferation and increased apoptosis in murine acute lung injury. Crit Care Med 33:2350–2357
46. Fukatsu K, Sakamoto S, Hara E et al (2005) Gut ischemia–reperfusion affects gut mucosal immunity: a possible mechanism for infectious complications after severe surgical insults. Crit Care Med 34:182–187
47. Osterberg J, Ljungdahl M, Haglund U (2006) Influence of cyclooxygenase inhibitors on gut immune cell distribution and apoptosis rate in experimental sepsis. Shock 25:147–154
48. van Saene HKF (2008) The history of SDD. In: an der Voort PHJ, van Saene HKF (eds) Selective digestive decontamination in intensive care medicine. Springer, Milan, pp 1–35

Classification of Microorganisms According to Their Pathogenicity

3

M. A. de la Cal, E. Cerdà, A. Abella
and P. Garcia-Hierro

3.1 Introduction

Isenberg wrote in 1988: "A modern clinical microbiologist who asks what is a pathogen and what is meant by virulence will meet with derision and probably be declared heretic, bereft of his or her senses" [1]. He expressed the difficulties in defining the concepts of pathogenicity and virulence, which have changed and are still changing with the growing number of infectious diseases in the hospital setting and in the immunocompromised host.

It is accepted that infection is the result of the interaction between the host, the microorganism, and the environment. Pathogenicity (Table 3.1) [2–4] is not only an intrinsic quality of microorganisms but the consequence of some properties of the microorganisms and the host. For example, coagulase-negative staphylococcus has been considered an avirulent, opportunistic organism and not a true pathogen [5], but the increasing number of bacteremias due to this organism in recent decades has emphasized its pathogenicity and virulence. The ability of coagulase-negative staphylococcus to induce disease increases when a patient's defense mechanisms are altered. Freeman et al. [6] emphasized that the fivefold increase of coagulase-negative staphylococcus bacteremia found in a neonatal care unit from 1975 to 1982 was mainly attributable to an increase in the number of children with a birth weight <1,000 g. Thus, the separation of pathogenicity, defense mechanisms, and type of infection is only justified for didactic reasons. Some terms routinely used by physicians working in intensive care units (ICUs) describe many aspects involved in pathogenicity:

M. A. de la Cal (✉)
Department of Intensive Care Medicine,
Hospital Universitario de Getafe, Getafe, Spain
e-mail: mcal@ucigetafe.com

Table 3.1 Glossary of terms

Term	Definition
Pathogenicity	The ability of microorganisms to induce disease, which may be assessed by disease-carriage ratios
Virulence[a]	The severity of the disease induced by microorganisms. In epidemiological studies virulence may be assessed by mortality or morbidity rates and the degree of communicability
Reservoir	The place where the organism maintains its presence, metabolizes, and replicates
Source	The place from which the infectious agent passes to the host. In some cases, the reservoir and the source are the same, but not always
Infection	A microbiologically proven clinical diagnosis of inflammation
Carriage[b]	Permanent (minimally 1 week) presence of the same strain in any concentration in body sites normally not sterile (oropharynx, external nares, gut, vagina, skin)
Abnormal carrier state	The abnormal carrier state exists when the isolated microorganism is not a constituent of normal flora (i.e., aerobic Gram-negative bacilli and methicillin-resistant *Staphylococcus aureus*) [3]
Colonization[b]	The presence of microorganisms in an internal organ that is normally sterile (e.g., lower airways, bladder). The diagnostic sample yields less than a predetermined level of CFU/ml of diagnostic sample [3]

CFU colony-forming units
[a] Some authors [4] consider virulence a synonym of pathogenicity
[b] Some authors [2] define colonization as the permanent presence of a micro-organism in or on a host without clinical expression. Carrier state is the condition of an individual colonized with a specific organism. These definitions do not take the sterility of colonized sites in normal individuals into consideration

1. Intrinsic characteristics of bacteria, i.e., Gram's stain; aerobic–anaerobic requirements for growth; antibiotic sensitivity–resistance patterns.
2. Quantitative criteria for defining some infections, i.e., pneumonia associated with mechanical ventilation or urinary tract infection. For instance, the probability of having pneumonia is higher if the quantitative culture of a protected brush catheter sample yields 10^4 colony forming units (CFU) instead of 10^3 CFU. Even the significance of the quantitative culture is different if the patient is neutropenic. These criteria are related to the classic concept of infective dose, which is the estimated dose of an agent necessary to cause infection.
3. Sites of isolation when evaluating the clinical significance of a culture. For instance, *Staphylococcus aureus* may colonize the external nares without any evidence of disease, but its presence in a fresh surgical wound may indicate colonization or infection.

4. Community—versus hospital—versus ICU-acquired flora, which recognizes that the relationship between the different species, the host, and the environment induces changes in the microbial habitat.
5. Carriage, colonization, and infection, which defines some possible host states according to the significance of the presence of microorganisms in different organs.
6. Exogenous, primary endogenous, and secondary endogenous infections, which describe a pathogenetic model based on some epidemiological criteria. In this chapter we address the concept of pathogenicity and the epidemiological aspects of microorganisms in clinical practice.

3.2 Magnitude of the Problem

Surveillance of microorganisms in the oropharynx and respiratory and digestive tracts in ICU patients has provided an essential basis for our understanding of infectious diseases in the ICU:
- patients' flora change after hospital admission, and this process is time dependent [7–9];
- in a high percentage of cases (70–100%) [7, 8, 10], infections were preceded by oropharyngeal or gut carriage with the same potentially pathogenic microorganism (PPM);
- digestive tract is usually the reservoir of antibiotic-resistant strains;
- different microorganisms found in the same patient show different abilities to induce infection, i.e., they have a different pathogenicity. Those observations imply two questions: Where is the flora? Which types of flora can be differentiated on an epidemiological basis?

3.2.1 Habitat

It is estimated that the human body consists of approximately 10^{13} cells, and hosts 10^{14}–10^{15} individual microorganisms [1]. These microorganisms can be divided into two groups: those that usually remain constant in their normal habitat (indigenous flora), and those that are accidentally acquired and that, after adherence to epithelial or mucosal surfaces, have to compete with other microorganisms and host defenses. The final outcome could be clearance or colonization of the new organisms.

Body areas that usually harbor microorganisms (Tables 3.2 and 3.3) [11] are skin, mouth, nasopharynx, oropharynx and tonsils, large intestine and lower ileum, external genitalia, anterior urethra, vagina, skin, and external ear. Nevertheless, the various anatomical sites suitable for microbiological habitats display overlapping boundaries and are subject to variation. Temporary habitats include larynx, trachea, bronchi, accessory nasal sinuses, esophagus, stomach and upper portions of the small intestine, and distal areas of the male and female genital organs [12]. Permanent colonization is often found in patients with some risks factors, i.e., chronic bronchitis [13].

Table 3.2 Microorganisms commonly found in healthy human body surfaces

Surface	Microorganism	Frequency of isolation
Skin	*Staphylococcus epidermidis*	4+
	Diphtheroids	3+
	Staphylococcus aureus	2+
	Streptococcus spp.	+
	Acinetobacter spp.	±
	Enterobacteriaceae	±
Mouth and throat	Anaerobic Gram-negative spp.	4+
	Anaerobic cocci	+
	Streptococcus viridans	4+
	Streptococcus pneumoniae	2+
	Streptococcus pyogenes	+
	Staphylococcus epidermidis	4+
	Neisseria meningitidis	+
	Haemophilus spp.	+
	Enterobacteriaceae	±
	Candida spp.	2+
Nose	*Staphylococcus epidermidis*	4+
	Staphylococcus aureus	2+
	Streptococcus pneumoniae	+
	Streptococcus pyogenes	+
	Haemophilus spp.	+
Large intestine (95% or more of species are obligate anaerobes)	Anaerobic Gram-negative spp.	4+
	Anaerobic Gram-positive spp.	4+
	Escherichia coli	4+
	Klebsiella spp.	3+
	Proteus spp.	3+
	Enterococcus spp.	3+
	Group B streptococci	+
	Clostridium spp.	3+
	Pseudomonas spp.	+
	Acinetobacter spp.	+
	Staphylococcus epidermidis	+
	Staphylococcus aureus	+
	Candida spp.	+

(continued)

Table 3.2 (continued)

Surface	Microorganism	Frequency of isolation
External genitalia and anterior urethra	Skin flora	4+
	Gram-negative anaerobic spp.	+
	Enterococcus spp.	+
	Enterobacteriaceae	±
Vagina	*Lactobacillus* spp.	4+
	Gram-negative anaerobic spp.	2+
	Enterococcus spp.	3+
	Enterobacteriaceae	1+
	Acinetobacter spp.	±
	Staphylococcus epidermidis	1+
	Candida spp.	1+

Relative frequency of isolation: 4+ almost always present, 3+ usually present, 2+ frequently present, + occasionally present, ± rarely present

3.2.2 Flora

Indigenous flora is very dynamic and reflects changes induced by environmental settings, medical treatments, and host and microbial characteristics. It is well accepted that normal individuals have normal indigenous flora (Tables 3.2 and 3.3) that represent the equilibrium reached between the normal hosts and the organisms. Quantitative estimation of different microorganisms found in human body surfaces helps us to understand pathogenicity, because it is often obvious that predominantly isolated microorganisms rarely induce disease. Anaerobes are a good example of organisms of low pathogenicity. They represent the highest percentage of microorganisms isolated per surface area but are only involved in a small proportion of infections.

Surveillance cultures performed in patients after hospital or ICU admission [7–9] demonstrate that flora changes over time. Carriage of aerobic Gram-negative bacilli (AGNB) *Pseudomonas* spp., *Klebsiella* spp., *Enterobacter* spp., *Acinetobacter* spp., *Serratia* and *Morganella* spp., and yeasts *Candida* spp. increases. This process of new organism acquisition is time dependent. For example, Kerver et al. [7] studied 39 intubated patients admitted to the ICU for more than 5 days, obtaining samples three times a week from the oropharynx, tracheal aspirate, urine, and feces. The prevalence of AGNB in the oropharyngeal cavity on admission was 23% and increased to 80% after 10 days. Similar figures were found for yeasts. In feces, the prevalence of AGNB other than *E. coli* was 20% and reached 79% on day 15. Yeasts were found in 13% of rectal swabs on admission and in 61% of samples on day 15. In 75.6% of infections, the same PPM was found in previous surveillance cultures [10]. This new flora comes into

Table 3.3 Quantitative cultures of healthy human surfaces

Surface	Microorganism	Percent carriers	CFU
Skin (per cm)	*Staphylococcus epidermidis*	100	10^5
	Anaerobes (*Propionibacterium acnes*)	100	10^3
Mouth and throat (per ml of saliva)	Anaerobic microorganisms	100	10^8
	Streptococcus viridans	100	10^6
	Streptococcus pneumoniae	30–60	$10^3 - 10^5$
	Haemophilus influenzae	30–80	$10^3 - 10^5$
	Moraxella catarrhalis	5	$10^3 - 10^5$
	Staphylococcus aureus	30	10^3
Large intestine (per gram of feces)	Anaerobic spp.	100	10^{12}
	Escherichia coli	100	$10^3 - 10^6$
	Enterococcus spp.	100	$10^3 - 10^6$
	Staphylococcus aureus	30	$10^3 - 10^5$
	Candida spp.	30	$10^3 - 10^5$
Vagina (per ml of vaginal fluid)	Aerobic spp.	100	10^8
	Anaerobic spp.	100	10^7

the human body from different animate (mostly patients and—uncommonly—health personnel) or inanimate (e.g., food; furniture) sources through different vehicles (e.g., hands; respiratory equipment). After being introduced, the new organisms adhere to surfaces and have to compete with preexisting flora and host defense barriers before a permanent carriage state is achieved. Apart from the severity of the underlying disease, parenteral antibiotic administration is the main mechanism that favors acquisition of hospital flora through selective pressure exerted against indigenous flora [14].

The boundaries between normal, community, and abnormal hospital flora are not always strict. Some groups of patients admitted to the hospital carry organisms, usually constituents of abnormal hospital flora. Alcoholism, diabetes, and chronic bronchitis are regarded as risk factors for carrying aerobic Gram-negative bacilli [13, 15] in the oropharynx and tracheobronchial tree, respectively.

3.3 Microorganism Classification According to Pathogenicity

Leonard et al. [16] attempted to quantitatively estimate intrinsic pathogenicity in a population of 40 infants admitted for at least 5 days to a neonatal surgical unit. The intrinsic pathogenicity index (IPI) for a y species was defined as:

$$IPI_y = \frac{\text{Number of patients infected by } y}{\text{Number of patients carrying } y \text{ in throat/rectum}}$$

The range of this index is 0–1. The highest IPI found was for *Pseudomonas* spp. (0.38). Other potential pathogens isolated had an IPI <0.1 (*Enterobacter* spp. 0.08; *S. aureus* 0.06; *Klebsiella* spp. 0.05; *E. coli* 0.05; *S. epidermidis* 0.03; *Enterococcus* spp. 0). This index provides useful information about the relative pathogenicity of different microorganisms in a specific population and could be used to design antibiotic policies, both prophylactic and therapeutic, in selected groups of patients in whom microbiological surveillance could be indicated (e.g., burn, severe trauma patients).

There are inherent limitations related to the small number of studied patients and the small number of infections (i.e., *S. aureus*: one infection over 17 colonizations), which can give an unreliable estimation of the IPI. Furthermore, the authors of the study suggested that the results should be interpreted taking into account technical aspects (definitions used; sites chosen for surveillance; microbiological techniques; result interpretation) and population characteristics, because IPI does not differentiate between the organism's intrinsic pathogenicity and other factors (host and environment) that allow their expression. The extreme alterations in host defense mechanisms in immunosuppressed patients is a good example of the different pathogenicity of microorganisms depending on the specific type of systemic immunosuppression, i.e., neutropenia or cellular (T lymphocyte) immune defect [17].

In general, the classification of microorganisms according to their pathogenicity is based on scales with few categories. Isenberg and D'Amato [12] classify organisms as commonly involved, occasionally involved, and rarely involved in disease production. Murray et al. [3] classify the pathogenicity of organisms as high, potential, and low. Categories in both classifications are not always equivalent. We found that the Murray et al. [3] classification (Table 3.4) is useful in ICU practice because it is best adapted to flora isolated in ICU patients and is more discriminatory between organisms of interest in the ICU. Another possible advantage is that this classification integrates other concepts of clinical epidemiology, such as community, or normal; and hospital, or abnormal, flora.

3.4 Antimicrobial Resistance as a Virulence Factor

Evaluation of the influence of antimicrobial resistance on mortality is difficult because of the requirement to adjust for underlying disease and illness severity. Recent literature suggests that the factor of immediate, adequate treatment plays an important role in evaluating the contribution of antimicrobial resistance to mortality [18–21]. Fagon et al. [22] found that in patients suspected of having ventilator-associated pneumonia, an invasive strategy based on the use of fiber-optic bronchoscopy improved the survival rate at day 14 ($p = 0.02$); 16.2% died in

Table 3.4 Classification of microorganisms based on their intrinsic pathogenicity

Intrinsic pathogenicity	Flora	Indigenous flora
Oropharynx: *Peptostreptococcus* spp., *Veillonella* spp., *Streptococcus viridans* Gut: *Bacteroides* spp., *Clostridium* spp., *Enterococcus* spp., *Escherichia coli* Vagina: *Peptostreptococcus* spp., *Bacteroides* spp., *Lactobacillus* spp. Skin: *Propionibacterium acnes*, coagulase-negative staphylococci, Community or normal microorganisms	Low pathogenic	Normal
Oropharynx: *Streptococcus pneumoniae, Haemophilus influenzae, Moraxella catarrhalis* Gut: *Escherichia coli* Oropharynx and gut: *Staphylococcus aureus, Candida* spp.	Potentially pathogenic	Normal
Hospital or abnormal microorganisms: *Klebsiella* spp., *Proteus* spp., *Enterobacter* spp., *Morganella* spp., *Citrobacter* spp., *Serratia* spp., *Pseudomonas* spp., *Acinetobacter* spp., MRSA	Potentially pathogenic	Abnormal
Epidemic microorganisms: *Neisseria meningitidis, Salmonella* spp.	Highly pathogenic	Abnormal

MRSA methicillin-resistant *Staphylococcus aureus*

the invasive management group and 25.8% in the clinical management group, i.e., a difference of 9.6%. This survival benefit can be explained by the fact that significantly more patients who did not undergo bronchoscopy received early, inadequate antimicrobial therapy (one patient died in the invasive group versus 24 in the control group; $p < 0.001$). The survival benefit was only transient, as the difference in mortality was no longer significant at day 28 ($p = 0.10$). Only a few of the evaluable studies adjusted mortality data for appropriate antimicrobial treatment, underlying disease, and illness severity.

3.4.1 Methicillin-Resistant S. aureus Versus Methicillin-Sensitive S. aureus

Of 31 bacteremia studies comparing mortality due to methicillin-resistant *S. aureus* (MRSA) and methicillin-sensitive *S. aureus* (MSSA) [23], only six adjusted for confounding factors, including adequate antibiotic therapy [24–29]. Three studies involving 401 patients found a significantly increased mortality rate, with odds ratios (OR) varying between 3 and 5.6. The other three studies, with a total of 1,385 patients, showed no significant difference. Only one study compared mortality due to MRSA in 86 bacteremic pneumonia patients and found no significant difference [30].

3.4.2 Vancomycin-Resistant Enterococci Versus Vancomycin-Sensitive Enterococci

Three studies in patients with positive blood cultures and that adjusted for appropriate antibiotic treatment are available [31–33]. Only one study in 106 patients reports a significantly higher mortality rate due to vancomycin-resistant enterococci (VRE), with an OR of 4.0 (1.2–13.3). The other two studies in a total of 467 patients failed to show a mortality rate difference.

3.4.3 Aerobic Gram-Negative Bacilli, Including Acinetobacter spp. and Pseudomonas aeruginosa

One study in 135 patients compared mortality rates in patients with infections due to piperacillin-resistant *P. aeruginosa* and patients with infections due to piperacillin-sensitive *P. aeruginosa* [34]. Mortality data were not adjusted for immediate, adequate antimicrobial therapy, as there was no difference in crude mortality. There are no data on *Acinetobacter* mortality, whether sensitive or resistant.

These data show that the association of antimicrobial resistance with mortality rate has not yet been appropriately evaluated. Evidence supports the concept that antibiotic resistance does not contribute to mortality.

3.5 Conclusions

Although the properties of the different microorganisms fail to explain completely their pathogenicity, it is clear that some characteristics do determine the different pathogenicity; for example, encapsulated pneumococci are more virulent than nonencapsulated pneumococci. Advances in molecular biology make it possible to characterize some virulence factors that allow microorganisms to overcome the set of obstacles to accomplish infection. These include selection of the niche and adherence to human body surfaces or medical devices (i.e., adhesins), competition with preexisting organisms in some cases, impairment of the host defense mechanism (i.e., antiphagocytic capsules; toxins), and production of tissue damage (i.e., toxins; enzymes). One report discusses the impact of critical illness on the expression of virulence in gut flora [35]. It has been hypothesized that gut bacteria change and become more virulent as the microorganisms sense that the host's capacity to control them is severely impaired. Identification of the virulent genes also provides a better understanding of the relationship between virulence factors and their clinical expression [36] and can be helpful in epidemiological studies, such as in determining transmission, carriage, colonization, and infection routes with specific microorganisms and the investigation of outbreaks [37–41].

References

1. Isenberg HD (1988) Pathogenicity and virulence: another view. Clin Microbiol Rev 1:40–53
2. Brachman PS (1992) Epidemiology of nosocomial infections. In: Bennett JV, Brachman PS (eds) Hospital infections, 3rd edn. Little Brown, Boston, pp 3–20
3. Murray AE, Mostafa SM, van Saene HKF (1991) Essentials in clinical microbiology. In: Stoutenbeek CP, van Saene HKF (eds) Infection and the anaesthetist, vol 5. Bailliere Tindall, London, pp 1–26
4. McCloskey RV (1979) Microbial virulence factors. In: Mandell GL, Douglas RG, Bennett IE (eds) Principles and practice of infectious diseases, vol 1, 1st edn. Wiley, New York, pp 3–11
5. Pfaller MA, Herwald LA (1988) Laboratory, clinical, and epidemiological aspects of coagulase-negative staphylococci. Clin Microbiol Rev 1:281–299
6. Freeman I, Platt R, Sidebottom DG et al (1987) Coagulase-negative staphylococcal bacteremia in the changing neonatal intensive care unit population. JAMA 258:2548–2552
7. Kerver AIH, Rommes IH, Mevissen-Verhage EAE et al (1987) Colonization and infection in surgical intensive care patients. Intensive Care Med 13:347–351
8. Leonard EM, van Saene HKF, Shears P, Walker I, Tam PKH (1990) Pathogenesis of colonization and infection in a neonatal surgical unit. Crit Care Med 18:264–269
9. van Saene HKF, Stoutenbeek CP, Zandstra DF, Gilberston A, Murray A, Hart CA (1987) Nosocomial infections in severely traumatized patient: magnitude of problem, pathogenesis, prevention and therapy. Acta Anaesthesiol Belg 38:347–356
10. van Saene HKF, Damjanovic V, Murray AE, de la Cal MA (1996) How to classify infections in intensive care units—the carrier state, a criterion whose time has come? J Hosp Infect 33:1–12
11. Tramont EC (1979) General or nonspecific host defense mechanisms. In: Mandell GL, Douglas RG, Bennett IE (eds) Principles and practice of infectious diseases, vol 1, 1st edn. Wiley, NewYork, pp 13–21
12. Isenberg HD, D'Amato RF (1990) Indigenous and pathogenic micro-organisms of humans. In: Mandell GL, Douglas RG, Bennett IE (eds) Principles and practice of infectious diseases, vol 1, 3rd edn. Churchill Livingstone, New York, pp 2–14
13. Jordan GW, Wong GA, Hoeprich PB (1976) Bacteriology of the lower respiratory tract as determined by fiberoptic bronchoscopy and transtracheal aspiration. J Infect Dis 134:428–435
14. van der Waaij D (1992) Selective gastrointestinal decontamination: history of recognition and measurement of colonization of the digestive tract as an introduction to selective gastrointestinal decontamination. Epidemiol Infect 109:315–326
15. Mackowiak PA, Martin RM, Smith LW (1979) The role of bacterial interference in the increased prevalence of oropharyngeal Gram-negative bacilli among alcoholics and diabetics. Am Rev Respir Dis 120:289–593
16. Leonard EM, van Saene HKF, Stoutenbeek CP, Walker I, Tam PKH (1990) An intrinsic pathogenicity index for micro-organisms causing infection in a neonatal surgical unit. Microb Ecol Health Dis 3:151–157
17. Shelhamer IH, Toews GB, Masur H et al (1992) Respiratory disease in the immunosuppressed patient. Ann Intern Med 117:415–443
18. Alvarez-Lerma F (1996) Modification of empiric antibiotic treatment in patients with pneumonia acquired in the intensive care unit. ICU-acquired pneumonia study group. Intensive Care Med 22:387–394
19. Luna CM, Vujacich P, Niederman MS et al (1997) Impact of BAL data on the therapy and outcome of ventilator-associated pneumonia. Chest 111:676–685

20. Iregui M, Ward S, Sherman G, Fraser VJ, Kollef MH (2002) Clinical importance of delays in the initiation of appropriate antibiotic treatment for ventilator associated pneumonia. Chest 122:262–268
21. Valles J, Rello J, Ochagavia A, Garnacho J, Alcala MA (2003) Community-acquired bloodstream infection in critically ill adult patients: impact of shock and inappropriate antibiotic therapy on survival. Chest 123:1615–1624
22. Fagon JY, Chastre J, Wolff M et al (2000) Invasive and noninvasive strategies for management of suspected ventilator associated pneumonia. A randomized trial. Ann Intern Med 132:621–630
23. Cosgrove SE, Sakoulas G, Perencevich EN, Schwaber MJ, Karchmer AW, Carmeli Y (2003) Comparison of mortality associated with methicillin-resistant and methicillin-susceptible *Staphylococcus aureus* bacteremia: a meta-analysis. Clin Infect Dis 36:53–59
24. Conterno LO, Wey SB, Castelo A (1998) Risk factors for mortality in *Staphylococcus aureus* bacteremia. Infect Control Hosp Epidemiol 19:32–37
25. Romero-Vivas J, Rubio M, Fernández C, Picazo JJ (1995) Mortality associated with nosocomial bacteremia due to methicillin-resistant *Staphylococcus aureus*. Clin Infect Dis 21:1417–1423
26. Harbarth S, Rutschmann O, Sudre P, Pittet D (1998) Impact of methicillin resistance on the outcome of patients with bacteremia caused by *Staphylococcus aureus*. Arch Intern Med 158:182–189
27. Soriano A, Martínez JA, Mensa J et al (2000) Pathogenic significance of methicillin resistance for patients with *Staphylococcus aureus* bacteremia. Clin Infect Dis 30:368–373
28. Mylotte JM, Tayara A (2000) *Staphylococcus aureus* bacteremia: predictors of 30-day mortality in a large cohort. Clin Infect Dis 31:1170–1174
29. Topeli A, Unal S, Akalin HE (2000) Risk factors influencing clinical outcome in *Staphylococcus aureus* bacteraemia in a Turkish University Hospital. Int J Antimicrob Agents 141:57–63
30. González C, Rubio M, Romero-Vivas J, González M, Picazo JJ (1999) Bacteremic pneumonia due to *Staphylococcus aureus*: a comparison of disease caused by methicillin-resistant and methicillin-susceptible organisms. Clin Infect Dis 29:1171–1177
31. Garbutt JM, Ventrapragada M, Littenberg B, Mundy LM (2000) Association between resistance to vancomycin and death in cases of *Enterococcus faecium* bacteremia. Clin Infect Dis 30:466–472
32. Vergis EN, Hayden MK, Chow JW et al (2001) Determinants of vancomycin resistance and mortality rates in enterococcal bacteremia. A prospective multicenter study. Ann Intern Med 135:484–492
33. Lodise TP, McKinnon PS, Tam VH, Rybak MJ (2002) Clinical outcomes for patients with bacteremia caused by vancomycin-resistant enterococcus in a level 1 trauma center. Clin Infect Dis 34:922–929
34. Trouillet JL, Vuagnat A, Combes A, Kassis N, Chastre J, Gibert C (2002) *Pseudomonas aeruginosa* ventilator-associated pneumonia: comparison of episodes due to piperacillin-resistant versus piperacillin-susceptible organisms. Clin Infect Dis 34:1047–1054
35. Alverdy JC, Laughlin RS, Wu L (2003) Influence of the critically ill state on host-pathogen interactions within the intestine: gut-derived sepsis redefined. Crit Care Med 31:598–607
36. Relman DA, Falkow S (1990) A molecular perspective of microbial pathogenicicty. In: Mandell GL, Douglas RG, Bennett IE (eds) Principles and practice of infectious diseases, vol 1, 3rd edn. Churchill Livingstone, New York, pp 25–32
37. Emori TG, Gaynes RG (1993) An overview of nosocomial infections, including the role of the microbiology laboratory. Clin Microbiol Rev 6:428–442
38. Neish AS (2002) The gut microflora and intestinal epithelial cells: a continuing dialogue. Microbes Infect 4:309–317
39. Guarner F, Malagelada JR (2003) Gutflora in health and disease. Lancet 361:512–519

40. D'Agata EMC, Venkataran L, De Girolami P, Burke P, Eliopoulos GM, Karchmer AW, Samore MH (1999) Colonisation with broad-spectrum cephalosporin-resistant Gram-negative bacilli in intensive care units during a non-outbreak period: prevalence, risk factors and rate of infection. Crit Care Med 27:1090–1095
41. Safdar N, Maki DG (2002) The commonality of risk factors for nosocomial colonization and infection with antimicrobial-resistant *Staphylococcus aureus*, *Enterococcus* Gram-negative bacilli, *Clostridium difficile* and Candida. Ann Intern Med 136:834–844

Classification of ICU Infections

L. Silvestri, H. K. F. van Saene
and A. J. Petros

4.1 Introduction

Classifying infections is crucial in any infection surveillance program, particularly in the intensive care unit (ICU). Time cutoffs, generally 48 h, have been accepted to distinguish community- from hospital-acquired infections, including ICU-acquired infections [1]. However, many clinicians appreciate that an infection due to a microorganism carried by the patient on admission to the ICU and that develops 48 h of ICU stay cannot be considered as being a "true" ICU-acquired infection. Obviously, this infection is nosocomial, i.e., the infection occurs in the ICU, but the causative microorganism does not belong to the ICU microbial ecology, as the patient imported the microorganism in her/his admission flora. A different classification of ICU infections is based on knowledge of the patient's carrier state [2]. This approach allows the distinction between primary (imported) and secondary carriage of potentially pathogenic microorganisms (PPMs) as well as between endogenous and exogenous infections.

This chapter compares the traditional approach with the concept of carrier state for classifying infections, mainly pneumonia, in critically ill patients.

L. Silvestri (✉)
Department of Emergency, Unit of Anesthesia and Intensive Care,
Presidio Ospedaliero di Gorizia, Gorizia, Italy
e-mail: lucianosilvestri@yahoo.it

4.2 Traditional Approach and Carrier-State Classification of ICU Infection

4.2.1 Traditional Approach

There are two standard means of classifying infections: the Gram-staining technique, which groups both microorganisms and infections into Gram-negative and Gram-positive categories; and incubation time, which distinguishes community from nosocomial infections. The in vitro staining method is still used to distinguish Gram-positive from Gram-negative bacteria and to classify microorganisms and ICU infections. However, there is no correlation between the Gram reaction of a particular microorganism and its pathogenicity (Chap. 3). For example, among Gram-positive cocci present in the oropharynx of critically ill ICU patients, such as enterococci, coagulase-negative staphylococci (CNS), viridans streptococci, methicillin-sensitive *Staphylococcus aureus* (MSSA) and *Streptococcus pneumoniae*, only MSSA and *S. pneumoniae* generally cause lower airway infections, suggesting a different pathogenicity among Gram-positive bacteria. Similarly, mortality rates are higher in ICU patients with a lower airway infection due to *Pseudomonas aeruginosa* than with *Haemophilus influenzae*, both of which are aerobic Gram-negative bacilli (AGNB) [3].

Studies on the prevalence of infections in the ICU include the usual definition of hospital-acquired infections (i.e., nosocomial) issued by the Centers for Disease Control and Prevention (CDC) [4]: "for an infection to be defined as nosocomial there must be no evidence that the infection was present or incubating at the time of hospital admission." Based on this definition, in the early 1990s, the European Prevalence of Infection in Intensive Care (EPIC) study distinguished each infection as one of the following [5]:

- community acquired: an infection occurring in the community and manifest on admission to the ICU;
- hospital acquired: an infection manifest on admission to the ICU and deemed to be related to the present hospital admission;
- ICU acquired: an infection originating in the ICU but not clinically manifest at the time of ICU admission.

The EPIC study showed that approximately 45% of enrolled patients were infected; nearly half (46%) of them acquired their infection in the ICU. The vagueness of this classification prompted investigators to adopt incubation times in order to improve the distinction between infections acquired in the community and/or hospital/ward from those acquired during the patient's ICU stay. Arbitrary time cutoffs varying between 24 h and 7 days [6–14] were chosen to distinguish ICU from non-ICU infections. Italian authors introduced early-onset and late-onset concepts in accordance with a cutoff of 4 days [13, 15] and emphasized that infections developing in the first 4 days could not be considered as ICU acquired [16]. Interestingly, 15 years after the EPIC study [5], the authors of the EPIC II study [17] did not focus their analysis on infection classification because they were concerned that it might be difficult to distinguish between community-, hospital-, and ICU-acquired infections. This concept was also embraced by the CDC, which recently dismissed the previous classification as obsolete and replaced it with the term healthcare-associated infection rather than nosocomial [18]. CDC defined healthcare-associated infection as "a localized or systemic condition resulting from an adverse reaction to the presence of an infectious agent(s) or its toxin(s), without any evidence that the infection was present or incubating at the time of admission to the acute care setting." Notwithstanding, the time cutoff method has not been completely withdrawn, and the following classification of pneumonia in the ICU is still in use [19–21]:

- community-acquired pneumonia (CAP): pneumonia present at hospital/ICU admission in patients who do not meet the criteria for healthcare-associated pneumonia (HCAP);
- HCAP: pneumonia present at hospital/ICU admission in patients with risk factors of multidrug-resistant pathogens because of prior contact with a health care environment (at least one of the following risk factors: hospitalization for ≥ 2 days in an acute care facility within 180 days of infection, residence in a nursing home or long-term care facility, antibiotic therapy, chemotherapy, wound care within 30 days of current infection, hemodialysis treatment at a hospital or clinic, home infusion therapy or home wound care, family member with infection due to multidrug-resistant bacteria, significant immune suppression);
- hospital-acquired pneumonia (HAP): pneumonia occurring typically ≥ 48 h after hospital admission in a nonintubated patient;
- ventilator-associated pneumonia (VAP): pneumonia occurring typically ≥ 48 h after hospital admission and endotracheal intubation and/or mechanical ventilation that was not present before intubation.

This "alphabet soup" of pneumonia, i.e., CAP, HCAP, HAP and VAP, is increasingly complex [22]. The definitions reflect the assumption that all pneumonias occurring after 48 h of ICU stay are acquired in the unit and are due to microorganisms transmitted via careers' hands, and this substantially magnifies the problem of defining ICU-acquired infections.

4.2.2 Carrier-State Approach

The traditional approach has been challenged by the carrier state concept [2]. Carriage or carrier state exists when the same strain is isolated from at least two consecutive surveillance samples (e.g., throat and rectal swabs) from an ICU patient, at any concentration, over a period of at least 1 week [23]. A surveillance set comprises throat and rectal swabs taken on admission and twice weekly afterward (e.g., Monday and Thursday). Diagnostic or clinical samples are samples from internal organs that are normally sterile, such as lower airways, blood,

Table 4.1 Classification of infections occurring in the ICU

Infection	PPMs	Timing	Frequency (%)	Preventing maneuver
Primary endogenous	6 normal 9 abnormal	<1 week	55	Parenteral antibiotics
Secondary endogenous	9 abnormal	>1 week	30	Enteral antibiotics in throat and gut; hygiene
Exogenous	9 abnormal	Any time during ICU stay	15	Topical antibiotics and hygiene

PPMs potentially pathogenic microorganisms
Normal PPMs: *S. pneumoniae, H. influenzae, Moraxella catarrhalis, Candida albicans, S. aureus, Escherichia coli*; abnormal PPMs: *Klebsiella, Proteus, Morganella, Enterobacter, Citrobacter, Serratia, Acinetobacter, Pseudomonas* species and methicillin-resistant *S. aureus*

bladder and skin lesions and are only taken on clinical indication with the aim of microbiologically proving a diagnosis of inflammation, either generalized or local [23]. Knowledge of the carrier state, together with diagnostic cultures, allows the distinction between the three types of infection occurring in the ICU [2, 24] (Table 4.1):

1. Primary endogenous infections are the most frequent infections in the ICU; the incidence varies between 50% and 85%, depending on the population studied and their degree of immunosuppression. They are caused by both normal and abnormal PPMs imported into the ICU by the patient in the admission flora. These episodes of infection generally occur early, during the first week of ICU stay. *S. pneumoniae, H. influenzae* and *S. aureus* are the etiological agents in previously healthy individuals requiring intensive care following an acute event, such as (surgical) trauma, pancreatitis, acute hepatic failure and burns. Abnormal AGNB can cause primary endogenous infections in patients with previous chronic underlying disease, such as severe chronic obstructive pulmonary disease, following acute deterioration of the underlying disease. Adequate parenteral antibiotics given immediately on admission to the ICU reduce the incidence of primary endogenous infection.
2. Secondary endogenous infections are invariably caused by one or more of eight abnormal AGNB as well as methicillin-resistant *S. aureus* (MRSA), accounting for one-third of all ICU infections. This type of infection, in general, occurs after 1 week in the ICU. These PPMs are first acquired in the oropharynx and subsequently in the gut. The topical application of nonabsorbable antimicrobials polymyxin E/tobramycin/amphotericin B has been shown to control secondary endogenous infection.
3. Exogenous infections are caused by abnormal hospital PPMs (15%) and may occur at any time during the patient's stay in the ICU. Typical examples are *Acinetobacter* lower airway infection following the use of contaminated

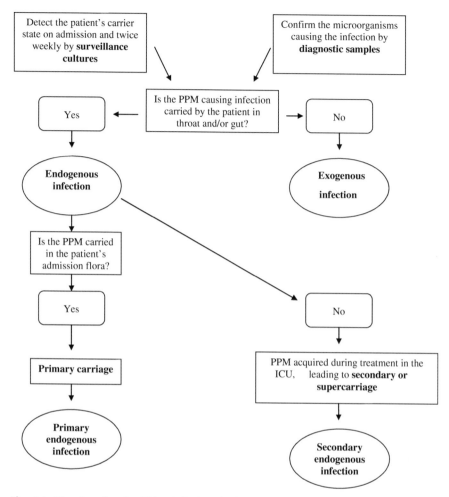

Fig. 4.1 Flowchart for classifying infections in the ICU using knowledge of the carrier state (*PPM* potentially pathogenic microorganism)

ventilation equipment, cystitis caused by *Serratia* associated with urinometers, or a MRSA tracheobronchitis in a tracheostomized patient. Surveillance samples are negative for microorganisms that readily appear in diagnostic samples. High levels of hygiene and topical antibiotics are required to control these infections.

According to this criterion, only secondary endogenous and exogenous infections are labeled ICU-acquired infections, whereas primary endogenous infections are considered to be imported infections. Figure 4.1 depicts infection classification based on knowledge of the carrier state.

4.3 Evidence Behind Time and Carriage Classification Systems of ICU Infections

4.3.1 Time Classification

Evidence that infections occurring on or at a specific time after ICU admission are attributable solely to microorganisms transmitted via careers' hands—and hence acquired during the ICU stay—is limited. Classifications based on time have been developed following the common experience of specific incubation times associated with highly pathogenic microorganisms due to their high intrinsic pathogenicity (or virulence) [25]. However, patients requiring intensive care develop infections with PPMs, including MRSA and AGNB and with low-level pathogens such as CNS and enterococci, due to the severity of their illness and associated immunosuppression [26]. The severity of illness rather than microorganism virulence is the most important factor for the conversion of the normal into the abnormal carrier state and will determine the time at which a potential or a low-level pathogen will cause infection.

According to the pathogenesis of ICU-acquired infections, PPM acquisition is followed by carriage and overgrowth of that microorganism before colonization and infection of an internal organ occurs. Undoubtedly, this process takes more than 2–4 days. Accordingly, a lower respiratory tract infection due to a PPM already carried in the throat and/or gut on admission and that develops in a ventilated trauma patient after 3, 4 or even 10 days from ICU admission, cannot be considered as ICU acquired. The concept of early- and late-onset infection, mainly pneumonia, remains accepted in general [21, 27]. Moreover, early-onset nosocomial pneumonia is believed to be due primarily to normal flora, such as *H. influenzae*, MSSA and *S. pneumoniae*, whereas late-onset nosocomial pneumonia is mainly caused by higher-level antibiotic-resistant AGNBs, such as *P. aeruginosa*, *Acinetobacter* species, or MRSA [28]. These statements are not generalizable to all ICU populations; patients with chronic underlying diseases, such as diabetes, alcoholism, chronic obstructive pulmonary disease and liver disease, may carry abnormal flora on ICU admission, including AGNB and/or MRSA, in the throat and gut. This is why some authors found no difference in microorganisms between early- and late-onset infections [28]. Moreover, it is unknown what is the best cut-off time by which to separate early- from late-onset pneumonia, as it is unknown how long it takes to develop pneumonia after aspiration of microorganisms [27]. Therefore, many clinicians, in prolonging the cutoff time, implicitly recognized the inaccuracy of the time classification method to determine whether an infection was imported or was really nosocomial [13, 14, 28].

4.3.2 Carriage Classification

In contrast, knowledge of the carrier state at the time of admission and throughout the ICU stay is indispensable in distinguishing infections due to imported PPMs (i.e., primary endogenous) from infections due to bacteria acquired on the unit (i.e., secondary endogenous and exogenous). Only secondary endogenous and exogenous infections are true ICU-acquired infections, as the origin of the causative bacteria is outside the ICU patient—in the ICU environment. In the case of the secondary endogenous infections, the microorganism acquired in the unit goes through a digestive tract phase, but this does not apply to exogenous infections.

Six studies prospectively evaluated the accuracy of the 48-h time cutoff using carriage as the gold standard (Table 4.2) [29–34]. More than 2,000 patients with 1,000 infection episodes were evaluated; 71% of all infection episodes were classified as nosocomial, as they occurred after 48 h. In contrast, using the carrier state criterion, of the 1,000 infection episodes, 612 (61%) were due to bacteria imported into the ICU, whereas 388 (39%) of all infections were caused by microorganisms transmitted in the unit via careers' hands. This figure was similar, or even higher in the pediatric population [31, 33, 34]. Moreover, two cohort studies assessed the time cutoff that was most in line with the carrier-state concept [30, 33]: a period ranging from 7 to 10 days (depending on the population studied) identified more accurately ICU-acquired infections than did the 48-h cutoff, although time was a less reliable method of identifying imported and ICU-acquired infections.

4.4 Impact of Time and Carrier-State Classification of ICU Infections

Although the CDC introduced a new classification of infections in which the concept that infections may originate from endogenous or exogenous sources [18], the 48-h time cutoff is still used to distinguish different types of infections, namely, pneumonia [19]. This approach implies that most pneumonias occurring in the ICU are nosocomial due to microorganisms transmitted via careers' hands, except pneumonias established in the first 2 days. The 48-h time cutoff is also responsible for blaming staff for almost all infections occurring in the ICU, for initiating expensive transmission investigations, and for reinforcing handwashing to control transmission. However, community-acquired and healthcare-associated infections, which are present or incubating at the time of ICU admission, cannot be prevented by handwashing [35].

These concepts are in contrast to data from the six previous studies [29–34]. Table 4.2 shows that 61% of all ICU infections are primary endogenous, i.e., due to microorganisms not related to the ICU ecology, and develop during the first week of ICU stay. The remaining 39% are true ICU-acquired infections and develop after 1 week in the unit. Handwashing cannot be expected to control primary endogenous infections, as it fails to clear oropharyngeal and gastrointestinal carriage of PPMs present in the patient on arrival at the ICU. Being inherently active solely on transmission, handwashing cannot reduce the major infection problem of primary endogenous infection, as transmission is not involved in this type of infection [35]. Additionally, handwashing does not influence the

Table 4.2 Classification of ICU infections using the 48-h time cutoff compared with carrier-state criteria

Author	No. of patients	No. of infection episodes	Classification of infection episodes				Nosocomial (48-h cutoff) [n (%)]
			Carriage				
			Primary endogenous [n (%)]	Secondary endogenous [n (%)]	Exogenous [n (%)]	Total secondary endogenous and exogenous [n (%)]	
Murray et al. [29]	21	12	6 (50)	6 (50)	0	6 (50)	9 (75)
Silvestri et al. [30]	117	74	44 (60)	17 (23)	13 (17)	30 (40)	59 (80)
Petros et al. [31]	52	18	15 (85)	2 (10)	1 (5)	3 (15)	15 (83)
de la Cal et al. [32]	56	37	21 (57)	14 (38)	2 (5)	16 (43)	30 (81)
Silvestri et al. [33]							
Adult	130	27	14 (52)	10 (37)	3 (11)	13 (48)	19 (70)
Pediatric	400	40	32 (80)	4 (10)	4 (10)	8 (20)	26 (65)
Sarginson et al. [34]	1,241	792	480 (61)	42 (5)	270 (34)	312 (39)	547 (69)
Total	2,017	1,000	612 (61)	95 (9)	293 (30)	388 (39)	705 (71)

For each study, the same episodes of infection are classified both with the carrier-state concept and with the traditional 48-h cutoff. ICU-acquired, secondary endogenous and exogenous infections based on knowledge of the carrier state; nosocomial, infection episodes of the previous columns reclassified using the traditional 48-h time cutoff. The two columns on the right show comparison between the two types of classifications

patient's immune status. Detecting primary endogenous infection as the major infection problem in the ICU avoids blaming health-care workers for most ICU infection, for which they are not responsible, and prevents unnecessary expensive cross-infection investigations. Finally, in strictly identifying the primary endogenous and the nosocomial problem of secondary endogenous and exogenous infections, surveillance of both infection and carriage allows the intensivist to start with the appropriate prevention measures, including selective decontamination of the digestive tract (SDD) [24].

4.5 Conclusions

Most ICU infections are due to microorganisms carried by the patient on admission to the unit. The difference in philosophy between the traditionalists and those who advocate the carriage-state method for classifying ICU infections is that the former focus on preventing transmission of all microorganisms via careers' hands in order to control all Gram-positive and Gram-negative infections occurring after 2 days of ICU stay. However, we believe that ICU patients may benefit from an infection control program that includes surveillance of both carriage and infection. In detecting abnormal carriage and overgrowth, surveillance cultures are indispensable for identifying a subset of patients at high risk of infection. Awareness of carriage in long-stay patients can provide more insights into the epidemiology of infection. The true nosocomial infection problem (i.e., secondary endogenous and exogenous infections) is detected easily and early. A regular audit of patients with nosocomial infections only may be useful, as the combination of secondary endogenous and exogenous infections may highlight a transmission problem in the ICU.

References

1. Spencer RC (1996) Definitions of nosocomial infections: surveillance of nosocomial infections. Bailliere's Clin Infect Dis 3:237–252
2. van Saene HKF, Damjanovic V, Murray AE et al (1996) How to classify infections in intensive care units—the carrier state, a criterion whose time has come? J Hosp Infect 33:1–12
3. Park DR (2005) The microbiology of ventilator associated pneumonia. Respir Care 50:742–763
4. Garner JS, Jarvis WR, Emori TG et al (1988) CDC definitions for nosocomial infections, 1988. Am J Infect Control 16:128–140
5. Vincent J-L, Bihari DJ, Suter PM et al (1995) The prevalence of nosocomial infection in intensive care units in Europe. JAMA 274:639–644
6. McGowan JE, Barnes MW, Finland M (1975) Bacteremia at Boston city hospital: occurrence and mortality during 12 selected years (1965–1972), with special reference to hospital-acquired cases. J Infect Dis 132:316–335
7. Potgieter PD, Hammond JMJ (1992) Etiology and diagnosis of pneumonia requiring ICU-admission. Chest 101:199–203

8. Estes RJ, Meduri GV (1995) The pathogenesis of ventilator-associated pneumonia. I. Mechanisms of bacterial transcolonization and airway inoculation. Intensive Care Med 21:365–383
9. Pugin J, Auckenthaler R, Lew DP, Suter PM (1991) Oropharyngeal decontamination decreases incidence of ventilator-associated pneumonia: a randomized, placebo-controlled, double-blind clinical trial. JAMA 265:2704–2710
10. Chevret S, Hemmer M, Carlet J, Langer M (1993) Incidence and risk factors of pneumonia acquired in intensive care units: results from a multicenter prospective study on 996 patients. Intensive Care Med 19:256–264
11. Rolando N, Gimson A, Wade J et al (1993) Prospective controlled trial of selective parenteral and enteral antimicrobial regimen in fulminant liver failure. Hepatology 17:196–201
12. Korinek AM, Laisne MJ, Nicolas MH et al (1993) Selective decontamination of the digestive tract in neurosurgical intensive care units patients—a double-blind, randomized, placebo-controlled study. Crit Care Med 21:1466–1473
13. Langer M, Cigada M, Mandelli M et al (1987) Early onset pneumonia: a multicenter study in intensive care units. Intensive Care Med 13:342–346
14. Trouillet JL, Chastre J, Vuagnat A et al (1998) Ventilator-associated pneumonia caused by potentially drug-resistant bacteria. Am J Respir Crit Care Med 157:531–539
15. Antonelli M, Moro ML, D'Errico RR et al (1996) Early and late onset bacteremia have different risk factors in trauma patients. Intensive Care Med 22:735–741
16. Mandelli M, Mosconi P, Langer M et al (1986) Is pneumonia developing in patients in intensive care always a typical "nosocomial" infection? Lancet 2:1094–1095
17. Vincent JL, Rello J, Marshall J et al (2009) International study of the prevalence and outcomes of infection in intensive care units. JAMA 302:2323–2329
18. Horan TC, Andrus M, Dudeck MA (2008) CDC/NHSN surveillance definition of health care-associated infection and criteria for specific types of infections in the acute care setting. Am J Infect Control 36:309–332
19. Morrow LE, Kollef MH (2010) Recognition and prevention of nosocomial pneumonia in the intensive care unit and infection control in mechanical ventilation. Crit Care Med 38(Suppl 8):S352–S362
20. Masterton RG, Galloway A, French G et al (2008) Guidelines for the management of hospital-acquired pneumonia in the UK: report of the working party on hospital-acquired pneumonia of the British Society for antimicrobial chemotherapy. J Antimicrob Chemother 62:5–34
21. Niederman MS, Craven DE, Bonten MJ et al (2005) Guidelines for the management of adults with hospital-acquired, ventilator-associated, and healthcare-associated pneumonia. Am J Respir Crit Care Med 171:388–416
22. Anand L, Kollef MH (2009) The alphabet soup of pneumonia: CAP, HAP, HCAP, NHAP, VAP. Semin Respir Crit Care Med 30:3–9
23. Sarginson RE, Taylor N, van Saene HKF (2001) Glossary of terms and definitions. Curr Anaesth Crit Care 12:2–5
24. van Saene HKF, Petros AJ, Ramsay G, Baxby D (2003) All great truths are iconoclastic: selective decontamination of the digestive tract moves from heresy to level 1 truth. Intensive Care Med 29:677–690
25. Gorbach SL, Bartlett JG, Blacklow NR (1998) Infectious diseases, 2nd edn. Saunders, Philadelphia
26. Leonard EM, van Saene HKF, Stoutenbeek CP et al (1990) An intrinsic pathogenicity index for microorganisms causing infection in a neonatal surgical unit. Microbiol Ecol Health Dis 3:151–157
27. Torres A, Ewig S, Lode H et al (2009) Defining, treating and preventing hospital acquired pneumonia: European perspective. Intensive Care Med 35:9–29
28. Gastmeier P, Sohr D, Geffers C et al (2009) Early- and late-onset pneumonia: is this still a useful classification? Antimicrob Agents Chemother 53:2714–2718

29. Murray AE, Chambers JJ, van Saene HKF (1998) Infections in patients requiring ventilation in intensive care: application of a new classification. Clin Microb Infect 4:94–102
30. Silvestri L, Monti-Bragadin C, Milanese M et al (1999) Are most ICU infections really nosocomial? a prospective observational cohort study in mechanically ventilated patients. J Hosp Infect 42:125–133
31. Petros AJ, O'Connell M, Roberts C et al (2001) Systemic antibiotics fail to clear multiresistant Klebsiella from a pediatric intensive care unit. Chest 119:862–866
32. de la Cal MA, Cerda E, Garcia-Hierro P et al (2001) Pneumonia in severe burns: a classification according to the concept of the carrier state. Chest 119:1160–1165
33. Silvestri L, Sarginson RE, Hughes J et al (2002) Most nosocomial pneumonias are not due to nosocomial bacteria in ventilated patients: prospective evaluation of the accuracy of the 48 h time cut-off using carriage as the gold standard. Anaesth Intensive Care 30:275–282
34. Sarginson R, Taylor N, Reilly N et al (2004) Infection in prolonged pediatric critical illness: a prospective four year study based on knowledge of the carrier state. Crit Care Med 32:839–847
35. Silvestri L, Petros AJ, Sarginson RE et al (2005) Handwashing in the intensive care unit: a big measure-with modest effects. J Hosp Infect 59:175–179

Gut Microbiology: Surveillance Samples for Detecting the Abnormal Carrier State in Overgrowth

H. K. F. van Saene, G. Riepi, P. Garcia-Hierro, B. Ramos and A. Budimir

5.1 Introduction

Critical illness impacts all organ systems, such as lungs, heart and gut. The gut also includes the vast living microbial tissue of the indigenous, mainly anaerobic, flora. This enormous bacterial tissue is embedded in the mucous layer and covers the inner wall of the gut. Amongst the aerobic Gram-negative bacilli (AGNB), only the indigenous *Escherichia coli* is carried by healthy people in the gut. Critical illness converts the normal carrier state of *E. coli* into carriage of abnormal AGNB, including *Klebsiella*, *Enterobacter* and *Pseudomonas* species [1], and methicillin-resistant *Staphylococcus aureus* (MRSA) [2]. It is hypothesised that receptors for AGNB and MRSA are constitutively expressed on the mucosal lining but are covered by a protective layer of fibronectin in the healthy mucosa. Significantly increased levels of salivary elastase have been shown to precede AGNB carriage in the oropharynx in post-operative patients and the elderly [3, 4]. It is probable that in individuals with both acute and chronic underlying illness, activated macrophages release elastase into mucosal secretions, thereby denuding the protective fibronectin layer. It is thought that this possible mechanism is a deleterious consequence of the inflammatory response encountered during and after illness. Critical illness profoundly impacts body flora in two ways: it induces qualitative changes from normal to abnormal flora [1, 2], as well as quantitative changes from low- to high-grade carriage or gut overgrowth defined as $\geq 2+$ or $\geq 10^5$ potential pathogens per millilitre of saliva and/or gram of faeces [5]. Overgrowth concentrations of both normal and abnormal flora in surveillance samples are frequently found on

H. K. F. van Saene (✉)
Institute of Ageing and Chronic Diseases, University of Liverpool,
Duncan Building, Liverpool, UK
e-mail: nia.taylor@liv.ac.uk

admission to the intensive care unit (ICU), accounting for the large percentage of primary endogenous infections [6, 7] (Table 4.1). Abnormal flora is often acquired during treatment in the ICU. Acquisition invariably leads to abnormal carriage due to critical illness. Most iatrogenic interventions in the patient requiring intensive care, including mechanical ventilation, promote quantitative changes from low- to high-grade carriage or overgrowth. Gut protection using H_2 antagonists and antimicrobials are commonly applied in the critically ill. H_2 antagonists increase gastric pH, thereby impairing the gastric acidity barrier [8]. Antimicrobials that are active against the indigenous, mainly anaerobic, flora, which are excreted via bile into the gut, may disturb gut ecology [9]. Integrity of both physiology and flora is essential for the individual's defence against AGNB carriage. Impairment of these two factors promotes overgrowth of abnormal, potentially pathogenic, microorganisms (PPM), such as AGNB in concentrations of $\geq 2+$ or $\geq 10^5$ colony forming units (CFU) per millilitre or gram of faeces.

Gut overgrowth of abnormal flora is not only a marker of critical illness, but it harms the patient, as it is a disease in itself. In addition, gut overgrowth of abnormal flora has a major epidemiological impact on the other patients in the ICU as well as on the ICU environment.

5.2 Clinical Impact of Gut Overgrowth

Gut overgrowth harms the critically ill in four ways:
1. *Immunosuppression*. Overgrowth of abnormal AGNB (and associated endotoxin) impairs systemic immunity due to generalised inflammation following absorption of AGNB and/or endotoxin [10];
2. *Inflammation*. Overgrowth of abnormal AGNB and/or endotoxin has been shown to lead to cytokinaemia and inflammation of major organ systems [11];
3. *Infection*. There is a quantitative relationship between surveillance and diagnostic samples; as soon as there is overgrowth in surveillance samples, the diagnostic samples become positive, which is the first stage in the development of infection [12];
4. *Antimicrobial resistance*. The abnormal carrier state in overgrowth concentrations guarantees increased spontaneous mutation, leading to polyclonality and antibiotic resistance [13].

5.3 Epidemiological Impact of Gut Overgrowth

The higher the salivary and faecal concentrations of AGNB and MRSA, the higher the possibility of PPM transmission via carer's hands [14, 15]. PPM acquisition invariably leads to carriage, as the critically ill are unable to clear the acquired AGNB and MRSA. Carriers of abnormal bacteria in overgrowth shed these microorganisms into the environment and determine the contamination level of the inanimate environment, including beds, tables, telephones and floors [16, 17].

5.4 Definitions

5.4.1 Surveillance Samples

Surveillance samples are defined as samples obtained from body sites where PPM may potentially be carried, i.e. the digestive tract, comprising oropharyngeal and rectal cavities [18]. Surveillance cultures should be distinguished from surface and diagnostic samples.

5.4.2 Surface Samples

Surface samples are taken from the skin, such as axilla, groin and umbilicus, and from the nose, eye and ear. They do not belong to a surveillance sampling protocol because positive surface swabs merely reflect the oropharyngeal and rectal carrier states.

5.4.3 Diagnostic Samples

Diagnostic samples are from internal organs that are normally sterile, such as lower airways, blood, bladder, and skin lesions. They are only taken on clinical indication. The endpoint of diagnostic samples is clinical, as they aim to prove microbiologically a clinical diagnosis of inflammation, both generalised and/or local.

5.5 Endpoints of Surveillance Samples

The aim of obtaining surveillance cultures is to determine the microbiological endpoint of the abnormal—in overgrowth concentrations—carrier state. Carriage or a carrier state exists when the same bacterial strain is isolated from at least two consecutive surveillance samples of the ICU patient in any concentration over a period of at least 1 week. Carriage implies persistent presence of a PPM and is distinguished from acquisition or transient presence. Persistent presence is the forerunner and virtually always precedes overgrowth ($\geq 2+$ or $\geq 10^5$) [5–7]. Surveillance samples are not useful for diagnosing infection of lungs, blood, bladder, or wounds. Diagnostic samples are required for this purpose.

5.6 Sampling for Surveillance Purposes

5.6.1 Which Patients?

Only the most critically ill patients require intensive microbiological monitoring using surveillance samples to detect the abnormal carrier state of AGNB and MRSA in overgrowth concentrations. Due to the severity of their illness, these patients require intensive care, including mechanical ventilation, for a minimum of

3 days. Critical illness related carriage in overgrowth [CIRCO] is often present on admission. In general, they have impaired gut motility and, hence, are at high risk of developing throat and gut overgrowth during treatment on ICU.

5.6.2 What Samples?

A surveillance programme for this type of patient includes samples from both oropharynx and gut. Potential pathogens carried in the throat and gut cause pneumonia and septicaemia, respectively [19]. These two serious infections are responsible for a high rate of mortality. Potential pathogens present in overgrowth in the throat and gut are implicated in transmission via the hands of carers, in particular, in outbreak situations. A throat and rectal swab are taken to detect oropharyngeal and gut carriage of AGNB and MRSA. Rectal swabs must be coated with stool. As MRSA has an affinity for the skin, skin is sampled only if lesions are present.

5.6.3 When?

Surveillance sets are obtained on admission and thereafter twice weekly (e.g. Monday, Thursday) throughout the ICU treatment to distinguish carriage due to PPM imported in the admission flora (import; primary carriage) from carriage due to ICU-associated PPM in the oropharynx or gut acquired during treatment in ICU (nosocomial; secondary; super carriage).

5.7 Microbiological Procedures

Throat and rectal swabs are processed qualitatively and semiquantitatively to detect the level of carriage of the two types of target microorganisms: AGNB and MRSA [20]. Two solid-media, MacConkey (AGNB) and a staphylococcal (MRSA) agar, are inoculated using the four-quadrant method (Fig. 5.1). Each swab is streaked onto the two solid media. All cultures are incubated aerobically at 37°C. The MacConkey plate is examined after one night, the plate for MRSA after 2 nights. A semiquantitative estimation is made by grading growth density on a scale of 1+ to 4+, as follows (Table 5.1): growth in the first quadrant of the solid plate 1+ ($>10^3$ CFU/ml), in the second quadrant 2+ ($>10^5$ CFU/ml), in the third quadrant 3+ ($>10^7$ CFU/ml) and on the entire plate 4+ ($>10^9$ CFU/ml). Macroscopically distinct colonies are isolated in pure culture. Standard methods for identification, typing, and sensitivity patterns are used for all microorganisms.

5.8 Interpretation of Surveillance Samples

Surveillance cultures allow the intensive care specialist to distinguish normal from abnormal carrier state, overgrowth from low-level carriage and endogenous from exogenous infections in combination with diagnostic samples.

5 Gut Microbiology

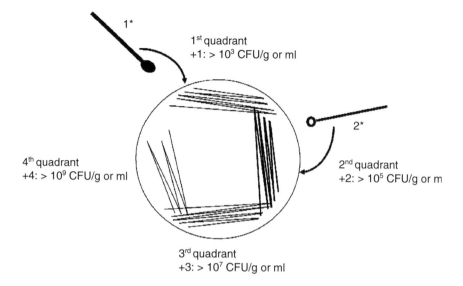

1* Inoculation of solid medium (1st quadrant)
2* Diluting using different loops

Fig. 5.1 Processing surveillance swabs using the four quadrant method

Table 5.1 Comparison of surveillance (throat/rectal) swabs and (salivary/faecal) specimens for detecting the carriage level (growth density) of aerobic Gram-negative bacilli and methicillin-resistant *Staphylococcus aureus* (MRSA)

Four-quadrant method: semiquantitative swab method	Growth density	Dilution series: quantitative specimen method
1+	Low	10^3
2+	Moderate	10^5
3+	High	10^7
4+	Very high	10^9

Moderate growth density, i.e. ≥ 2 or $\geq 10^5$ colony forming units, reflects overgrowth

5.8.1 Normal Versus Abnormal Carriage

Surveillance swabs processed for one group of target microorganisms, AGNB, using an inexpensive MacConkey agar plate, yield a positive or negative result after 18 h of incubation. AGNB, including *E. coli,* are uncommon in the oropharynx, whereas healthy people carry their own indigenous *E. coli* in the intestine in concentrations varying between 10^3 and 10^6 CFU/ml or gram of faeces. There are no other AGNB, including *Klebsiella, Proteus, Morganella, Enterobacter, Citrobacter, Serratia, Acinetobacter* and *Pseudomonas* species, in either the throat or gut. Interpreting the staphylococcal plate requires 2 nights of incubation. About one-third of the healthy population carries methicillin-sensitive *S. aureus*. MRSA isolation is always abnormal.

5.8.2 Low-Level Carriage Versus Overgrowth

Oropharyngeal and intestinal overgrowth is defined as $\geq 2+$ or $\geq 10^5$ microorganisms per millilitre of saliva and/or gram of faeces and is distinguished from low-grade carriage of $<2+$ or $<10^5$ microorganisms [5–7]. Individuals with a chronic disease, such as chronic obstructive pulmonary disease, generally carry abnormal flora in low concentrations once the forced expiratory volume in 1 s (FEV_1) is <50% [21]. The low-level carrier status is mainly due to the presence of clearing mechanisms, such as swallowing, chewing and peristalsis. However, patients who require mechanical ventilation for a minimum of 3 days generally have CIRCO on admission and often develop it during treatment in ICU [20]. Gut overgrowth harms the critically ill, as it causes immunosuppression [10], inflammation [11], infection [12] and resistance [13].

5.8.3 Primary Versus Secondary (Super) Carriage

Knowledge of the carrier state at the time of admission (primary carriage) and subsequently during treatment in the ICU (secondary or super carriage) is crucial for managing infection in the unit.

5.8.3.1 Primary Carriage
Primary carriage of potential pathogens is defined as the carrier state of potential pathogens present in the admission flora, i.e. imported into the ICU. The potential pathogens include both normal and abnormal potential pathogens.

5.8.3.2 Secondary (Super) Carriage
Secondary carriage of potential pathogens is defined as the carrier state of potential pathogens not present in the admission flora but acquired later and subsequently carried during treatment in the ICU. Potential pathogens are invariably abnormal bacteria, including AGNB and MRSA.

Primary and secondary (super) infections are preceded by primary endogenous and secondary (super) carriage in overgrowth concentrations, respectively [5–7]. Exogenous infections are caused by potential pathogens not carried at all. In general, exogenous infections are due to abnormal bacteria (Table 5.2).

Hygiene measures will only have an impact on infections due to externally transmitted microorganisms, e.g. secondary endogenous (super) and exogenous infection [22]. A primary endogenous infection caused by a potential pathogen imported by the patient into the ICU in the admission flora can only be managed effectively with knowledge of the carrier state. It is obvious that hand hygiene fails to eradicate carriage of potential pathogens in throat and gut detected by surveillance samples on admission.

To detect resistance at an early stage, surveillance cultures are more sensitive than diagnostic cultures. Eighteen percent of critically ill patients carried AGNB resistant to ceftazidime in their admission flora. Diagnostic cultures detected these resistant

Table 5.2 Carriage classification of severe infections of lower airways and blood

Infection	PPM	Timing	Frequency(%)	Manoeuvre
Primary endogenous	6 normal; 9 abnormal	<1 week	55	Parenteral antimicrobials
Secondary endogenous	9 abnormal	>1 week	30	Hygiene and enteral antimicrobials
Exogenous	9 abnormal	Anytime during ICU treatment	15	Hygiene and topical antimicrobials

PPM, potentially pathogenic microorganism; *6 normal PPM*, *Streptococcus pneumoniae*, *Haemophilus influenzae*, *Moraxella catarrhalis*, *Candida albicans*, *Staphylococcus aureus*, *Escherichia coli*; *9 abnormal PPM*, *Klebsiella*, *Enterobacter*, *Citrobacter*, *Proteus*, *Morganella*, *Serratia*, *Acinetobacter*, *Pseudomonas* species and methicillin-resistant *Staphylococcus aureus* (MRSA)

bacteria in only 5% of these patients [23]. A recent study from Trieste [7] reports resistance figures of 8% in diagnostic cultures compared with 22% in surveillance cultures. This difference is highly likely to be due to the observation that overgrowth in the throat and gut is necessary to make diagnostic cultures positive [24].

However, information provided by surveillance cultures of throat and rectum enables the intensivist to implement isolation and to reinforce hygiene measures as soon as possible following admission. Two recent studies show that MRSA and ceftazidime-resistant AGNB were identified in 23.8% and 52.1% of patients, respectively, within the first 72 h of admission to the ICU [6, 25].

5.9 Role of Surveillance Samples in Infection Control in the ICU Patient

Recent studies using surveillance cultures of throat and rectum to detect carrier state demonstrate that only infections occurring after 1 week of ICU stay are due to microbes transmitted via the hands of health-care workers [26–30]. The incidence varies between 15% and 45% depending on illness severity. Microorganisms related to the ICU environment are first acquired in the oropharynx. In the critically ill, oropharyngeal acquisition invariably leads to secondary carriage. The subsequent build up to digestive tract overgrowth, which can then result in colonisation of normally sterile internal organs, takes a few days. Finally, it is the degree of immunosuppression of the ICU patient that determines the day of colonization, leading to an established secondary endogenous or super infection. The other type of ICU infection is the exogenous infection [31–33] due to breaches of hygiene. Causative bacteria are also acquired in the unit but are never present in patient throat and/or gut flora. For example, long-stay patients, particularly those who receive a tracheostomy in respiratory units, are at high risk of exogenous lower-airway infections. Purulent lower-airway secretions yield a microorganism that has never been previously carried by the patient in the digestive tract flora, or indeed in their oropharynx. Although both the tracheostomy and the oropharynx are equally accessible for bacterial entry, the tracheotomy tends to be the entry site for bacteria that colonise/infect the lower airways.

However, primary endogenous infections cause the major infection problems, and the microorganisms involved do not bear any relation to ICU ecology [34, 35]. A recent study compared the traditional 48 h cutoff and the criterion of the carrier state and found that the time cutoff significantly overestimated the magnitude of the nosocomial problem [30]. This approach to the carrier state may be more useful for interhospital comparison, as only infections due to microorganisms acquired in the different units are compared, independent of illness severity.

In identifying the right population with primary endogenous infections, classification using the carrier state avoids blaming staff for all infections occurring after 48 h for which they are not responsible. Knowledge of carrier status thus prevents fruitless investigation of apparent cross-infection episodes. Secondly, without surveillance samples, exogenous infections are impossible to recognise, at least at an early stage when only diagnostic samples such as tracheal aspirate, urine and blood have been tested. Finally, knowledge of the carrier state using surveillance cultures on admission and twice weekly is an effective strategy for early identification of carriers of multidrug-resistant microorganisms—including AGNB such as *A. baumannii* [7, 36], MRSA [6, 24] and vancomycin-resistant enterococci [37]—both on admission and during ICU stay. Surveillance cultures, in particular of the oropharynx, that become positive for a PPM during ICU stay reveal ongoing transmission and an impending outbreak long before the diagnostic samples yield the outbreak strain [38]. This surveillance strategy optimises targeted infection control interventions—including (1) hand hygiene, (2) isolation, (3) personal protective equipment and (4) care of patient equipment—to control transmission from one patient-carrier to another patient via carer's hands.

5.10 Future Lines of Research on Surveillance Samples in the ICU Patient

Most infection surveillance programmes include all patients admitted to the ICU, whether they stay a few days or 2 weeks [39, 40]. Including a large number of relatively short-stay patients with a low risk of infection tends to dilute total rates of infection by increasing the size of the denominator. However, whereas low percentages look good to the hospital manager, they do not allow room for improvement, i.e. detecting a significant reduction in infection rate following the introduction of an intervention [39]. We believe that critically ill patients benefit from a surveillance programme of both infection and of carriage [41, 42], in particular, in combination with selective decontamination of the digestive tract (SDD) [43–45].

References

1. Johanson WG, Pierce AK, Sanford JP (1969) Changing pharyngeal bacterial flora of hospitalized patients. Emergence of Gram-negative bacilli. New Engl J Med 281:1137–1140
2. Chang FY, Singh N, Gayowski T et al (1998) *Staphylococcus aureus* nasal colonization in patients with cirrhosis: prospective assessment of association with infection. Infect Control Hosp Epidemiol 19:328–332
3. Dal Nogare AR, Toews GB, Pierce AK (1987) Increased salivary elastase precedes Gram-negative bacillary colonization in post-operative patients. Am Rev Respir Dis 135:671–675
4. Palmer LB, Albulak K, Fields S et al (2001) Oral clearance and pathogenic oropharyngeal colonization in the elderly. Am J Respir Crit Care Med 164:464–468
5. van Saene HKF, Damjanovic V, Murray AE, de la Cal MA (1996) How to classify infections in intensive care units—the carrier state, a criterion whose time has come? J Hosp Infect 33:1–12
6. Viviani M, van Saene HKF, Dezzoni R et al (2005) Control of imported and acquired methicillin-resistant *Staphylococcus aureus* [MRSA] in mechanically ventilated patients: a dose response study of oral vancomycin to reduce absolute carriage and infection. Anaesth Intensive Care 33:361–372
7. Viviani M, van Saene HK, Pisa F et al (2010) The role of admission surveillance cultures in patients requiring prolonged mechanical ventilation in the intensive care unit. Anaesth Intensive Care 38:325–335
8. Hillman KM, Riordan T, O'Farrell SM, Tabaqchali S (1982) Colonization of the gastric contents in critically ill patients. Crit Care Med 10:444–447
9. Vollaard EJ, Clasener HAL (1994) Colonization resistance. Antimicrob Agents Chemother 38:409–414
10. Deitch EA, Xu DZ, Qi L, Berg RD (1993) Bacterial translocation from the gut impairs systemic immunity. Surgery 104:269–276
11. Baue AE (1993) The role of the gut in the development of multiple organ dysfunction in cardiothoracic patients. Ann Thoracic Surg 55:822–829
12. van Uffelen R, van Saene HKF, Fidler V et al (1984) Oropharyngeal flora as a source of bacteria colonizing the lower airways in patients on artificial ventilation. Intensive Care Med 10:233–237
13. van Saene HKF, Taylor N, Damjanovic V, Sarginson RE (2008) Microbial gut overgrowth guarantees increased spontaneous mutation leading to polyclonality and antibiotic resistance in the critically ill. Curr Drug Targ 9:419–421
14. Riley TV, Webb SAR, Cadwallader H et al (1996) Outbreak of gentamicin-resistant *Acinetobacter baumanii* in an intensive care unit: clinical, epidemiological and microbiological features. Pathology 28:359–363
15. Lin MY, Hayden MK (2010) Methicillin-resistant *Staphylococcus aureus* and vancomycin-resistant enterococcus: recognition and prevention in intensive care units. Crit Care Med 38(suppl 8):S335–S344
16. Go ES, Urban C, Burns J et al (1994) Clinical and molecular epidemiology of *Acinetobacter* infections sensitive only to polymyxin B and sulbactam. Lancet 344:1329–1332
17. Bocher S, Skov RL, Knudsen MA et al (2010) The search and destroy strategy prevents spread and long-term carriage of MRSA: results from follow-up screening of a large ST22 (E-MRSA) 15 outbreak in Denmark. Clin Microb Infect 16:1427–1434
18. Damjanovic V, van Saene HKF, Weindling AM (1994) The multiple value of surveillance cultures: an alternative view. J Hosp Infect 28:71–78
19. Silvestri L, van Saene HKF, Zandstra DF et al (2010) Selective decontamination of the digestive tract reduces multiple organ failure and mortality in critically ill patients: systematic review of randomized controlled trials. Crit Care Med 38:1370–1376
20. van Saene HKF, Damjanovic V, Alcock SR (2001) Basics in microbiology for the patient requiring intensive care. Curr Anaesth Crit Care 12:6–17

21. Mobbs KJ, van Saene HKF, Sunderland D, Davies PDO (1999) Oropharyngeal Gram-negative bacillary carriage in chronic obstructive pulmonary disease: relation to severity of disease. Respir Med 93:540–545
22. Silvestri L, Petros AJ, Sarginson RE et al (2005) Handwashing in the intensive care unit: a big measure with modest effects. J Hosp Infect 59:172–179
23. D'Agata EM, Venkataraman L, DeGirolami P et al (1999) Colonization with broad-spectrum cephalosporin-resistant gram-negative bacilli in intensive care units during a nonoutbreak period: prevalence, risk factors, and rate of infection. Crit Care Med 27:1090–1095
24. de la Cal MA, Cerda E, van Saene HKF et al (2004) Effectiveness and safety of enteral vancomycin to control endemicity of methicillin-resistant *Staphylococcus aureus* in a medical/surgical intensive care unit. J Hosp Infect 56:175–183
25. Toltzis P, Yamashita T, Vilt L et al (1997) Colonization with antibiotic-resistant Gram-negative organisms in a pediatric intensive care unit. Crit Care Med 25:538–544
26. Murray AE, Chambers JJ, van Saene HKF (1998) Infections in patients requiring ventilation in intensive care: application of a new classification. Clin Microbiol Infect 4:94–102
27. Silvestri L, Monti Bragadin C, Milanese M et al (1999) Are most ICU-infections really nosocomial? A prospective observational cohort study in mechanically ventilated patients. J Hosp Infect 42:125–133
28. Petros AJ, O'Connell M, Roberts C et al (2001) Systemic antibiotics fail to clear multi-drug-resistant *Klebsiella* from a pediatric ICU. Chest 119:862–866
29. de la Cal MA, Cerda E, Garcia-Hierro P et al (2001) Pneumonia in patients with severe burns. A classification according to the concept of the carrier state. Chest 119:1160–1165
30. Silvestri L, Sarginson RE, Hughes J et al (2002) Most nosocomial pneumonias are not due to nosocomial bacteria in ventilated patients. Evaluation of the accuracy of the 48 h time cut-off using carriage as the gold standard. Anaesth Intensive Care 30:275–282
31. Hammond JMJ, Potgieter PD, Saunders GL et al (1992) Double blind study of selective decontamination of the digestive tract in intensive care. Lancet 340:5–9
32. Morar P, Singh V, Makura Z et al (2002) Differing pathways of lower airway colonization and infection according to mode of ventilation (endotracheal versus tracheostomy). Arch Otolaryngol Head Neck Surg 128:1061–1066
33. Morar P, Makura Z, Jones AS et al (2000) Topical antibiotics on tracheostoma prevents exogenous colonization and infection of lower airways in children. Chest 117:513–518
34. Stoutenbeek CP (1989) The role of systemic antibiotic prophylaxis in infection prevention in intensive care by SDD. Infection 17:418–421
35. Sirvent JM, Torres A, El-Ebiary M et al (1997) Protective effect of intravenously administered cefuroxime against nosocomial pneumonia in patients with structural coma. Am J Respir Crit Care Med 155:1729–1734
36. Corbella X, Pujol M, Ayats J et al (1996) Relevance of digestive tract colonization in the epidemiology of nosocomial infections due to multiresistant *Acinetobacter baumannii*. Clin Infect Dis 23:329–334
37. Hendrix CW, Hammond JMJ, Swoboda SM et al (2001) Surveillance strategies and impact of vancomycin-resistant enterococcal colonization and infection in critically ill patients. Ann Surg 233:259–265
38. Chetchotisakd P, Phelps CL, Hartstein AI (1994) Assessment of bacterial cross-transmission as a cause of infections in patients in intensive care units. Clin Infect Dis 18:929–937
39. Kollef MH, Sherman G, Ward S, Fraser VJ (1999) Inadequate antimicrobial treatment of infections. Chest 115:462–474
40. Richards MJ, Edwards JR, Culver DH et al (1999) Nosocomial infections in medical intensive care units in the United States. Crit Care Med 27:887–892
41. Langer M, Carretto E, Haeusler EA (2001) Infection control in ICU: back (forward) to surveillance samples? Intensive Care Med 27:1561–1563
42. Silvestri L, van Saene HKF (2002) Surveillance of carriage. Minerva Anestesiol 68(Suppl 1):S179–S182

43. de Jonge E, Schultz MJ, Spanjaard L et al (2003) Effects of selective decontamination of the digestive tract on mortality and acquisition of resistant bacteria in intensive care: a randomised controlled trial. Lancet 362:1011–1016
44. de Smet AM, Kluytmans JA, Cooper BS et al (2009) Decontamination of the digestive tract and oropharynx in ICU patients. N Engl J Med 360:20–31
45. Liberati A, D'Amico R, Pifferi S et al (2009) Antibiotic prophylaxis to reduce respiratory tract infections and mortality in adults receiving intensive care. Cochrane Database Syst Rev CD000022

Part II
Antimicrobials

Systemic Antibiotics

A. R. De Gaudio, S. Rinaldi and C. Adembri

6.1 Introduction

Systemic antibiotics remain the main causative therapy for critically ill patients with infection. This chapter aims to provide a clinical review of the antibiotics available for systemic administration in the intensive care unit (ICU). Pharmacological and microbiological factors that affect antimicrobial administration regimen in the critical patient are also discussed.

As new drugs have been developed to overcome antimicrobial resistance, bacteria acquired new kinds of resistance in the endless war for survival. The opportunity of using appropriate pharmacokinetic/pharmacodynamic (PK/PD) parameters to optimize dosing in order not only to cure patients but also to reduce the spreading of resistance is therefore becoming imperative, as there are now fewer new therapeutic options than in the past.

Bacteria have the capacity to adapt to a wide range of conditions. Any strategy aimed at destroying bacterial flora has resulted in a dramatic failure. It is likely that in the future, the definitive answer to infectious diseases will stand not only on the development of new antibiotics but also in immunomodulating strategies. The goal of the intensivist challenged with an infectious disease will include turning the relationship between bacterial flora and the host from infection back to symbiosis.

C. Adembri (✉)
Department of Medical and Surgical Critical Care,
Section of Anesthesiology and Intensive Care, University of Florence,
Azienda Ospedaliero-Universitaria Careggi, Florence, Italy
e-mail: chiara.adembri@unifi.it

6.2 The Puzzle of Antimicrobial Activity

Antimicrobial activity is the result of many variables that fit together in the clinical setting just as in a puzzle (Table 6.1), as it depends on the PD properties of the antibiotic, the specific bacterial strain, the infection site, and the setting in which the antimicrobial drug challenges the microorganism [1–3]. In the ICU, infections are often caused by multiresistant strains and develop in patients who have coexistent multiple organ dysfunction and impaired immune function, a clinical setting in which optimal antimicrobial therapy (in terms of both activity spectrum and administration dose and modality) is essential to improve outcome.

One of the main goals of antimicrobial therapy is that the antimicrobial reaches and remains in the site of infection in a sufficient concentration and for a sufficient time. Regarding the pharmacological action of antimicrobials (that is, killing activity), this may be concentration dependent or time dependent [4]. Concentration-dependent antibiotics kill bacteria at a greater rate and to a greater extent with increasing antibiotic concentrations, whereas time-dependent antibiotics kill bacteria at the same rate and to the same extent once an appropriate concentration threshold has been achieved. Aminoglycosides, fluoroquinolones, clarithromycin, azalides, ketolides, and metronidazole are considered concentration-dependent antimicrobial drugs, whereas glycopeptides, clindamycin, natural macrolides, β-lactams, linezolid, and quinupristin-dalfopristin are considered time-dependent drugs. These differences in PD activity should result in different dosing regimens for time- and concentration-dependent antibiotics.

Besides these PD considerations, the bactericidal activity of antimicrobial agent is influenced by several factors correlated with infection site, including antibiotic diffusion, local pH, bacterial load, phase of bacterial growth, and oxygen tension. In recent years, antibiotic penetration into the infection site has become one of the main factors that should be taken into account when choosing an antibiotic regimen. Linezolid and fluoroquinolones penetrate well into the lungs, and their use in nosocomial pneumonia is associated with a significant clinical success rate. Vancomycin has a poor lung penetration, and many clinical failures of this drug in pneumonia due to strains sensitive to this antimicrobial may derive from its poor lung disposition.

Several studies regarding the inoculum effect considered the effect of the bacterial load on the minimal inhibitory concentration (MIC) of several antibiotics. Standard laboratory inoculum for MIC determination is around 10^5 CFU/ml. The presence of the inoculum effect is defined as an eightfold or greater increase in MIC on testing, with an inoculum as high as 10^7–10^8 CFU/ml, with higher inoculum better reflecting most clinical settings. Aztreonam, piperacillin, cefotaxime, and cefoxitin show a significant inoculum effect against susceptible strains. A significant inoculum effect is associated with β-lactams with prevalent inhibition of penicillin-binding protein 3(PBP3) because, in the setting of a high inoculum, bacteria proliferation slows and they produce less PBP3. Moreover, the inoculum effect is present when a bacterium produces an enzyme able to destroy the tested antibiotic, because the enzymes

Table 6.1 Pieces of the antimicrobial activity puzzle

Variables influencing antimicrobial effectiveness
Pharmacodynamic properties — Concentration dependency / Time dependency
Antibiotic penetration into the infection site
pH and oxygen tension at the infection site
Vascularization at the infection site
Phase of bacterial growth
Inoculum effect
Endotoxin release
Postantibiotic effect

released from the dead cells inactivate the antibiotic, which is why the combination with β-lactamase inhibitors may prevent the inoculum effect observed with many β-lactams. Among the clinical conditions mimicking a high inoculum are endocarditis, meningitis, septic arthritis, osteomyelitis, abscesses, and deep-seated infections. In these conditions, antibiotics without an inoculum effect have been demonstrated to be more effective.

Regarding the bactericidal activity of antibiotics, another important factor is the presence or absence of a postantibiotic effect (PAE). PAE is the ability of an antimicrobial drug to exert a persistent inhibitory effect on microorganism growth after the drug has been completely removed. Usually, antibiotics with a main time-dependent activity lack a significant PAE, although differences among the different classes do exist. β-lactams, for example, show a significant PAE only against Gram-positive organisms, although carbapenems may have a sustained PAE against aerobic Gram-negative bacilli (AGNB). Agents that interfere with protein or DNA synthesis, such as fluoroquinolones and aminoglycosides, usually show a sustained PAE, mainly against AGNB. The PAE is unique to the pathogen and is generally longer in vivo than in vitro. For example, PAE duration for aminoglycosides ranges from 0.5 to 8 h depending on the bacterial strain, the MIC, the duration of exposure, and the relative concentration of the aminoglycoside. The PAE may decrease with multiple dosing [1–3].

6.3 The Frame of the Puzzle: Critical Illness

Assuming antimicrobial activity is like a puzzle with many important pieces, critical illness is like the frame of this puzzle, representing the context in which antimicrobial activity challenges microorganisms. But it is not a passive frame, because it continuously interacts with antimicrobial activity in many ways. In fact, pathophysiological changes in critical illness affect antibiotic PK variables, with possible effects on antibiotic efficacy and clinical outcomes. Critical illness often changes the volume of distribution (Vd) and clearance (CL) of antibiotics, parameters usually correlated to the hydrophilicity and lipophilicity of the antibiotic molecule. During sepsis, vascular endothelium derangement results in maldistribution of blood flow and increased capillary permeability, with fluid shifts from the intravascular compartment to the interstitial space [5, 6]. This usually increases the Vd of hydrophilic drugs, decreasing their plasma concentration. A similar effect on Vd of hydrophilic drugs is caused by mechanical ventilation, hypoalbuminemia, extracorporeal circuits, postsurgical drains, and burns. Lipophilic drugs typically have a large Vd because of their partitioning into adipose tissue or into cells. Therefore, the increase in Vd resulting from third spacing is considered insignificant [7, 8].

Drug-elimination half-life ($T_{1/2}$) is indirectly related to antibiotic CL and directly related to its Vd and is therefore reduced with an increased drug CL and increased with an increased Vd. In critically ill patients, cardiovascular support with intravenously administered fluids, vasopressors, and inotropes sustains a hyperdynamic state that, in the absence of significant organ dysfunction, increases renal perfusion and creatinine clearance (CrCl) of hydrophilic antibiotics. It follows that dose adjustment for hydrophilic antibiotics can be guided by CrCl [9].

Protein binding is a factor that may influence the Vd and CL of many antibiotics with high protein-binding affinity (such as ceftriaxone, oxacillin, teicoplanin). In hypoalbuminemic states, as commonly occur in critically ill patients, these drugs may have a 100% increased CL and Vd. With further deterioration in the patient's health status, significant myocardial depression can occur, which leads to a decrease in organ perfusion and failure of the microvascular circulation until multiple-organ dysfunction syndrome occurs, with renal and/or hepatic dysfunction. In this phase of critical illness, there is usually a decreased antibiotic CL and prolonged $T_{1/2}$. Finally, antibiotic penetration at the target site is impaired in patients with septic shock, being 5–10 times lower than in healthy volunteers [7].

The above-mentioned causes of altered PKs in the ICU septic patients require specific dosing strategies in this special patient population. Ongoing evaluations of sickness severity can facilitate timely adjustment of antibiotic dosing [9]. Specific consideration regarding each class of antibiotics is necessary when they are used in critically ill patients.

6.3.1 Aminoglycosides

The kill characteristic of aminoglycosides is concentration dependent. Aminoglycosides often have increased Vd in critically ill patients, which can result in a decreased maximum concentration (C_{max}). Vd has been shown to increase proportionally with increasing sickness severity. Because of their narrow therapeutic index, maximal weight-based once-day dosing is required to achieve adequate C_{max}:MIC ratios. PK variability and potential for adverse effects mandates monitoring plasma aminoglycoside concentrations. Once-daily administration appears to be as effective as multiple doses per day but with reduced risks of toxicity. Therefore, multiple doses per day should only be considered for treating endocarditis or in neutropenic patients [7, 8].

6.3.2 β-Lactams

The β-lactam antibiotics are generally hydrophilic molecules, renally cleared, with moderate-to-low protein binding (although ceftriaxone has high protein binding). An improved PD profile in critically ill patients is obtained with either more frequent dosing or extended or continuous infusions. This mode of administration is especially useful in critically ill patients with high glomerular filtration rate or increased Vd. The superiority of continuous infusions of β-lactam antibiotics in comparison with intermittent administration is supported by the fact that the former administration modality theoretically favors the achievement of the optimal PD target. Reduced mortality from extended infusions (4 h infusion every 8 h) of piperacillin–tazobactam has been shown in critically ill patients with *Pseudomonas aeruginosa* infection [10]. In critical illness, carbapenems develop increased Vd and higher CL. Extended infusion of these drugs seems to be appropriate in critical patients because optimal activity requires time above MIC >40%.

6.3.3 Glycopeptides

Glycopeptides are relatively hydrophilic drugs, with PD properties not completely elucidated. It remains unclear whether AUC/MIC or time >MIC is the target parameter to optimize activity. The benefit of continuous infusion, especially against methicillin-resistant *Staphylococcus aureus* (MRSA), seems significant, although data require further confirmation. Nonrenal CL of vancomycin occurs in critical patients with acute renal failure. Therefore, empirical dosing based on CrCl data with subsequent therapeutic drug monitoring of C_{min} plasma concentrations (15–20 mg/L) are recommended because of the risk of nephrotoxicity with higher C_{min} (>20 mg/L) concentrations.

6.3.4 Fluoroquinolones

Fluoroquinolones are lipophilic antibiotics with extensive distribution and excellent penetration into neutrophils and lymphocytes. Their Vd is minimally affected in the critically ill patient. Fluoroquinolones display concentration-dependent kill characteristics but also some time-dependent effects. A C_{max}/MIC ratio of 10 seems to be the critical variable in predicting bacterial eradication, but in critically ill patients, an area under the concentration–time curve (AUC)/MIC >125 in case of Gram-negative infection and >30 in case of Gram-positive infection is also fundamental to achieve successful clinical outcome and to avoid the emergence of resistant bacterial strains.

6.3.5 Linezolid

Linezolid is quite lipophilic, and it distributes widely into tissues and is mostly metabolized hepatically before being cleared renally. No dose adjustment seems to be necessary in renal or hepatic dysfunction. The killing characteristic is time dependent, being optimal when the time above MIC is >40–80%. In critical patients, linezolid shows an increased Vd and CL, requiring appropriate dose adjustment.

6.3.6 Tigecycline

Tigecycline is a lipophilic glycylcycline eliminated by biliary excretion. Its killing characteristic is time dependent, but the AUC/MIC ratio is the target parameter for efficacy because of its PAE. Critical illness does not seem to affect its PKs significantly, but further clinical studies specifically performed in this patient population are needed to confirm this.

6.3.7 Daptomycin

Daptomycin is a concentration-dependent antibiotic, and PK parameters that best predict its efficacy are C_{max}/MIC and AUC/MIC. Daptomycin is eliminated primarily by glomerular filtration; people receiving daptomycin should be monitored for skeletal muscle damage. Doses higher than those initially suggested (4 mg/kg once daily) are necessary in severely ill or ICU patients.

6.3.8 Colistin

The polymyxin antibiotics are hydrophilic molecules with predominantly concentration-dependent bacterial killing activity. Patient dosing should follow patient weight and renal dysfunction considerations because of the risk of nephrotoxicity [7].

6.4 Time-Dependent Antibiotics

Time-dependent antibiotic activity is correlated to T > MIC; that is, the duration of time that antibiotic concentrations exceed the minimum inhibitory concentration [1]. Larger doses increase the efficacy of these antibiotics, extending the time during which the drug remains above the effective concentration rather than increasing its absolute concentration. PD studies led to a shift of dosage regimens toward more fragmented doses or even continuous infusion. The results of many clinical studies recommend exceeding the MIC by 2–5 times for between 40 and 100% of the dosage interval when using time-dependent antibiotics. This time should probably be further extended when using antibiotics that are highly protein bound (>90%) [2].

Strategies to keep drug concentrations above the MIC for a longer period include: multiple doses given frequently, administration in a continuous infusion, use of agents with long serum half-lives, use of agents with active metabolites, choice of agents with the lowest MIC toward the causative microorganism, and concomitant administration of antibiotic elimination inhibitors (i.e., probenecid).

6.5 Concentration-Dependent Antibiotics

PD parameters predicting the performance of concentration-dependent antibiotics are: AUC_{0-24}/MIC (ratio of AUC during a 24-h dosing period to MIC) and C_{max}/MIC (ratio of maximum serum antibiotic concentration to MIC). In experimental studies, a C_{max}/MIC ratio above at least 8–10 was required to optimize bactericidal activity of concentration-dependent antibiotics [1].

Clinical studies demonstrated a correlation between higher aminoglycoside peak levels and improved clinical outcome. The dosage of aminoglycosides in case of a once-daily strategy should be 5–7 mg/kg for gentamicin and tobramycin and 15–30 mg/kg for amikacin. These dosages have been selected to reach a C_{max}/MIC ratio of 10 considering the usual MIC for susceptible *P. aeruginosa* strains. With this causative pathogen, tobramycin is preferred because it usually has a lower MIC. In patients with decreased renal function, the interval between doses should be lengthened, but doses should not be decreased, so that a high C_{max}/MIC ratio is maintained and an appropriate drug-free period thus allowed [1, 2].

Also for fluoroquinolones, many studies confirmed the importance of a C_{max}/MIC ratio >10 as an important predictor of antimicrobial effect and clinical outcome. Regarding the effect of the AUC_{0-24}/MIC ratio on the antimicrobial activity of fluoroquinolones, a ratio >100 seems to optimize fluoroquinolone activity, whereas a lower AUC_{0-24}/MIC ratio is associated with an increased risk of antimicrobial resistance development. Improper dosing regimens of fluoroquinolones that do not produce AUC_{0-24}/MIC ratios >100 or C_{max}/MIC ratios >8–10 may increase the risk of resistance in AGNB [1]. Also new macrolides (clarithromycin, azalides, ketolides), colistin, and daptomycin have a concentration-dependent activity.

6.6 Tissue Penetration of Antibiotics

An important factor in determining a successful therapeutic response to antimicrobial drugs is maintaining the level of free antibiotic in extravascular fluid above the MIC of the infecting organism [1, 3, 8]. Extravascular distribution, tissue binding, and free drug concentration of an antibiotic can be predicted from serum kinetics and serum protein binding [11].

Serum protein binding of antimicrobial drugs may have important consequences on their action. In particular, high serum protein binding can reduce antimicrobial activity, tissue distribution, and elimination of antibiotics. Binding $\geq 80\%$ have the potential to significantly reduce free drug levels and affect therapeutic efficacy [2]. The extent of protein binding is a major factor determining active drug concentration in serum and most extravascular fluids. As a general rule, agents with minimal protein binding penetrate tissues better than those that are highly protein bound, although the latter might be excreted much faster. Among drugs that are $<80-85\%$ protein bound, differences appear to be of slight clinical importance [11]. The concentration of several plasma proteins can be altered by many factors, including stress, surgery, liver or kidney dysfunction, and pregnancy. In such circumstances, the free-drug concentration may increase if the antimicrobial drug has high protein binding. Antibiotic penetration into tissues is related to the amount of antibiotic not protein bound.

The ability of antibiotics to penetrate can be evaluated using the ratio of the AUC for antibiotic in the peripheral site to that of serum. Penetration into fibrin and lymph follows Fick's law of diffusion. The antibiotic present in the serum penetrates into peripheral tissues after lag times [1, 3, 10]. Drug concentration in tissues is generally lower than in serum; peaks may occur simultaneously or shortly after the maximal levels are reached in serum, and for most antibiotics, elimination from the extravascular component is slower than from serum.

The relationship between protein binding, tissue penetration, and excretory mechanisms has been widely studied, especially for third-generation cephalosporins. These derivatives seem to penetrate adequately into the cerebrospinal fluid and appear to be appropriate agents for treating meningitis [11]. Generally, the fluoroquinolones have a low degree of plasma protein binding, with excellent tissue penetration and high concentrations, as reflected by their particularly large apparent Vd [11].

6.7 Inactivation of Antibiotics

This mechanism of resistance is common for many antibiotics, including β-lactams and aminoglycosides [12, 13]. Inactivation of β-lactam antibiotics requires specific bacterial enzymes. Currently, more than 300 β-lactamase enzymes have been described, and they can be divided in four different functional groups (1–4). Group 1 includes β-lactamases that confer resistance to all classes of β-lactams, except carbapenems, and that are not inhibited by clavulanic acid. They can be either chromosomal or plasmid encoded. Group 2 includes β-lactamases susceptible to inhibition due to clavulanic acid, and they are divided in six subgroups. Subgroup 2a includes staphylococcal and enterococcal penicillinases. Subgroup 2b includes broad spectrum β-lactamases of AGNB strains but also extended spectrum β-lactamases. Subgroup 2c includes carbenicillin hydrolyzing β-lactamases. Subgroup 2d includes cloxacillin hydrolyzing enzymes. Subgroup 2e includes cephalosporinases. Subgroup 2f includes β-lactamases active on carbapenems. Group 3 includes metallo-beta-lactamases with activity against carbapenems and all β-lactam classes except monobactams. Group 4 includes the other β-lactamases not included in the previous groups [12].

Extended spectrum β-lactamases (ESBL) are β-lactamase able to hydrolyze the extended-spectrum cephalosporins, including third-generation compounds. Antibiotics susceptible to ESBL include cefotaxime, ceftazidime, aztreonam, and other expanded-spectrum cephalosporins, whereas imipenem is usually resistant. These enzymes are encoded also in plasmids containing genes for aminoglycoside resistance, trimethoprim–sulfamethoxazole, and often fluoroquinolones. ESBL are often present in *Escherichia coli* or *Klebsiella pneumoniae* but can be transferred to *Proteus mirabilis, Citrobacter, Serratia,* and other AGNB [12]. Every *E. coli* and *K. pneumoniae* with reduced susceptibility to these drugs or to aztreonam should be considered at risk of possessing these enzymes. Treating infections caused by ESBL-producing strains is difficult due to the high risk of concomitant resistance to aminoglycosides, trimethoprim–sulfamethoxazole, and fluoroquinolones. Carbapenems are the agents of choice against ESBL-producing bacteria because they are highly stable against β-lactamase hydrolysis [12].

Inactivation is by far the most important mechanism of acquired microbial resistance toward aminoglycosides in clinical practice. Aminoglycosides may become the substrate of several microbial enzymes that may phosphorylate, adenylate, or acetylate specific hydroxyl or amino groups. Phosphorylation is the main mechanism of inactivation for aminoglycosides, it is determined by either Gram-positive or AGNB strains, and it results in complete inactivation of aminoglycosides. Some aminoglycosides are resistant to phosphorylation due to the presence of side chains, such as amikacin, or the absence of specific hydroxyl groups, such as tobramycin and gentamicin. Aminoglycoside-inactivating enzymes are often encoded in plasmids that are especially common in hospital environments. Pharmacological strategies to inhibit aminoglycoside-inactivating enzymes are under evaluation.

6.8 Relationship Between Antibiotics and Endotoxins

Bacterial endotoxins are thought to play a fundamental role in the pathogenesis of sepsis and septic shock. Bacterial growth and death is associated with the release of variable amounts of endotoxins outside the bacteria. Antibiotic therapy may increase the release of endotoxins that trigger the septic response by binding to specific receptors upon mononuclear phagocytes, endothelial cells, and polymorphonuclear leucocytes [14–17]. This effect has been studied for several agents, including β-lactams, glycopeptides, aminoglycosides, and fluoroquinolones.

Regarding β-lactams, different patterns of endotoxin release seem to be correlated with the inhibition of different PBPs. In particular, inhibition of PBP1a and 1b results in a massive bactericidal activity against AGNB associated with bacterial wall molecule degradation. These changes lead to production of spheroplasts that undergo immediate bacteriolysis. In AGNB, PBP2 inhibition results in spheroid elements osmotically stable but unable to proliferate, and thus increases bacterial mass. Conversely, inhibition of PBP3 located in bacterial septa prevents separation of the proliferating bacteria, resulting in long filaments that are vital syncytia resistant to lysis but able to produce and release endotoxins. Carbapenems, ceftriaxone, cefepime, and β-lactams in combination with β-lactamase inhibitors inhibit PBP2 and 3 in AGNB. Therefore, they have a rapid bactericidal activity without increments of bacterial mass and are associated with poor endotoxin release. Ceftazidime, ticarcillin, and cefoxitin inhibit PBP3 and, at high concentrations, PBP1; they have a slower bactericidal activity associated with a slight increase in bacterial mass and a moderate release of endotoxins. Piperacillin, monobactams, cefuroxime, and cefotaxime inhibit mainly PBP3, resulting in slow bactericidal activity associated with an increase in bacterial mass and endotoxin release [17].

Glycopeptides induce bacteriolysis and release endotoxins, but the lipid part of the endotoxin is inactivated by these antibiotics. Fluoroquinolones result in a slightly greater endotoxin release than do carbapenems, as they cause DNA damage associated with the inhibition of cellular division that produces bacterial filaments able to release endotoxins. Besides the role of antibiotic therapy in endotoxin release, they may have also endotoxin-neutralizing properties that may inhibit the effects of endotoxin [18]. Antibiotics with endotoxin-neutralizing properties are polycationic molecules that can link the polyanionic moieties of lipopolysaccharides, including polymyxins, teicoplanin, and aminoglycosides [14, 15]. In experimental studies, polymyxin B resulted in reduced endotoxin shock, pyrogenicity, Shwartzman reaction, and endotoxin lethality [15]. Teicoplanin shows an endotoxin-neutralizing property that results in reduced levels of tumor necrosis factor (TNF)-α and interleukin (IL)-1 after endotoxin stimulation.

Antibiotics inhibiting protein synthesis result in a lower release of endotoxins than the agents acting on the cell wall. Aminoglycosides inhibit endotoxin synthesis, and although they favor endotoxin release, they neutralize them chemically by binding their anionic moieties. In this regard, variable effects have been observed for different compounds of this class of antibiotics: tobramycin seems to be the most effective in neutralizing endotoxins.

6.9 Respect for Ecology: A Prerequisite for a Safe Antibiotic Therapy

The relationship between the microbes and host is not just a fight between two contenders [19]. Ecological studies show symbiosis in the microbial communities of the skin and mucous membranes. In these ecosystems, the resident microorganisms play an important physiological role with mutualistic relationships, protection from infections included [20, 21]. The normal microflora acts as a barrier against carriage of potentially pathogenic microorganisms and against overgrowth of opportunistic microorganisms (colonization resistance) [21, 22]. For this protective effect to occur, great stability of these ecosystems is fundamental [22]. Administration of antimicrobial agents interferes with the ecological balance between host and normal microflora.

The impact of antibiotics on normal intestinal flora has been widely studied. The gastrointestinal tract is a complex ecosystem that may be altered by antibiotic administration, resulting clinically in diarrhea and fungal infections that usually cease after treatment. Pseudomembranous colitis is an example of the deleterious effects of antimicrobial therapy that disturbs the normal ecologic balance of the bowel flora, leading to an abnormal proliferation of *Clostridium difficile*. The effects of antibiotics on oropharyngeal and skin microflora may be important as well. Antibiotic therapy may cause alterations in skin microbial flora with a decline in the number of bacteria—mostly anaerobic bacteria [23]. Moreover, exposure to antibiotics often results in selection of antibiotic-resistant organisms that can transfer resistance to other microorganisms. By using antimicrobial agents that do not alter the level of resistance of colonizing microorganisms, the risk of emergence and spread of resistant strains is reduced [20, 21].

Respect for the individual's ecology should be a prerequisite for every antibiotic policy, and the use of antibiotics with little or no impact on the normal flora should always be encouraged. Antibiotics that are not active against the indigenous bacteria in the mouth and intestine and are not excreted to a significant degree via the intestine, saliva, or skin are therefore preferred [20, 21]. First generation β-lactams, aminoglycosides, and polymyxins are favorable from an ecological point of view.

6.10 De-Escalation Therapy

In addition to treating infections, antibiotic use contributes to the emergence of resistance among potentially pathogenic microorganisms. Therefore, avoiding unnecessary antibiotic use and optimizing antimicrobial agent administration will help improve patient outcomes while minimizing further pressures for resistance [24]. Antibiotic administration guidelines/protocols developed locally or by national societies suggest avoiding unnecessary administration [25, 26].

Severe infections, including pneumonia and bacteremia, remain a major cause of morbidity and mortality among hospitalized patients. Clinical evidence suggests that failure to quickly treat these infections with an adequate initial antibiotic regimen is associated with greater patient morbidity and mortality. Delays of 24–48 h in initiating adequate treatment are associated with increased mortality rates. Appropriate therapy should be instituted as soon as sepsis is suspected in critically ill patients [27]. During recent decades, the types of pathogens have significantly changed, with shifts from AGNB to Gram-positive multi-drug-resistant organisms requiring appropriate empirical regimens. Although early and appropriate therapy are the best predictors of positive outcome, the microorganism causing the infection is frequently not known at the time antimicrobial therapy is initiated [28]. This has led to the development of a novel paradigm guiding empirical antimicrobial therapy administration for patients with serious infections, called antibacterial de-escalation therapy. This is an approach to antibacterial use that attempts to balance the need to provide appropriate, initially broad antibacterial treatment while limiting the emergence of antibacterial resistance. Resistance is minimized by narrowing the antibacterial regimen once the pathogens and their susceptibility profiles are known and by employing the shortest course of therapy [29]. De-escalation antimicrobial therapy should be tailored to critically ill patients according to their clinical status, illness severity, and suspicion of sepsis or nosocomial pneumonia [25]. Risk stratification should be employed to identify patients at high risk of infection with antibiotic-resistant bacteria (prior treatment with antibiotics during hospitalization; prolonged hospital stay; and presence of invasive devices, e.g., central venous catheters, endotracheal tubes, urinary catheters). Patients at high risk for infection with resistant bacteria should be treated initially with an appropriate combination of antibiotics. This approach must be modified if specific microorganisms are excluded based on examination of appropriate clinical specimens. Delays in de-escalating unnecessary antibiotic treatment are harmful, as they promote emergence of resistant bacterial pathogens. Decreasing the overall duration of empirical and potentially unnecessary antibiotic use reduces the incidence of hospital-acquired superinfections attributed to antibiotic-resistant microorganisms [24].

6.11 Main Classes of Systemic Antibiotics

Systemic antibiotics include drugs commonly used in the ICU, such as β-lactams; drugs to be used under specific indications, such as aminoglycosides, glycopeptides, fluoroquinolones, and macrolides; and drugs used only for multi-drug-resistant microorganisms, including *streptogramins*, linezolid, colistin, advanced-generation cephalosporins, glycylcycline, and daptomycin (Table 6.2).

Table 6.2 Main systemic antibiotic used in ICU and their spectrum of antimicrobial activity

Class	Drug	S. spp.	E. spp.	SA	MRSA	HA	NM	AGNB	PA	Anaerobes G+	Anaerobes G−
Penicillin	Penicillin G	S	S	R	R	R	S	R	R	S	R
Penicillinase-resistant Penicillin	Oxacillin	S	R	S	R	R	R	R	R	R	R
	Nafcillin	S	R	S	R	R	R	R	R	R	R
Aminopenicillin	Amoxicillin	S	S	R	R	S/R	S	S/R	R	S	R
	Ampicillin	S	S	R	R	S/R	S	S/R	R	S	R
Carboxy-penicillin	Ticarcillin	S	S	R	R	S/R	S	S	S	S	R
	Carbenicillin	S	S	R	R	S/R	S	S	S	S	R
Ureidopenicillins	Piperacillin	S	S	R	R	S/R	S	S	S	S	R
	Mezlocillin	S	S	R	R	S/R	S	S	S	S	R
Cephalosporin I° 1st generation	Cefazolin	S	R	S	R	S	R	R	R	R	R
	Cephalothin										
Cephalosporin II° 2nd generation	Cefoxitin	S	R	S	R	S	S	S/R	R	S	S
	Cefuroxime										
Cephalosporin III° 3rd generation	Ceftriaxone	S	R	S	R	S	S	S	S/R	S	R
	Ceftazidime	S	R	S	R	S	S	S	S	S	R
Cephalosporin IV° 4th generation	Cefepime	S	R	S	R	S	S	S	S	R	R
Advanced-generation Cephalosporin	Ceftobiprole	S	S	S	S	S	S	S	S	S	R
	Ceftaroline	S	S	S	S	S	S	S	S	S	R
Carbapenem	Imipenem	S	S/R	S	R	S	S	S	S	S	S
Monobactam	Aztreonam	R	R	R	R	S	S	S	S	R	R

(continued)

Table 6.2 (continued)

β-lactam + β lactam inhibitors	Amoxicillin + clavulanate	S	S	S	R	S	S	S	R	S	S
	Piperacillin + tazobactam	S	S	S	R	S	S	S	S	S	S
Aminoglycosides	Tobramycin	R	R/S	S	RR	S	S	S	S	R	R
	Amikacin	R	R/S	S	RR	S	S	S	S	R	R
Fluoroquinolone II° 2nd generation	Ciprofloxacin	R	R	S	R	S	S	S	S	R	R
	Ofloxacin	R	R	S	R	S	S	S	S	R	R
Fluoroquinolone III° 3rd generation	Levofloxacin	S	R/S	S	R	S	S	S	S	S	R
	Moxifloxacin	S	R/S	S	R	S	S	S	S	S	R
Macrolides I° 1st generation	Erythromycin	S	S	S	R	R	S	R	R	R	R
Macrolides III° 3rd generation	Clarithromycin.	S	S	S	R	S	S	S	S	S	R
	Azithromycin	S	S	S		S	S	S	S	S	R
Macrolides IV° 4th generation	Telithromycin	S	S	S	R	S	S	S	S	S	R
Glycopeptides	Vancomycin	S	S	S	S	R	R	R	R	R	S
	Teicoplanin	S	S	S	S	R	R	R	R	S	R
Polymyxin	Colistin	R	R	R	R	S	S	S	S	S	S
Oxazolidones	Linezolid	S	S	S	S	R	R	R	R	R	R
Streptogramins	Dalfopristin	S	S	S	S	R	R	R	R	S	S
	Quinupristin	S	S	S	S	R	R	R	R	S	S
Lipopeptides	Daptomycin	S	S	S	S	R	R	R	R	S	R
Glycylcycline	Tigecycline	S	S	S	S	S	S	S	S	S	S

S. spp. Streptococcus spp., *E. spp. Enterococcus* spp., *SA Staphylococcus aureus*, *MRSA* methicillin-resistant *S aureus*, *HI Haemophilus influenzae*, *NM Neisseria meningitidis*, *AGNB* aerobic Gram-negative bacilli, *PA Pseudomonas aeruginosa*, *S* sensitive, *R* resistant

6.11.1 β-Lactams

The basic structure of these antibiotics is a β-lactam ring to which is attached a side chain [17].

6.11.1.1 Mechanism of Action
These drugs act by inhibiting the synthesis of the bacterial cell wall due to selective acylation of specific membrane proteins (the so-called PBPs). There are several PBPs with different affinities for different β-lactam antibiotics. PBP1a and 1b include the transpeptidases involved in peptidoglycan synthesis. Other PBPs maintain the rodlike shape or are involved in septum formation at division [17].

6.11.1.2 Mechanism of Resistance
- intrinsic low affinity of PBPs;
- development of high molecular weight PBPs with decreased affinity for antibiotics;
- enzymatic disruption by β-lactamases;
- changes in permeability to the antibiotic or extrusion from the target site.

6.11.1.3 Side Effects
- hypersensitivity reactions (maculopapular rash, urticarial rash, fever, bronchospasm, vasculitis, serum sickness, exfoliative dermatitis); cross-reactions with different molecules of the same class do occur;
- exfoliative dermatitis and exudative erythema multiforme of either the erythematopapular or vesiculobullous type constitute the characteristic Stevens–Johnson syndrome;
- bone marrow depression with granulocytopenia;
- hepatitis.

6.11.2 Penicillin G

6.11.2.1 Spectrum of Activity
Active against most anaerobic microorganisms (except *Bacteroides fragilis*): *Borrelia burgdorferi*, *Treponema pallidum*, *B. anthracis*. Syphilis, actinomycosis, and anthrax can be treated successfully with penicillin G. It may be still also useful in meningococcal and clostridial infections [17].

6.11.2.2 Pharmacological Properties
The $T_{1/2}$ of penicillin G is within 30 min, it is rapidly eliminated from the body, mainly by the kidney (10% by glomerular filtration and 90% by tubular secretion); a small amount is excreted in the bile.

6.11.3 Penicillinase-Resistant Penicillins (Nafcillin, Oxacillin, Cloxacillin, Dicloxacillin)

6.11.3.1 Spectrum of Activity
These are resistant to staphylococcal penicillinase and remain useful despite the increasing incidence of methicillin-resistant (MR) microorganisms, a term that denotes resistance to all penicillinase-resistant penicillins and cephalosporins. MRSA contains a high molecular weight PBP (PBP2) with a very low affinity for β-lactams. Fifty percent of *S. epidermidis* strains are resistant to the penicillinase-resistant penicillins by the same mechanism. The daily dose of oxacillin for adults is 2–4 g divided into four doses [17].

6.11.3.2 Pharmacological Properties
All these congeners are bound to plasma albumin (approximately 90%); none is removed from the circulation to a significant degree by hemodialysis. They are rapidly excreted by the kidney, with half-lives between 30 and 60 min. Intervals between doses of oxacillin, cloxacillin, and dicloxacillin do not have to be altered for patients with renal failure.

6.11.4 Aminopenicillins (Ampicillin, Amoxicillin)

6.11.4.1 Spectrum of Activity
Active against Gram-positive and Gram-negative bacteria. Many pneumococcal isolates are resistant to ampicillin. *Haemophilus influenzae, Enterococcus* spp., and the viridans group of streptococci usually are inhibited by ampicillin. Many strains of *Neisseria gonorrhoeae, E. coli, P. mirabilis, Salmonella, Shigella*, and *Enterobacter* are now resistant. Most strains of *Pseudomonas, Klebsiella, Serratia, Acinetobacter*, and indole-positive *Proteus* also are resistant to this group of penicillins. The combination with a β-lactamase inhibitor, such as clavulanic acid or sulbactam, markedly expands the spectrum of activity of these drugs. Aminopenicillins are useful in upper respiratory tract infections (sinusitis, otitis media, acute exacerbations of chronic bronchitis, and epiglottitis) caused by *Streptococcus pyogenes, S. pneumoniae*, and *H. influenzae* [17].

6.11.4.2 Pharmacologic Properties
Ampicillin and amoxicillin are used at doses of 1–4 g per day every 6 h. Their half-time is around 80 min. Dose adjustment is required in case of renal dysfunction. About 20% protein bound in plasma. Ampicillin is excreted in the bile, amoxicillin in the urine.

6.11.5 Carboxypenicillins (Carbenicillin, Ticarcillin)

6.11.5.1 Spectrum of Activity
Active against some isolates of *P. aeruginosa* and *Proteus* that are resistant to aminopenicillins. They are not active against *S. aureus*. Carbenicillin use may cause excessive Na^+ intake with congestive heart failure; it may also interfere with platelet function. Ticarcillin is associated with fewer side effects [17].

6.11.6 Ureidopenicillins (Mezlocillin, Piperacillin)

6.11.6.1 Spectrum of Activity
These are active against *P. aeruginosa* and *Klebsiella* spp. [27]. They are neutralized by β-lactamases. Ureidopenicillins are important agents for treating patients with serious infections, such as bacteremia, pneumonia, and burns, caused by AGNB.

6.11.6.2 Pharmacologic Properties
The usual adult dosage is 6–18 g per day divided into 4–6 doses. These drugs are excreted in bile to a significant degree [27].

6.11.7 Cephalosporins

6.11.7.1 Mechanism of Action
These drugs inhibit bacterial cell-wall synthesis in a similar manner to that provoked by β-lactams.

6.11.7.2 Spectrum of Action
Cephalosporins are not active against the following microorganisms: MRSA, MR coagulase-negative staphylococci (MRCNS), *Enterococcus* spp., *Listeria monocytogenes*, *Legionella pneumophila*, *C. difficile*, *Stenotrophomonas maltophilia*, *Campylobacter jejuni*, and *Acinetobacter* spp. [28].

6.11.7.3 Mechanisms of Resistance
- inability to reach the sites of action;
- alterations in PBPs, especially PBP1a and 2x;
- β-lactamases—cephalosporins have variable susceptibility to β-lactamase; cefazolin is more susceptible than cephalothin, cefoxitin, cefuroxime [28].

6.11.7.4 Side Effects
- hypersensitivity reactions (maculopapular rash, anaphylaxis, bronchospasm, urticaria); patients allergic to penicillins may manifest cross-reactivity to cephalosporins;

- nephrotoxicity, although less than the aminoglycosides or polymyxins;
- diarrhea and alcohol intolerance;
- serious bleeding related to either hypoprothrombinemia, thrombocytopenia, and/or platelet dysfunction.

6.11.7.5 Classification

Classification of cephalosporins by generations is based on general features of their antimicrobial activity [28]:

- First-generation cephalosporins—include cephalothin, cefazolin, cephalexin, cephradine, and cefadroxil. They have good activity against Gram-positive bacteria with the exception of enterococci, MRSA, and MRCNS, and relatively modest activity against Gram-negative microorganisms. Most oropharyngeal anaerobes are sensitive, but the *B. fragilis* group is usually resistant. Cephalothin is the most resistant to staphylococcal β-lactamase and is effective in severe staphylococcal infections.
- Second-generation cephalosporins—including cefamandole, cefoxitin, cefaclor, loracarbef, cefuroxime, cefotetan, and cefprozil, have somewhat increased activity against AGNB (*Enterobacter*, *Proteus*, and *Klebsiella* spp.), but are less active than the third-generation agents. A subset of second-generation agents including cefoxitin and cefotetan are active against *B. fragilis*.
- Third-generation cephalosporins—include cefotaxime, ceftizoxime, ceftriaxone, cefixime, cefpodoxime, cefoperazone, and ceftazidime. They are less active than first-generation agents against Gram-positive cocci, but they are much more active against the Enterobacteriaceae, including β-lactamase-producing strains. A subset of third-generation agents (ceftazidime and cefoperazone) also is active against *P. aeruginosa*. Ceftriaxone has a $T_{1/2}$ of about 8 h, so it can be used once or twice daily. More than half the drug can be recovered from the urine; the remainder appears to be eliminated by biliary secretion. Ceftazidime has a better activity than cefoperazone or piperacillin against *Pseudomonas*.
- Fourth-generation cephalosporins—such as cefepime, have an extended spectrum of activity compared with the third generation, with increased resistance to β-lactamases. Fourth-generation agents may prove to have particular therapeutic usefulness for treating infections due to AGNB resistant to third-generation cephalosporins. Cefepime has greater activity than cefotaxime against Gram-negative bacteria (*H. influenzae*, *N. gonorrhoeae* and *N. meningitidis*). Regarding *P. aeruginosa*, cefepime is as active as ceftazidime and a higher activity against streptococci and *S. aureus*. It is not active against MRSA, penicillin-resistant pneumococci, enterococci, *B. fragilis*, or *L. monocytogenes*. Its serum $T_{1/2}$ is 2 h and it is renally excreted. Doses should be adjusted for renal failure. Cefepime has excellent penetration into CSF. Adult dosage is 2 g intravenously every 12 h.
- Advanced-generation cephalosporins—such as ceftobiprole and ceftaroline has been proposed for the treatment of complicated skin and skin structure infections and bacterial pneumonia [29]. Ceftobiprole has activity against aerobic Gram-negative bacilli, which extends to cefepime-sensitive *P. aeruginosa*, and activity against Gram-positive organisms, which includes methicillin-resistant

Staphylococcus aureus. Its most common side effects are nausea and dysgeusia. Ceftaroline is a novel, broad-spectrum, with antimicrobial activity against MRSA, *Streptococcus pneumonia* and respiratory Gram-negative pathogens such as *Moraxella catarrhalis* and H. influenzae. It is eliminated primarily by renal excretion, with a $T_{1/2}$ of approximately 3 h [29].

6.11.8 Carbapenems (Imipenem, Meropenem, Doripenem, Ertapenem)

6.11.8.1 Mechanism of Action
Mechanism of action is similar to that of other β-lactams; very resistant to hydrolysis by most β-lactamases [30].

6.11.8.2 Spectrum of Activity
These are active against aerobic and anaerobic microorganisms: streptococci, enterococci (excluding *Enterococcus faecium* and non-β-lactamase-producing penicillin-resistant strains), staphylococci, *Listeria*, Enterobacteriaceae, many strains of *Pseudomonas* and *Acinetobacter*, and all anaerobes, including *B. fragilis*. On the other hand, MRSA and methicillin-resistant MRCNS, as well as *S. maltophilia*, are resistant to carbapenems [30]. Doripenem may offer slightly more activity against selected pathogens, as it seems to resist attack by carbapenem-hydrolyzing β-lactamases such as imipenem-hydrolyzing β-lactamase Sme1. Therefore, empiric therapy with doripenem may be useful when multidrug resistance is suspected. Ertapenem is a unique member of this class; it lacks activity against Pseudomonas and Enterococcus, but it has a favorable PK profile.

6.11.8.3 Pharmacological Properties
Imipenem is hydrolyzed rapidly by a dipeptidase of the proximal renal tubule, which is inhibited by cilastatin. Imipenem has a $T_{1/2}$ of about 1 h, and 70% is recovered in the urine. Dosage should be modified for patients with renal insufficiency. Meropenem does not require coadministration with cilastatin because it is not sensitive to renal dipeptidase.

6.11.8.4 Side Effects
- nausea and vomiting are the most common;
- seizures have been noted, especially with imipenem when high doses are given to patients with central nervous system lesions and to those with renal insufficiency.

6.11.9 Monobactams (Aztreonam)

6.11.9.1 Mechanism of Action
These antibiotics interact with PBP to form long, filamentous bacterial structures.

6.11.9.2 Spectrum of Activity
Gram-positive bacteria and anaerobic organisms are naturally resistant. On the other hand, activity against Enterobacteriaceae, *P. aeruginosa*, *H. influenzae*, and gonococci is good. Monobactams are resistant to many β-lactamases.

6.11.9.3 Pharmacological Properties
The usual adult dose is 2 g every 6–8 h. The $T_{1/2}$ is 1.7 h, and most of the drug is recovered unaltered in the urine.

6.11.10 β-Lactams Combined with β-Lactamase Inhibitors

β-lactamase inhibitors bind to β-lactamases and inactivate them. They are mostly active against plasmid-encoded β-lactamases, including the extended-spectrum ESBL, but are inactive against type I chromosomal β-lactamases of AGNB. β-lactamase inhibitors include clavulanic acid, sulbactam, and tazobactam [12]. Clavulanic acid has been combined with amoxicillin and ticarcillin with extension of the antimicrobial activity to β-lactamase-producing strains of staphylococci, *H. influenzae*, gonococci, and *E. coli*. Sulbactam is usually combined with ampicillin; tazobactam has been combined with piperacillin. Although this combination extends its spectrum of activity, it does not enhance that against *P. aeruginosa*, as resistance is due to either chromosomal β-lactamases or decreased permeability of piperacillin into the periplasmic space due to either porin protein OprD loss or multidrug efflux system upregulation.

6.11.11 Aminoglycosides (Gentamicin, Tobramycin, Amikacin)

These drugs are used primarily to treat infections caused by AGNB [31].

6.11.11.1 Mechanism of Action
Aminoglycosides interact with the 30S ribosomal subunit, with inhibition of protein synthesis. They have a concentration-dependent effect and have a PAE.

6.11.11.2 Spectrum of Activity
The antibacterial activity of aminoglycosides includes AGNB. Kanamycin, as with streptomycin, has a more limited spectrum compared with other aminoglycosides and should not be used against *Serratia* spp. or *P. aeruginosa*. They have little activity against anaerobic microorganisms, and their action against most Gram-positive bacteria is limited. *S. pneumoniae* and *S. pyogenes* are resistant. Both gentamicin and tobramycin are active against *S. aureus* and *S. epidermidis*. However, staphylococci become rapidly gentamicin resistant during exposure to the drug.

6.11.11.3 Clinical Use

Gentamicin, tobramycin, amikacin, and netilmicin can be used for treating AGNB infections, including urinary tract infections, bacteremia, infected burns, osteomyelitis, pneumonia, peritonitis, and otitis caused by *P. aeruginosa*, *Enterobacter*, *Klebsiella*, *Serratia*, and other species resistant to less toxic antibiotics. Penicillins and aminoglycosides must never be mixed in the same flask because penicillin inactivates the aminoglycoside. An aminoglycoside in combination with a β-lactam is indicated for empirical therapy of pneumonia acquired in the ICU. Combination therapy is also recommended for treating pneumonia caused by *P. aeruginosa*. Aminoglycosides are ineffective for treating *S. pneumoniae*. They are very useful, however, in cases of enterococcal endocarditis. In granulocytopenic patients infected by *P. aeruginosa*, antipseudomonal penicillin administration in combination with aminoglycosides is recommended [31].

6.11.11.4 Mechanism of Resistance
- mutations affecting proteins in the bacterial ribosome;
- impaired transport of the drug into the bacteria;
- acquisition of plasmids coding for aminoglycoside-metabolizing enzymes, such as phosphoryl, adenyl, or acetyl transferases.

6.11.11.5 Pharmacologic Properties

There is negligible binding (<5%) of aminoglycosides to plasma albumin. They have poor penetration in most cells, in the central nervous system, and into respiratory secretions. Aminoglycosides are excreted almost entirely by glomerular filtration. Their $T_{1/2}$ in plasma are similar and vary between 2 and 3 h in patients with normal renal function. A linear relationship exists between plasma creatinine concentration and $T_{1/2}$ of aminoglycosides. Gentamicin and tobramycin are used at the adult dosage of 3–5 mg/kg per day. Amikacin is used at 15 mg/kg. Its spectrum of antimicrobial activity is the broadest of the group, and it is resistant to aminoglycoside-inactivating enzymes. Routine aminoglycoside plasma concentration monitoring is strongly recommended to confirm that drug concentrations are in the therapeutic range [31].

6.11.11.6 Side Effects

Side effects are vestibular, cochlear, and renal toxicity, and rarely, neuromuscular blockade. Ototoxicity and nephrotoxicity are more frequent in patients with elevated drug concentrations in plasma. Ototoxicity is largely irreversible, resulting from progressive destruction of vestibular or cochlear sensory cells. Nephrotoxicity—usually reversible—is the result of marked accumulation of aminoglycosides in the proximal tubular cells. Once-daily administration reduces nephrotoxicity because it can saturate the tubular cells, with no reduction in efficacy [31].

6.11.12 Fluoroquinolones

6.11.12.1 Mechanism of Action
Fluoroquinolones inhibit two enzymes involved in bacterial DNA synthesis: DNA gyrase and topoisomerase IV [32, 33].

6.11.12.2 Generational Classification
First-generation drugs comprises nonfluorinated compounds, including nalidixic acid, pipemidic acid, and cinoxacin; second-generation compounds include norfloxacin, enoxacin, pefloxacin, ofloxacin, lomefloxacin, and ciprofloxacin; third-generation compounds include levofloxacin, gatifloxacin, and moxifloxacin [32].

6.11.12.3 Spectrum of Activity
Second-generation quinolones are rapidly bactericidal on *E. coli* and various species of *Salmonella*, *Shigella*, *Enterobacter*, *Campylobacter*, and *Neisseria*. Ciprofloxacin and levofloxacin have good activity against non-multi-drug-resistant strains of *P. aeruginosa*. Third-generation quinolones are highly active against pneumococci and enterococci, though they have low activity against *P. aeruginosa* strains. Several intracellular bacteria are inhibited by fluoroquinolones (*Chlamydia*, *Mycoplasma*, *Legionella*, *Brucella*, and *Mycobacterium*). Most anaerobic microorganisms are resistant to quinolones but sensitive to third-generation compounds [32].

6.11.12.4 Clinical Use
Norfloxacin is useful for urinary tract infections only. The major limitation of second-generation quinolones for treating community-acquired pneumonia and bronchitis is their poor activity against *S. pneumoniae*. For these infections, third-generation derivatives are highly effective. However, fluoroquinolones have in vitro activity against other common respiratory pathogens, including *H. influenzae*, *M. catarrhalis*, *S. aureus*, *M. pneumoniae*, *C. pneumoniae*, and *L. pneumophila*. Mild to moderate respiratory exacerbations due to *P. aeruginosa* in patients with cystic fibrosis have responded to orally administered fluoroquinolone therapy. Third-generation quinolones are indicated for infections caused by *L. pneumophila*, *C. pneumoniae*, and *M. pneumoniae*. MRSA is generally resistant to fluoroquinolones [33].

6.11.12.5 Mechanism of Resistance
- alterations in the drug target enzymes (DNA gyrase or topoisomerase mutations);
- bacterial expression of membrane-associated efflux pumps [32].

6.11.12.6 Pharmacologic Properties
Quinolones are widely distributed in body tissues. Serum $T_{1/2}$ ranges from 3 to 5 h for norfloxacin and ciprofloxacin, 7–8 h for gatifloxacin and levofloxacin,

and 10–12 h for pefloxacin and moxifloxacin. Concentrations of quinolones in urine, kidney, lung and prostate tissue; stool, bile, macrophages, and neutrophils are higher than serum levels. Concentrations in CSF are lower than in serum. Elimination routes differ: renal clearance predominates for ofloxacin, lomefloxacin, levofloxacin, and gatifloxacin; pefloxacin and nalidixic acid are predominantly eliminated nonrenally. Dose adjustments in patients with renal insufficiency are generally required, except for pefloxacin and moxifloxacin. None of the agents is efficiently removed by peritoneal or hemodialysis.

6.11.12.7 Side Effects
- nausea, abdominal discomfort;
- headache, dizziness;
- rarely: hallucinations, delirium, and seizures, especially if associated with non-steroidal anti-inflammatory drugs;
- rashes, including photosensitivity;
- arthralgias and joint swelling have developed in children.

6.11.13 Macrolides

6.11.13.1 Generational Classification
First-generation macrolide is erythromycin; second generation is represented by spiramycin; third generation is clarithromycin and azithromycin, fourth generation corresponds to ketolides [34, 35].

6.11.13.2 Mechanism of Action
Macrolides interact with the peptidyl transferase center in the 50S ribosomal subunit.

6.11.13.3 Spectrum of Activity
Erythromycin is most effective against aerobic Gram-positive cocci and bacilli. Some staphylococci are sensitive to erythromycin, but resistant strains are frequently encountered in hospitals. Many other Gram-positive bacilli, including *C. perfringens* and *Corynebacterium diphtheriae,* are sensitive. Erythromycin is not active against most AGNB. However, it retains activity against other Gram-negative organisms, including *N. meningitidis* and *N. gonorrhoeae*, and is effective against *M. pneumoniae, L. pneumophila,* and *C. trachomatis.* Clarithromycin is more potent than erythromycin against streptococci and staphylococci. Azithromycin generally is less active than erythromycin against Gram-positive organisms and is more active than either erythromycin or clarithromycin against *H. influenzae.* It is highly active against *M. catarrhalis, Chlamydia* spp., *M. pneumoniae, L. pneumophila, B. burgdorferi, Fusobacterium* spp., and *N. gonorrhoeae* [24]. Telithromycin is the first ketolide antibiotic; it is used for treating community-acquired respiratory tract infections and has high activity against many common

and atypical/intracellular respiratory pathogens, including macrolide-lincosamide-streptogramin (MLSB)-resistant strains. It has more in vitro activity against Gram-positive aerobes than the other macrolides. It is inactive against Enterobacteriaceae, non-fermentative Gram-negative bacilli, and *A. baumannii* [32]. Macrolides are not active against MRSA [35].

6.11.13.4 Mechanism of Resistance
- modifies the 50S ribosomal subunit;
- produces inactivating enzymes;
- decreases bacterial influence of the drug;
- increases bacterial efflux of the drug.

6.11.13.5 Pharmacologic Properties
Erythromycin protein binding is approximately 70–80%. It is concentrated in the liver and excreted in the bile, with a plasma elimination $T_{1/2}$ of 1.6 h. Clarithromycin distributes widely throughout the body and achieves high intracellular concentrations; its protein binding ranges from 40 to 70%. It is metabolized in the liver and is eliminated by renal and nonrenal mechanisms, with $T_{1/2}$ of 3–7 h. Clarithromycin is usually given at an adult dosage of 250 or 500 mg twice daily. Azithromycin reaches high concentrations within cells, including phagocytes. Its protein binding is low (51%), and the antibiotic undergoes some hepatic metabolism to inactive metabolites, even if biliary excretion is the major elimination route, with $T_{1/2}$ of 68 h that allows a once-daily regimen of 500 mg. Telithromycin is metabolized hepatically and is eliminated primarily through the feces. It shows good penetration into respiratory tissues, with concentration above mean MIC 90 s for common respiratory pathogens in bronchial mucosa and epithelial lining fluid. Macrolides have been reported to cause clinically significant drug interactions, potentiating the effects of astemizole, carbamazepine, corticosteroids, cyclosporine, digoxin, ergot alkaloids, terfenadine, theophylline, triazolam, valproate, and warfarin. Telithromycin should be used cautiously in combination with simvastatin, midazolam, theophylline, and digoxin [34, 35].

6.11.13.6 Side Effects
- allergic skin eruptions;
- cholestatic hepatitis;
- epigastric distress with abdominal cramps, nausea, vomiting, and diarrhea;
- cardiac arrhythmias, including QT prolongation with ventricular tachycardia.

6.11.14 Glycopeptides (Vancomycin and Teicoplanin)

6.11.14.1 Mechanism of Action
Glycopeptides bind to the D-alanyl-D-alanine terminus of cell-wall precursor units, inhibiting transglycosylase and transpeptidase enzymes that are necessary for bacterial-wall synthesis. They are rapidly bactericidal for dividing bacteria [36, 37].

6.11.14.2 Spectrum of Activity

Gram-positive bacteria such as *S. aureus* and *S. epidermidis*, including methicillin-resistant strains, are usually sensitive. Strains with MIC >1 mg/L, which include glycopeptide intermediate *S. aureus* (GISA) are now spreading, requiring other antimicrobial agents. Synergism between vancomycin and gentamicin or tobramycin has been demonstrated in vitro against *S. aureus*, including methicillin-resistant strains. *S. pyogenes*, *S. pneumoniae*, and viridans streptococci are highly susceptible, as are most strains of *Enterococcus* spp. Glycopeptides are not generally bactericidal for *Enterococcus* spp., and the addition of a synergistic aminoglycoside might be necessary to produce a bactericidal effect. *Corynebacterium*, *Actinomyces*, and *Clostridium* spp. are sensitive [38, 39].

6.11.14.3 Mechanism of Resistance

These drugs express an enzyme that modifies the cell-wall precursor so that it no longer binds vancomycin (*Enterococci*). Three clinically important types of resistance have been described for vancomycin. The Van-A-inducible phenotype confers resistance to both teicoplanin and vancomycin. The Van-B phenotype tends to confer a lower level of resistance to vancomycin but not to teicoplanin. The Van-C constitutive phenotype confers resistance to vancomycin only [40].

6.11.14.4 Pharmacological Properties

Vancomycin has a serum elimination $T_{1/2}$ of about 6 h, and approximately 55% is bound to plasma protein. It appears in various body fluids, including CSF when the meninges are inflamed, bile, and pleural, pericardial, synovial, and ascitic fluids. It scarcely penetrates the lungs. More than 90% of an injected dose is excreted by glomerular filtration. The dose for adults is 30 mg/kg per day. The best way to divide this dose (every 6 or 12 h) and the best administration modality (intermittent administration vs continuous infusion) have not been established. Dosage adjustments must be made in cases of renal failure. Teicoplanin is a mixture of six closely related compounds. It is highly bound by plasma proteins (90–95%) and has an extremely long serum elimination $T_{1/2}$ (up to 100 h). Dosage in adults is 6–30 mg/kg per day. As with vancomycin, teicoplanin doses must be adjusted in patients with renal insufficiency [39].

6.11.14.5 Side Effects

- hypersensitivity reactions produced by vancomycin (macular skin rashes, chills, fever);
- nephrotoxicity and ototoxicity (less frequent with teicoplanin);
- rapid intravenous infusion may cause erythematous or urticarial reactions, flushing (red-neck or red-man syndrome), tachycardia, and hypotension [39].

6.11.15 Polymyxins (Polymyxin E or Colistin and Polymyxin B)

6.11.15.1 Mechanism of Action
Polymyxins interact with phospholipids and disrupt their structure [41, 42].

6.11.15.2 Mechanism of Resistance
There is reduced influx of the drug across the bacterial wall into the cell membrane [39].

6.11.15.3 Spectrum of Activity
AGNB, including *Enterobacter*, *E. coli*, *Klebsiella*, *Citrobacter*, *A. baumannii*, and *P. aeruginosa*. *Proteus*, *Morganella*, *Serratia* are intrinsically resistant.

6.11.15.4 Clinical Use
Used to treat multi-drug-resistant nosocomial infections from AGNB. Aerosol administration of the parenteral preparation has also been used as an adjuvant in patients with severe *Pseudomonas* and *A. pneumonia* [43].

6.11.15.5 Side Effects
- nephrotoxicity.

6.11.16 Oxazolidinones

Linezolid is the first member (and at present the only available molecule) of a new class of antibiotics known as oxazolidinones [44, 45].

6.11.16.1 Mechanism of Action
Oxazolidinones prevent formation of the fmet-total RNA:messenger RNA:30S subunit ternary complex with ribosomal protein synthesis inhibition.

6.11.16.2 Spectrum of Activity
Linezolid is active against nosocomial infections involving Gram-positive organisms, including MRSA, multi-drug-resistant strains of *S. pneumoniae*, and vancomycin-resistant *E. faecium* (VRE) [44].

6.11.16.3 Mechanism of Resistance
Linezolid-resistant VRE has been isolated, especially in immunosuppressed patients [44].

6.11.16.4 Side Effects
- thrombocytopenia and myelosuppression;
- elevated liver and pancreatic enzymes;
- pseudomembranous colitis;

- diarrhea, nausea, and vomiting;
- headache and dizziness;
- monoamine oxidase inhibition.

6.11.16.5 Pharmacologic Properties

Linezolid is widely distributed in the respiratory tract, with plasma protein binding of 30%. About one-third of the dose is eliminated in the urine, with elimination $T_{1/2}$ of about 6.5 h. Dosage for most indications is 600 mg (iv or po) every 12 h. There appears to be no need for renal dose adjustment. Linezolid has a monoamine oxidase (MAO) inhibitor action. Therefore, precautions should be followed to avoid potentially serious food–drug or drug–drug interactions with other MAO inhibitors [44].

6.11.17 Streptogramins (Streptogramin A-Dalfopristin and Streptogramin B-Quinupristin)

These drugs are available in an injectable combination in a ratio of 70:30 [46, 47].

6.11.17.1 Mechanism of Action

Binding to 23S RNA of the 50S ribosomal subunit, where they cause dissociation of peptidyl-tRNA from the ribosome [46].

6.11.17.2 Spectrum of Activity

These antibiotics are active against Gram-positive bacteria, including multi-drug-resistant strains of staphylococci, pneumococci, and enterococci. They are inactive against *E. faecalis* but effective against VRE. They are as active as vancomycin against MRSA [45].

6.11.17.3 Mechanism of Resistance

- enzymatic modification through virginiamycin acetyltransferases;
- efflux pump;
- alteration of the 50S ribosomal subunit.

6.11.17.4 Side Effects

- reversible arthralgias, myalgias;
- peripheral venous irritation.

6.11.17.5 Pharmacologic Properties

These medications are metabolized by liver enzymes, including CYP450. The postantibiotic effect and their PK characteristics allow dosing at 8–12-h intervals. A potential for drug interactions exists because they inhibit the cytochrome P450-3A4 enzyme system.

6.11.18 Lipopeptides (Daptomycin)

6.11.18.1 Mechanism of Action
Action is via plasma membrane alteration without penetrating into the cytoplasm. Inhibiting the production of protein has also been reported [48].

6.11.18.2 Spectrum of Activity
S. aureus, S. pyogenes, S. agalactiae, group C and G β-hemolytic streptococci, E. faecalis, MRSA and VRE [48] are responsive to lipopeptides

6.11.18.3 Pharmacologic Properties
Daptomycin is eliminated primarily by glomerular filtration, with a $T_{1/2}$ of 0.9–1.4 h. The level of protein binding is 90%. Daptomycin demonstrates concentration-dependent killing action and produces in vivo PAEs of 4.8–10.8 h. Under conditions of high inoculum, daptomycin is highly effective. The intravenous adult dose is 4–6 mg/kg once a day.

6.11.18.4 Side Effects
- gastrointestinal disorders;
- injection-site reactions;
- fever;
- dizziness;
- rash;
- people receiving daptomycin should be monitored for muscle pain or weakness, and blood tests measuring creatine phosphokinase levels should be monitored.

6.11.19 Glycylcycline (Tigecycline)

6.11.19.1 Mechanism of Action
Tigecycline inhibits protein translation by binding to the 30S ribosomal subunit and blocking entry of amino-acyl tRNA molecules into the A site of the ribosome [49, 50].

6.11.19.2 Spectrum of Activity
Gram-positive pathogens, including methicillin-resistant MRSA and S. epidermidis (MRSE), VRE, Gram-negative pathogens, and anaerobic pathogens. Pseudomonas is usually resistant [51].

6.11.19.3 Mechanism of Resistance
Tigecycline resistance in some bacteria (e.g., Acinetobacter strains) is associated with multi-drug-resistant efflux pumps.

6.11.19.4 Clinical Use
This drug is used to treat complicated skin and skin-structure infections, complicated intra-abdominal infections, and bacterial pneumonia.

6.11.19.5 Pharmacologic Properties
Tigecycline is not extensively metabolized, and is eliminated by biliary/fecal excretion (60%) and in urine (33%). Its $T_{1/2}$ is 27 h and protein binding of 80%. Both AUC and time > MIC correlates with efficacy, but the AUC/MIC ratio is likely the primary PK/PD determinant of efficacy because tigecycline exhibits time-dependent bacterial killing properties in combination with a moderate-to-prolonged postantibiotic effect [51].

6.11.19.6 Side Effects
- nausea, vomiting, diarrhea, abdominal pain, and headache are the most common (>5%);
- anaphylactic reactions;
- hepatic dysfunction and failure (transaminases should be monitored);
- discoloration of the teeth if used during tooth development;
- photosensitivity;
- antianabolic action, with increased blood urea nitrogen, acidosis, and hyperphosphatemia.

References

1. Gunderson BW, Ross GH, Ibrahim KH, Rotschafer JC (2001) What do we really know about antibiotic pharmacodynamics? Pharmacotherapy 21:302s–318s
2. Mehrota R, De Gaudio R, Palazzo M (2004) Antibiotic pharmacokinetic and pharmacodynamic considerations in critical illness. Int Care Med 30:2145–2156
3. Kollef MH (2001) Optimizing antibiotic therapy in the intensive care unit setting. Crit Care 5:189–195
4. Ambrose PG, Bhavnani SM, Rubino CM et al (2007) Pharmacokinetics-pharmacodynamics of antimicrobial therapy: it's not just for mice anymore. Clin Infect Dis 44:79–86
5. Pea F, Viale P (2009) Bench-to-bedside review: appropriate antibiotic therapy in severe sepsis and septic shock–does the dose matter? Crit Care 13:214
6. Kumar A (2009) Optimizing antimicrobial therapy in sepsis and septic shock. Crit Care Clin 25:733–751
7. Roberts JA, Lipman J (2009) Pharmacokinetic issues for antibiotics in the critically ill patient. Crit Care Med 37:840–851
8. Figueiredo Costa S (2008) Impact of antimicrobial resistance on the treatment and outcome of patients with sepsis. Shock 30:23–29
9. Lipman J, Boots R (2009) A new paradigm for treating infections: "go hard and go home". Crit Care Resusc 11:276–281
10. Lodise TP Jr, Lomaestro B, Drusano GL (2007) Piperacillin-tazobactam for Pseudomonas aeruginosa infection: clinical implications of an extended-infusion dosing strategy. Clin Infect Dis 44(3):357–363
11. Barbour A, Scaglione F, Derendorf H (2010) Class-dependent relevance of tissue distribution in the interpretation of anti-infective pharmacokinetic/pharmacodynamic indices. Int J Antimicrob Agents 35:431–438

12. Drawz SM, Bonomo RA (2010) Three decades of beta-lactamase inhibitors. Clin Microbiol Rev 23:160–201
13. Novelli A, Mini E, Mazzei T (2004) Pharmacological interactions between antibiotics and other drugs in the treatment of lower respiratory tract infections. Eur Respir Mon 28:1–26
14. Nagaoka I, Hirota S, Niyonsaba F et al (2001) Cathelicidin family of antibacterial peptides CAP18 and CAP11 inhibit the expression of TNF-alpha by blocking the binding of LPS to CD14(+) cells. J Immunol 167:3329–3338
15. Zhang L, Dhillon P, Yan H et al (2000) Interactions of bacterial cationic peptide antibiotics with outer and cytoplasmic membranes of *Pseudomonas aeruginosa*. Antimicrob Agents Chemother 44:3317–3321
16. Tsuzuki H, Tani T, Ueyama H, Kodama M (2001) Lipopolysaccharide: neutralization by polymyxin B shuts down the signaling pathway of nuclear factor kappa B in peripheral blood mononuclear cells, even during activation. J Surg Res 100:127–134
17. Suárez C, Gudiol F (2009) Beta-lactam antibiotics. Enferm Infecc Microbiol Clin 27(2):116–129 Article in Spanish
18. Augusto LA, Decottignies P, Synguelakis M et al (2003) Histones: a novel class of lipopolysaccharide-binding molecules. Biochemistry 42:3929–3938
19. Sullivan A, Edlund C, Nord CE (2001) Effect of antimicrobial agents on the ecological balance of human microflora. Lancet Infect Dis 1:101–114
20. Klein G (2003) Taxonomy, ecology and antibiotic resistance of enterococci from food and the gastro-intestinal tract. Int J Food Microbiol 88:123–131
21. Tannock GW (2001) Molecular assessment of intestinal microflora. Am J Clin Nutr 73(Suppl 2):410S–414S
22. Dunne C (2001) Adaptation of bacteria to the intestinal niche: probiotics and gut disorder. Inflamm Bowel Dis 7:136–145
23. Brook I (2000) The effects of amoxicillin therapy on skin flora in infants. Pediatr Dermatol 17:360–363
24. Antonelli M, Mercurio G, Di Nunno S, Recchioni G, Deangelis G (2001) De-escalation antimicrobial chemotherapy in critically ill patients: pros and cons. J Chemother 1:218–223
25. Doğan O, Gülmez D, Hasçelik G (2010) Effect of new breakpoints proposed by Clinical and Laboratory Standards Institute in 2008 for evaluating penicillin resistance of *Streptococcus pneumoniae* in a Turkish University Hospital. Microb Drug Resist 16:39–41
26. Feldman C (2004) Clinical relevance of antimicrobial resistance in the management of pneumococcal community-acquired pneumonia. J Lab Clin Med 143:269–283
27. Goosen H (2003) Susceptibility of multi-drug-resistant *Pseudomonas aeruginosa* in intensive care units: results from the European MYSTIC study group. Clin Microbiol Infect 9:980–983
28. Kahlmeter G (2008) Breakpoints for intravenously used cephalosporins in Enterobacteriaceae—EUCAST and CLSI breakpoints. Clin Microbiol Infect 14:169–174
29. Bazan JA, Martin SI, Kaye KM (2009) Newer beta-lactam antibiotics: doripenem, ceftobiprole, ceftaroline, and cefepime. Infect Dis Clin North Am 23:983–996
30. Baughman RP (2009) The use of carbapenems in the treatment of serious infections. J Intensive Care Med 24:230–241
31. Smith CA, Baker EN (2002) Aminoglycoside antibiotic resistance by enzymatic deactivation. Curr Drug Targets Infect Disord 2:143–160
32. Viale P, Pea F (2003) What is the role of fluoroquinolones in intensive care? J Chemother 15(Suppl 3):5–10
33. Blondeau JM (2004) Fluoroquinolones: mechanism of action, classification, and development of resistance. Surv Ophthalmol 49(Suppl 2):S73–S78
34. Labro MT (2004) Macrolide antibiotics: current and future uses. Expert Opin Pharmacother 5:541–550
35. Ackermann G, Rodloff AC (2003) Drugs of the 21st century: telithromycin (HMR 3647)—the first ketolide. J Antimicrob Chemother 51:497–511
36. Malabarba A, Ciabatti R (2001) Glycopeptide derivatives. Curr Med Chem 8:1759–1773

37. Esposito S, Noviello S (2003) What is the role of glycopeptides in intensive care? J Chemother 15(Suppl 3):11–16
38. Parenti F, Schito GC, Courvalin P (2000) Teicoplanin chemistry and microbiology. J Chemother 12(Suppl 5):5–14
39. Harding I, Sorgel F (2000) Comparative pharmacokinetics of teicoplanin and vancomycin. J Chemother 12(Suppl 5):15–20
40. Lundstrom TS, Sobel JD (2000) Antibiotics for Gram-positive bacterial infections. Vancomycin, teicoplanin, quinupristin/dalfopristin, and linezolid. Infect Dis Clin North Am 14:463–474
41. Rocha JL, Kondo W, Baptista MI et al (2002) Uncommon vancomycin-induced side effects. Braz J Infect Dis 6:196–200
42. Beringer P (2001) The clinical use of colistin in patients with cystic fibrosis. Curr Opin Pulm Med 7:434–440
43. Tsubery H, Ofek I, Cohen S et al (2002) Modulation of the hydrophobic domain of polymyxin B nonapeptide: effect on outer-membrane permeabilization and lipopolysaccharide neutralization. Mol Pharmacol 62:1036–1042
44. Diekema DJ, Jones RN (2001) Oxazolidinone antibiotics. Lancet 358:1975–1982
45. Paradisi F, Corti G, Messeri D (2001) Antistaphylococcal (MSSA, MRSA, MSSE, MRSE) antibiotics. Med Clin North Am 85:1–17
46. De Gaudio AR, Di Filippo A (2003) What is the role of streptogramins in intensive care? J Chemother 15(Suppl 3):17–21
47. Hershberger E, Donabedian S, Konstantinou K, Zervos MJ (2004) Quinupristin-dalfopristin resistance in Gram-positive bacteria: mechanism of resistance and epidemiology. Clin Infect Dis 38:92–98
48. Devasahayam G, Scheld WM, Hoffman PS (2010) Newer antibacterial drugs for a new century. Expert Opin Investig Drugs 19:215–234
49. Zuckerman JM, Qamar F, Bono BR (2009) Macrolides, ketolides, and glycylcyclines: azithromycin, clarithromycin, telithromycin, tigecycline. Infect Dis Clin North Am 23:997–1026
50. Barton E, MacGowan A (2009) Future treatment options for Gram-positive infections–looking ahead. Clin Microbiol Infect 15:17–25
51. Bouza E (2009) New therapeutic choices for infections caused by methicillin-resistant *Staphylococcus aureus*. Clin Microbiol Infect 15:44–52

Systemic Antifungals

C. J. Collins and Th. R. Rogers

7.1 Introduction

Since approximately 2005, there have been important developments in antifungal therapy relevant to managing invasive fungal infections (IFIs) in intensive care unit (ICU) patients. We now have a new triazole—posaconazole—and two new echinocandins—anidulafungin and micafungin—to add to the previous repertoire of systemic antifungals for treating IFIs. There has been much debate on how best to use systemic antifungals in patients at high risk of candidaemia/invasive candidiasis, with studies and reviews addressing the issues of antifungal prophylaxis, empirical and pre-emptive therapy, and treating documented infection. Unfortunately, the one area that has not progressed significantly is diagnosis. There are developments with nonculture diagnostic methods, such as detecting circulating beta-D-glucan, and polymerase chain reaction (PCR) for detecting candidiasis and some other mycoses, but none has yet become firmly incorporated into established care pathways. Surveillance studies of candidaemia show that *Candida albicans* continues to be the most common cause, followed by *C. glabrata* and *C. parapsilosis*. A worrying development is resistance to echinocandins, especially in *C. glabrata,* but the impact of this in clinical practice is not clear. Invasive aspergillosis (IA) has been reported in ICU patients outside of the traditional immunocompromised risk groups. The incidence appears quite variable between units, but it is not so common that it needs to be factored in when considering empirical therapy unless the ICU involved has experienced an increase in cases or the patient is in a recognised risk group. The older agents have been addressed in previous editions of this book [1]; we therefore concentrate on the newer antifungals in this edition.

C. J. Collins (✉)
Clinical Microbiology, Trinity College Dublin, Dublin,
Leinster, Republic of Ireland
e-mail: collinc6@tcd.ie

7.2 Antifungal Drugs

7.2.1 Posaconazole

Posaconazole (Noxafil) is a structural analogue of itraconazole. It is licensed in Europe for first-line treatment of oropharyngeal candidiasis in patients who have severe disease or are immunocompromised. Unlike under the US Food and Drug Administration (FDA) license, it may be used for those with refractory IFIs or with IFIs and who are intolerant of first-line antifungals. It is also approved for IFI prophylaxis in severely immunocompromised patients, e.g., haematopoietic stem-cell transplantation (HSCT) recipients with graft versus host disease (GVHD) who are at high risk for IFIs and in patients with acute myelogenous leukaemia (AML) or myelodysplastic syndrome (MDS) who are at high risk for IFIs.

7.2.1.1 Spectrum of Activity

Posaconazole is active against all organisms covered by the other triazoles, including fluconazole-resistant *Candida* spp., but it is also active against members of the Zygomycetes [2]. It is fungistatic against many of the common *Candida* spp., including *C. albicans*, but is generally fungicidal against *Aspergillus* spp. [2].

7.2.1.2 Pharmacological Properties

Posaconazole is available only as an oral suspension. The bioavailability is variable but is considerably increased when taken with fatty meals. The dosing varies according to indication: 200 mg three times daily for prophylaxis against IFIs; 100 mg twice daily for treating oropharyngeal candidiasis; 400 mg twice daily for treating oropharyngeal candidiasis refractory to other azoles. There are no dose adjustments required for renal or liver impairment. It is highly protein bound (>/=99%). Although it is not metabolised by CYP enzymes, it has been found to significantly decrease the activity of the CYP3A4 isoenzyme, resulting in interactions with drugs that are metabolised via this pathway. Also, coadministration with phenytoin, rifabutin (increased clearance of both) or cimetidine (may decrease absorption) is not recommended unless the benefits outweigh the risks. It is eliminated primarily unchanged and has no microbiologically active metabolites. Posaconazole is generally well tolerated, with gastrointestinal symptoms such as nausea, abdominal pain and diarrhoea being the most common adverse effects.

7.2.1.3 Clinical Experience

Posaconazole is mainly used as a prophylactic agent against IFI in severely immunocompromised patients. Based on two large antifungal prophylaxis studies [3, 4] it has received an A-I grade recommendation from the Infectious Diseases Society of America (IDSA) for prophylaxis in HSCT recipients with GVHD who are at high risk for IA and in patients with AML or MDS who are at high risk for IA [5]. In a study of salvage therapy for IA in which controls were historical and had mostly received amphotericin B, the response rates overall were superior for posaconazole, irrespective of the *Aspergillus* spp. [6]. In two studies and a case report including a review of the literature, posaconazole as salvage therapy for zygomycosis was evaluated with encouraging results [7–9]. However, there are no data yet supporting its use as first-line therapy for IA, and this may have to await the development of an intravenously administered formulation. Posaconazole has also been investigated as treatment for other mould infections in immunocompromised patients, with similarly encouraging results [2, 10].

So far, clinical experience of using posaconazole in ICU patients appears to be restricted to small case report series [11]. Due to the lack of an intravenously administered formulation, therapeutic drug monitoring may be required in patients with invasive fungal disease. Studies to date are limited on its value, but one small series in critical care patients has shown that serum concentrations >0.5 mg/l are more likely to achieve therapeutic success [12].

7.2.2 Echinocandins and Pneumocandins

Caspofungin, anidulafungin and micafungin are now approved for treating invasive *Candida* infections. In the 2009 IDSA guidelines for managing candidiasis, echinocandins along with fluconazole received a grade A-I recommendation for treating candidaemia in non-neutropenic patients, with the expert panel favouring echinocandins in those with moderate to severe illness or with recent azole exposure [13]. They also received a grade A-II recommendation for the initial treatment of candidaemia in neutropenic patients and a grade B-III recommendation for the treatment of *C. glabrata*. Although head-to-head studies among the three approved echinocandins are limited [14], overall, there have been no significant differences found in their clinical efficacy [15], although there are pharmacokinetic and pharmacodynamic differences [16].

7.2.3 Caspofungin

Caspofungin (Cancidas) was reviewed in the last edition of this series [1]. It was the first echinocandin to be approved for clinical use in Europe and is the first and only member of this group to be licensed by the European Medicines Agency (EMEA) and the FDA for treating patients with invasive *Aspergillus* infections refractory to other therapy. It has also been licensed as empirical therapy for presumed fungal infections in febrile, neutropenic patients and for treating invasive candidiasis. It is also the only echinocandin with both an FDA and EMEA license for therapeutic use in the paediatric population.

Standard dosing is a 70-mg loading dose followed by 50 mg daily. Dosing in the paediatric population is based on the patient's body surface area (BSA). High-dose therapy with caspofungin was recently evaluated primarily for safety.

Betts et al. [17] undertook a double-blind comparison of caspofungin 150 mg daily with standard dosing in patients diagnosed with invasive candidiasis at a sterile site. This higher dose was well tolerated. There were insufficient patients in the study to draw any conclusion on the possibility of superior efficacy of the higher dose regimen. Liver function tests should be monitored during caspofungin treatment, especially when it is prescribed concomitantly with cyclosporine.

7.2.4 Micafungin

Micafungin (Mycamine) was synthesised by chemical modification of an environmental mould *Coleophoma empedri*. It is approved by both the EMEA and FDA for treating invasive and oesophageal candidiasis. It is also approved by both for the prophylaxis of *Candida* infections in patients undergoing HSCT. It has not yet been approved for use in *Aspergillus* infections. Only the EMEA has licensed its use in the paediatric population.

7.2.4.1 Spectrum of Activity
Micafungin appears to be similar to caspofungin in terms of spectrum of activity.

7.2.4.2 Pharmacological Properties
Micafungin, like the other members of this class, is available only as an intravenously administered formulation. Dosing varies according to indication: 100 mg once daily for treating invasive *Candida* infections; 150 mg once daily for treating oesophageal candidiasis; 50 mg once daily for prophylaxis against *Candida* infections. A loading dose is not required, and no dosage adjustments dependent on renal or liver indices are required, including for patients on dialysis. However, its use in severe hepatic impairment is not recommended, as no data are available. Micafungin is generally well tolerated, with the most common side effects being fever, headache, gastrointestinal symptoms and electrolyte and haematological disturbances. The liver function tests should be monitored during treatment. It is highly protein bound. Monitoring for toxicity due to increased serum concentrations of sirolimus, nifedipine and itraconazole should be performed when these are co-prescribed with micafungin. Preclinical data in rats raised some concerns regarding micafungin and the development of hepatic neoplasms, although the relevance of this to human use is not clear. This has prompted the EMEA to refer to this potential risk in its product information sheet and advises that micafungin should only be used if other antifungals are not appropriate.

7.2.4.3 Clinical Experience
In two separate double-blind, randomised non-inferiority studies, activity of micafungin (100 mg/day) versus liposomal amphotericin B (3 mg/kg/day) and micafungin (100 or 150 mg/day) versus caspofungin (70 mg on day 1 followed by 50 mg/day) was compared for treating candidaemia and invasive candidiasis in

predominantly non-neutropenic patients [18, 19]. Micafungin, at the studied doses, was found to be as effective as the two other agents but was associated with fewer adverse events when compared with liposomal amphotericin B. In a post-hoc analysis of data from the study comparing micafungin with liposomal amphotericin B, the therapeutic efficacy of micafungin was lower in ICU patients when compared with non-ICU patients. However, multivariate regression analysis suggested that this was related only to Acute Physiology and Chronic Health Evaluation II (APACHE II) score, and mortality at either days 8 or 30 was lower in patients with low APACHE II scores [20].

Micafungin has been compared in a randomised, double-blind trial with liposomal amphotericin B for treating candidaemia and other forms of invasive candidiasis in a young paediatric population. Rates of treatment success were similar with a lower overall rate of adverse events associated with micafungin [21]. Clinical trials have shown that, at the appropriate dosage (i.e., 100 and 150 mg/day), micafungin efficacy is comparable with that of fluconazole (200 mg/day) for treating endoscopically and culture-proven oesophageal candidiasis, with no significant differences in safety and tolerability [22, 23]. In a randomised controlled study of antifungal prophylaxis in an adult and paediatric population following HSCT, patients were randomised to receive either micafungin (50 mg or 1 mg/kg/day) or fluconazole (400 mg or 8 mg/kg/day) [24]. Where success was defined as the absence of IFI through the end of therapy and at the end of the 4-week period after treatment, overall micafungin efficacy was superior to that of fluconazole (80.0% in the micafungin arm vs. 73.5% in the fluconazole arm, a statistically significant finding). So far, there are relatively limited clinical data on micafungin therapy for aspergillosis. In a prospective, open-label, noncomparative study, micafungin was evaluated in patients with probable or proven IA and found to be efficacious and safe [25]. However, the numbers treated with micafungin only were small.

7.2.5 Anidulafungin

Anidulafungin (Eraxis, Ecalta) is also a semisynthetic cyclic lipopeptide synthesised from a fermentation product of *A. nidulans*. It is approved by the EMEA for treating invasive candidiasis in non-neutropenic adult patients. It has not yet been approved for use in *Aspergillus* infections, nor has it received a license for use in the paediatric population either in the USA or Europe. It has been approved by the FDA for treating candidaemia and other forms of *Candida* infections (intra-abdominal abscess and peritonitis) and oesophageal candidiasis.

7.2.5.1 Spectrum of Activity

Anidulafungin appears to be similar to caspofungin and micafungin in terms of spectrum of activity.

7.2.5.2 Pharmacological Properties

This has recently been reviewed [26]. Anidulafungin, as with the other members of this class, is available only for intravenous administration. For treating candidaemia, intra-abdominal or peritoneal candidiasis, a loading dose of 200 mg on day 1 is required, followed by a maintenance dose of 100 mg once daily thereafter. For treating oesophageal candidiasis, loading and maintenance doses are 100 and 50 mg once daily, respectively. It is not metabolised in the body but is slowly chemically degraded and excreted into the intestine in an inactive form. No dose adjustment is required in either hepatic or renal failure, including for patients on dialysis. There are no serious drug interactions to date. Overall, it has a good safety profile, but liver function should be monitored during treatment.

7.2.5.3 Clinical Experience

Anidulafungin (200 mg on day 1, then 100 mg/day) was compared to intravenously administered fluconazole (400 mg/day) in a double-blind, randomised trial of invasive candidiasis in mostly non-neutropenic patients [27]. In the modified intention-to-treat group analysis, the global response rate (clinical and microbiological) at the end of intravenous therapy significantly favoured anidulafungin (however, the study had a number of limitations). The frequency and types of adverse events were similar in the two groups. Anidulafungin (100 mg on day 1, 50 mg once daily maintenance) was compared with fluconazole (200 mg/day) in a randomised double-blind trial in patients with oesophageal candidiasis [28]. In an intent-to-treat analysis, the rate of endoscopic success for anidulafungin was found not to be inferior to that for fluconazole. The safety profiles were similar. However, recurrence rates at the 2-week follow-up visit were higher for anidulafungin.

7.2.6 Combination Antifungal Therapy

Until recently, the mechanism of action of antifungal drugs was based mostly on activity on the fungal cell membrane, such as for amphotericin B and triazoles. Therefore, the benefit of a combination of antifungals that both acted on the cell membrane was debatable. However, the echinocandins act at a different site, i.e., the fungal cell wall, so arguments for combination therapy, such as an echinocandin and a polyene or an echinocandin and an azole, make more theoretical sense. Unfortunately, high-quality clinical data on combination antifungal therapy is limited. Recommendations for their use are often based on in vitro data, animal studies and limited clinical experience. The IDSA published guidelines on treating various fungal infections and recommended combination therapy in some instances [5, 13, 29–33]. For *Candida* spp. infections, combination therapy is recommended for treating some forms of invasive infection but not for candidaemia. A combination of amphotericin B and flucytosine is recommended by the IDSA as first-line therapy for central nervous system infections, endocarditis, endophthalmitis, urinary fungal balls, infected pacemakers, intracardiac devices and ventricular assist devices and as second-line therapy for pyelonephritis [13]. Combinations such as amphotericin B and flucytosine, amphotericin B and fluconazole, and fluconazole and flucytosine may be used for treating cryptococcal infection [30].

For initial primary IA therapy, combination therapy is not routinely recommended. However, addition of a second agent may be considered as part of salvage therapy when a primary agent is failing [5]. For endemic mycoses, combination therapy is again not routinely recommended. However, combination therapy with amphotericin B and an azole has been used to treat coccidioidomycosis, especially when infection is widespread or there is single-agent failure [32].

Consensus guidelines for treating rare mould infections, such as zygomycosis, are not available and are much needed. Combination therapy has been used to treat some of these infections, but there are very limited clinical data to support definite strategies of management.

7.3 Antifungal Susceptibility Testing

Data on antifungal susceptibility is important for patient management and—as there is only a limited number of classes of antifungal agents available—for surveillance of drug resistance. Epidemiological data and guidelines, such as those provided by the IDSA for treating invasive candidiasis, may be used to guide initial therapy. However, antifungal susceptibility testing provides additional data on local epidemiology and may provide valuable information for decisions regarding ongoing therapy in terms of the safest, most efficacious and cost-effective agent. There have been major developments in antifungal susceptibility testing in recent years, with several automated or semiautomated commercial systems and methods based on the disk-diffusion technique now available, providing simple, flexible and affordable procedures in the clinical laboratory [34]. Some of these commercial methods (e.g., E test) correlate well with reference procedures.

Minimum inhibitory concentration (MIC) breakpoints have traditionally divided an organism into three categories of susceptibility to a drug (susceptible, intermediate and resistant), with these breakpoints determined using epidemiological, in vitro, pharmacokinetic/pharmacodynamic and clinical data. For some fungi, the Clinical Laboratories Standard Institute (CLSI) has replaced the intermediate category with a category labelled susceptible–dose dependent (S-DD), whereby an antifungal would be expected to work with maximisation of dose and bioavailability. Committees in Europe [e.g., The European Committee on Antimicrobial Susceptibility Testing (EUCAST)] and the US (CLSI) are responsible for developing reproducible methods of antimicrobial susceptibility testing and for setting interpretative breakpoints, with efforts being made to align these for a consistent approach. These are continuously reviewed and are subject to change. Unlike breakpoints for antibacterial antibiotics, where much more clinical and in vitro data are available to set these breakpoints, there is still much work to be done in setting interpretative breakpoints for all antifungal agents against all clinically relevant fungi. For example, whereas there are standard guidelines with interpretative breakpoints for several antifungal agents versus *Candida* spp. [35], there are still no interpretative criteria for any antifungal agent versus *Cryptococcus neoformans*. However, based on current in vitro and clinical data, the activities of the antifungal agents currently in use are known for many of the common IFIs (Table 7.1).

7.4 Impact of Changing Epidemiology of Invasive Mycoses in Intensive Care

Since the last edition of this book [1], there have been further epidemiological studies to determine what the predominant fungal infections are, and in particular, the frequency of candidaemia/candidiasis is in intensive care practice [36]. Differences in the reported incidence of candidaemia between European countries have been noted, although there is no clear explanation for this [37]. *C. albicans* continues to account for about half of all documented cases, although improved microbiological investigation has meant that other *Candida* spp. are being more reliably identified. In a recent Italian study [38], the incidence of candidaemia and distribution of the causative species were recorded for 1999–2007 in an 18-bed mixed medical and surgical ICU. The incidence rate was 1.42 episodes/10,000 patient days/year. Overall, *C. albicans* accounted for 46% of isolates and other *Candida* spp. 54%, mainly *C. parapsilosis* (22%) and *C. glabrata* (13%).

Data from the 2008–2009 SENTRY Antimicrobial Surveillance Program on nosocomial *Candida* bloodstream infections showed that *C. glabrata* was the second most commonly isolated *Candida* spp. after *C. albicans* and was associated with the highest frequency of resistance to both fluconazole and other triazoles (range 5.1–7.7%) and the echinocandins (range 3.2–5.1%) [39].

7.5 Relationship Between Treating Invasive Candidiasis/ Candidaemia and Outcome

Several recent studies assessed the relationship between patient survival, time of starting antifungal therapy and its appropriateness following candidaemia documentation. In a Canadian study, administering "adequate" empirical antifungal therapy—defined as giving an adequate dose of antifungal drug to which the identified pathogen was shown to be susceptible in vitro—was associated with a significant decrease in mortality rate [40]. When assessing the appropriateness of empirical antibiotic therapy in septic patients admitted to the ICU, Garnacho-Montero et al. [41] found that fungal infection was an independent variable related to inappropriate therapy, which in turn was a predictor of

Table 7.1 Comparison of the major antifungal agents used to treat fungal infections in the intensive care unit

Class	Polyenes			
Generic name	Amphotericin B deoxycholate ("conventional")	Amphotericin B colloidal dispersion	Liposomal amphotericin B	Amphotericin B lipid complex
Trade name(s)	Fungizone Fungilin	Amphocil (Eur) Amphotec (US)	AmBisome	Abelcet
Main spectrum of activity (relative clinical and in vitro activity)				
Candida spp.				
C. albicans	++			
C. glabrata	++			
C. tropicalis	++			
C. parapsilosis	++			
C. krusei	+			
Cryptococcus neoformans	++			
Trichosporon spp.	+			
Aspergillus spp.				
A. fumigatus	++			
A. flavus	++			
A. terreus	±			
A. niger	++			
A. nidulans	–			
Zygomycetes	±			
Fusarium spp.	+			
S. prolificans	–			
S. apiospermum	–			

(continued)

Table 7.1 (continued)

	Polyenes			
Class				
Generic name	Amphotericin B deoxycholate ("conventional")	Amphotericin B colloidal dispersion	Liposomal amphotericin B	Amphotericin B lipid complex
Trade name(s)	Fungizone Fungilin	Amphocil (Eur) Amphotec (US)	AmBisome	Abelcet
Indication (Please refer to specific licensed indications and full prescribing information according to jurisdiction; adults only unless specified)	*Fungizone*: Systemic fungal infections *Fungilin*: Oral and perioral fungal infections	*Amphocil*: Severe systemic or deep mycoses where toxicity and renal failure preclude use of conventional amphotericin *Amphotec* Invasive aspergillosis in patients not responding to conventional amphotericin or where toxicity or renal impairment precludes conventional amphotericin	AmBisome: 1. Severe systemic or deep mycoses where toxicity (especially nephrotoxicity) precludes use of conventional amphotericin 2. Suspected or proven infection in febrile neutropenic patients unresponsive to broad-spectrum antibacterials	Abelcet: 1. Severe invasive candidiasis 2. Severe systemic fungal infections in patients not responding to conventional amphotericin or to other antifungal drugs or where toxicity or renal impairment precludes conventional amphotericin, including invasive aspergillosis, cryptococcal meningitis and disseminated cryptococcosis in HIV patients
Routes of administration (labelled and unlabelled routes)	*Fungizone*: IV, neb, IT, bladder irrigation *Fungilin*: topical	IV, neb	IV, neb	IV, neb
PO dose (Adult only)	NA	NA	NA	NA

(continued)

Table 7.1 (continued)

Class	Polyenes			
Generic name	Amphotericin B deoxycholate ("conventional")	Amphotericin B colloidal dispersion	Liposomal amphotericin B	Amphotericin B lipid complex
Trade name(s)	Fungizone Fungilin	Amphocil (Eur) Amphotec (US)	AmBisome	Abelcet
IV dose (Adult only)	0.7–1 mg/kg OD	3–7.5 mg/kg OD	3–5 mg/kg OD	5 mg/kg OD
Dose adjustment if renal impairment	No			
Dose adjustment if liver impairment	No			
TDM recommended	No			
Main side effects	Infusional toxicity and nephrotoxiciy more common with the conventional form. Hypokalaemia disturbance headache, fever, rigors, hypotension, tachypnoea			
Drug interactions	Renal toxicity may indirectly affect the action of othr drugs			

(continued)

Table 7.1 (continued)

Class	Azoles			
Generic name	Fluconazole	Itraconazole	Voriconazole	Posaconazole
Trade name(s)	Diflucan Trican	Sporanox	Vfend	Noxafil
Main spectrum of activity (relative clinical and in vitro activity)				
Candida spp.				
C. albicans	++	++	++	++
C. glabrata	±	+	+	+
C. tropicalis	++	++	++	++
C. parapsilosis	++	++	++	++
C. krusei	+	±	+	+
Cryptococcus neoformans	−	+	++	++
Trichosporon spp.	++	N	N	N
Aspergillus spp.				
A. fumigatus	−	++	++	++
A. flavus	−	++	++	++
A. terreus	−	++	++	++
A. niger	−	++	++	++
A. nidulans	−	++	++	++
Zygomycetes	−	±	−	+
Fusarium spp.	−	−	±	+
S. prolificans	−	N	N	N
S. apiospermum	−	±	+	N

(continued)

7 Systemic Antifungals

Table 7.1 (continued)

Class	Azoles			
Generic name	Fluconazole	Itraconazole	Voriconazole	Posaconazole
Trade name(s)	Diflucan Trican	Sporanox	Vfend	Noxafil
Indication (Please refer to specific licensed indications and full prescribing information according to jurisdiction; adults only unless specified)	Generic: 1. Vaginal candidiasis and candidal balanitis 2. Mucosal candidiasis 3. Fungal skin infections 4. Invasive candidal infections including candidaemia and disseminated candidiasis 5. Cryptococcal infections including meningitis 6. Prevention of relapse of cryptococcal meningitis in AIDS patients 7. Prevention of fungal infections in immuno-compromised patients	Generic: 1. Oropharyngeal candidiasis 2. Vulvovaginal candidiasis 3. Fungal skin infections 4. Onychomycosis 5. Histoplasmosis 6. Systemic aspergillosis, candidiasis and cryptococcosis including cryptococcal meningitis where other antifungal drugs are inappropriate or ineffective 7. Maintenance in AIDS patients to prevent relapse of underlying fungal infection 8. Prophylaxis in haematological malignancy or if undergoing BMT	Generic: 1. Invasive aspergillosis 2. Serious infections caused by *S. apiospermum*, *Fusarium* spp., or invasive fluconazole-resistant *Candida* spp. (including *C. krusei*)	Noxafil (EMEA) 1. Prophylaxis of invasive fungal infections in: - those receiving remission-induction chemotherapy AML or MDS expected to result in prolonged neutropenia and who are at high risk of developing invasive fungal infections - HSCT recipients who are undergoing high-dose immunosuppressive therapy for GVHD and who are at high risk of developing invasive fungal infections 2. Severe oropharyngeal candidiasis or if immuno-compromised 3. Salvage therapy for invasive aspergillosis, fusariosis, chromoblastomycosis, mycetoma and coccidioidomycosis in patients refractory to or intolerant of first-line therapy with other antifungal agents FDA: not licensed for indication number 3

(continued)

Table 7.1 (continued)

Class	Azoles			
Generic name	Fluconazole	Itraconazole	Voriconazole	Posaconazole
Trade name(s)	Diflucan Trican	Sporanox	Vfend	Noxafil
Routes of administration (labelled and unlabelled routes)	PO, IV	PO, IV, topical mouth	PO, IV	PO
PO dose[a] (Adult only)	1. 150 mg single dose 2. 50–100 mg OD 3. 50 mg OD 4. 400–800 mg OD 5. 400–800 mg OD 6. 200 mg OD 7. 50–400 mg OD	1. 100–200 mg OD 2. 200 mg BD for 1 day 3. 100 mg OD to 200 mg BD 4. 200 mg OD 5. 200 mg OD/BD 6. 100–200 mg OD/BD 7. 200 mg OD/BD 8. 5 mg/kg daily in 2 divided doses	>40kg: 400 mg BD/day, then 200–300 mg BD <40kg 200 mg BD/day, then 100–150 mg BD	1. 200 mg TDS 2. 200 mg/day, then 100 mg OD 3. 400 mg BD with food; 200 mg QDS without food
IV dose[a] (Adult only)	4. 400–800 mg OD 5. 400–800 mg OD 6. 200 mg OD 7. 50–400 mg OD	5. and 6. 200 mg BD for 2 days, then 200 mg OD	6 mg/kg BD for 24hrs, then 3–4 mg/kg BD	NA
Dose adjustment if renal impairment	Yes	Yes	Oral formulation if possible	No

(continued)

Table 7.1 (continued)

Class	Azoles			
Generic name	Fluconazole	Itraconazole	Voriconazole	Posaconazole
Trade name(s)	Diflucan Trican	Sporanox	Vfend	Noxafil
Dose adjustment if liver impairment	No	No	Yes	No
TDM recommended	No	Yes[b]	Yes[b]	Yes[b]
Main side effects	GI disturbance, abnormal LFTs	GI disturbance especially nausea and diarrhoea	Hallucinations, Transient visual disturbance, raised creatinine, photosensitivity	GI disturbance, abnormal LFTs, headache, fever, rigors
Drug interactions	Few	Numerous Inhibits CYP3A4	Numerous Inhibits CYP3A4 Also interacts with CYP 2C19	Some Inhibits CYP3A4

(continued)

Table 7.1 (continued)

Class	Echinocandins		
Generic name	Caspofungin	Micafungin	Anidulafungin
Trade name(s)	Cancidas	Mycamine	Ecalta (Eur) Eraxis (US)
Main spectrum of activity (relative clinical and in vitro activity)			
Candida spp.			
C. albicans	++	++	++
C. glabrata	++	++	++
C. tropicalis	++	++	++
C. parapsilosis	+	+	+
C. krusei	++	++	++
Cryptococcus neoformans	−	−	−
Trichosporon spp.	−	−	−
Aspergillus spp.			
A. fumigatus	+	+	+
A. flavus	+	+	+
A. terreus	+	+	+
A. niger	+	+	+
A. nidulans	+	+	+
Zygomycetes	−	−	−
Fusarium spp	−	−	−
S. prolificans	−	−	−
S. apiospermum	−	−	−

(continued)

Table 7.1 (continued)

Class	Echinocandins		
Generic name	Caspofungin	Micafungin	Anidulafungin
Trade name(s)	Cancidas	Mycamine	Ecalta (Eur) Eraxis (US)
Indication (Please refer to specific licensed indications and full prescribing information according to jurisdiction; adults only unless specified)	*Cancidas:* (EMEA) 1. Invasive candidiasis in adult or paediatric patients 2. Invasive aspergillosis in adult or paediatric patients who are refractory to or intolerant of first line therapy with other antifungal agents 3. Empirical therapy for presumed fungal infections in febrile, neutropenic adult or paediatric patients	*Mycamine:* (EMEA) *Adults >16 years:* 1. Invasive candidiasis 2. Oesophageal candidiasis 3. Prophylaxis of *Candida* infection in patients undergoing allogeneic HSCT or patients expected to have neutropenia for >10 days *In children <16 years:* 1. Invasive candidiasis 2. Prophylaxis of *Candida* infection in patients undergoing allogeneic HSCT or expected to have neutropenia >10 days FDA: not licensed in the paediatric population for prophylaxis of *Candida* infection in patients expected to have neutropenia >10 days	*Ecalta:* (EMEA) Treatment of invasive candidiasis in adult non-neutropenic patients *Eraxis:* 1. Oesophageal candidiasis 2. Candidaemia and other forms of *Candida* infections, including abdominal abscesses and peritonitis
Routes of administration (labelled and unlabelled routes)	IV	IV	IV
PO dose (Adult only)	NA	NA	NA

(continued)

Table 7.1 (continued)

Class	Echinocandins		
Generic name	Caspofungin	Micafungin	Anidulafungin
Trade name(s)	Cancidas	Mycamine	Ecalta (Eur) Eraxis (US)
IV dose[a] (Adult only)	1., 2., and 3 70 mg/day, then 50 mg OD If >80kg, 70 mg OD	>40kg: 1. 100–200 mg OD 2. 150 mg OD 3. 50 mg OD <40kg: 1. 2 mg/kg/day 2. 3 mg/kg/day 3. 1 mg/kg/day	*Ecalta:* 200 mg/day, then 100 mg OD *Eraxis:* 1. 100 mg/day, then 50 mg OD 2. 200 mg/day, then 100 mg OD
Dose adjustment if renal impairment	No	No	No
Dose adjustment if liver impairment	Yes	No	No
TDM recommended	No	No	No

Table 7.1 (continued)

Class	Echinocandins		
Generic name	Caspofungin	Micafungin	Anidulafungin
Trade name(s)	Cancidas	Mycamine	Ecalta (Eur) Eraxis (US)
Main side effects	Hypotension, peripheral oedema, tachycardia, fever, chills, headache, rash, hypokalaemia, GI disturbance, abnormal LFTs, phlebitis, infusion reactions, anaemia	Fever, headache, hypokalaemia, hypomagnesaemia, GI disturbance, neutropenia, thrombocytopenia	Hypokalaemia, GI disturbance, abnormal LFTs
Drug interactions	Cyclosporine, tacrolimus, rifampicin	Few Monitor for toxicity due to sirolimus, nifedipine and itraconazole if co-prescribed	Few

S. Scedosporium, *spp* species, *−* no activity, *±* slight activity, *+* modest activity, *++* good activity, *N* no data, *Eur* Europe, *US* United States, *EMEA* European Medicines Agency, *FDA* US Food and drug administration, *BMT* bone marrow transplantation, *IV* intravenous, *neb* nebulised, *IT* intrathecal, *PO* oral, *NA* not applicable, *OD* once daily, *BD* twice daily, *TDS* three times daily, *QDS* four times daily, *TDM* therapeutic drug monitoring, *GI* gastrointestinal, *LFTs* liver function tests, CYP3A4, Cytochrome P450 3A4 enzyme, CYP2C19, Cytochrome P450 2C19 enzyme.

[a] Where revelant, the doses categorised numerically correspond to the numerically categorised indications in the 'Indication' section
[b] In immunocompromised patients with invasive mycoses

in-hospital mortality. Morrell et al. [42] found that in cases of candidaemia, a > 12-h delay in starting antifungal therapy after the time the first positive blood culture sample was drawn was an independent predictor of mortality rate by multiple logistic regression analysis. Collectively, these and related studies have drawn into focus the way in which antifungal agents are being used in ICUs and how prescribing practice might be improved.

7.6 Approaches to Antifungal Therapy in Intensive Care

How best to utilise systemic antifungal agents in ICU patients is the subject of ongoing debate [43]. The challenges faced by intensivists and microbiologists are to identify which patients are most at risk for invasive candidiasis, to determine at what point it is appropriate to start antifungal therapy in a critically ill patient and which antifungal agent to use.

It is now accepted that antifungals can be prescribed in one of several ways. Firstly, there is prophylaxis, a practice that is more established in neutropenic haematological malignancy patients. There are less convincing supportive data in the ICU population. In considering what a preventive strategy should include, Pfaller and Diekema [35] remind practitioners of the need to educate staff on the importance of hand washing, optimal central vascular catheter care and prudent antibiotic prescribing to prevent nosocomial candidiasis. They also reviewed meta-analyses of published antifungal prophylaxis trials. The incidence of invasive candidiasis was reduced in all meta-analyses by between 50 and 80%; three of the five studies showed that the mortality rate was reduced while there was no apparent overall increase in antifungal drug resistance. Despite these encouraging results, the authors [35] suggest that further controlled trials are needed to identify subsets of patients who would benefit most from prophylaxis and also to emphasise the need to assess the efficacy of echinocandins, as earlier studies predominantly evaluated fluconazole.

In the study of Bassetti et al. [38], stopping the use of prophylactic fluconazole in their ICU resulted in a significant reduction in candidaemia caused by non-albicans *Candida* spp., and there was no change in the incidence of invasive candidiasis. Although studies showing that antifungal prophylaxis in ICU patients reduced the number of IFIs, the effect on mortality rate and the overall benefits of this strategy are not established. For reasons such as cost, concern about antifungal resistance and drug-related adverse events, antifungal prophylaxis should only be considered for selected high-risk patients.

Antifungal prophylaxis has received a grade B–I recommendation from the IDSA for patients at highest risk (>10% risk of invasive candidiasis) in ICUs with high rates of invasive candidiasis (compared with normal rates of 1–2%) [13]. Fluconazole 400 mg (6 mg/kg) daily is recommended for such patients in this setting. However, accurately identifying patients at >10% risk needs further refining, as yet there is no universally agreed-upon risk prediction algorithm that takes account of risk factors such as previous abdominal surgery, broad-spectrum antibiotic therapy, presence of an intravascular catheter and number of sites colonised with *Candida* spp. A 2007 Cochrane review of the use of prophylactic systemic antifungal agents in very-low-birth-weight infants cautiously found that prophylactic fluconazole reduces the rates of invasive fungal infection but with no statistically significant effect on overall mortality rates [44]. The role of other prophylactic antifungals, such as orally administered nystatin and nebulised amphotericin, is less clear, especially for ICU patients.

Alternative strategies to prophylaxis are, firstly, empirical therapy, where the basis for giving antifungals is clinical evidence of fungal infection but without mycological documentation; and, secondly, pre-emptive therapy, a newer concept in which patients are identified for treatment according to predetermined risk factors combined with several surrogate markers of fungal disease before it is clinically evident [45]. Intensivists need to be cautious when interpreting microbiological culture results, for example, being careful not to equate the isolation of *Candida* spp. from respiratory samples with the presence of an infection. Many ventilated patients will have *Candida* spp. isolated from respiratory samples, reflecting the altered flora due to antibiotic selection. Some studies used colonisation indices as a basis for pre-emptive therapy, but many microbiology laboratories do not provide this service at the level equivalent to a clinical trial. Furthermore, *Candida* spp. identified in colonisation samples do not necessarily correlate with the species causing candidaemia; this appears to be especially the case for *C. glabrata* candidaemias [46].

An alternative is to use the clinical approach initially to decide which patients will receive antifungal treatment. Spellberg et al. [47] proposed an empirical therapy algorithm for known or suspected cases of disseminated candidiasis based on the patient's general clinical status. Haemodynamically stable patients are distinguished from those who unstable, the latter likely being those with either severe sepsis and organ dysfunction or septic shock [45]. It is not clear whether or not this is advocated for all such patients or limited to those in whom there may be some additional evidence, such as fungal colonisation and prior broad-spectrum antibiotic exposure. In the former, less seriously ill patient, the authors recommend fluconazole but prefer an echinocandin, an amphotericin B formulation, or voriconazole in the latter group. If the patient has colonisation with *C. glabrata* or *C. krusei*, they recommend not using fluconazole.

Fluconazole is an attractive option for initial empirical therapy because it has few side effects and is cheaper than the newer systemic antifungals. However, the response rates of treating candidaemia reported in the comparative clinical trials suggest that either amphotericin B or an echinocandin may be more efficacious, even though superior response rates in individual studies were not significantly different on statistical analysis [27, 48]. Zilberberg et al. [49] designed a decision model aimed at assessing the cost-effectiveness of using an echinocandin—in this case, micafungin—rather than fluconazole for empirical therapy of suspected ICU-acquired candidaemia. It was based on a hypothetical 1,000-patient cohort. A number of parameters were compared, including differences in mortality rates, drug costs and cost per quality adjusted life year (QALY). The authors concluded that preferred use of the echinocandin was cost effective. Their study builds on earlier analysis of the optimal choice of empirical therapy, which also favoured an echinocandin [50]. In an accompanying commentary to the Zilberberg study [49], Golan [51] suggests the study may have overestimated the benefits of micafungin compared with fluconazole and suggest further studies should be undertaken in this area.

For antifungal therapy of a documented case of candidaemia in the ICU, the IDSA guidelines [13] recommend either fluconazole or an echinocandin (AI grade) with some caveats: Liposomal amphotericin B (AmBisome) was found to be as effective as micafungin in a randomised double-blind trial [18], suggesting that it is an alternative option, although as with other amphotericin B formulations, a higher rate of treatment-related adverse events might be expected.

References

1. Cooke FJ, Rogers T (2005) Systemic antifungals. In: van Saene HKF, Silvestri L, de la Cal MA (eds) Infection control in the intensive care unit, 2nd edn. Springer, Berlin, pp 155–170
2. Schiller DS, Fung HB (2007) Posaconazole: an extended-spectrum triazole antifungal agent. Clin Ther 29:1862–1886
3. Ullmann AJ, Lipton JH, Vesole DH et al (2007) Posaconazole or fluconazole for prophylaxis in severe graft-versus-host disease. N Engl J Med 356:335–347
4. Cornely OA, Maertens J, Winston DJ et al (2007) Posaconazole vs. fluconazole or itraconazole prophylaxis in patients with neutropenia. N Engl J Med 356:348–359
5. Walsh TJ, Anaissie EJ, Denning DW et al (2008) Treatment of aspergillosis: clinical practice guidelines of the Infectious Diseases Society of America. Clin Infect Dis 46:327–360
6. Walsh TJ, Raad I, Patterson TF et al (2007) Treatment of invasive aspergillosis with posaconazole in patients who are refractory to or intolerant of conventional therapy: an externally controlled trial. Clin Infect Dis 44:2–12
7. Greenberg RN, Mullane K, van Burik JA et al (2006) Posaconazole as salvage therapy for zygomycosis. Antimicrob Agents Chemother 50:126–133
8. van Burik JA, Hare RS, Solomon HF et al (2006) Posaconazole is effective as salvage therapy in zygomycosis: a retrospective summary of 91 cases. Clin Infect Dis 42:e61–e65
9. Page RL 2nd, Schwiesow J, Hilts A (2007) Posaconazole as salvage therapy in a patient with disseminated zygomycosis: case report and review of the literature. Pharmacotherapy 27:290–298
10. Zoller E, Valente C, Klepser ME (2010) Development, clinical utility, and place in therapy of posaconazole for prevention and treatment of invasive fungal infections. Drug Des Devel Ther 4:299–311
11. Strorzinger D, Lichtenstern C, Weigand MA et al (2011) Posaconazole as part of the antifungal armamentarium in the intensive care unit-case reports from a surgical ICU. Mycoses 54(suppl 1):45–48
12. Shields RK, Clancy CJ, Vadnerkar A et al (2010) Posaconazole serum concentrations among cardiothoracic transplant recipients: factors impacting levels and correlation with clinical response. Antimicrob Agents Chemother 55(3):1308–1311
13. Pappas PG, Kauffman CA, Andes D et al (2009) Clinical practice guidelines for the management of candidiasis: 2009 update by the Infectious Diseases Society of America. Clin Infect Dis 48:503–535

14. Pappas PG, Rotstein CM, Betts RF et al (2007) Micafungin versus caspofungin for treatment of candidemia and other forms of invasive candidiasis. Clin Infect Dis 45:883–893
15. Vazquez JA (2010) Invasive fungal infections in the intensive care unit. Semin Respir Crit Care Med 31:79–86
16. Wagner C, Graninger W, Presterl E et al (2006) The echinocandins: comparison of their pharmacokinetics, pharmacodynamics and clinical applications. Pharmacology 78:161–177
17. Betts RF, Nucci M, Talwar D et al (2009) A multicenter, double-blind trial of a high-dose caspofungin treatment regimen versus a standard caspofungin treatment regimen for adult patients with invasive candidiasis. Clin Infect Dis 48:1676–1684
18. Kuse ER, Chetchotisakd P, da Cunha CA et al (2007) Micafungin versus liposomal amphotericin B for candidaemia and invasive candidosis: a phase III randomised double-blind trial. Lancet 369:1519–1527
19. Pappas PG, Rotstein CM, Betts RF et al (2007) Micafungin versus caspofungin for treatment of candidemia and other forms of invasive candidiasis. Clin Infect Dis 45:883–893
20. Dupont BF, Lortholary O, Ostrosky-Zeichner L et al (2009) Treatment of candidemia and invasive candidiasis in the intensive care unit: *post hoc* analysis of a randomized, controlled trial comparing micafungin and liposomal amphotericin B. Crit Care 13:R159
21. Queiroz-Telles F, Berezin E, Leverger G et al (2008) Micafungin versus liposomal amphotericin B for pediatric patients with invasive candidiasis. Pediatr Infect Dis 27:820–826
22. de Wet N, Llanos-Cuentas A, Suleiman J et al (2004) A randomized, double-blind, parallel-group, dose-response study of micafungin compared with fluconazole for the treatment of esophageal candidiasis in HIV-positive patients. Clin Infect Dis 39:842–849
23. de Wet NT, Bester AJ, Viljoen JJ et al (2005) A randomized, double blind, comparative trial of micafungin (FK463) vs. fluconazole for the treatment of oesophageal candidiasis. Aliment Pharmacol Ther 21:899–907
24. van Burik JA, Ratanatharathorn V, Stepan DE et al (2004) Micafungin versus fluconazole for prophylaxis against invasive fungal infections during neutropenia in patients undergoing hematopoietic stem cell transplantation. Clin Infect Dis 39:1407–1416
25. Denning DW, Marr KA, Lau WM et al (2006) Micafungin (FK463), alone or in combination with other systemic antifungal agents, for the treatment of acute invasive aspergillosis. J Infect 53:337–349
26. Perkhofer S, Lass-Florl C (2009) Anidulafungin and voriconazole in invasive fungal disease: pharmacological data and their use in combination. Expert Opin Investig Drugs 18:1393–1404
27. Reboli AC, Rotstein C, Pappas PG et al (2007) Anidulafungin versus fluconazole for invasive candidiasis. N Engl J Med 356:2472–2482
28. Krause DS, Simjee AE, van Rensburg C et al (2004) A randomized, double-blind trial of anidulafungin versus fluconazole for the treatment of esophageal candidiasis. Clin Infect Dis 39:770–775
29. Kauffman CA, Bustamante B, Chapman SW et al (2007) Clinical practice guidelines for the management of sporotrichosis: 2007 update by the Infectious Diseases Society of America. Clin Infect Dis 45:1255–1265
30. Perfect JR, Dismukes WE, Dromer F et al (2010) Clinical practice guidelines for the management of cryptococcal disease: 2010 update by the Infectious Diseases Society of America. Clin Infect Dis 50:291–322
31. Chapman SW, Dismukes WE, Proia LA et al (2008) Clinical practice guidelines for the management of blastomycosis: 2008 update by the Infectious Diseases Society of America. Clin Infect Dis 46:1801–1812
32. Galgiani JN, Ampel NM, Blair JE et al (2005) Coccidioidomycosis. Clin Infect Dis 41:1217–1223
33. Wheat LJ, Freifeld AG, Kleiman MB et al (2007) Clinical practice guidelines for the management of patients with histoplasmosis: 2007 update by the Infectious Diseases Society of America. Clin Infect Dis 45:807–825

34. Cuenca-Estrella M, Rodriguez-Tudela JL (2010) The current role of the reference procedures by CLSI and EUCAST in the detection of resistance to antifungal agents in vitro. Expert Rev Anti Infect Ther 8:267–276
35. Pfaller MA, Diekema DJ (2007) Epidemiology of invasive candidiasis: a persistent public health problem. Clin Microbiol Rev 20:133–163
36. Kett DH, Azoulay E, Echeverria PM et al. for the Extended Prevalence of Infection in the ICU Study (EPIC. II) Group of investigators (2010) Candida bloodstream infections in intensive care units: analysis of the extended prevalence of infection in an intensive care unit study. Crit Care Med 39(4):665-670
37. Lass-Florl C (2009) The changing face of epidemiology of invasive fungal disease in Europe. Mycoses 52:197–205
38. Bassetti M, Ansaldi F, Nicolini L et al (2009) Incidence of candidaemia and relationship with fluconazole use in an intensive care unit. J Antimicrob Chemother 64:625–629
39. Pfaller MA, Moet GJ, Messer SA et al (2010) Candida bloodstream infections: comparison of species distribution and antifungal resistance in community onset and nosocomial isolates in the SENTRY antimicrobial surveillance program (2008–2009). Antimicrob Agents Chemother 55(2):561–566
40. Parkins MD, Sabuda DM, Elsayed S et al (2007) Adequacy of empirical antifungal therapy and effect on outcome among patients with invasive *Candida* species infections. J Antimicrob Chemother 60:613–618
41. Garnacho-Montero J, Garcia-Garmendia JL, Barrero-Almodovar A et al (2003) Impact of adequate empirical antibiotic therapy on the outcome of patients admitted to the intensive care unit with sepsis. Crit Care Med 31:2742–2751
42. Morrell M, Fraser VJ, Kollef MH (2005) Delaying the empiric treatment of *Candida* bloodstream infection until positive blood culture results are obtained: a potential risk factor for hospital mortality. Antimicrob Agents Chemother 49:3640–3645
43. Cruciani M, Serpelloni G (2008) Management of *Candida* infections in the adult intensive care unit. Expert Opin Pharmacother 9:175–191
44. Clerihew L, Austin N, McGuire W (2007) Prophylactic systemic antifungal agents to prevent mortality and morbidity in very low birth weight infants. Cochrane Database Syst Rev (4):CD003850
45. Guery BP, Arendrup MC, Auzinger G et al (2009) Management of invasive candidiasis and candidemia in adult non-neutropenic intensive care unit patients. Part II: Treatment. Intensive Care Med 35:206–214
46. Troughton JA, Browne G, McAuley DF et al (2010) Prior colonisation with *Candida* species fails to guide empirical therapy for candidaemia in critically ill adults. J Infect 61:403–409
47. Spellberg BJ, Filler SG, Edwards JE Jr (2006) Current treatment strategies for disseminated candidiasis. Clin Infect Dis 42:244–251
48. Rex JH, Bennett JE, Sugar AM et al (1994) A randomized trial comparing fluconazole with amphotericin B for the treatment of candidemia in patients without neutropenia. N Engl J Med 331:1325–1330
49. Zilberberg MD, Kothan S, Shorr AF (2009) Cost-effectiveness of micafungin as an alternative to fluconazole empiric treatment of suspected ICU-acquired candidemia among patients with sepsis: a model simulation. Crit Care 13:R94
50. Golan Y, Wolf MP, Pauker SG et al (2005) Empirical anti-Candida therapy among selected patients in the intensive care unit: a cost effectiveness analysis. Ann Intern Med 143:857–869
51. Golan Y (2009) Empiric anti-*Candida* therapy for patients with sepsis in the ICU: how little is too little? Crit Care 13:180

Enteral Antimicrobials

8

M. Sánchez García, M. Nieto Cabrera, M. A. González Gallego and F. Martínez Sagasti

8.1 Introduction

Healthy individuals may carry one or more of the six potentially pathogenic microorganisms (PPM), considered either normal or community-acquired, in their upper [1, 2] and lower [3] gastrointestinal tract flora. These PPMs are *Streptococcus pneumoniae*, *Haemophilus influenzae*, *Moraxella catarrhalis*, *Staphylococcus aureus*, *Escherichia coli*, and *Candida albicans*. The presence of the opportunistic or abnormal aerobic gram-negative bacilli (AGNB), *Klebsiella*, *Enterobacter*, *Proteus*, *Morganella*, *Citrobacter*, *Serratia*, *Acinetobacter*, and *Pseudomonas* species, and of methicillin-resistant *S. aureus* (MRSA) in the oropharynx and gastrointestinal tract of healthy individuals is uncommon (see Chap. 2), although extended-spectrum beta-lactamases (ESBL) harboring Enterobacteriaceae, as well as MRSA, are increasingly being detected at hospital admission [4]. The nine abnormal bacteria are predominantly carried by patients with an underlying condition, either chronic or acute [5]. Illness severity and antibiotic use [3, 5, 6] are the most important factors in conversion of the normal to the abnormal carrier state. Carriage of abnormal flora invariably leads to high concentrations, i.e., abnormal bacteria overgrowth, in the throat and gut of the critically ill [7, 8]. Overgrowth is defined as $\geq 10^5$ of abnormal flora per milliliter of saliva and/or gram of feces [9]. In turn, intestinal overgrowth with AGNB is associated with systemic immune-system suppression [10, 11] and has also been shown to be an independent risk factor for endogenous infection, endotoxemia, emergence of resistance, transmission via hands of carers, and outbreaks.

M. Sánchez García (✉)
Servicio de Medicina Intensiva,
Hospital Clínico San Carlos Universidad Complutense,
Madrid, Spain
e-mail: msanchezga.hcsc@salud.madrid.org

8.2 Eradication and Control of Abnormal Flora Carriage and Overgrowth

8.2.1 Parenterally Administered Antimicrobials

The most commonly used parenterally antimicrobials have been shown to clear the three oropharyngeal microorganisms *S. pneumoniae, H. influenzae*, and *M. catarrhalis*. For example, cefotaxime is excreted into saliva in concentrations high enough to eradicate oropharyngeal carriage of these three community-acquired respiratory PPMs [12]. The failure rate in clearing *E. coli* from the gut is substantially due to the nonlethal fecal concentrations following excretion via bile and mucus [12, 13], although relatively high concentrations of 153 kg have been documented for ceftriaxone in human volunteers [14]. Systemic antifungals are not associated with significant eradication or prevention of yeast carriage in critically ill patients, as shown in a randomized controlled trial (RCT) of fluconazole [15]. Although penicillinase-resistant penicillins are widely regarded as the antistaphylococcal agents of choice, there are no accurate data on the clearance of methicillin-sensitive *S. aureus* (MSSA) carriage [16]. Effective eradication of MSSA from throat and gut has, however, been reported for intravenously administered (IV) cephradine [17].

Two grams of vancomycin IV produce concentrations of between 6 and 11 mg/kg of feces. Enteral administration, however, results in fecal levels between 3,000 and 24,000 µg/g of feces [18, 19]. These pharmacokinetic data may explain why systemic vancomycin fails to eradicate MRSA gut carriage. The same concept that salivary, fecal, and mucus concentrations are in general nonlethal for AGNB carried in the throat and gut applies to the commonly used systemic antimicrobials, including beta-lactams, aminoglycosides, and fluoroquinolones [20–22]. Even the newer and more potent carbapenems and the combination of beta-lactams and beta-lactamase inhibitors fail to clear AGNB, including *Pseudomonas* and *Acinetobacter* spp. [23, 24]. This emphasizes the importance of measuring drug levels at all relevant sites in addition to blood levels.

8.2.2 Enterally Administered Antimicrobials

Enterally administered antimicrobials are used to prevent and, if already present, eradicate carriage and overgrowth with abnormal bacteria, including AGNB and MRSA. Critically ill patients are unable to clear these opportunistic PPMs [8] due to their underlying disease. Only recovery from their acute condition promotes return to the normal carrier state [25]. Therefore, during the period of critical illness, enterally administered antimicrobials are required to combat gut overgrowth of abnormal flora.

Administration of nonabsorbable enterally administered antimicrobials is based on the experience that critically ill patients given parenterally administered antibiotics only have harmful gut overgrowth with abnormal flora [26]. Selective decontamination of the digestive tract (SDD), a maneuver based mainly on enteral administration of antimicrobials, is designed to convert the abnormal to the normal carrier state. The purpose of SDD is therefore to prevent, or eradicate if initially present, carriage and overgrowth of abnormal AGNB and MRSA. In addition, SDD is used to eradicate MSSA and yeasts, which are carried by varying percentages of healthy people. The overall aim of SDD using enterally administered antimicrobials is to reduce mortality and morbidity rates following recovery of systemic immunity [11, 27] by preventing endogenous infections, resistance, and outbreaks and reducing endotoxemia. A combination of nonabsorbable antimicrobials is given enterally, which leaves indigenous flora relatively undisturbed, believed to play a defensive role against abnormal bacterial carriage [28]. To qualify for selective elimination of abnormal flora, antimicrobials should fulfil four criteria:

1. adequate spectrum, covering AGNB, MRSA, MSSA and yeasts, while sparing indigenous, mostly anaerobic, flora as much as possible [28];
2. nonabsorbable, in order to achieve constant high intraluminal levels, which would be lowered by absorption [29];
3. minimal inactivation by salivary, fecal, and food compounds, and no degradation by fecal enzymes produced by indigenous anaerobic flora [30]; interactions between feces, bacteria, and decontaminating antimicrobials determining the microbiologically active fecal concentrations are of great importance in the ultimate outcome of SDD;
4. bactericidal, with low minimal bactericidal concentrations (MBC) for AGNB, MRSA, MSSA and yeasts, because there are no leucocytes in the human alimentary canal to assist antimicrobial decontamination [31].

The most commonly used protocol is a combination of polymyxin and tobramycin to clear AGNB and MSSA, amphotericin or nystatin to eradicate yeasts, and vancomycin in case of MRSA (Table 8.1) [32].

8.2.2.1 Polymyxins

Polymyxins given enterally are nonabsorbable [33] and cover AGNB, including ESBLs in general, as well as ESBLs conferring carbapenem resistance to enterobacteria [34, 35]. These compounds have excellent activity against *P. aeruginosa* and *Acinetobacter* spp., although not against *Proteus, Morganella,* or *Serratia* spp. Polymyxins are selective in that they are not active against the indigenous—mainly anaerobic—flora [36]. The mode of action is disruption of the bacterial cell wall, making the bacterial cell permeable and leading to cell death. This mechanism is independent of enzymatic systems [37], and acquired resistance against polymyxins is uncommon [38]. Polymyxins are inactivated to a moderate extent by proteins, fiber, food, cell debris, and salivary and fecal compounds, and should therefore be given in a relatively high daily dose of 400 mg of polymyxin E (300 mg of polymyxin B) [36]. Polymyxins should also be combined with an aminoglycoside due to the gap in activity against *Proteus, Morganella* and *Serratia* spp. The aminoglycoside should be active against *P. aeruginosa* because polymyxins lose activity against this common intensive care unit (ICU) bacterium

Table 8.1 Enterally administered antimicrobials for eradication of carriage of potential pathogens

Selective digestive decontamination		Total daily dose in four divided doses		
Target microorganisms		<5 years	5–12 years	>12 years
Oropharynx				
AGNB	Polymyxin E with tobramycin	2 g of 2% paste or gel		
Yeasts	Amphotericin B, or nystatin	2 g of 2% paste or gel		
MRSA	Vancomycin	2 g of 4% paste or gel		
Gut				
AGNB	Polymyxin E (mg)	100	200	400
	With tobramycin (mg)	80	160	320
Yeasts	Amphotericin B (mg)	500	1,000	2,000
	Nystatin (Units)	2×10^6	4×10^6	8×10^6
MRSA	Vancomycin (mg)	20–40/kg	20–40/kg	500–2,000

AGNB aerobic gram-negative bacilli, *MRSA* methicillin-resistant *Staphylococci aureus*

in the presence of feces. Polymyxins also neutralize endotoxin in the intestinal lumen by adsorption [39].

8.2.2.2 Aminoglycosides

Aminoglycosides have several ideal features cited above for enterally administered antimicrobials. They are active against a wide range of AGNB, including *P. aeruginosa*, have a potent bactericidal activity similar to polymyxins, and synergistic activity with polymyxins. Antipseudomonal aminoglycosides include gentamicin, tobramycin, and amikacin. They are nonabsorbable, and the bactericidal activity is by inhibiting protein synthesis. Tobramycin is the least inactivated by feces, followed by amikacin and gentamicin [40–42]. According to an older study [43] based on culture results, tobramycin is considered to be selective in terms of leaving the indigenous flora undisturbed in doses <500 mg a day. A recent investigation [8], ancillary to a randomized clinical trial [44], used more precise molecular quantification methods and found reductions in the *Faecalibacterium prausnitzii* group, which were attributed to enterally administered tobramycin. Although an important component of intestinal microbiota—*F. prausnitzii* seems to have several beneficial functions in the normal host—it is important to note that the study is potentially biased because it was performed in a very small subgroup, approximately 20%, of patients enrolled in one center and that, as recently shown by the same group [45], other factors, including nutrition type and systemic administration of antibiotics, may have been responsible for reductions in the *F. prausnitzii* group count. The clinical relevance of this finding in critically ill patients therefore remains to be elucidated. Blood levels of tobramycin and gentamicin have been monitored during SDD [46–48]. Aminoglycoside levels were undetectable in most patients. Low concentrations, <1 mg/l, were measured in ICU patients, particularly those with renal impairment. In a series of 19 patients under standard SDD doses and with severe, acute renal failure requiring continuous renal replacement therapy, tobramycin serum concentrations were ≤1 mg/l [49]. In three patients with concomitant bowel ischemia, serum levels ranged between 1.1 and 3.0 mg/l [49]. Although the three antipseudomonal aminoglycosides and polymyxins have a similar bactericidal activity, the total daily dose recommended for tobramycin is 320 mg, which is lower compared with the 400 mg for the polymyxins, which are inactivated to a moderate extent by fecal material. Aminoglycosides require the addition of polymyxins, as the emergence of aminoglycoside-neutralizing enzymes is not uncommon [50]. Polymyxins are thought to protect tobramycin from being inactivated by fecal enzymes.

Practically all ESBL-producing AGNB are sensitive to the enterally administered combination of polymyxin/tobramycin [51]. Although rare, some ESBL-producing AGNB, such as *Klebsiella* spp., may be resistant to tobramycin [52]. In this case, tobramycin may be replaced by an aminoglycoside active against such species, e.g., neomycin [53] or paromomycin [54]. Parenterally administered antimicrobials that disregard the patient's gut ecology may promote acquisition, carriage, and subsequent overgrowth of ESBL-producing AGNB [55, 56]. Tobramycin has also been found to reduce endotoxin release [57].

8.2.2.3 Polyenes

The two polyenes used as decontaminating agents are either amphotericin B or nystatin. They are fungicidal and highly selective, as fungi are the only PPM covered by polyenes. They bind to a sterol of the plasma membrane and alter the membrane permeability of the fungal cell, which leads to leakage of essential metabolites and finally to fungal cell lysis. Absorption of polyenes is minimal [47, 48], and emergence of resistance to them amongst yeasts and fungi is highly uncommon [58]. Fecal inactivation of polyenes is high, explaining the high daily dose of 2 g of amphotericin B and of 8×10^6 U of nystatin required for decontamination purposes [59, 60] (Table 8.1).

8.2.2.4 Glycopeptides

Of the two glycopeptides, vancomycin and teicoplanin, the most experience as decontaminating agents has been gathered for enterally administered vancomycin [19]. Vancomycin is active against MRSA but cannot be considered as a selective decontaminating agent as it covers the vast majority of the anaerobic *Clostridium* spp. Thus, SDD protocols do not routinely include enterally administered vancomycin because of its negative impact on the gut ecology. Enterally administered vancomycin is only recommended to eradicate MRSA carriage and overgrowth and should always be given in combination with polymyxin/tobramycin/amphotericin B (PTA) to offset the potential for AGNB and yeast overgrowth as a consequence of using a nonselective decontaminating agent [61]. The mode of action is bactericidal, as vancomycin is bound rapidly and irreversibly to cell walls of sensitive bacteria, thereby inhibiting cell-wall synthesis. Vancomycin absorption is rare [48]. Inactivation by proteins, fiber, food, and feces is substantial, hence the high daily dose of 2 g (Table 8.1).

8.3 Efficacy of Enterally Administered Polymyxin/ Tobramycin, Polyenes, and Vancomycin in Eradicating AGNB, Yeast, and MRSA Carriage and Overgrowth

Sixty randomized controlled trials (RCTs) evaluating SDD were conducted [62] between 1987 and 2010 (Chap. 13). The antibiotic combinations most frequently used were polymyxin/tobramycin and polymyxin/gentamicin, in approximately two-thirds and one-third of trials, respectively. Ten meta-analyses of RCTs on SDD all invariably show a significant reduction in infection, and five meta-analyses report a mortality rate reduction [63].

Surveillance cultures of the throat and rectum are an integral part of enterally administered antimicrobial protocols [64]. Monitoring the carrier state in the critically ill receiving antimicrobials enterally is essential, as only surveillance cultures allow monitoring of compliance and efficacy. SDD is considered to be effective only if surveillance samples show AGNB, MRSA, MSSA, and yeast eradication. In addition, comparison of microorganisms cultured in surveillance and diagnostic samples allows classification of ICU-acquired infections in endogenous, i.e., SDD failure, and exogenous, i.e., hygiene failure [64]. Surveillance samples were taken in most trials, predominantly twice-weekly throat and/or rectal swab, although only a few provided classification of the type of infections detected [65].

8.3.1 Aerobic Gram-Negative Bacilli (AGNB)

Most RCTs report effective clearance of AGNB carriage following polymyxin/ tobramycin administration. Reductions of AGNB in surveillance cultures can be detected within 2–3 days of starting SDD [65]. Abnormal carriage in the throat is eradicated within 3 days, whereas it takes 7 days for abnormal rectal carriage to be eradicated, depending on the return of peristalsis. A meta-analysis of the impact of SDD on AGNB carriage [66] shows impressive 87 and 85% reductions in oropharyngeal and rectal carriage, respectively. A recent study employing more sensitive molecular methods shows significant—more than tenfold—mean reduction in Enterobacteriaceae [8].

8.3.2 Yeasts

Data on yeast carriage show that enterally administered polyenes significantly reduce the odds ratio (OR) for carriage to 0.31 (0.18–0.54) [67]. More recent trials, such as one multicenter RCT enrolling 6,000 patients [44], confirm this effect.

8.3.3 MRSA

Six RCTs included vancomycin enterally but none analyzed the impact on MRSA carriage and infections [48, 68–72]. A 4% vancomycin gel applied in the lower cheeks was associated with a significantly reduced OR for oropharyngeal MRSA carriage to 0.25 (0.09–0.69) in one RCT [73]. A before–after study performed in a burn unit observed significant relative risk (RR) reductions >80% for acquisition of MRSA carriage and infection [74] after the introduction of routine enterally administered vancomycin, and a prospective nonrandomized study performed in a medical/surgical unit revealed similar findings [75]. The recent detection of an outbreak of linezolid-resistant but vancomycin-susceptible MRSA [76] implies a potential application for prevention and control of this type of problem with topical vancomycin.

Seven studies report fecal levels of one or more decontaminating agents polymyxin, tobramycin, gentamicin, amphotericin B, nystatin, and vancomycin [19, 43, 59, 60, 77–79]. Compared with polymyxin, tobramycin was less inactivated by fecal material. In one study, fecal specimens contained tobramycin levels of at least 100 mg/L feces following the daily intake of 300 mg of tobramycin [43]. In another study, individuals taking 600 mg of tobramycin daily showed >500 mg/L of fecal sample [77]. Polymyxin is moderately inactivated by mucosal cells, fiber and feces, and hence the variation in fecal drug levels. Polymyxin was not detected in one-third of individuals who took 600 mg of polymyxin daily [78]. One-third had fecal levels >1,000 mg/L of feces, whereas the remaining individuals showed polymyxin levels between 16 and 1,000 mg/L of feces. Tobramycin at a daily dose of 320 added to 400 mg of polymyxin is the most commonly used combination for eradicating AGNB carriage and overgrowth due to its synergism and relatively less fecal inactivation [80]. Vancomycin inactivation by fecal material is high. In one study, vancomycin po was given in doses of 2 g daily for 7 days, and the mean concentration in 25 stool samples obtained during treatment was $3,100 \pm 400$ µg/g (range of 905–8,760 µg/g) [26]. Fecal concentrations of polymyxin E and gentamicin were measured in 38 stool samples obtained from 15 patients [79]. The levels of both were <20 µg/ml of feces in ten stools. The remaining 28 samples showed fecal polymyxin E levels of 94 ± 174 mg/L (median 42 µg/ml, range 0–1,055 mg/L) and gentamicin levels of 466 ± 545 mg/L (median 196 mg/L, range 0–2,098 µg/ml). Inactivation of polyenes, including amphotericin B and nystatin, by fecal material is high. Daily doses of 2,000 mg of amphotericin B or 8×10^6 U of nystatin were associated with fecal levels of 60 and 20 mg/L of feces, respectively [59, 60].

Most parenterally administered antimicrobials do not act upon gut flora. However, fluoroquinolones including ciprofloxacin have been shown to possess the pharmacokinetic characteristic of transintestinal secretion [81]. A substantial amount of intravenously administered ciprofloxacin is excreted via mucus rather than via bile (15 vs. 1%), leading to high fecal ciprofloxacin concentrations. The mean fecal level of ciprofloxacin was 108.7 mg/L of feces following parenteral administration of a daily dose of 400 mg of ciprofloxacin [81].

The antifungal 5-flucytosine is a small molecule that also possesses the pharmacokinetic property of transintestinal secretion, i.e., 10% of systematically administered 5-flucytosine is excreted via mucus into the gut [82]. The good penetration of flucytosine into most body tissues and fluids has been ascribed to its high water solubility, low molecular weight, and low protein binding properties. These features of ciprofloxacin and 5-flucytosine can be useful in critically ill patients in whom rectal swabs remain positive for AGNB and yeasts following 1 week of polymyxin/tobramycin/amphotericin B treatment. Failure of the classic PTA protocol may be due to AGNB and yeasts already translocated into the gut-associated lymphoid tissue on admission and hence escape the intraluminal lethal activity of nonabsorbable PTA. Three days of high intravenous doses of ciprofloxacin or 5 flucytosine has been shown to assist effective SDD as measured by surveillance samples negative for AGNB and yeasts in patients with inflamed gut.

Apart from monitoring efficacy and compliance of enterally administered antimicrobials, surveillance samples, in particular rectal swabs, provide the unique method of detecting antimicrobial resistance at an early stage, allowing prompt treatment adjustment. In three RCTs [22, 70, 83], throat and rectal swabs were also cultured on agar plates containing 2 mg/l of polymyxin, 4 mg/l of tobramycin, and 6 mg/l of vancomycin. For example, *Proteus* and *Serratia* spp. intrinsically resistant to polymyxins may become resistant to tobramycin. There are reports that describe the enteral use of amikacin [84] and paromomycin [29] replacing tobramycin to eradicate tobramycin-resistant *Proteus* and *Serratia*, respectively.

8.4 Impact on Clinical and Epidemiological Endpoints of Abnormal Flora Eradication Using Enterally Administered Antimicrobials

8.4.1 Infectious Morbidity and Attributable Mortality

Infection-control policies that include SDD have four fundamental features [64]:
1. enterally administered antimicrobials to decontaminate the gastrointestinal tract; they are combined with an oropharyngeal decontamination procedure using a paste or gel containing 2% PTA; the aim of administering oropharyngeal and intestinal nonabsorbable antimicrobials is preventing secondary endogenous infections;
2. antibiotics given parenterally immediately upon admission to control primary endogenous infections;
3. hygiene to control exogenous infections;
4. surveillance samples to monitor the SDD protocol.

The two most complete meta-analyses demonstrate that enterally administered polymyxins with tobramycin or gentamicin significantly reduce AGNB infections [85, 86]. Enterally administered polyenes significantly reduced both the number of patients with yeast infections and episodes of yeast infections in 42 of 54 RCTs evaluating the efficacy of antifungal polyenes as part of SDD [67]. Lower-airway infections due to MRSA were significantly reduced in the RCT using 4% vancomycin gel [73], as well as in two open trials employing both a 4% vancomycin paste and vancomycin enterally [74, 75].

The most compelling evidence that infection is responsible for increased mortality derives from RCTs of SDD. Several trials of large enough sample size [22, 44, 70] documented a significant absolute mortality-rate reduction in patients receiving the prophylactic regimen and a significantly reduced RR for developing pneumonia of 0.20 (0.07–0.58) and bloodstream infections of 0.38 (0.17–0.83) [70]. Whereas it is possible that these clinical benefits of SDD arise from reasons other than preventing both early primary endogenous and late secondary endogenous infections—e.g., reduced absorption of gut endotoxin—the most plausible interpretation of these recent data is that infection is responsible for a relative increase in risk of ICU mortality rates of 20–40%. A recent trial found a lower mortality risk in both medical and surgical patients and in all severity groups [22].

8.4.2 Endotoxemia

AGNBs present as overgrowth in the gut are the major source of endotoxin in the human body. Up to 10 mg of fecal endotoxin per gram of feces has been measured in critically ill patients with AGNB gut overgrowth [87]. For example, gut ischemia at the time of cardiac surgery and liver transplantation promotes transmural migration or translocation of AGNB present in concentrations of $\geq 10^5$/g of feces [88]. Most translocating AGNB are killed by macrophages of gut-associated lymphoid tissue, including the liver, which maintains bloodstream sterility. However, the subsequent release of endotoxin may spill over into the bloodstream and often lead to fluctuating levels of endotoxemia [89]. The enterally administered combination of polymyxin/tobramycin has been shown to significantly reduce fecal endotoxin load by a factor of 10^4 [90]. Five RCTs evaluated the impact of SDD on endotoxemia: three during cardiopulmonary bypass surgery [91–93] and two in liver transplant patients [94, 95]. Two trials reported a significant reduction following SDD [91, 92]; three trials failed to show a difference [93–95]. The cardiac patients received enterally administered polymyxin/tobramycin 3 days preoperatively in the two positive studies. In the negative cardiac study, tobramycin was replaced by neomycin, a poor antiendotoxin agent [96, 97]. In the two liver transplant studies, polymyxin/tobramycin was started 12 h preoperatively and postoperatively only [98].

8.4.3 Antimicrobial Resistance

The most frequently used argument against the SDD strategy, and also a sincere concern of some intensivists, is that the routine use of SDD may promote the development of bacterial resistance or select resistant PPMs. This type of reasoning directly derives from the well-known fact that extensive systemic antibiotic use is associated with induction of resistance and selection of resistant microorganisms, sometimes with dramatic reductions in therapeutic options [35, 76]. Mechanisms contributing to an increase in the number of patients who carry resistant microorganisms are: (1) admission to the ICU of patients already carriers of resistant microorganisms; (2) selection and induction or mutation of resistant microorganisms following antibiotic pressure; (3) transmission of resistant microorganisms while in the ICU. Effective control of carriage/overgrowth using antimicrobials enterally guarantees control of the import of resistance, control of induction or mutation at the gut level, and significantly reduced transmission due to the reduced number of carriers combined with a lower level of carriage of resistant microorganisms (Chaps. 12 and 28).

The most extensive meta-analyses demonstrate the virtual absence of any reported resistance, with all assessed RCTs being free of this problem and of subsequent superinfections and/or epidemics of multiresistant strains [85, 86].

In one multicenter RCT from Madrid [65], MRSA carriage but not infection was significantly greater in the test group. An immediately posttrial observational study in 100 consecutive patients receiving SDD (enterally administered antimicrobial regimen: polymyxin E-gentamicin-amphotericin B, without vancomycin) showed a progressive significant reduction from 27.6 to 8% and ruled out a causal relationship [65]. The coordinating ICU of the trial has been using SDD in long-term (>48 h) intubated patients for >20 years now, without significant resistance problems. This accords with data from four SDD studies in which the endpoint of resistance was evaluated over periods of 2, 2.5, 6 and 7 years [84, 99–102], whereas two studies evaluating the emergence of resistant microorganisms following SDD discontinuation failed to show any negative effect [102, 103]. Two trials designed to evaluate the effect of SDD on mortality and resistance rate showed both significant mortality-rate reductions [22, 44] and demonstrated significant reductions in carriage of resistant bacteria. The trial comparing patients on an SDD unit versus patients receiving parenterally administered antibiotic-only approach in a different ICU showed significantly fewer carriers of multiresistant AGNB and *P. aeruginosa* in the SDD unit than in the control unit [22]. A multicenter trial enrolling 6,000 patients also showed significant reductions in ceftazidime-resistant AGNB and *P. aeruginosa* [44].

A follow-up study in patients in hospital wards after discharge from the ICU performed in two of the 13 participating centers detected an increased incidence of infections in patients who had been in the SDD test group [104]. Per 100 surgical procedures, the incidences of respiratory tract and blood-stream infections were similar between the control and the decontaminated groups. The global increase in infection was mainly due to, presumably exogenous, surgical site infections, 18 of 26 of which were superficial and 15 had no or negative cultures.

Another ancillary study of this trial [105] evaluated the influence of SDD on bacterial resistance in point prevalence cultures obtained during the trial from all concomitant ICU patients not enrolled in the trial. The study confirms that SDD not only reduces resistant AGNB carriage in individual patient [8, 22, 44] but protects other patients not receiving SDD probably by reducing transmission

[105]. This beneficial effect has been known for many years [106] and explains why the efficacy of SDD increases with higher "prevalence" of the maneuver, i.e., during routine use in all eligible patients or without a simultaneous placebo control group during trials. After SDD discontinuation, significant increases in some resistance markers were detected (ceftazidime), although not in others (ciprofloxacin, tobramycin). Resistance levels remained stable over the next 12 months without SDD [105]. The various sources of bias for the results of this are appropriately addressed by the authors in the discussion section of their manuscript.

Six RCTs conducted in ICUs in which MRSA was endemic at the time of the study showed a trend toward higher MRSA colonization [65] or infection rates in patients receiving SDD [107–112]. MRSA, by design, is not covered by SDD antimicrobials. Inevitably, SDD exerts selective pressure on this PPM. Hence, proponents of SDD have always accepted this possibility and proposed an SDD strategy consisting of surveillance cultures to detect MRSA overgrowth in carriers, combined with vancomycin administered either oropharyngeally [73, 113] or oropharyngeally and enterally to control MRSA overgrowth [74, 75]. When there is a serious clinical MRSA problem, this approach can be used as a prophylactic policy in all high-risk groups. These patients should receive PTA combined with enterally administered vancomycin on admission, and throat and rectal swabs should be taken during the entire ICU stay. With an incidence of less than one event per week, SDD that includes vancomycin enterally can be commenced as treatment if swabs prove positive [114].

8.4.4 Transmission of Abnormal Flora Via Hands of Carers

The high density of *S. aureus*, both methicillin sensitive and resistant, in the oropharynx and gut promotes skin carriage and hand and environmental contamination. Quantitative studies from the early 1950s demonstrated that *S. aureus* overgrowth in the nasal cavity leads to skin carriage of *S. aureus* in 44% of individuals, but only in 16% if the level of contamination of nasal secretions was $<10^5$ *S. aureus* [115]. Airborne dissemination was also a function of the number of microorganisms present in the nose. However, similar research from the late 1950s demonstrated that the weight of microorganisms released to the environment by the fecal carrier greatly exceeded that of organisms released by the nasal carrier [116, 117]. Twenty years later, the importance of fecal carriage of MRSA in children was shown from air contamination studies during nappy changing, when patients who were fecal carriers yielded the same type from the air [118]. More recently, gut overgrowth of MRSA was shown to be associated with a significant amount of MRSA dispersed from the perianal site into clothing and bedding and hence into the environment [119]. Long-stay patients invariably have overgrowth in their throat and gut of $>10^9$ potential pathogens per milliliter of saliva or gram of feces [7]. Washing a patient or changing a nappy may lead to hand contamination of health-care workers to levels of $>10^6$ PPM/cm^2 of finger surface [120]. For hand hygiene to be effective, a disinfecting agent such as 0.5% chlorhexidine in 70% alcohol is required, and the procedure must take at least 2 min. Under these circumstances, contamination levels are lowered at most by 10^4 microorganisms, still leaving up to 10^2 per cm^2 of finger surface [121]. These quantitative data show that the intervention of hand disinfection in a busy ICU with a few long-stay patients can only ever hope to reduce transmission but never abolish it [122]. From an SDD perspective, even under the hypothetical circumstances of completely clearing hand contamination, hand hygiene could never exert an influence on the major infection problem of primary endogenous infection with a magnitude of between 60 and 85% of all infections (Chap. 5). The intervention of hand disinfection also fails to clear oropharyngeal and gastrointestinal carriage and/or overgrowth of PPM present on arrival. However, high standards of hygiene, including hand disinfection, are part of the SDD infection-control protocol. This protocol aims to reduce the level of hand contamination below which transmission occurs. It is possible to achieve these low levels, as the enterally administered antimicrobials eradicate throat and gut carriage of PPM and substantially reduce overall levels of PPM density on the patient's skin. In this way, handwashing becomes more effective in controlling transmission of PPM and subsequent endogenous and exogenous infections.

8.4.5 Outbreaks

Observations on the characteristics of infection outbreaks show that once approximately half the ICU population carries the outbreak strain in overgrowth concentrations of minimally 3+ on the semiquantitative culturing scale [123], spread via the hands of carers is impossible to prevent, and an outbreak is difficult to avoid. Dissemination of AGNB invariably occurs whether there is oropharyngeal or intestinal overgrowth [53, 106]. In ICUs with ongoing endemicity of multiresistant *Klebsiella* [53, 124], *C. parapsilosis* [125], and MRSA [61, 75], reinforcement of conventional hygiene measures, including hand disinfection, invariably failed to stop the outbreaks. The introduction of enterally administered antimicrobials was reported to be successful in controlling AGNB, yeast, and MRSA outbreaks in five reports [53, 61, 75, 124, 125]. In a French study, patients were randomized and given antimicrobials either enterally or not enterally [53]. Fecal carriage of the ESBL-producing *Klebsiella* strain was cleared in 50% of patients, and the outbreak was under control within 8 weeks. In a Manchester, UK, ICU all patients received SDD, and a *Klebsiella* outbreak was stopped within 3 weeks [124]. Similarly, gut carriage/overgrowth is the main source of *Candida* and MRSA, which are then transmitted via the hands of health-care workers [61, 75, 125]. On a Liverpool, UK, neonatal ICU, enterally administered nystatin was given as treatment to neonates who were identified to carry the outbreak strain of *C. parapsilosis*, and the outbreak was controlled within 14 weeks [125]. Enterally administered vancomycin added to the classic SDD was an effective outbreak control measure in Italian [61] and Spanish [75] ICUs with MRSA endemicity. In the Spanish study, enterally administered vancomycin given as prophylaxis to all patients at high risk was more effective in controlling endemicity compared with when administered to confirmed carriers only. The main concerns about its prophylactic use is vancomycin-resistant enterococci (VRE) [126]. Vancomycin resistance among low-level pathogens such as enterococci is an endemic problem in ICUs in the USA.

SDD, including enterally administered vancomycin, has been evaluated in five European studies in mechanically ventilated patients [61, 73, 75, 113, 127]. None of the studies report an increased infection rate due to VRE. They evaluated SDD including vancomycin in ICUs without VRE history, and in one study VRE was imported into the unit but no change in policy was required, as rapid and extensive spread did not occur [75]. Recent literature shows that parenterally administered antibiotics that do not respect the patient's gut ecology rather than high doses of enterally administered vancomycin promote the emergence of VRE in the gut [128, 129].

8.5 Conclusions

SDD using enterally administered antimicrobials is now an evidence-based protocol. It is the best-ever evaluated intervention in intensive care medicine for reducing infectious morbidity and mortality. It is inexpensive and without side effects in terms resistance emergence. In intensive care units (ICUs) using enterally administered antimicrobials, gut carriage of potential pathogens, both sensitive and resistant, is significantly reduced with SDD. However, hand disinfection as a general hygiene procedure is still valuable and can be expected to be more effective in ICUs where all long-stay patients are successfully decontaminated and are thus free from aerobic gram-negative bacilli (AGNB), yeast, and *Staphylococcus aureus* overgrowth, This subsequently reduces hand contamination and, consequently, the chance of transmission. SDD is the gold standard to which new maneuvers of infection control should be compared.

References

1. Aas JA, Paster BJ, Stokes LN et al (2005) Defining the normal bacterial flora of the oral cavity. J Clin Microbiol 43(11):5721–5732
2. Preza D, Olsen I, Willumsen T et al (2009) Diversity and site-specificity of the oral microflora in the elderly. Eur J Clin Microbiol Infect Dis 28(9):1033–1040
3. Raum E, Lietzau S, von Baum H et al (2008) Changes in *Escherichia coli* resistance patterns during and after antibiotic therapy: a longitudinal study among outpatients in Germany. Clin Microbiol Infect 14(1):41–48
4. Friedmann R, Raveh D, Zartzer E et al (2009) Prospective evaluation of colonization with extended-spectrum beta-lactamase (ESBL)-producing Enterobacteriaceae among patients at hospital admission and of subsequent colonization with ESBL-producing Enterobacteriaceae among patients during hospitalization. Infect Control Hosp Epidemiol 30(6):534–542
5. Tacconelli E, De Angelis G, Cataldo MA et al (2009) Antibiotic usage and risk of colonization and infection with antibiotic-resistant bacteria: a hospital population-based study. Antimicrob Agents Chemother 53(10):4264–4269

6. Rodriguez-Bano J, Alcala J, Cisneros JM et al (2009) *Escherichia coli* producing SHV-type extended-spectrum beta-lactamase is a significant cause of community-acquired infection. J Antimicrob Chemother 63(4):781–784
7. van Saene HK, Taylor N, Donnell SC et al (2003) Gut overgrowth with abnormal flora: the missing link in parenteral nutrition-related sepsis in surgical neonates. Eur J Clin Nutr 57(4):548–553
8. Benus RF, Harmsen HJ, Welling GW et al (2010) Impact of digestive and oropharyngeal decontamination on the intestinal microbiota in ICU patients. Intensive Care Med 36(8):1394–1402
9. Husebye E (1995) Gastrointestinal motility disorders and bacterial overgrowth. J Intern Med 237(4):419–427
10. Marshall JC, Christou NV, Meakins JL (1988) Small-bowel bacterial overgrowth and systemic immunosuppression in experimental peritonitis. Surgery 104(2):404–411
11. Horton JW, Tan J, White DJ et al (2004) Selective decontamination of the digestive tract attenuated the myocardial inflammation and dysfunction that occur with burn injury. Am J Physiol Heart Circ Physiol 287(5):H2241–H2251
12. Alcock SR (1990) Short-term parenteral antibiotics used as a supplement to SDD regimens. Infection 18(suppl 1):S14–S18
13. Sompolinsky D, Yaron V, Alkan WJ (1967) Microbiological changes in the human fecal flora following the administration of tetracyclines and chloramphenicol. Am J Proctol 18(6):471–478
14. Pletz MW, Rau M, Bulitta J et al (2004) Ertapenem pharmacokinetics and impact on intestinal microflora, in comparison to those of ceftriaxone, after multiple dosing in male and female volunteers. Antimicrob Agents Chemother 48(10):3765–3772
15. Garbino J, Lew DP, Romand JA et al (2002) Prevention of severe *Candida* infections in nonneutropenic, high-risk, critically ill patients: a randomized, double-blind, placebo-controlled trial in patients treated by selective digestive decontamination. Intensive Care Med 28(12):1708–1717
16. Chang FY, Peacock JE Jr, Musher DM et al (2003) *Staphylococcus aureus* bacteremia: recurrence and the impact of antibiotic treatment in a prospective multicenter study. Medicine (Baltimore) 82(5):333–339
17. van Saene R, Fairclough S, Petros A (1998) Broad- and narrow-spectrum antibiotics: a different approach. Clin Microbiol Infect 4(1):56–57
18. Geraci JE, Heilman FR, Nicolson DR et al (1956) Some laboratory and clinical experiences with a new antibiotic, vancomycin. Proc Staff Meet Mayo Clin 31(21):564–582
19. Tedesco F, Markham R, Gurwith M et al (1978) Oral vancomycin for antibiotic-associated pseudomembranous colitis. Lancet 2(8083):226–228
20. D'Agata EM, Venkataraman L, DeGirolami P et al (1999) Colonization with broad-spectrum cephalosporin-resistant gram-negative bacilli in intensive care units during a nonoutbreak period: prevalence, risk factors, and rate of infection. Crit Care Med 27(6):1090–1095
21. Petros AJ, O'Connell M, Roberts C et al (2001) Systemic antibiotics fail to clear multidrug-resistant Klebsiella from a pediatric ICU. Chest 119(3):862–866
22. De Jonge E, Schultz MJ, Spanjaard L et al (2003) Effects of selective decontamination of digestive tract on mortality and acquisition of resistant bacteria in intensive care: a randomised controlled trial. Lancet 362(9389):1011–1016
23. Corbella X, Montero A, Pujol M et al (2000) Emergence and rapid spread of carbapenem resistance during a large and sustained hospital outbreak of multiresistant Acinetobacter baumannii. J Clin Microbiol 38(11):4086–4095
24. Toltzis P, Yamashita T, Vilt L et al (1998) Antibiotic restriction does not alter endemic colonization with resistant gram-negative rods in a pediatric intensive care unit. Crit Care Med 26(11):1893–1899

25. Ketai LH, Rypka G (1993) The course of nosocomial oropharyngeal colonization in patients recovering from acute respiratory failure. Chest 103(6):1837–1841
26. van Saene HK, Petros AJ, Ramsay G, Baxby D (2003) All great truths are iconoclastic: selective decontamination of the digestive tract moves from heresy to level 1 truth. Intensive Care Med 29(5):677–690
27. Yao YM, Lu LR, Yu Y et al (1997) Influence of selective decontamination of the digestive tract on cell-mediated immune function and bacteria/endotoxin translocation in thermally injured rats. J Trauma 42(6):1073–1079
28. van der Waaij D (1992) History of recognition and measurement of colonization resistance of the digestive tract as an introduction to selective gastrointestinal decontamination. Epidemiol Infect 109(3):315–326
29. Bodey GP (1981) Antibiotic prophylaxis in cancer patients: regimens of oral, nonabsorbable antibiotics for prevention of infection during induction of remission. Rev Infect Dis 3(suppl):S259–S268
30. van Saene HK, Stoutenbeek CP (1987) Selective decontamination. J Antimicrob Chemother 20(4):462–465
31. Harris JC, Dupont HL, Hornick RB (1972) Fecal leukocytes in diarrheal illness. Ann Intern Med 76(5):697–703
32. Stoutenbeek CP (1989) Topical antibiotic regimen. In: van Saene HK, Stoutenbeek CP, Lawin P, Ledingham IM (eds) Infection control by selective decontamination. Springer, Heidelberg, pp 95–101
33. Guyonnet J, Manco B, Baduel L et al (2010) Determination of a dosage regimen of colistin by pharmacokinetic/pharmacodynamic integration and modeling for treatment of G.I.T. disease in pigs. Res Vet Sci 88(2):307–314
34. Nordmann P, Cuzon G, Naas T (2009) The real threat of Klebsiella pneumoniae carbapenemase-producing bacteria. Lancet Infect Dis 9(4):228–236
35. Kumarasamy KK, Toleman MA, Walsh TR et al (2010) Emergence of a new antibiotic resistance mechanism in India, Pakistan, and the UK: a molecular, biological, and epidemiological study. Lancet Infect Dis 10(9):597–602
36. van Saene JJ, van Saene HK, Tarko-Smit NJ, Beukeveld GJ (1988) Enterobacteriaceae suppression by three different oral doses of polymyxin E in human volunteers. Epidemiol Infect 100(3):407–417
37. Sogaard H (1982) The pharmacodynamics of polymyxin antibiotics with special reference to drug resistance liability. J Vet Pharmacol Ther 5(4):219–231
38. Hawser SP (2010) Susceptibility of Klebsiella pneumoniae clinical isolates from 2007 to 2009 to colistin and comparator antibiotics. Int J Antimicrob Agents 2010 36(4):383–384
39. Danner RL, Joiner KA, Rubin M et al (1989) Purification, toxicity, and antiendotoxin activity of polymyxin B nonapeptide. Antimicrob Agents Chemother 33(9):1428–1434
40. Veringa EM, van der Waaij D (1984) Biological inactivation by faeces of antimicrobial drugs applicable in selective decontamination of the digestive tract. J Antimicrob Chemother 14(6):605–612
41. van Saene JJ, van Saene HK, Stoutenbeek CP, Lerk CF (1985) Influence of faeces on the activity of antimicrobial agents used for decontamination of the alimentary canal. Scand J Infect Dis 17(3):295–300
42. Hazenberg MP, Pennock-Schroder AM, van de Merwe JP (1985) Binding to and antibacterial effect of aztreonam, temocillin, gentamicin and tobramycin on human faeces. J Hyg (Lond) 95(2):255–263
43. Mulder JG, Wiersma WE, Welling GW, van der WD (1984) Low dose oral tobramycin treatment for selective decontamination of the digestive tract: a study in human volunteers. J Antimicrob Chemother 13(5):495–504
44. de Smet AM, Kluytmans JA, Cooper BS et al (2009) Decontamination of the digestive tract and oropharynx in ICU patients. N Engl J Med 360(1):20–31

45. Benus RF, van der Werf TS, Welling GW et al (2010) Association between Faecalibacterium prausnitzii and dietary fibre in colonic fermentation in healthy human subjects. Br J Nutr 29:1–8
46. Cavaliere F, Sciarra M, Crociani E et al (1988) Serum levels of tobramycin during selective decontamination of the gastrointestinal tract. Minerva Anestesiol 54(5):223–226
47. Zobel G, Kuttnig M, Grubbauer HM et al (1991) Reduction of colonization and infection rate during pediatric intensive care by selective decontamination of the digestive tract. Crit Care Med 19(10):1242–1246
48. Gaussorgues P, Salord M, Sirodot M et al (1991) Efficacité de la décontamination digestive sur la survenue des bactériémies nosocomiales chez les patients sous ventilation méchanique et recevant des betamimétiques. Réanimation Soins Intensifs Médecin d'Urgence 7:169–174
49. Mol M, van Kan HJ, Schultz MJ, De Jonge E (2008) Systemic tobramycin concentrations during selective decontamination of the digestive tract in intensive care unit patients on continuous venovenous hemofiltration. Intensive Care Med 34(5):903–906
50. Smith CA, Baker EN (2002) Aminoglycoside antibiotic resistance by enzymatic deactivation. Curr Drug Targets Infect Disord 2(2):143–160
51. Rodriguez-Bano J, Navarro MD, Romero L et al (2006) Clinical and molecular epidemiology of extended-spectrum beta-lactamase-producing *Escherichia coli* as a cause of nosocomial infection or colonization: implications for control. Clin Infect Dis 42(1): 37–45
52. Al Naiemi N, Heddema ER, Bart A et al (2006) Emergence of multidrug-resistant gram-negative bacteria during selective decontamination of the digestive tract on an intensive care unit. J Antimicrob Chemother 58(4):853–856
53. Brun-Buisson C, Legrand P, Rauss A et al (1989) Intestinal decontamination for control of nosocomial multiresistant gram-negative bacilli. Study of an outbreak in an intensive care unit. Ann Intern Med 110(11):873–881
54. Abecasis F, Kerr S, Sarginson RE et al (2007) Comment on: emergence of multidrug-resistant gram-negative bacteria during selective decontamination of the digestive tract on an intensive care unit. J Antimicrob Chemother 60(2):445
55. Hoyen CK, Pultz NJ, Paterson DL et al (2003) Effect of parenteral antibiotic administration on establishment of intestinal colonization in mice by *Klebsiella pneumoniae* strains producing extended-spectrum beta-lactamases. Antimicrob Agents Chemother 47(11):3610–3612
56. Martins IS, Pessoa-Silva CL, Nouer SA et al (2006) Endemic extended-spectrum beta-lactamase-producing *Klebsiella pneumoniae* at an intensive care unit: risk factors for colonization and infection. Microb Drug Resist 12(1):50–58
57. Sjolin J, Goscinski G, Lundholm M et al (2000) Endotoxin release from *Escherichia coli* after exposure to tobramycin: dose-dependency and reduction in cefuroxime-induced endotoxin release. Clin Microbiol Infect 6(2):74–81
58. Vanden Bossche H, Dromer F, Improvisi I et al (1998) Antifungal drug resistance in pathogenic fungi. Med Mycol 36(Suppl 1):119–128
59. Hofstra W, Vries-Hospers HG, van der WD (1979) Concentrations of nystatin in faeces after oral administration of various doses of nystatin. Infection 7(4):166–170
60. Hofstra W, de Vries-Hospers HG, van der Waaij D (1982) Concentrations of amphotericin B in faeces and blood of healthy volunteers after the oral administration of various doses. Infection 10(4):223–227
61. Silvestri L, Milanese M, Oblach L et al (2002) Enteral vancomycin to control methicillin-resistant *Staphylococcus aureus* outbreak in mechanically ventilated patients. Am J Infect Control 30(7):391–399
62. Silvestri L, van Saene HK, Zandstra DF et al (2010) Impact of selective decontamination of the digestive tract on multiple organ dysfunction syndrome: systematic review of randomized controlled trials. Crit Care Med 38(5):1370–1376

63. Silvestri L, van Saene HK, Folla L, Milanese M (2010) Selective digestive decontamination is superior to oropharyngeal chlorhexidine in preventing pneumonia and reducing mortality in critically ill patients. J Bras Pneumol 36(2):270–272
64. Baxby D, van Saene HK, Stoutenbeek CP, Zandstra DF (1996) Selective decontamination of the digestive tract: 13 years on, what it is and what it is not. Intensive Care Med 22(7):699–706
65. Sánchez García M, Cambronero Galache JA, Lopez DJ et al (1998) Effectiveness and cost of selective decontamination of the digestive tract in critically ill intubated patients. A randomized, double-blind, placebo-controlled, multicenter trial. Am J Respir Crit Care Med 158(3):908–916
66. Silvestri L, van Saene HK, Casarin A et al (2008) Impact of selective decontamination of the digestive tract on carriage and infection due to gram-negative and gram-positive bacteria: a systematic review of randomised controlled trials. Anaesth Intensive Care 36(3):324–338
67. Silvestri L, van Saene HK, Milanese M, Gregori D (2005) Impact of selective decontamination of the digestive tract on fungal carriage and infection: systematic review of randomized controlled trials. Intensive Care Med 31(7):898–910
68. Bergmans DC, Bonten MJ, Gaillard CA et al (2001) Prevention of ventilator-associated pneumonia by oral decontamination: a prospective, randomized, double-blind, placebo-controlled study. Am J Respir Crit Care Med 164(3):382–388
69. Korinek AM, Laisne MJ, Nicolas MH et al (1993) Selective decontamination of the digestive tract in neurosurgical intensive care unit patients: a double-blind, randomized, placebo-controlled study. Crit Care Med 21(10):1466–1473
70. Krueger WA, Lenhart FP, Neeser G et al (2002) Influence of combined intravenous and topical antibiotic prophylaxis on the incidence of infections, organ dysfunctions, and mortality in critically ill surgical patients: a prospective, stratified, randomized, double-blind, placebo-controlled clinical trial. Am J Respir Crit Care Med 166(8):1029–1037
71. Pugin J, Auckenthaler R, Lew DP, Suter PM (1991) Oropharyngeal decontamination decreases incidence of ventilator-associated pneumonia. A randomized, placebo-controlled, double-blind clinical trial. JAMA 265(20):2704–2710
72. Schardey HM, Joosten U, Finke U et al (1997) The prevention of anastomotic leakage after total gastrectomy with local decontamination. A prospective, randomized, double-blind, placebo-controlled multicenter trial. Ann Surg 225(2):172–180
73. Silvestri L, van Saene HK, Milanese M et al (2004) Prevention of MRSA pneumonia by oral vancomycin decontamination: a randomised trial. Eur Respir J 23(6):921–926
74. Cerda E, Abella A, de La Cal MA et al (2007) Enteral vancomycin controls methicillin-resistant *Staphylococcus aureus* endemicity in an intensive care burn unit: a 9-year prospective study. Ann Surg 245(3):397–407
75. de la Cal MA, Cerda E, van Saene HK et al (2004) Effectiveness and safety of enteral vancomycin to control endemicity of methicillin-resistant *Staphylococcus aureus* in a medical/surgical intensive care unit. J Hosp Infect 56(3):175–183
76. Sanchez Garcia M, De la Torre MA, Morales G et al (2010) Clinical outbreak of linezolid-resistant *Staphylococcus aureus* in an intensive care unit. JAMA 303(22):2260–2264
77. Bodey GP (1980) Absorption of tobramycin after chronic oral administration. Curr Ther Res 28:394–401
78. Gotoff SP, Lepper MH, Fiedler MA (1965) Treatment of salmonella carriers with colistin sulfate. Am J Med Sci 249:399–403
79. Misset B, Kitzis MD, Conscience G et al (1994) Mechanisms of failure to decontaminate the gut with polymixin E, gentamicin and amphotericin B in patients in intensive care. Eur J Clin Microbiol Infect Dis 13(2):165–170
80. Stoutenbeek CP, van Saene HK (1990) Infection prevention in intensive care by selective decontamination of the digestive tract. J Crit Care 5:137–156

81. Krueger WA, Ruckdeschel G, Unertl K (1999) Elimination of fecal Enterobacteriaceae by intravenous ciprofloxacin is not inhibited by concomitant sucralfate—a microbiological and pharmacokinetic study in patients. Infection 27(6):335–340
82. Daneshmend TK, Warnock DW (1983) Clinical pharmacokinetics of systemic antifungal drugs. Clin Pharmacokinet 8(1):17–42
83. Winter R, Humphreys H, Pick A et al (1992) A controlled trial of selective decontamination of the digestive tract in intensive care and its effect on nosocomial infection. J Antimicrob Chemother 30(1):73–87
84. Stoutenbeek CP, van Saene HK, Zandstra DF (1987) The effect of oral non-absorbable antibiotics on the emergence of resistant bacteria in patients in an intensive care unit. J Antimicrob Chemother 19(4):513–520
85. D'Amico R, Pifferi S, Leonetti C et al (1998) Effectiveness of antibiotic prophylaxis in critically ill adult patients: systematic review of randomised controlled trials. BMJ 316(7140):1275–1285
86. Liberati A, D'Amico R, Pifferi S (2009) Antibiotic prophylaxis to reduce respiratory tract infections and mortality in adults receiving intensive care. Cochrane Database Syst Rev (4):CD000022
87. van Saene HK, Stoutenbeek CP, Faber-Nijholt R, van Saene JJ (1992) Selective decontamination of the digestive tract contributes to the control of disseminated intravascular coagulation in severe liver impairment. J Pediatr Gastroenterol Nutr 14(4):436–442
88. Fink MP, Mythen MG (1999) The role of gut-derived endotoxin in the pathogenesis of multiple organ dysfunction. In: Brade H, Opal SM, Vogel SN, Morrison DC (eds) Endotoxin in health and disease. Dekker, New York, pp 855–864
89. Cohen J (2000) The detection and interpretation of endotoxaemia. Intensive Care Med 26(Suppl 1):S51–S56
90. van Saene JJ, Stoutenbeek CP, van Saene HK et al (1996) Reduction of the intestinal endotoxin pool by three different SDD regimens in human volunteers. J Endotoxin Res 3:337–343
91. Martinez-Pellus AE, Merino P, Bru M et al (1993) Can selective digestive decontamination avoid the endotoxemia and cytokine activation promoted by cardiopulmonary bypass? Crit Care Med 21(11):1684–1691
92. Martinez-Pellus AE, Merino P, Bru M et al (1997) Endogenous endotoxemia of intestinal origin during cardiopulmonary bypass. Role of type of flow and protective effect of selective digestive decontamination. Intensive Care Med 23(12):1251–1257
93. Bouter H, Schippers EF, Luelmo SA et al (2002) No effect of preoperative selective gut decontamination on endotoxemia and cytokine activation during cardiopulmonary bypass: a randomized, placebo-controlled study. Crit Care Med 30(1):38–43
94. Bion JF, Badger I, Crosby HA et al (1994) Selective decontamination of the digestive tract reduces gram-negative pulmonary colonization but not systemic endotoxemia in patients undergoing elective liver transplantation. Crit Care Med 22(1):40–49
95. Maring JK, Zwaveling JH, Klompmaker IJ et al (2002) Selective bowel decontamination in elective liver transplantation: no improvement in endotoxaemia, initial graft function and post-operative morbidity. Transpl Int 15(7):329–334
96. Oudemans-van Straaten HM, van Saene HK, Zandstra DF (2003) Selective decontamination of the digestive tract: use of the correct antibiotics is crucial. Crit Care Med 31(1):334–335
97. Schippers EF, van Dissel JT (2003) Selective gut decontamination. Crit Care Med 31(11):2715–2716
98. van Saene HK, Silvestri L, Bams JL et al (2003) Selective decontamination of the digestive tract: use in liver transplantation is evidence based. Crit Care Med 31(5):1600–1601
99. Hammond JM, Potgieter PD (1995) Long-term effects of selective decontamination on antimicrobial resistance. Crit Care Med 23(4):637–645

100. Leone M, Albanese J, Antonini F et al (2003) Long-term (6-year) effect of selective digestive decontamination on antimicrobial resistance in intensive care, multiple-trauma patients. Crit Care Med 31(8):2090–2095
101. Tetteroo GW, Wagenvoort JH, Bruining HA (1994) Bacteriology of selective decontamination: efficacy and rebound colonization. J Antimicrob Chemother 34(1): 139–148
102. Ochoa–Ardila ME et al (2011) Long-term use of selective decontamination of the digestive tract does not increase antibiotic resistance: a 5-year prospective cohort study. Intensive Care Med 37:1458
103. Saunders GL, Hammond JM, Potgieter PD et al (1994) Microbiological surveillance during selective decontamination of the digestive tract (SDD). J Antimicrob Chemother 34(4): 529–544
104. de Smet AM, Hopmans TE, Minderhoud AL et al (2009) Decontamination of the digestive tract and oropharynx: hospital acquired infections after discharge from the intensive care unit. Intensive Care Med 35(9):1609–1613
105. Oostdijk EA, de Smet AM, Blok HE et al (2010) Ecological effects of selective decontamination on resistant gram-negative bacterial colonization. Am J Respir Crit Care Med 181(5):452–457
106. Bonten MJ, Gaillard CA, Johanson WG Jr et al (1994) Colonization in patients receiving and not receiving topical antimicrobial prophylaxis. Am J Respir Crit Care Med 150(5 Pt 1):1332–1340
107. Gastinne H, Wolff M, Delatour F et al (1992) A controlled trial in intensive care units of selective decontamination of the digestive tract with nonabsorbable antibiotics. The french study group on selective decontamination of the digestive tract. N Engl J Med 326(9):594–599
108. Hammond JM, Potgieter PD, Saunders GL, Forder AA (1992) Double-blind study of selective decontamination of the digestive tract in intensive care. Lancet 340(8810): 5–9
109. Ferrer M, Torres A, Gonzalez J et al (1994) Utility of selective digestive decontamination in mechanically ventilated patients. Ann Intern Med 120(5):389–395
110. Wiener J, Itokazu G, Nathan C et al (1995) A randomized, double-blind, placebo-controlled trial of selective digestive decontamination in a medical-surgical intensive care unit. Clin Infect Dis 20(4):861–867
111. Lingnau W, Berger J, Javorsky F et al (1997) Selective intestinal decontamination in multiple trauma patients: prospective, controlled trial. J Trauma 42(4):687–694
112. Verwaest C, Verhaegen J, Ferdinande P et al (1997) Randomized, controlled trial of selective digestive decontamination in 600 mechanically ventilated patients in a multidisciplinary intensive care unit. Crit Care Med 25(1):63–71
113. Sánchez M, Mir N, Canton R et al (1997) The effect of topical vancomycin on acquisition, carriage and infection with methicillin-resistant *Staphylococcus aureus* in critically ill patients (abstract). 37th Interscience Conference on Antimicrobial Agents and Chemotherapy (ICAAC) (28 Sept–1 Oct) Toronto.
114. van Saene HK, Weir WI, de La Cal MA et al (2004) MRSA—time for a more pragmatic approach? J Hosp Infect 56(3):170–174
115. White A (1961) Relation between quantitative nasal cultures and dissemination of staphylococci. J Lab Clin Med 58:273–277
116. Brodie J, Kerr MR, Sommerville T (1956) The hospital *Staphylococcus*; a comparison of nasal and faecal carrier states. Lancet 270(6906):19–20
117. Greendyke RM, Constantine HP, Agruder GB, Dean DC, Gardner JH, Morgan HR et al (1958) Staphylococci on a medical ward, with special reference to fecal carriers. Am J Clin Pathol 30(4):318–322
118. Hone R, Keane CT, Fitzpatrick S (1974) Faecal carriage of *Staphylococcus aureus* in infantile enteritis due to enteropathic *Escherichia coli*. Scand J Infect Dis 6(4):329–332

119. Brady LM, Thomson M, Palmer MA, Harkness JL (1990) Successful control of endemic MRSA in a cardiothoracic surgical unit. Med J Aust 152(5):240–245
120. Salzman TC, Clark JJ, Klemm L (1967) Hand contamination of personnel as a mechanism of cross-infection in nosocomial infections with antibiotic-resistant *Escherichia coli* and *Klebsiella-Aerobacter*. Antimicrobial.Agents Chemother 7:97–100
121. Nystrom B (1983) Optimal design/personnel for control of intensive care unit infection. Infect Control 4(5):388–390
122. Crossley K, Landesman B, Zaske D (1979) An outbreak of infections caused by strains of *Staphylococcus aureus* resistant to methicillin and aminoglycosides. II. Epidemiologic studies. J Infect Dis 139(3):280–287
123. Viviani M, van Saene HK, Dezzoni R et al (2005) Control of imported and acquired methicillin-resistant *Staphylococcus aureus* (MRSA) in mechanically ventilated patients: a dose-response study of enteral vancomycin to reduce absolute carriage and infection. Anaesth Intensive Care 33(3):361–372
124. Taylor ME, Oppenheim BA (1991) Selective decontamination of the gastrointestinal tract as an infection control measure. J Hosp Infect 17(4):271–278
125. Damjanovic V, Connolly CM, van Saene HK et al (1993) Selective decontamination with nystatin for control of a *Candida* outbreak in a neonatal intensive care unit. J Hosp Infect 24(4):245–259
126. Rice LB (2001) Emergence of vancomycin-resistant enterococci. Emerg Infect Dis 7(2):183–187
127. Sánchez M, Mir N, Cantón R et al (1997) Incidence of carriage and colonization pattern of vancomycin-resistant *enterococcus* (VRE) in intubated patients (Pts) receiving topical vancomycin (V) (abstract). 37th Interscience Conference on Antimicrobial Agents and Chemotherapy (ICAAC)
128 Stiefel U, Paterson DL, Pultz NJ et al (2004) Effect of the increasing use of piperacillin/tazobactam on the incidence of vancomycin-resistant enterococci in four academic medical centers. Infect Control Hosp Epidemiol 25(5):380–383
129. Salgado CD, Giannetta ET, Farr BM (2004) Failure to develop vancomycin-resistant Enterococcus with oral vancomycin treatment of Clostridium difficile. Infect Control Hosp Epidemiol 25(5):413–417

Part III
Infection Control

Evidence-Based Infection Control in the Intensive Care Unit

9

J. Hughes and R. P. Cooke

9.1 Introduction

The rate of healthcare-associated infections (HCAIs) is higher in the intensive care unit (ICU) patients than in the general hospital population, mainly due to its unique environment where the most severely ill patients are brought together in one unit [1]. This increases patients' susceptibility to HCAIs, particularly with multi-drug-resistant pathogenic microorganisms (MDRPMs). Risk factors for HCAIs include antimicrobials, and invasive devices such as peripheral and central intravenous catheters, urinary catheters, endotracheal tubes, tracheostomy, and surgical and chest drains [2]. Due to the amount of patient-care contact in the ICU environment, the risk of HCAIs is further increased. With the often urgent nature of ICU interventions, suboptimal compliance with infection prevention and control (IPC) practices can occur [3].

As a result of the high priority given to quality management, clinical governance and patient safety, HCAIs rates are increasingly in the political and public spotlight. In the UK, trusts are held accountable by the 2008 Health Act. Code of Practice for the Prevention and Control of Health Care Associated Infections [4]. In addition, from 2009, trusts had to register with the Care Quality Commission, a new regulatory body that has enforcement powers against noncompliant organisations [5].

To achieve sustainable reductions in HCAIs in the ICU, the support, commitment and engagement of all healthcare workers (HCWs), both clinical and nonclinical, are essential [6]. Though no single action on its own will guarantee

---

J. Hughes (✉)
Infection Prevention and Control, 5 Boroughs Partnership NHS
FoundationTrust/University of Chester Warrington,
Winwick, Warrington, UK
e-mail: Julie.hughes@5bp.nhs.uk

Table 9.1 Classification of the US Centre for Disease Control guidelines

Category	Application
IA	Strongly recommended for implementation and then supported by well-designed experimental, clinical or epidemiological studies
IB	Strongly recommended for implementation and then supported by certain experimental, clinical or epidemiological studies and a strong theoretical rationale
IC	Required for implementation, as mandated by federal and/or state regulation or standard
II	Suggested for implementation and then supported by suggestive clinical or epidemiological studies or a theoretical rationale
No recommendation/ unresolved issue	Practices for which insufficient evidence or no consensus regarding efficacy exist

effective results, adherence to IPC practices is one of the best means of minimising HCAIs [7].

Universally accepted standards for IPC include hand hygiene, use of personal protective equipment (PPE), patient isolation, care of equipment and environmental cleanliness [7, 8]. The role of invasive devices, antibiotics and surveillance-related policies are discussed in Chaps. 10 and 11. Although there are a number of studies on the benefits of such IPC measures, the evidence base is often questionable or lacking [9]. However, several studies and reviews have tried to address this issue [10–12]. In 2010, the European Centre for Disease Prevention and Control (ECDC) convened a group of experts to discuss patient safety and infection prevention and control to formulate risk-based strategies and evidence-based measures for effective HCAI reduction [13].

9.2 Evidence-Based Practice in the ICU

Evidence-based practice (EBP) should enable HCWs to be confident that their interventions are informed by a sound knowledge base. Clinical care guidelines provide key principles for good practice and ensure that practices can be standardised and auditable [9–14]. Therefore, the following review and recommendations are based on guidance provided by the US Centre for Disease Control (CDC) (Table 9.1), the UK Department of Health Epic 2: National Evidence-Based Guidelines for Preventing Healthcare-Associated Infections in Hospitals and the World Health Organisation (WHO) [11, 12, 15]. Although some of the evidence for prevention and control is based on studies in the general hospital population (Table 9.2), many interventions to prevent and control HCAIs, in particular, methicillin-resistant *Staphylococcus aureus* (MRSA), were pioneered initially in the ICU, being a reflection of the magnitude of the problem across the entire patient population [16]. Therefore, adherence to infection prevention and control EBP will affect not only the ICU but the rest of the healthcare facility (Table 9.3).

Table 9.2 Recommendations for hand hygiene (*HCWs* healthcare workers; classification of the US Centre for Disease Control guidelines)

Recommendation	Level of evidence
When hands are visibly dirty or contaminated with proteinaceous material or are visibly soiled with blood or other body fluids, wash hands with water and either a nonantimicrobial or an antimicrobial soap	IA
If hands are not visibly soiled, use an alcohol-based hand rub for routinely decontaminating hands in all other clinical situations described	IC
Decontaminate hands after contact with a patient's intact skin (e.g. when taking a pulse or blood pressure and lifting)	IB
Decontaminate hands after contact with body fluids or excretions, mucous membranes, nonintact skin and wound dressings if hands are not visibly soiled	IA
Decontaminate hands after removing gloves	IB
Before eating and after using a restroom, wash hands with water and either a nonantimicrobial or antimicrobial soap	IB
No recommendation can be made regarding the routine use of non-alcohol-based hand rubs for hand hygiene in healthcare settings	Unresolved issue
When decontaminating hands with an alcohol-based hand rub, apply product to palm of one hand and rub hands together, covering all surfaces of hands and fingers, until hands are dry	IB
When washing hands with soap and water, wet hands first with water, apply an amount of product recommended by the manufacturer to hands, and rub hands together vigorously for at least 15 s, covering all surfaces of the hands and fingers. Rinse hands with water and dry thoroughly with a disposable towel. Use paper towel to turn off the faucet	IB
Provide personnel with efficacious hand-hygiene products that have low irritancy potential, particularly when these products are used many times per shift. This recommendation applies to products used for hand antisepsis before and after patient care in clinical areas and to products used for surgical hand antisepsis by surgical personnel	IB
Do not add soap to a partially empty soap dispenser. This practice of "topping up" dispensers can lead to a bacterial contamination of the soap	IA
Provide HCWs with hand lotions or creams to minimise the occurrence of irritant contact dermatitis associated with hand antisepsis or handwashing	IA
As part of a multidisciplinary programme to improve hand-hygiene adherence, provide HCWs with a readily accessible alcohol-based hand-rub product	IA
To improve hand-hygiene adherence among personnel who work in areas in which high workloads and high intensity of patient care are anticipated, make an alcohol-based hand rub available at the entrance to all patient rooms or at the bedside, in other convenient locations and in individual pocket-sized containers to be carried by HCWs	IA

HCW healthcare workers

Table 9.3 Recommendations for protective clothing and care of equipment and environment

Recommendation	Level of evidence
Select protective equipment on the basis of a risk assessment of microorganism transmission	II
Gloves Wear gloves (clean, nonsterile gloves are adequate) when touching blood, body fluids, secretions, excretions and contaminated items. Put on clean sterile gloves just before touching mucous membranes and nonintact skin. Change gloves between tasks and procedures on the same patient after contact with material that may contain a high concentration of microorganisms. Remove gloves promptly after use, before touching noncontaminated items and environmental surfaces and before going to another patient, and decontaminate hands immediately to avoid transfer of microorganisms to other patients or environments	IB
Face and eye protection Wear a mask or a face shield to protect mucous membranes of the eyes, nose and mouth during procedures and patient-care activities that are likely to generate splashes or sprays of blood, body fluids, secretions or excretions	IB
Gown Wear a gown (a clean, nonsterile gown is adequate) to protect skin and prevent soiling of clothing during procedures and patient-care activities that are likely to generate splashes or sprays of blood, body fluids, secretions or excretions. Select a gown that is appropriate for the activity and amount of fluid likely to be encountered. Remove a soiled gown as promptly as possible, and wash hands to avoid transfer of microorganisms to other patients or environments	IB
Isolation Place in a private room a patient who contaminates the environment or who does not (or cannot be expected to) assist in maintaining appropriate hygiene or environmental control. If a private room is not available, consult with infection-control professionals regarding patient placement or other alternatives	IB
Patient-care equipment Handle used equipment soiled with blood, body fluids, secretions or excretions in a manner that prevents skin and mucous-membrane exposure, clothing contamination and microorganism transfer to other patients and environments. Ensure that reusable equipment is not used for the care of another patient until it has been cleaned and reprocessed appropriately. Ensure that single-use items are discarded properly	IB
Environmental control Ensure that the hospital has adequate procedures for the routine care, cleaning and disinfecting of environmental surfaces, beds, bedrails, bedside equipment and other frequently touched surfaces, and ensure that these procedures are being followed. Handle, transport, and process used linen soiled with blood, body fluids, secretions or excretions in a manner that prevents skin and mucous-membrane exposure and clothing contamination and that avoids microorganism transfer to other patients and environments	IB

9.3 Five Main IPC Manoeuvres

9.3.1 Hand Hygiene

Hand washing is often referred to as the single most important means of preventing HCAIs [11, 12, 15, 16]. The UK epic2: Guidelines for Preventing Healthcare Associated Infections in NHS Hospitals in England suggest that effective hand decontamination can significantly reduce infection rates in high-risk areas such as the ICU [11]. However, there is no supporting level 1 evidence, (i.e. randomised controlled trials), as ethical approval for such studies would be not possible. The available evidence is based on expert consensus opinion and several observational epidemiological studies [11, 12, 15]. WHO guidelines on hand hygiene identify "Five Moments for Hand Hygiene" [12]. Hands must be decontaminated and dried thoroughly immediately before each direct patient contact/care episode and after any activity or contact that can result in hands becoming contaminated, such as contact with patient-care equipment and their immediate environment.

Many guidelines and studies review a variety of differing products for hand decontamination, with some studies suggesting that soap and water is as effective as antimicrobial-based hand-washing products [11]. Alcohol-based hand rubs (ABHRs) are highly popular in ICUs but alone are not effective in removing physical dirt of soiling, with some studies suggesting that they are not deemed as effective in removing spore-forming bacteria such as *Clostridium difficile,* although other studies repute this [17]. Some studies have also shown that once alcohol gel has evaporated, a residue is left that can be deposited in the environment and which may facilitate growth of organisms such as *Acinetobacter* species [18]. To combat these problems, newer gels with an aloe vera base and containing copper-based biocidal formulations are being trialled that may also be less irritating to HCWs hands [19].

Most studies fail to find compelling evidence for the general use of one hand contaminant agent over another. However, all infer that HCW's acceptability and effective hand hygiene techniques and adequate drying are the most essential factors when selecting products to promote compliance with hand washing. In Europe, there are a set of standards, referred to as European Norms (EN), which are laboratory tests that any product needs to pass before it can be marketed. Therefore, any product chosen should comply with EN standards [20].

Hand decontamination is often poorly performed, and several studies demonstrate that compliance can be suboptimal [11, 12, 21], particularly by some physicians. The various reasons for this include availability of hand-decontamination facilities, selection of harsh hand-care products, workload and HCW attitudes. ICUs should always have enough easily accessible hand-wash basins, the recommended ratio being 1 to 1 per ICU bed in the UK. The increased availability of ABHRs has also been found to improve compliance [12], as have regular hand-decontamination training sessions/audits and feedback to all ICU staff [11, 12, 21]. Reinforcing the importance of physicians, in particular, as positive role models to influence behaviour could also help, as they are often the main leads for ICU. Hand-decontamination policies should also ensure that no jewellery, including watches and rings (other than a plain wedding band) are worn, nails are kept short and acrylic/false fingernails and nail polish are prohibited [11, 12]. Clinical staff should wear short sleeves (or long sleeves rolled up to above the elbow) when performing patient-care procedures. In the UK, this is referred to as the principle of "bare below the elbow" [22]. However, although hand hygiene is the cornerstone of IPC, it is nonetheless not a stand-alone procedure and should be part of a multifaceted approach [23].

9.4 Personal Protective Equipment (PPE)

PPE includes the use of aprons, gowns, gloves, eye protection and face masks and should be easily accessible to all HCWs. Employers have a duty to provide PPE for staff who in turn have to wear PPE to comply with health and safety guidelines, such as the Personal Protective Equipment Regulations (1992), which are compulsory in some countries, e.g. the UK [24]. However, wearing PPE should always be based on a patient- and task-risk assessment.

Gloves are one of the most effective barriers against microorganisms, although studies have shown both lack of understanding and poor compliance with glove use [11, 15, 25]. This includes gloves being worn when not required or worn for prolonged periods with hands not being washed following glove removal. Gloves can also cause adverse skin reactions and skin sensitivity [11, 25]. Sterile gloves should be worn for all invasive procedures and contact with nonintact skin. Nonsterile gloves are suitable for all other procedures. Gloves should also be single-use items and discarded immediately after each activity, followed by hand decontamination [25].

Disposable plastic aprons are just as effective as gowns in most situations. However, where there is a possibility of contamination of the HCW's clothing with blood or body fluids, it is recommended that disposable plastic aprons are worn. Gowns are only required where there is a risk of gross contamination of splashing, such as in major burn patients or severe trauma, or when dealing with biohazard group 4 pathogens (e.g. Lassa fever) [11, 15, 26]. HCWs should also have access to facial and eye protection. Personal respiratory protection is required when caring for patients with serious infections, such as tuberculosis pandemic flu when aerosol-generating procedures are performed [26, 27]. The choice of mask/respirator will depend on the level and extent of protection required. Eye protection and visors should be worn when there is a risk of body-fluid contamination to the face or eyes.

9.5 Isolation

In addition to standard IPC precautions, further procedures (i.e. side-room isolation) should be implemented if a patient is identified as carrying a highly transmissible microbe. Several studies have demonstrated that isolation precautions are effective in achieving a significant reduction in transmission, particularly in relation to glycopeptide-resistant enterococci, *C. difficile*, respiratory syncytial virus (RSV), MRSA, chickenpox and *Acinetobacter* [11, 15, 16, 27–29]. However, some studies have disputed the role of isolation in preventing MRSA transmission [30]. Nonetheless, current guidance suggest isolating or cohorting most patients with transmissible infections wherever possible. Furthermore, these precautions should be commenced on suspicion without awaiting microbiological confirmation [11, 15, 31–33]. Isolating patients may also be difficult due to the lack of single rooms. In this event, a risk assessment with the infection prevention and control team (IPCT) should be undertaken, and procedures should be simple to implement and follow [34].

9.6 Patient-Care Equipment

Patient-care equipment such as ventilators, humidifiers, analysers and transducers have all been implicated in ICU and anaesthesia-associated outbreaks [1, 21, 35], particularly where equipment is shared between patients. Common procedures and device-related infections are discussed within Chap. 11.

9.6.1 High-Risk Items

High-risk items include invasive devices in contact with a break in the skin or with mucous membranes, or those introduced into a sterile body area, such as surgical instruments, catheters, prosthetic devices etc. These items require sterilisation, but if that is not practically achievable, e.g. in the case of flexible endoscopes, then high-level disinfection.

9.6.2 Intermediate Risk

These include items in contact with intact mucous membranes or body fluids, are contaminated with particularly virulent or readily transmissible organisms, or items to be used on highly susceptible patients or sites, e.g. endoscopes and respiratory equipment require disinfection.

9.6.3 Low-Risk Items

These items are those in contact with normal or intact skin, e.g. thermometers, stethoscopes, washbowls, toilets and bedding. Cleaning and drying is usually sufficient, but disinfecting is required in the case of a patient with a known infection risk, e.g. MRSA.

9.6.4 Minimal-Risk Items

Minimal-risk items are items that do not come into contact with the patient, such as floors and surfaces. Cleaning and drying is usually adequate unless in an outbreak situation. Equipment used for invasive procedures should be decontaminated after being used on every patient, not only on those known to be infected. Equipment such as stethoscopes and thermometers should be designated to individual patients wherever possible. When dedicated equipment is not practical, e.g. portable X-ray and ultrasound machines, staff should ensure that such equipment is decontaminated between patients. Policies should ensure that all staff receive training and are aware of their roles and responsibilities in relation to decontamination. The policy should also ensure close liaison with procurement officers and the IPC team when purchasing any new equipment.

9.7 Patient-Care Environment

Although the ICU patient's surrounding is classed as low risk, a clean environment provides the background for good standards of hygiene as well as maintaining patient, staff and visitor confidence [1]. In the UK, the ICU environment is categorised as a high-risk area under the Standards of Environmental Cleanliness in Hospitals Guidelines [36]. When considering the role of the environment in the ICU, the design of the unit should ensure that there is adequate space between beds to allow easy access for staff and equipment [37, 38]. Furniture and fixtures should be kept to a minimum and be of materials that are easy to clean. A suitable area should also be designated for safe storage of equipment. "Dirty" and "clean" areas should be separate so that no mixing of equipment occurs, and clinical waste should be stored where there is no risk of transporting waste through clean or patient areas. Despite the pressure for ICU beds, ICU mangers should maintain close liaison with domestic services staff to maintain standards.

9.8 Audit and Surveillance

As stated the IPC, manoeuvres referred to should be used in conjunction and are rarely stand alone. Therefore, it is often a challenge to gauge exactly which manoeuvres reviewed reduce HCAIs, and the evidence should be viewed in light of this. However, to ensure compliance with IPC and monitor HCAIs, it is essential that there are effective audit and surveillance systems in place to monitor HCAIs [6–8, 39, 40].

The Saving Lives High Impact Interventions (HIIs), launched in the UK in 2005, are practical EBP tools to audit practice and compliance and help reduce HCAI [6–8]. These are based on a care-bundle approach and have been implemented by many ICUs in the UK. There are several available, e.g. care of invasive devices such as peripheral, central venous and urinary catheters, reducing

9 Evidence-Based Infection Control in the Intensive Care Unit   153

surgical-site infections, reducing the risk of *C. difficile* and cleaning and decontamination of the environment.

In relation to surveillance the rapid rise in the rate of bacterial antibiotic resistance in ICU patients is well recognised [41]. Four key organism groups warrant regular surveillance in the ICU setting, as highlighted by the National Nosocomial Infections Surveillance (NNIS) system report in MDRPMs in US ICUs [42]. These include MRSA, vancomycin-resistant *Enterococcus faecium* (VRE), *Pseudomonas aeruginosa* resistant to carbapenems or fluoroquinolones and Enterobacteriaceae resistant to third-generation cephalosporins [including production of extended-spectrum beta-lactamases (ESBLs)]. ICU screening protocols for MRSA and VRE are well established through infection control; guidelines for ESBL surveillance are lacking.

Many factors contribute to the high incidence of nosocomial infections in the ICU and associated poor patient outcomes. Though most studies have come from industrialised countries, the rates of infection in developing countries may be higher [43]. This relates particularly to the use of invasive devices, the use of which should be linked to an ICU audit programme. Such a programme should look at not only infection rates but mortality rates, length of ICU stay and hospital costs.

Indwelling devices, such as central venous catheters (VCs), Foley catheters and endotracheal tubes, bypass natural host defence mechanisms and predispose to infection. The Surveillance and Control of Pathogens of Epidemiological Importance (SCOPE) database found that 51% of all catheter-associated blood-stream infections (CR-BSIs) in 49 US hospitals occurred in the ICU. CR-BSI rates per 1,000 catheter days for a variety of vascular devices were listed in the report [44]. A recent systematic review indicated that CR-BSIs per 1,000 catheter days range from 0.5 for peripheral VCs to 1.6 for long-term central VCs, 1.7 for arterial catheters, 2.1 for peripherally inserted central VCs and 2.7 for short-term central VCs [45]. EPIC guidelines recommend using antimicrobial-impregnated central VC if short-term CR-BSI rates are high despite introducing a comprehensive strategy to reduce rates [11].

The highest risk for nosocomial pneumonia is in patients on mechanical ventilation [i.e. ventilator-associated pneumonia (VAP)], which has been the most studied form of nosocomial pneumonia. ICUs should therefore identify cases of VAP and collect data on the number of ventilator-associated days on a routine basis.

Catheter-associated urinary tract infection (UTI) is overall the most common nosocomial infection. In the ICU setting, auditing infection per 1,000 catheter days will allow a rational approach for using urinary catheters impregnated with either antimicrobial or antiseptic agents.

9.9   Use of the Microbiology Laboratory by the ICU

The purpose of a microbiology laboratory is to provide an accurate and clinically relevant service in a timely manner. In the context of ICU, this must be available 7 days per week. Whenever possible, every effort should be made to obtain specimens prior to starting antibiotic therapy, especially by taking two independent blood cultures from septic patients.

Prompt transport to the laboratory is equally essential. Once local criteria are agreed upon, this can usually be by means of a pneumatic tube system directly to the microbiology laboratory. The ICU must also be supported by good information technology access to microbiology reports. This should be complemented by daily ward rounds involving a consultant in microbiology or infectious diseases.

In certain circumstances, point-of-care microbiology testing in the ICU may offer a more rapid response service. For MRSA screening, this may have a number of advantages, but it must be offset against local MRSA prevalence, standard laboratory turnaround times and equipment/staff consumable cost [46].

Selective decontamination of the digestive tract (SDD) is an antimicrobial strategy that reduces the incidence of severe infections of lower airways and blood by eradicating throat and gut carriage of normal and abnormal flora. Sixty randomised controlled trials (RCTs) and 11 meta-analyses demonstrated that SDD confers protection against severe infections of lower airways and blood [47]. Despite the optimism regarding SDD, it has not been used widely in the ICU setting, principally due to anxiety in the emergence of antibiotic-resistant bacteria [48]. Hence, in units that wish to perform SDD, a bacteriological protocol for gut-surveillance cultures as opposed to diagnostic cultures is recommended. SDD is discussed in Chap. 13.

9.10 Summary and Conclusions

In this chapter, recommendations for EBP IPC practice and strategies have been made following review of the literature. However, to ensure best practice, ICUs should also be adequately staffed, as many studies demonstrate the detrimental effect of poor staffing-to-patient ratios and increased workload [49, 50]. Good IPC practices in the ICU rely on strong medical and nursing leadership plus good multidisciplinary working practices. It also needs to be recognised that IPC in the ICU patient must be practised slightly differently from the non-ICU patient. Hence, specific IPC policies and procedures for the ICU should be drawn up. These should be underpinned by audit and surveillance to demonstrate that they are working effectively, and they should be reviewed by the multidisciplinary group on a regular basis.

References

1. Cooper M (2009) Prevention of infection in special wards and departments–critical care units. In: Fraise AP, Bradley C (eds) Ayliffe's control of healthcare-associated infection, 5th edn. Hodder Arnold, Kent
2. Fraise AP, Bradley C (eds) (2009) Ayliffe's control of healthcare-associated infection, 5th edn. Hodder Arnold, Kent UK
3. Department of Health (2006) Infection prevention and control in adult critical care reducing the risk of infection through best practice. Department of Health, London

4. Department of Health (2009) The health and social care act 2008: code of practice for the NHS on the prevention and control of health care associated infections and related guidance. Department of Health, London
5. Care Quality Commission (2008) Registering with the Care Quality Commission in relation to healthcare associated infection. Guidance for trust 2009/10. Care Quality Commission, London
6. Department of Health (2006) Saving lives: a delivery programme to reduce healthcare associated infection, including MRSA screening for methicillin-resistant *Staphylococcus aureus* (MRSA) colonisation: a strategy for NHS trusts: a summary of best practice. Department of Health, London
7. Department of Health (2006) Going further faster: implementing the saving lives delivery programme sustainable change for cleaner safer care. Department of Health, London
8. Department of Health (2008) Clean safe care reducing infections and saving lives. Department of Health, London
9. Ayliffe GJ (2000) Evidence-based practises in infection control. Br J Infect Control 1(4):5–9
10. NICE (2004) Guideline development methods: information for national collaborating centres and guideline developers. National Institute for Health and Clinical Excellence (updated 2005)
11. Pratt RP, Pellowe CM, Wilson JA et al (2007) epic2: national evidence-based guidelines for preventing healthcare-associated infections in hospitals in England. J Hosp Infect 65S:S1–S64
12. World Health Organization (2009) Patient safety a world alliance for safer health care. WHO guidelines on hand hygiene in health care. First global patient safety challenge clean care is safer care. WHO, Geneva
13. European centre for disease prevention and control (2010) meeting report: expert consultation on healthcare-associated infection prevention and control. ECDC Stockholm
14. Harbour R, Miller JA (2001) A new system for grading recommendations in evidence-based guidelines. BMJ 323:334–336
15. Siegel JD, Rhineheart E, Jackson M, Chiarello L (2007) Guideline for isolation precautions: preventing transmission of infectious agents in healthcare settings. The Healthcare Infection Control Practices Advisory Committee. Available at http://www.cdc.gov/ncidod/dhqp/pdf/guidelines/isolation2007.pdf. Accessed Jun 2011
16. Humphreys H (2008) Can we do better in controlling and preventing methicillin-resistant *Staphylococcus aureus* (MRSA) in the intensive care unit (ICU)? Eur J Clin Micro Infect Dis 27(6):409–413
17. Boyce JM, Ligi C, Kohan C et al (2006) Lack of association between the increased incidence of *Clostridium difficile*-associated disease and the increasing use of alcohol-based hand rubs. Infect Control Hosp Epidemiol 27(5):479–483
18. Edwards J, Patel G, Wareham DW (2007) Low concentrations of commercial alcohol hand rubs facilitate the growth of and secretion of extracellular proteins by multidrug-resistant strains of *Acinetobacter baumannii*. J Med Micro 56:1595–1599
19. Hall TJ, Wren MWD, Wareham DW et al (2010) Effect of the dried residues of two hand gels on the survival of methicillin–resistant *Staphylococcus aureus* and *Acinetobacter calcoaceticus-baumannii*. J Inf Prev 11(3):70–72
20. Fraise A, Bradley C (2007) Decontamination of equipment, the environment and the skin. In: Fraise AP, Bradley C (eds) Ayliffe's control of healthcare-associated infection, 5th edn. Hodder Arnold, Kent
21. Pittet D, Simon A, Hugonnet S (2004) Hand hygiene among physicians: performance, beliefs, and perceptions. Ann Intern Med 141:11–18
22. Department of Health (2010) Uniform and workwear: guidance on uniform and workwear policies for NHS employers. Department of Health, London
23. Silvestri L, Petros AJ, Sarginson RE et al (2005) Review: handwashing in the intensive care unit: a big measure with modest effects. J Hosp Inf 59:172–179
24. Health and Safety Executive (1992) The personal protective equipment at work regulations guidance on regulations. The Stationery Office, London

25. Infection Control Nurses Association (2002) Protective clothing: principles and guidance. Fitwise, Bathgate
26. Ho PL, Tang XP, Seto WH (2003) SARS: hospital infection control and admission strategies. Respirology 8:S41–S45
27. Humphreys H (2007) Control and prevention of healthcare-associated tuberculosis: the role of respiratory isolation and personal respiratory protection. J Hosp Inf 66(1):1–5
28. Trautmann M, Pollitt A, Loh U et al (2007) Implementation of an intensified infection control program to reduce MRSA transmission in a German tertiary care hospital. Am J Infect Control 35(10):643–649
29. Raineri E, Crema L, De Sivestri A et al (2007) Methicillin-resistant *Staphylococcus aureus* in an intensive care unit: a 10 year analysis. J Hosp Infect 67(4):308–315
30. Cepeda JA, Whitehouse T, Cooper B et al (2005) Isolation of patients in single rooms or cohorts to reduce spread of MRSA in intensive-care units: prospective two-centre study. Lancet 36(945):295–304
31. Farr BM, Bellingan G (2004) Pro/con clinical debate: isolation precautions for all intensive care unit patients with methicillin-resistant Staphylococcus aureus colonisation are essential. Crit Care 8(3):153–156
32. Groothuis J, Bauman J, Malinoski F, Eggleston M (2008) Strategies for prevention of RSV nosocomial infection. J Perinatol 28(5):319–323
33. Kappstein I, van der Muhlen K, Meschzan D et al (2009) Prevention of transmission of methicillin-resistant Staphylococcus aureus (MRSA) infection: standard precautions instead of isolation: a 6-year surveillance in a university hospital. Chirurg 80(1):49–61
34. Kilpatrick C, Prieto J, Wigglesworth N (2008) Single room isolation to prevent transmission of infection: development of a patient journey tool to support safe practice. Br J Inf Control 9(6):19–25
35. King TA, Cooke RPD (2005) Cleaning, disinfection and sterilisation. In: Darcy AJ, Diba A (eds) Ward's anaesthetic equipment, 5th edn. Elsevier, London
36. National Patient Safety Agency (2007) The national specifications for cleanliness in the NHS, London. NHS/NPSA. Available at www.npsa.nhs.uk/health/currentprojects/nutrition/cleaning. Accessed Jun 2011
37. Dettenkofer M, Seegers S, Antes G et al (2004) Does the architecture of hospital facilities influence infection rates? A systematic review. Infect Control Hosp Epidemiol 25(1):21–25
38. Estates NHS (2005) Health building note 57: facilities for critical care. The Stationery Office, London
39. McGingle KL, Gourlay ML, Buchanan IB (2008) The use of active surveillance cultures in adult intensive care units to reduce methicillin-resistant *Staphylococcus aureus*-related morbidity, mortality, and costs: a systematic review. Clin Infect Dis 46(11):1717–1725
40. Aragon D, Sole ML (2006) Implementing best practice strategies to prevent infection in the ICU. Crit Care Clin N Am 18(4):441–452
41. Ahern JW, Alston WK (2009) Use of longitudinal surveillance data to assess the effectiveness of infection control in critical care. Infect Control Hosp Epidemiol 30(11):1109–1112
42. National Nosocomial Infections Surveillance (2000) NNIS system report, data summary from January 1992–April. Am J Infect Control 28:429
43. Depuydt PO, Blot SI, Benoit DD et al (2006) Antimicrobial resistance in nosocomial bloodstream infection associated with pneumonia and the value of systematic surveillance cultures in an adult intensive care unit. Crit Care Med 34(3):653–659
44. Wisplinghoff H, Bischoff T, Tallent SM (2004) Nosocomial bloodstream a prospective nationwide surveillance study. Clin Infect Dis 39:309–317
45. Maki DG, Kluger DM, Crivich CJ (2006) The risk of bloodstream infection in adults with different intravascular devices: a systematic review of 200 published prospective studies. Mayo Clin Pro 23006:1159–1171
46. Cunningham R, Jenks B, Northwood J (2007) Effect of MRSA transmission of rapid PCR testing of patients admitted to critical care. J Hosp Infect 65:24–38

47. Silvestri L, van Saene HK, Casarin A (2008) Impact of selective decontamination of the digestive tract on carriage and infection due to Gram-negative and Gram-positive bacteria: a systematic review of randomised controlled trials. Anaesth Intensive Care 36:324–338
48. Oostdijk EA, de Smet AM, Blok HE et al (2010) Ecological effects of selective decontamination on resistant Gram-negative bacterial colonization. Am J Respir Crit Care Med 181(5):452–457
49. Stone PW, Mooney-Kane C, Larson EL (2007) Nurse working conditions and patient safety outcomes. Med Care 45(6):571–578
50. Hugonnet S, Chevrolet JC, Pittet D (2007) The effect of workload on infections in critically ill patients. Crit Care Med 35(11):76–81

Device Policies

10

A. R. De Gaudio, A. Casini and A. Di Filippo

10.1 Introduction

This chapter presents a summary of the latest guidelines for preventing infections in intensive care units (ICUs), particularly regarding ventilation-associated pneumonia (VAP), catheter-related bloodstream infections (CRBSI), and catheter-associated urinary tract infections (UTI). Recent clinical trials were evaluated to investigate the latest products, procedures, and treatments aimed at preventing infections in ICUs. A summary table is provided, describing the most recent acquisitions and their effectiveness (Table 10.1).

10.2 Ventilation-Associated Pneumonia

The 2004 guidelines for preventing VAP indicate the existence of fundamental principles that possess level 1A evidence [1, 2]. These principles include educating all workers about health epidemiology and VAP control procedures, instructing them on how to effectively use various techniques, and continuous technique updating through regular audits. The guidelines advise thorough cleaning of all equipment (sterilization when possible, or high-level disinfection), with attention to complete rinsing with sterile water, drying, and packaging. The ventilation circuit should not be changed routinely on the basis of duration of use if used on a single patient; rather, the circuit should be changed only when it is visibly dirty or mechanically malfunctioning. When removing the condensation tube, healthcare workers' hands must be cleaned with soap and water or alcohol-based

---

A. Di Filippo (✉)
Department of Critical Care Section of Anaesthesia,
c/o Careggi Teaching Hospital,
University of Florence, Firenze, Italy
e-mail: adifilippo@unifi.it

Table 10.1 Recent advances in preventing intensive care patient infections and their effectiveness assessed by large clinical trials

Method	Study contents	Efficacy	Reference
Ventilation-associated pneumonia			
Oral cavity decontamination	Chlorhexidine (0,2%) versus potassium permanganate	Not effective	[3]
	Saline versus chlorhexidine 2% versus chlorhexidine 2% + colistin 2%	Effective	[4]
	Chlorhexidine (0,2%) gel	Not Effective	[5]
	Povidone iodine versus saline	Effective	[6]
	Electric toothbrushes versus chlorhexidine	Not effective	[7]
Endotracheal secretion removal	Washing with isotonic saline	Effective	[8]
	Closed tracheal suction system versus open system	Not effective	[9]
Subglottic continuous suction		Effective	[10]
Materials	Polyurethane versus polyvinyl chloride tube	Effective	[11]
	Polyurethane cuff and subglottic suction tube versus polyvinyl tube with no subglottic suction	Effective	[12]
Cuff inflation control	Automatic	Not effective	[13]
	Low-pressure and low-volume inflating cuff	Effective	[14]
	Cuff lubrication	Effective	[15]
Silver-coated endotracheal tube	Preliminary study	Effective	[16]
	NASCENT study	Effective	[17]
Humidification device	Humidification method	Not effective	[18]
	Humidification method	Not effective	[19]
	Antibacterial filters	Not effective	[20]
Tracheotomy	Early tracheotomy	Not effective	[21]
	Early tracheotomy	Effective	[22]
Mechanical ventilation mode	Prophylactic PEEP	Effective	[23]
Patient positioning	Prone position	Not effective	[24, 25]
Selective decontamination of the digestive tract		Effective	[26]

(continued)

Table 10.1 (continued)

Method	Study contents	Efficacy	Reference
Catheter-related bloodstream infections			
Medicated catheters	Catheters with silver–platinum–carbon versus catheters with rifampicin–minocycline	Effective but not different	[29]
	Catheters with chlorhexidine and sulfadiazine versus standard catheters	Effective	[30]
	Silver-impregnated versus standard multilumen catheters	Not effective	[31]
Catheter tunneling	Long-stay medicated catheter versus tunneled catheter	Effective	[32]
Site chosen	Jugular versus femoral	Not effective	[33]
Medication	Chlorhexidine versus povidone iodine alcohol	Effective	[34]
	Chlorhexidine for daily hygiene	Effective	[35]
	Chlorhexidine-impregnated wipes	Effective	[36]
Urinary tract infections			
Medicated catheters	Nitrofurazone-impregnated versus silicone catheters	Effective	[38]
	Hydrophilic catheters	Not effective	[39]
Antibiotic prophylaxis	Trimethoprim/sulfamethoxazole in three doses	Effective	[40]

NASCENT North American Silver-Coated Endotracheal Tube investigation group

disinfectants. Nebulizers should only be used with sterile liquid and should be placed with the most aseptic maneuver possible.

To prevent infection transmission from person to person, contaminated hands should be frequently and thoroughly washed with water and soap (antimicrobial or nonantimicrobial) or with an alcoholic antiseptic solution. This procedure must be performed before and after any contact with intubated or tracheostomized patients, as well as before and after contact with any respiratory device. It is also recommended to wear gloves for handling respiratory secretions or contaminated objects and to change gloves and decontaminate hands between contact with different patients and between contact with a contaminated body site and the respiratory tract.

To prevent inhalation of gastric content, it is good practice to remove all devices, such as endotracheal, tracheostomy, or enteral feeding tubes when clinical indications are absent. When the patient's condition permits, orotracheal intubation should be preferred over nasotracheal intubation. Enteral tube placement should be routinely controlled to prevent enteral nutrition-combined inhalation. Postoperative pneumonia can be prevented by directing high-risk patients to breathe deeply and ambulate as soon as possible. Indeed, this education would benefit all postsurgery patients.

Recent clinical trials investigated the main methods for preventing VAP and found that poor oral hygiene in patients undergoing mechanical ventilation is often associated with secondary colonization of the respiratory tract, leading to subsequent development of pneumonia. This observation implies that proper oral hygiene should reduce VAP incidence; however, the existence of highly resistant microorganisms makes the benefit of this strategy unclear.

Multiple strategies are used to decontaminate the oral cavity. For example, Panchabhai et al. compared chlorhexidine (CHX) 0.2% with a control solution of 0.01% potassium permanganate in a prospective randomized trial [3]. Oral hygiene was performed twice daily on 512 patients admitted to ICUs. Statistical analysis indicated that the VAP incidence was not correlated with oral hygiene using CHX or potassium permanganate. Mortality, seen as a secondary outcome, occurred at rates of 34.8% for CHX-treated patients and 28.3% for the control group. However, the VAP incidence was lower (7.4%) 3 months after treatment compared with 3 months before (21.7%), regardless of treatment type. Therefore, oral hygiene seems to act as a protective factor against VAP development independently of the pharmacological agent employed [3].

Koeman et al. conducted a randomized double-blind trial of 385 patients divided into three groups: 130 placebo-treated patients, 127 treated with CHX 2%, and 128 treated with CHX 2% + colistin 2% [4]. The daily risk of VAP was reduced in both treatment groups compared with placebo: 65% [hazard ratio (HR) = 0.352; 95% confidence interval (CI), 0.160–0.791; $p = 0.012$] for CHX and 55% (HR = 0.454; 95% CI, 0.224–0.925; $p = 0.030$) for CHX/COL. The combination of colistin (COL) with CHX resulted in a significant reduction in colonization by Gram-positive and Gram-negative endotracheal and oral microorganisms [4]. However, in a multicenter prospective double-blind trial conducted in 228 patients undergoing mechanical ventilation for at least 5 days, oral CHX gel decontamination was not associated with significant decreases in VAP incidence, hospitalization duration, or mortality, nor was it effective against multi-drug-resistant microorganisms (*Pseudomonas aeruginosa*, *Acinetobacter*, Enterobacteriaceae) [5].

The use of povidone iodine for oral decontamination seems to be related to reduced development of secondary infections. Regular use was associated with a significant reduction in the incidence of VAP in a prospective randomized study conducted on 98 patients with severe head trauma who underwent mechanical ventilation for at least 48 h [6]. In this study, 36 patients were treated with povidone iodine, 31 with saline, and the rest with simple secretion aspiration; VAP incidence was 8, 39, and 42%, respectively. There were no statistically significant differences in duration of hospitalization or intra-ICU mortality among the groups [6].

Effective VAP reduction due to the use of electric toothbrushes is still controversial. In a recent prospective trial conducted on 147 patients intubated for more than 48 h, Pobo et al. demonstrated that the use of electric toothbrushes did not significantly reduce VAP development compared with 0.12% CHX oral hygiene [7].

Removing endotracheal secretions appears to be a primary step in preventing VAP and can be carried out continuously or at scheduled intervals. Periodic secretion aspiration after instilling isotonic saline seems to reduce VAP incidence in patients with tracheotomies. A randomized trial of 262 patients admitted to ICUs revealed that VAP incidence was significantly lower in patients in whom aspiration was performed following administered isotonic saline (23.5 vs. 10.8%, $p < 0.008$), with a relative risk of 54% (95% CI = 18–74%). In contrast, the incidence of atelectasis and endotracheal tube obstruction was similar in both groups [8]. Secretion aspiration can be performed with closed or open systems. No significant difference in VAP prevention was found in a randomized study of 443 patients, 210 treated with a closed tracheal suction system and 233 with an open system [9]. However, continuous subglottic secretion aspiration can reduce the use of antimicrobial agents and the incidence of VAP in patients undergoing cardiac surgery [10].

For patients undergoing mechanical ventilation via endotracheal tube placement, special attention must be paid to the material used to build the device and the integrity of the structures of the device itself. These patients experience an increased risk of nosocomial pneumonia, and microsubglottic contaminated secretions are among the leading causes of VAP.

A polyurethane-cuffed tube may prevent VAP onset. For example, Poelaert et al. in a study of 134 postcardiac surgery patients, showed that the incidence of pneumonia during early postoperative mechanical ventilation was significantly reduced when a polyurethane tube was used compared with a polyvinyl chloride tube [11]. These results were corroborated by Lorente et al. in a randomized study of 280 patients. VAP incidence was 22.1% in the patient group ($n = 140$) with conventional polyvinyl chloride endotracheal tubes with no subglottic aspiration compared with 7.9% ($p < 0.001$) in patients with polyurethane cuff tubes and subglottic continuous suction. These devices appear to reduce the incidence of VAP whether used early or late [12].

Automated devices more accurately assess adherence of the endotracheal tube cuff; however, available data suggest that this is not sufficient to significantly reduce VAP occurrence [13]. In addition, studies in animal models have shown that cuff inflation performed at low pressures and low volumes may reduce the risk of inhalation, especially during tracheotomy. This situation cannot be true in cases of selective intubation or when the positioning of the endotracheal tube excludes areas of lung ventilation [14]. Cuff lubrication reduces fluid outflow during thoracic surgery [15].

Endotracheal tubes coated with silver appear to contribute to VAP prevention. A preliminary study demonstrated reduced airway bacterial colonization [16]. These data were partly confirmed by the 2003 North American Silver-Coated Endotracheal Tube (NASCENT) investigation group study of patients undergoing mechanical ventilation >24 h. Data analysis from bronchoalveolar lavage showed that VAP onset was delayed and its incidence reduced compared with the control group [17].

Even circuit components used for ventilation and humidification of the gas mixtures administered to patients can serve as a source of bacterial contamination, prompting the onset of pneumonia. However, the likelihood of this occurrence is in dispute. A study of an unselected population of 369 ICU patients who underwent mechanical ventilation >48 h demonstrated that VAP onset was not related to the device types used to humidify the gas mixture [18]. Similar results emerged from another study conducted on 181 patients [19]. Moreover, bacterial filters do not appear to be involved in reducing VAP incidence. Bacterial filters used in a group of 230 patients undergoing mechanical ventilation >24 h did not reduce the prevalence of respiratory infections associated with mechanical ventilation [20].

Tracheotomy is commonly performed in patients undergoing mechanical ventilation over shorter and longer periods. An early tracheotomy may reduce the duration of mechanical ventilation and the incidence of respiratory tract infections, as well as improve patient comfort and reduce respiratory dead space. Evidence also exists to the contrary. Early tracheotomy (within 8 days) in a small group (60) of trauma patients was unable to reduce ventilation duration, pneumonia frequency, or ICU hospitalization compared with a control group in which the tracheotomy was performed $\geq$28 days after the acute event [21]. However, a prospective study of 62 patients with isolated severe head trauma showed that early tracheostomy shortened mechanical ventilation duration after VAP onset [22].

The mode of mechanical ventilation also appears to play a role in preventing VAP, but the use of positive end-expiratory pressure (PEEP) seems to be an issue. PEEP effectiveness was recently studied in 131 mechanically ventilated patients with chest radiographs and Horowitz indexes >250 [23]. The primary outcome was intra-ICU mortality and secondary outcomes were VAP, acute respiratory distress syndrome (ARDS), barotrauma, occurrence of atelectasis, and development of hypoxemia. The application of prophylactic PEEP in ventilated hypoxemic patients did not reduce the number of hypoxemia episodes or the VAP incidence [23].

Placing the patient undergoing mechanical ventilation in the prone position appears to be associated with reduced gastric content aspiration and VAP incidence. However, there is a lack of data on large-scale clinical studies that validate the effectiveness and feasibility of this strategy. For example, a multicenter prospective study conducted on ICU patients on mechanical ventilation showed that the prone position is not easily achieved and its effectiveness is therefore probably negative [24]; these data were also confirmed in children [25].

The role of selective decontamination (SDD) of the digestive tract is controversial with regards to VAP. De la Cal et al. employed a randomized double-blind study of 107 patients with severe burns at high risk of inhalation to assess whether SDD could reduce the incidence of infections, morbidity, and mortality in critically ill patients. Statistical analysis demonstrated that the treatment was able to reduce mortality and incidence compared with a control group [26].

10.3 Catheter-Related Bloodstream Infections

Given the incidence and clinical impact of catheter-related bloodstream infections (CRBSI) (5.3 per 1,000 catheter days), practical guidelines for their prevention were proposed based on type-A evidence [27, 28]. For example, educating medical staff is encouraged regarding indications for using vascular catheters, proper device insertion and maintenance, and careful surveillance of control measures to prevent infection. Testing knowledge and guideline compliance should be conducted, as well as management of staff who insert catheters, ensuring an adequate number of nurses on duty. Monitoring catheter insertion sites visually or by palpation through the intact dressing is important, depending on the clinical situation of the individual patient. If patients exhibit tenderness at the insertion site without an obvious source of infection, with or without fever, the dressing should be removed to examine the site. It is important to observe correct procedures with regard to hand hygiene by washing hands with conventional antiseptic soap and water or an alcohol-based gel. Hand hygiene must be performed before and after palpating the insertion site, as well as before and after insertion, replacement, or medication. The use of gloves does not eliminate the need for hand hygiene.

It is important to maintain an aseptic technique during the insertion of intravenous catheters and dressings. Indeed, gloves should be cleaned or sterilized before inserting an intravascular catheter. Wearing clean gloves when inserting catheters is acceptable, as is not touching the peripheral access site after application of skin antiseptics; sterile gloves should be worn for inserting arterial catheters or central lines. Clean or sterile gloves should also be worn when changing dressings.

Skin disinfection must be done with an appropriate antiseptic before inserting the catheter and during dressing changes. Although it is preferable to use CHX 2%, povidone iodine can be used with 70% alcohol. The antiseptic must be allowed to air dry; povidone must remain on the skin for at least 2 min, or longer if not completely dry. The dressing to be applied over the catheter insertion site should be of sterile gauze or semipermeable dressings and be transparent. The dressing should be replaced when wet, nonadhesive, or visibly soiled. Topical antibiotics should not be used on the insertion site to avoid fungal infections and microbial resistance.

Catheter type and insertion technique and site should be chosen for the lowest risk of complications for the therapy type and expected duration. Any catheter that is no longer essential should be promptly removed. In adults, it is necessary to replace peripheral venous catheters at least every 72–96 h to prevent phlebitis. Short-term central venous catheters (CVCs) should be replaced if there are signs of infection at the insertion site; they should not be used in guide-wire techniques to replace catheters in patients with suspected CRBSI.

Administration sets must be frequently replaced at a minimum time interval of 72 h unless a CRBSI is suspected or documented. The infusion sets used to administer blood (or its derivatives) or lipid emulsions should be replaced within

24 h of starting the infusion. If injections are performed, taps must first be disinfected, and all taps not in use should be covered. Contaminated fluids must not be administered; it is therefore recommended that parenteral nutrition be prepared aseptically in the pharmacy. It is also not recommended to use in-line filters for preventing infections, as administering systemic antibiotic prophylaxis routinely before insertion or during use of an intravascular catheter adequately prevents colonization.

Devices with as few lines as possible should be selected for patient management. Catheters impregnated with antimicrobial or antiseptic are best choices if they remain in place >5 days and if the infection rate remains high in the ward after using a global strategy. The risks and benefits of placing a CVC in the recommended site must be weighed, comparing the reduction of infectious complications and mechanical complications. Subclavian access is recommended for reducing infection in nontunneled catheters, and using the jugular or femoral vein is recommended regarding CVC dialysis (to avoid venous stasis). An episode of fever should not lead to changing these devices, as a clinical evaluation will determine whether to remove the catheter if infection is evidenced elsewhere or if the cause is not infectious. Routine exchange by guidewire should not be used to prevent infections; this technique should be reserved for cases of catheter malfunction without signs of infection. Disposable peripheral arterial catheters should be used with monitoring systems and should not substitute for routine peripheral arterial catheters to prevent catheter infections.

Clinical trials have recently been used to assess various methods to prevent CRBSI. For example, using particular types of medicated catheters appeared to correlate with a reduced incidence of catheter-related infections. A randomized study of 646 catheterizations compared the effectiveness of silver–platinum–carbon antimicrobial catheters with rifampicin–minocycline medicated catheters. The former served as effective antimicrobials, but the proportions of catheter-related infections were extremely low in both groups (1.4% for silver–platinum–carbon catheters vs. 1.7% for medical catheters with rifampicin–minocycline) [29]. Rupp et al. initiated a multicenter randomized double-blind controlled study of 780 patients to compare the incidence of infections due catheters medicated with CHX and sulfadiazine versus standard catheters. The results suggested that medicated catheters are highly tolerated by the patient, with less colonization by pathogenic organisms at the time of removal. The main colonizing microorganisms were coagulase-negative staphylococci and other Gram-positive microorganisms. Noninfectious adverse events occurred in both groups with comparable frequencies [30]. However, a recent prospective multicenter randomized controlled study demonstrated that there was no effective reduction in the infection if multilumen CVCs or catheters impregnated with silver were used. In both groups of patients, the incidence of infections was high: 2.5% in the standard catheter group versus 2.7% in the multilumen silver-impregnated catheter group [31].

Tunneling catheters are often used to prevent colonization and subsequent infections related to long-standing catheters. Darouiche et al. showed that a group of patients with long-stay antimicrobial-medicated catheters experienced a lower incidence of catheter-related infections than patients with tunneled catheters (3.6 vs. 1.43 per 1,000 catheter days) [32].

The impact of the site of catheter insertion has not yet been determined in preventing catheter-related infections. In a recent multicenter randomized investigation, Parienti et al. studied the infection incidence in patients with CVCs, comparing femoral versus jugular access. The entire patient cohort was subjected to cycles of short-term dialysis. The risk of colonization (assessed per 1,000 catheter days) was similar in both groups: 40.8 for femoral access versus 35.7 for jugular access. However, a higher infection incidence occurred in patients with body mass index (BMI) >28.4 with femoral central venous access (50.9 femoral vs. 24.5 jugular). The risk of hematoma was highest when using jugular access [33].

Careful disinfection of the CVC insertion site may reduce the incidence of infection. Mimoz et al. conducted a randomized study of 538 CVCs with jugular and subclavian access, demonstrating that the use of CHX may represent a valid alternative to the use of povidone iodine alcohol. CHX was able to reduce the incidence of colonization by 50% ($p < 0.002$) for the same incidence of overt bacterial infection ($p < 0.09$) [34]. Bleasdale et al. confirmed these data in a randomized study, emphasizing that using CHX for daily patient hygiene can reduce the incidence of primary systemic infections [35]. Timsit et al. evaluated the effectiveness of using CHX-gluconate-impregnated sponges to reduce the incidence of infection originating from the catheter insertion site. The randomized controlled trial conducted in 3,778 catheters kept in place for an average of 6 days demonstrated that the use of medicated wipes with CHX reduced the incidence of infection [6].

10.4 Urinary Tract Infections

Several studies provide useful information regarding UTI prevention [2, 37]. These studies argue that UTI prevention occurs in surgical patients by limiting the use of bladder catheters to only those cases with real need. The necessity of the bladder catheter should be assessed on the basis of clinical circumstances, and the routine use of these devices is therefore not recommended. Indwelling urinary catheters are recommended in long-term-care patients for managing incontinence.

Closed drainage systems are recommended after aseptically inserting the urinary catheter; catheters should only be inserted under the appropriate indications and should be kept in place only as long as necessary. Use and duration should be minimized in all patients, especially in those at increased risk for UTI, such as women, the elderly, and patients with compromised immune systems. Aseptic insertion should be ensured; and hospital staff, patients, and family should be educated in the correct insertion technique. It is necessary to attain a free urine flow.

The risks and benefits of various catheterization approaches have also been assessed. If an intermittent catheterization is preferable, this technique should be performed at regular intervals to avoid bladder distension. When urinary catheter placement is indicated in surgical patients, it must be removed as soon as possible after surgery, preferably within 24 h, unless there are appropriate indications for continuous use. If UTI rate is not reduced after applying a comprehensive strategy (appropriate positioning and proper aseptic maintenance), using catheters impregnated with an antimicrobial or antiseptic should be considered. After inserting the catheter aseptically, maintaining a closed drainage system is recommended.

In the absence of specific clinical indications, the use of systemic antibiotics as routine UTI prophylaxis is not recommended. For UTI prevention, it is not necessary to clean the periurethral area when routine cleaning during daily hygiene is required. Replacing catheters or drainage bags at regular intervals is also not recommended. Catheter replacement should be based on clinical indications, such as infections, obstructions, or when the closed system is compromised. Disposable sterile gel is also recommended for catheter insertion. Medical staff and professionals who manage catheters should continue to take refresher courses and further education for insertion and removal of the maintenance device. Hand hygiene before catheter insertion or any manipulation of the catheter site or devices is mandatory.

Several recent clinical trials have been performed regarding the prevention of UTI. A randomized double-blind controlled study of 212 patients enrolled consecutively after traumatic events compared the UTI incidence in patients with silicone urinary catheters with patients with catheters impregnated with nitrofurazone. There were significantly fewer bacteriurias and fungurias associated with nitrofurazone-impregnated bladders than with the silicone urinary catheters (9.1 vs. 24.7%). The clinical significance of asymptomatic bacteria and fungi in urine was unclear, limiting the study [38]. However, the use of hydrophilic catheters in a randomized controlled trial for self-intermittent catheterization after spinal injury did not significantly reduce the UTI incidence compared with standard catheters [39].

Finally, the efficacy of prophylactic antibiotic therapy before bladder catheter removal was assessed. The prospective randomized study was conducted on 239 patients undergoing major abdominal surgery who were catheterized perioperatively; the usefulness and effectiveness of trimethoprim–sulfamethoxazole in three doses was evaluated. Urine cultures were taken before and 3 days after bladder catheter removal. Trimethoprim–sulfamethoxazole administration significantly reduced the incidence of symptomatic UTI if administered before catheter removal (4.9% of the analysis group vs. 21.6% in the control group, $p < 0.001$) [40].

10.5 Conclusions

Recent findings seem to confirm the effectiveness of certain procedures for infection prevention, particularly with regard to VAP. Oral-cavity decontamination, continuous subglottic secretion suction, early tracheotomy, SDD and, for high-risk patients, endotracheal tubes with silver were all shown to be useful in preventing VAP. Medicated catheters and CHX-based dressings were efficacious against CRBSI. UTIs were shown to be prevented through the use of medical catheters. All these procedures can be incorporated into departmental protocols for preventing nosocomial infections in ICUs.

References

1. Centers for Disease Control and Prevention (2004) Guidelines for preventing health-care-associated pneumonia, 2003: recommendations of CDC and the Healthcare Infection Control Practices Advisory Committee. MMWR 53(RR-3)
2. Di Filippo A, De Gaudio AR (2003) Device-related infections in critically ill patients. Part II: prevention of ventilator-associated pneumonia and urinary tract infections. J Chemother 15(6):536–542
3. Panchabhai TS, Dangayach NS, Krishnan A et al (2009) Oropharyngeal cleansing with 0.2% chlorhexidine for prevention of nosocomial pneumonia in critically ill patients: an open-label randomized trial with 0.01% potassium permanganate as control. Chest 135(5):1150–1156
4. Koeman M, van der Ven AJ, Hak E et al (2006) Oral decontamination with chlorhexidine reduces the incidence of ventilator-associated pneumonia. Am J Respir Crit Care Med 173(12):1348–1355
5. Fourrier F, Dubois D, Pronnier P et al (2005) Effect of gingival and dental plaque antiseptic decontamination on nosocomial infections acquired in the intensive care unit: a double-blind placebo-controlled multicenter study. Crit Care Med 33(8):1728–1735
6. Seguin P, Tanguy M, Laviolle B et al (2006) Effect of oropharyngeal decontamination by povidone-iodine on ventilator-associated pneumonia in patients with head trauma. Crit Care Med 34(5):1514–1519
7. Pobo A, Lisboa T, Rodriguez A, RASPALL Study Investigators et al (2009) A randomized trial of dental brushing for preventing ventilator-associated pneumonia. Chest 136(2): 433–439
8. Caruso P, Denari S, Ruiz SA et al (2009) Saline instillation before tracheal suctioning decreases the incidence of ventilator-associated pneumonia. Crit Care Med 37(1):32–38
9. Lorente L, Lecuona M, Martín MM et al (2005) Ventilator-associated pneumonia using a closed versus an open tracheal suction system. Crit Care Med 33(1):115–119
10. Bouza E, Pérez MJ, Muñoz P et al (2008) Continuous aspiration of subglottic secretions in the prevention of ventilator-associated pneumonia in the postoperative period of major heart surgery. Chest 134(5):938–946
11. Poelaert J, Depuydt P, De Wolf A et al (2008) Polyurethane cuffed endotracheal tubes to prevent early postoperative pneumonia after cardiac surgery: a pilot study. J Thorac Cardiovasc Surg 135(4):771–776
12. Lorente L, Lecuona M, Jiménez A et al (2007) Influence of an endotracheal tube with polyurethane cuff and subglottic secretion drainage on pneumonia. Am J Respir Crit Care Med 176(11):1079–1083
13. Valencia M, Ferrer M, Farre R et al (2007) Automatic control of tracheal tube cuff pressure in ventilated patients in semirecumbent position: a randomized trial. Crit Care Med 35(6): 1543–1549
14. Young PJ, Pakeerathan S, Blunt MC et al (2006) A low-volume, low-pressure tracheal tube cuff reduces pulmonary aspiration. Crit Care Med 34(3):632–639
15. Sanjay PS, Miller SA, Corry PR et al (2006) The effect of gel lubrication on cuff leakage of double lumen tubes during thoracic surgery. Anaesthesia 61(2):133–137

16. Rello J, Kollef M, Diaz E et al (2006) Reduced burden of bacterial airway colonization with a novel silver-coated endotracheal tube in a randomized multiple-center feasibility study. Crit Care Med 34(11):2766–2772
17. Kollef MH, Afessa B, Anzueto A et al (2008) Silver-coated endotracheal tubes and incidence of ventilator-associated pneumonia: the NASCENT randomized trial. JAMA 300(7):805–813
18. Lacherade JC, Auburtin M, Cerf C et al (2005) Impact of humidification systems on ventilator-associated pneumonia: a randomized multicenter trial. Am J Respir Crit Care Med 172(10):1276–1282
19. Boots RJ, George N, Faoagali JL et al (2006) Double-heater-wire circuits and heat-and-moisture exchangers and the risk of ventilator-associated pneumonia. Crit Care Med 34(3):687–693
20. Lorente L, Lecuona M, Málaga J et al (2003) Bacterial filters in respiratory circuits: an unnecessary cost? Crit Care Med 31(8):2126–2130
21. Barquist ES, Amortegui J, Hallal A et al (2006) Tracheostomy in ventilator dependent trauma patients: a prospective, randomized intention-to-treat study. J Trauma 60(1):91–97
22. Bouderka MA, Fakhir B, Bouaggad A et al (2004) Early tracheostomy versus prolonged endotracheal intubation in severe head injury. J Trauma 57(2):251–254
23. Manzano F, Fernández-Mondéjar E, Colmenero M et al (2008) Positive-end expiratory pressure reduces incidence of ventilator-associated pneumonia in nonhypoxemic patients. Crit Care Med 36(8):2225–2231
24. van Nieuwenhoven CA, Vandenbroucke-Grauls C, van Tiel FH et al (2006) Feasibility and effects of the semirecumbent position to prevent ventilator-associated pneumonia: a randomized study. Crit Care Med 34(2):396–402
25. Aly H, Badawy M, El-Kholy A et al (2008) Randomized, controlled trial on tracheal colonization of ventilated infants: can gravity prevent ventilator-associated pneumonia? Pediatrics 122(4):770–774
26. de La Cal MA, Cerdá E, García-Hierro P et al (2005) Survival benefit in critically ill burned patients receiving selective decontamination of the digestive tract: a randomized, placebo-controlled, double-blind trial. Ann Surg 241(3):424–430
27. Centers for Disease Control and Prevention (2002) Guidelines for the prevention of intravascular catheter-related infections. MMWR 2002 51(RR-10)
28. De Gaudio AR, Di Filippo A (2003) Device-related infections in critically ill patients. Part I: prevention of catheter-related bloodstream infections. I Chemother 15(5):419–427
29. Fraenkel D, Rickard C, Thomas P et al (2006) A prospective, randomized trial of rifampicin-minocycline-coated and silver-platinum-carbon-impregnated central venous catheters. Crit Care Med 34(3):668–675
30. Rupp ME, Lisco SJ, Lipsett PA et al (2005) Effect of a second-generation venous catheter impregnated with chlorhexidine and silver sulfadiazine on central catheter-related infections: a randomized, controlled trial. Ann Intern Med 143(8):570–580
31. Kalfon P, de Vaumas C, Samba D et al (2007) Comparison of silver-impregnated with standard multi-lumen central venous catheters in critically ill patients. Crit Care Med 35(4):1032–1039
32. Darouiche RO, Berger DH, Khardori N et al (2005) Comparison of antimicrobial impregnation with tunneling of long-term central venous catheters: a randomized controlled trial. Ann Surg 242(2):193–200
33. Parienti JJ, Thirion M, Mégarbane B et al (2008) Femoral vs jugular venous catheterization and risk of nosocomial events in adults requiring acute renal replacement therapy: a randomized controlled trial. JAMA 299(20):2413–2422
34. Mimoz O, Villeminey S, Ragot S et al (2007) Chlorhexidine-based antiseptic solution vs alcohol-based povidone-iodine for central venous catheter care. Arch Intern Med 167(19): 2066–2072
35. Bleasdale SC, Trick WE, Gonzalez IM et al (2007) Effectiveness of chlorhexidine bathing to reduce catheter-associated bloodstream infections in medical intensive care unit patients. Arch Intern Med 167(19):2073–2079

36. Timsit JF, Schwebel C, Bouadma L et al (2009) Chlorhexidine-impregnated sponges and less frequent dressing changes for prevention of catheter-related infections in critically ill adults: a randomized controlled trial. JAMA 301(12):1231–1241
37. Healthcare Infection Control Practices Advisory Committee (2009) Guideline for prevention of catheter-associated urinary tract infections. http://www.cdc.gov/ncidod/dhqp/pdf/guidelines/CAUTI_Guideline2009final.pdf. Accessed June 2011
38. Stensballe J, Tvede M, Looms D et al (2007) Infection risk with nitrofurazone-impregnated urinary catheters in trauma patients: a randomized trial. Ann Intern Med 147(5):285–293
39. Cardenas DD, Hoffman JM (2009) Hydrophilic catheters versus noncoated catheters for reducing the incidence of urinary tract infections: a randomized controlled trial. Arch Phys Med Rehabil 90(10):1668–1671
40. Pfefferkorn U, Lea S, Moldenhauer J et al (2009) Antibiotic prophylaxis at urinary catheter removal prevents urinary tract infections: a prospective randomized trial. Ann Surg 249(4):573–575

Antibiotic Policies in the Intensive Care Unit

11

H. K. F. van Saene, N. J. Reilly, A. de Silvestre and F. Rios

11.1 Introduction

Every intensive care unit (ICU) should have well-structured guidelines on the use of antimicrobial agents to guarantee that patients requiring intensive care receive appropriate antimicrobials for a relevant period to prevent and treat infections. These guidelines should meet the therapeutic needs of the consultants and allow the intensivist, clinical microbiologist, and pharmacist to monitor efficacy, toxicity—including allergy and diarrhea—and side effects, such as the emergence of resistant strains and subsequent outbreaks of superinfections. Calculation of infection rates is only feasible following implementation of an antibiotic policy. Apart from audit and research, antimicrobial guidelines aid educational programs and enable the clinical pharmacist to control drug expenditure.

11.2 Main Feature of Antibiotic Guidelines

The main feature of an antibiotic policy in the ICU is the use of a minimum of well-established antimicrobial agents that are associated with a minimum of side effects but also allow the control of the three patterns of ICU infections due to the 15 potentially pathogenic microorganisms (PPM) (Chaps. 3 and 5).

H. K. F. van Saene (✉)
Institute of Ageing and Chronic Disease, University of Liverpool,
Duncan Building, Liverpool, UK
e-mail: nia.taylor@liv.ac.uk

11.2.1 Antimicrobials Chosen on the Basis of Three Characteristics

11.2.1.1 Preserving Indigenous Flora

Control of the abnormal flora, including (potentially resistant) aerobic Gram-negative bacilli (AGNB) and methicillin-resistant *Staphylococcus aureus* (MRSA), by normal indigenous, mainly anaerobic, flora is termed microbial ecology [1]. Normal flora provides resistance to acquisition and subsequent carriage of PPM and constitutes the microbial component of the carriage defense (Chap. 2). Antimicrobial agents active against indigenous anaerobic flora and excreted into throat and gut via saliva, bile, and mucus in lethal concentrations, may suppress indigenous flora. Diarrhea and candidiasis are well known side effects of commonly used antibiotics. Disregarding ecology by using antimicrobial agents leads to an impaired microbial factor of carriage defense and promotes abnormal AGNB [2] and MRSA [3] overgrowth, as well as *Clostridium difficile* [4] and vancomycin-resistant enterococci (VRE) [5]. Narrow-spectrum antimicrobials can be defined as those that only cover the 15 aerobic PPM, leaving indigenous normal flora more or less intact [6]. Broad-spectrum antimicrobials are not only active against the 15 disease-causing PPM but affect the normal indigenous anaerobic flora that contributes to physiology rather than infection. From an ecological perspective, ampicillin, amoxicillin, and flucloxacillin are antimicrobials with a broader spectrum than that of cephradine and cefotaxime [7–11]. Metronidazole, although active against anaerobes, does not affect indigenous flora, as it is readily neutralized following biliary excretion [12]. The most recent, ever-more potent, antimicrobials, such as ceftriaxone, generally belong to the group of ecology-disregarding antimicrobials that predispose to, e.g., AGNB, MRSA, and yeast overgrowth and subsequent superinfection [3, 13–17] (Table 11.1).

11.2.1.2 Limiting the Emergence of Resistant Microbes by Using Antimicrobials with the Lowest Resistance Potential

If resistance occurs during drug development or clinical trials or within 2 years of general use, the antibiotic has a high resistance potential [18]. Ceftazidime-, ciprofloxacin-, and imipenem-resistant *Pseudomonas aeruginosa* were reported during clinical trials and early after introduction for general use [19–21]. Antimicrobials with little or no resistance potential include cephradine, piperacillin, cefotaxime, amikacin, and meropenem (Table 11.2) [21–24]. Three observations have emerged from this historical experience: (1) each antibiotic class has one or more antimicrobials capable of causing antibiotic resistance, but this is not a class phenomenon; antibiotic resistance is agent specific; (2) resistance is not related to duration of use; and (3) resistance is not related to volume of use.

The underlying mechanisms explaining the difference between antibiotics with a high and a low resistance potential are not fully understood but are thought to be based on specific antibiotic-resistance mechanisms. For example, among the aminoglycosides, only gentamicin has been associated with widespread *P. aeruginosa*

Table 11.1 Classification of parenterally administered antimicrobials based on respect for ecology

Indigenous flora friendly	Indigenous flora suppressing
Challenge studies in volunteers	
Cephradine, cefotaxime	Ampicillin, amoxicillin
Comparative studies in patients	
Cephradine, penicillin	Amoxicillin, Ampicillin
Observational studies in patients	
Gentamicin, tobramycin, amikacin, polymyxins, polyenes, metronidazole	Flucloxacillin, amoxicillin + clavulanic acid, piperacillin + tazobactam, ceftriaxone, ciprofloxacin, carbapenems, macrolides

Table 11.2 Classification of parenteral antimicrobials based on the potential for resistance

Low resistance	High resistance
Piperacillin	Ampicillin
Cephradine	Ceftazidime
Cefotaxime	Gentamicin
Cefepime	Ciprofloxacin
Amikacin	Imipenem
Levofloxacin	
Meropenem	

resistance, but amikacin continues to be effective against most gentamicin-resistant *P. aeruginosa*. Gentamicin is an aminoglycoside that is highly susceptible to inactivation by a variety of enzymes at six different loci on the gentamicin molecule, but amikacin has only one such vulnerable point [25]. Substituting amikacin for gentamicin decreased gentamicin-resistant *P. aeruginosa* when amikacin was used in the same volume as gentamicin, and no subsequent resistance problems developed. Some institutions with renewed gentamicin susceptibility to *P. aeruginosa* returned to using gentamicin as the major hospital aminoglycoside (i.e., rotating formularies) [26]. Predictably, gentamicin-resistant *P. aeruginosa* isolates returned to previous levels and were perpetuated as long as gentamicin was the primary aminoglycoside used in the hospital and ICU. Some people believe that these aminoglycoside lessons of the past should be applied to the problems of *P. aeruginosa* resistant to ceftazidime, ciprofloxacin, and imipenem. Substitution of cefepime, levofloxacin, and meropenem for ceftazidime, ciprofloxacin, and imipenem may decrease or even eliminate resistant *P. aeruginosa* from the ICU environment [27–29]. According to the concept of low and high resistance potential of antimicrobial agents, the key to controlling antibiotic resistance is agent related and is not class, duration, or volume associated.

11.2.1.3 Controlling Inflammation by Using Antimicrobials with Anti-Endotoxin/Inflammation Properties

Lipopolysaccharide (LPS), or endotoxin, is the major component of the outer membrane of AGNB and is thought to be a key molecule in the induction of generalized inflammation. LPS causes the production and release from host effector cells of various proinflammatory cytokines and other mediators of inflammation, such as nitric oxide and prostaglandins. The degree to which these mediators are released depends, in part, on the amount of LPS that is presented to CD14-bearing effector cells, such as monocytes, macrophages, and polymorphonuclear leukocytes. Therefore, it is possible that factors affecting the amount of LPS released in vivo may modulate the inflammatory response associated with AGNB infection. Several in vitro and animal studies show that antimicrobial agents may differentially release LPS from AGNB [30, 31]. They also demonstrated that antibiotics associated with substantial release of endotoxin generate higher levels of proinflammatory cytokines and suggested that using antimicrobials associated with the release of lower amounts of LPS leads to lower levels of cytokinemia and better outcome. Carbapenems, such as imipenem and meropenem, release a small amount of endotoxin, whereas third-generation cephalosporins, such as ceftazidime and cefotaxime, are associated with far greater release of endotoxin [32]. Three clinical trials failed to support this hypothesis that differential antibiotic-induced endotoxin release is of clinical significance, as there were no significant differences in clinical parameters (temperature, blood pressure, or heart rate) or plasma endotoxin and cytokine levels [33–35].

Fluoroquinolones, such as ciprofloxacin, release substantial amounts of endotoxin compared with the aminoglycosides gentamicin and tobramycin and with the polymyxins E (colistin) and B [36, 37]. Although not active against AGNB, glycopeptides, including teicoplanin [38] and vancomycin [39]; and polyenes, such as amphotericin B [40], have been shown to downregulate LPS-induced cytokine release (Table 11.3).

Classifying antimicrobials using these three criteria of flora friendliness, low resistance potential, and anti-inflammation propensity is not evidence based, i.e., not evaluated in randomized trials. However, despite the lack of level 1 evidence, we found the available data compelling and difficult to ignore in selecting antimicrobials for our antibiotic policy.

Using a limited number of antimicrobial agents allows the control of the 15 potential pathogens implicated in the three types of ICU infections. The main antimicrobial groups are:
1. β-lactams, i.e., antibiotics with a β-lactam ring in their structure, such as penicillins and cephalosporins;
2. aminoglycosides, e.g., tobramycin;
3. polymyxins, e.g., polymyxin E or colistin;

Table 11.3 Classification of antimicrobials based on their anti-inflammation propensities

Inflammation controlling	Inflammation promoting
Aminoglycosides	Beta-lactams
Glycopeptides	Cefotaxime
Polymyxins	Ceftazidime
Polyenes	Fluoroquinolones
Carbapenems	Ciprofloxacin

4. glycopeptides, e.g., vancomycin;
5. polyenes, such as amphotericin B.

All these agents are lethal to microorganisms. Polymyxins, glycopeptides, and polyenes have a rapid action on the microbial cell membrane. β-lactams interfere with the cell-wall synthesis, a slower mechanism of action. Aminoglycosides inhibit protein synthesis but still kill microbes in the rest phase. These differences in mechanism of action may explain why aminoglycosides and polyenes are more toxic to the ICU patient than are β-lactams when parenterally administered. Table 11.4 shows the spectrum of activity of the five main antimicrobial groups according to the minimal bactericidal concentration (MBC) for the 15 PPMs. The MBC of an antimicrobial agent is defined as the amount of the antimicrobial (milligram per liter) required to establish irreversible inhibition in the test tube without the support of the killing activity of leukocytes of the ICU patient. Leukocytes of the critically ill are thought to be less effective in killing PPM than those of a healthy population [41]. Antimicrobial agents with an MBC of 1 mg/l for PPM are in general suitable for clinical use. Nontoxic antibiotics, such as the β-lactams, are ideal for systemic administration, and high doses (50–100 mg/kg per day) can be given. The more toxic agents, such as polymyxins and the polyenes, can be safely applied enterally and topically in high doses. Polyenes given parenterally are toxic, and the daily doses are in the order of milligrams (1.5 mg/kg per day for amphotericin B). Aminoglycosides and glycopeptides, although toxic, are administered systemically in lower doses (5–25 mg/kg per day).

11.3 Antimicrobial Use for Both Prophylaxis and Therapy

Antimicrobial administration in the ICU falls into three categories: parenteral, enteral nonabsorbable, and topical.

11.3.1 Parenterally Administered Antimicrobials

Parenteral administration is aimed at preventing and, if already present, eradicating colonization/infection of internal organs, including lungs, and bladder, as well as in the bloodstream. Systemic prophylaxis is generally accepted in surgery

Table 11.4 Spectrum of activity of the commonly used antimicrobial agents for the 15 potential pathogens expressed by the minimal bactericidal concentration (MBC) (milligrams per liter)

PPM	Antimicrobial agents							
	Penicillin G	Cephradine	Cefotaxime	Ceftazidime	Aminoglycosides, e.g., tobramycin	Polymyxins, e.g., polymyxin E	Glycopeptides, e.g., vancomycin	Polyenes, e.g., amphotericin B
Normal								
S. pneumoniae	0.1		0.2	(2)				
H. influenzae			0.06	0.2				
M. catarrhalis			1	1	1			
E. coli			0.02	0.2	0.2	0.1		
S. aureus		1	1	(8.0)	0.2		0.05	
Candida spp.								0.05
Abnormal								
Klebsiella spp.			0.1	0.1	0.1	0.1		
Proteus spp.			0.1	0.1	0.2			
Morganella spp.			0.1	0.1	0.2			
Citrobacter spp.			0.3	0.3	0.1	0.1		
Enterobacter spp.			0.2	0.2	0.1	0.1		
Serratia spp.			1	1	0.2			
Acinetobacter spp.			(8)	(8)	0.1	0.1		
Pseudomonas spp.			–	0.1	0.1	0.5		
MRSA							1.0	

PPM potentially pathogenic microorganisms, *MRSA* methicillin-resistant *Staphylococcus aureus*

[42]. The aim is to achieve a tissue concentration at the time of the surgical trauma in order to prevent wound infections. Patients who require intensive care due to an acute trauma or worsening of the underlying disease invariably receive invasive devices, including ventilation tube, urinary catheter, and intravascular lines. These interventions are well-known risk factors for lower airway, bladder, and bloodstream infections in the ICU patient whose immunoparalysis is at its nadir during the first week of admission. This is the time during which primary endogenous infections occur. Only the immediate parenteral administration of antimicrobials can prevent this type of infection and early therapy of an already incubating primary endogenous infection. If the primary endogenous infection is the indication for ICU admission, parenterally administered antimicrobials are required to treat the established infection. The philosophy that preventing infection is always better than cure dictates the immediate systemic administration of antibiotics to a critically ill patient requiring mechanical ventilation. Hence, systemically administered cefotaxime is an integral part of the concept of the prophylactic protocol of selective decontamination of the digestive tract (SDD) [43].

The criteria for parenteral administration include flora friendliness and low resistance potential (after excretion into throat and gut via saliva, bile, and mucus) and anti-inflammation propensity. In addition, the pharmacokinetic properties should include a high excretion in the target organs and, in particular, in bronchial secretions. The ratio of the antimicrobial level in the target organ and the MBC (Table 11.4) determines the efficacy against a particular microorganism (Chap. 7). Protein binding should be minimal. Parenterally administered antimicrobials require a good safety profile in terms of allergy, nephro- and ototoxicity, and influence on hemostasis. Finally, the target PPM is a criterion of paramount importance for choosing an antimicrobial to be administered parenterally. Primary endogenous infections are caused by both normal, e.g., *Streptococcus pneumoniae*, *Haemophilus influenzae*, and *S. aureus*, and abnormal potential pathogens, including AGNB and MRSA. General health before ICU admission influences the carrier state (Chap. 2). Previously, healthy individuals such as trauma, burn, acute liver, and pancreatitis patients only carry normal potential pathogens, whereas patients with chronic underlying diseases, including chronic obstructive pulmonary disease, diabetes, and alcoholism, may carry AGNB and MRSA. It is obvious that patients referred to the ICU from other hospitals or wards are highly likely to be carriers of abnormal potential pathogens. Taking these criteria into consideration, there are only a few antimicrobials suitable for prophylaxis. The first- and second-generation β-lactams cover the normal potential pathogens but are less effective against the abnormal AGNB. Cefotaxime, a third-generation cephalosporin, has an adequate spectrum toward both normal and abnormal AGNB, with the exception of *P. aeruginosa* and *Acinetobacter* spp. Ceftazidime adequately covers AGNB but at the expense of *S. aureus*. Cefepime may be a suitable alternative for ceftazidime. Three randomized SDD trials used the fluoroquinolones ciprofloxacin and ofloxacin as systemic prophylaxis despite inadequate cover of *S. pneumoniae* [44–46]. Most SDD studies employed cefotaxime as the parenterally administered antimicrobial. Many patients admitted to a medical/

surgical ICU receive perioperative prophylaxis. This surgical prophylaxis may be replaced by cefotaxime as soon as SDD is started. In patients in whom prosthetic material has been implanted, an appropriate endocarditis prophylaxis should also be given. It is not uncommon that patients in a generalized inflammatory state on ICU admission receive an aminoglycoside to control inflammation, in addition to cefotaxime.

Colonization of the lower airways, particularly with *S. aureus*, MRSA, *P. aeruginosa*, and *Aspergillus fumigatus*, may persist despite adequate systemic therapy. Cephradine, vancomycin, polymyxin E, cefotaxime, ceftazidime, gentamicin, tobramycin, and amphotericin B can be nebulized to achieve higher antibiotic concentrations in the lower airways. The ventilation tube is often contaminated and has to be changed and replaced by a new tube following nebulization. Surveillance swabs of the oropharynx are required to monitor therapy efficacy. Chapter 22 discusses in detail the fundamental features of infection therapy:
1. sterilizing the infected internal organ using parenterally administered antibiotic(s);
2. eliminating the source with enterally administered antibiotics;
3. removing or changing the invasive device;
4. evaluating therapeutic efficacy using surveillance samples.

11.3.2 Enterally Administered Nonabsorbable Antimicrobials

The purpose of enterally administered nonabsorbable antimicrobials is to prevent, or if already present, eradicate abnormal flora carriage and overgrowth from throat and gut. The abnormal carrier state always precedes secondary endogenous infections. Whereas parenterally administered antimicrobials are required to control primary endogenous infections, enterally administered nonabsorbable antibiotics are used to prevent secondary endogenous infections [47]. The commonly used decontaminating agents are polymyxin E, tobramycin, amphotericin B, or nystatin and vancomycin. They all fulfil the three requirements of narrow spectrum or ecology friendliness, low resistance potential, and anti-inflammation properties. Additionally, they are nonabsorbable in order to achieve high salivary and fecal concentrations, and—as all antimicrobials—are inactivated by fiber, cells, and fecal material to varying extents. Tobramycin and polymyxin are minimally and moderately inactivated, respectively. The polyenes and vancomycin require high oral doses due to a high inactivation rate (Chap. 8). For decontaminating agents to be effective, a minimal contact time of 15 min is required between antimicrobial agent and an abnormal potential pathogen. This contact time is no problem in the stomach and gut due to the ileus and is guaranteed by the application of a paste or a gel in the oropharynx. High failure rates of orally administered sprays and rinses of antimicrobials have been reported (Chap. 27). Apart from nystatin, all antimicrobials used for SDD are administered parenterally despite their toxicity. Toxicity is a lesser problem following enterally administered administration, even in high doses. Chapter 8 discusses the significant reductions in AGNB, yeast, and MRSA carriage following enteral use of polymyxin/tobramycin, polyenes, and vancomycin. Interestingly, among the 15 target PPMs, *P. aeruginosa*, *Candida* spp., and MRSA are less easy to completely clear from the throat and/or gut. It is not uncommon that surveillance swabs yield their very low concentrations even during long-term SDD. Apparently, reducing overgrowth to very-low-growth densities is sufficient to control infection, resistance, and transmission [48, 49].

11.3.3 Topically Administered Antimicrobials

Topically administered antimicrobials are intended to prevent and, if already present, eradicate colonization/infection of abnormal flora from wounds in which plastic devices may be present, such as a tracheostoma and gastrostoma. Wounds, in particular burn wounds, are prone to potential acquisition and subsequent exogenous colonization/infection with pathogens, such as *P. aeruginosa* and MRSA, without previous carriage in the digestive tract. Gels including AquaForm and IntraSite are highly suitable for topical application of antimicrobials to burn wounds [50]. The concentration of, for example, polymyxin E or vancomycin is in general 2%. Each application has to be preceded by wound debridement and cleaning with a disinfecting agent, such as 2% taurolin, to remove necrotic tissue that may inactivate polymyxin E or vancomycin. The transparent gels allow careful inspection of wound healing and granulating tissue. Tracheostoma and gastrostoma are artificially created long-term wounds kept open by plastic devices. Potential pathogens, such as *P. aeruginosa* and non-*aeruginosa*, *A. baumannii*, and *S. aureus*, both methicillin-sensitive and -resistant, have an intrinsic affinity for plastic. Colonization/infection of exogenous origin is not uncommon in patients with tracheostoma and/or gastrostoma. As it is virtually impossible to sterilize plastic using parenterally administered agents, the devices must be removed and the wounds cleaned with taurolin. A thin layer of a paste containing 2% polymyxin E and/or vancomycin is applied to the stoma before a new device is put in. Obviously, preventing colonization/infection of tracheostoma and gastrostoma using the paste twice daily throughout ICU treatment is preferred to having to treat colonization/infection [51].

11.4 Efficacy in Relation to Antimicrobial Therapy Duration

11.4.1 Parenterally Administered Antimicrobials

Preventing primary endogenous infection is the main reason for parenteral administration of antimicrobials, being one of the crucial components of the SDD protocol. Supplementary prophylaxis is the second reason [52], i.e., cover while establishing SDD on mucosal surfaces, cover for procedurally released microorganisms, and elimination from mucosal surfaces of PPM resistant to enterally administered antimicrobials (e.g., *S. pneumoniae* is resistant to polymyxins, aminoglycosides, and polyenes).

The duration of parenterally administered prophylaxis as an integral part of SDD depends on the type of carrier state, i.e., normal versus abnormal. The maximum period of parenterally administered prophylaxis is 5 days for patients with abnormal flora. The oropharynx and gut (not rectal cavity) are expected to be free from abnormal AGNB and MRSA within 3 days of enterally administered antimicrobials. In patients who were previously healthy, a shorter period of 3 or even 2 days has been shown to be effective [53].

According to the guidelines of the American Thoracic Society, lower airway infections due to normal potential pathogens, including *H. influenzae* and *S. aureus*, should be treated for 7–10 days, whereas episodes caused by *P. aeruginosa* and *Acinetobacter* spp. should be treated for at least 14–21 days [54]. The guidelines are based on expert opinion. There is only one randomized controlled trial evaluating whether a short course of intravenously administered antimicrobial therapy of 1 week is as effective as a prolonged treatment ≥2 weeks [55]. These investigators showed that there is no evidence to support an antibiotic course exceeding 1 week. A third approach for determining antibiotic therapy duration is the use of inflammation markers, including C-reactive protein (CRP). Five prospective studies show that a course of appropriate antimicrobials of <1 week results in significant improvement in clinical, radiographic, and microbiological parameters [56–60]. There is no evidence to support the superiority of a 2-week course of intravenously administered antibiotics for >1 week, which prompted us to implement a parenterally administered antibiotic policy of 5 days, followed by careful evaluation of patients' clinical, radiographic, and microbiological parameters [61, 62].

11.4.2 Enterally Administered Antimicrobials

Enterally administered antimicrobials using a paste or gel and a suspension into the throat and gut, respectively, is indicated as long as the patient is immunoparalyzed, i.e., at high risk of acquiring abnormal flora and subsequently of developing an infection. SDD is generally given throughout the ICU treatment or, in practice, until extubation.

There is general consensus that long-term use of enterally administered polymyxin E/tobramycin/amphotericin B (PTA) in the correct concentrations in throat and gut abolishes oropharyngeal and gastric carriage, respectively, of the target PPM within a few days. Eradication of rectal carriage appears to depend on the presence of peristalsis and may vary until the patient produces feces [63].

11.4.3 Topically Administered Antimicrobials

Three days of topical application of PTA and/or vancomycin into wounds or tracheostoma or gastrostoma has been shown to eradicate the potential pathogens using daily sampling [50, 51]. Preventing colonization/infection of wounds and stomas obviously requires topical application throughout the ICU treatment [51].

11.5 Endpoints of Antimicrobial Policies

A new antimicrobial agent launched by the pharmaceutical industry or a new antibiotic policy implemented in the ICU should be assessed using four main endpoints, including morbidity, mortality, antimicrobial resistance, and costs (Table 11.5). The pharmaceutical industry is not often able to provide that information. If the superinfection rate associated with a particular antimicrobial is known, that figure is often diluted by the number of all patients enrolled in all studies, whether community-, hospital-, or ICU-based, as denominator. Superinfection rates are invariably higher in critically ill patients requiring intensive care, including the need for mechanical ventilation, compared with patients staying in wards. The more severely ill the patient population studied, the higher the superinfection rate. Mortality rate should be assessed following immediate administration of the antimicrobial(s), as the delay of adequate therapy is associated with increased mortality rates [64, 65]. Immediate administration of an antimicrobial agent always implies an empirical decision in the absence of any knowledge of the causative microorganism, although, of course, reasonable assumptions can be made depending upon disease presentation [62]. Presence of normal potential pathogens in admission flora is highly likely if the patient was previously healthy (trauma, burn, acute liver failure, and pancreatitis patients). Patients with chronic underlying diseases, including alcoholism, chronic obstructive pulmonary disease, and diabetes, often import abnormal potential pathogens in their flora on admission. Patients referred from other hospitals or from wards are generally ill and may bring abnormal bacteria associated with the hospital ecology into the ICU. Surveillance samples of throat and rectum taken at the time of admission may help identify normal versus abnormal carrier state. These samples are also required to assess the impact of an antibiotic on the patient's ecology and to monitor secondary or supercarriage of resistant bacteria. This information is invariably missing for most new antibiotics or antibiotic policies. New antibiotics are also recommended for 10 or more days and are always more expensive than the older antimicrobials that are often out of patent and inexpensive.

Our antimicrobial policy using the above criteria is shown in Chap. 17. A prospective, observational, cohort study was performed for 4 years (1999–2003) to assess efficacy, side-effects, and costs of this antibiotic policy. Only critically ill children requiring 4 or more days of intensive care were included in the epidemiological descriptive study [66]. This study group represents the sicker patients with longer pediatric ICU stays. Approximately two thirds of pediatric ICU admissions did not meet the 4-day stay entry criterion for the study and are thus not included in the denominator for infection rates. Short-stay patients have a low

Table 11.5 Endpoints of antimicrobial policies

Desired endpoints
Efficacy: clinical endpoints
• reduction in infectious morbidity (superinfection)
• reduction in mortality following the immediate administration of empirical antimicrobial
Safety: microbiological endpoints (using surveillance samples)
• impact on ecology: yeasts, *Clostridium difficile* (diarrhea)   • antimicrobial resistance: supercarriage of aerobic Gram-negative bacilli, methicillin-resistant *Staphylococcus aureus*, vancomycin-resistant enterococci
Costs
• duration: an antimicrobial course of <1 week is as good as that of ≥2 weeks
• is the newer, more expensive, antimicrobial superior than the older, less expensive one, in terms of efficacy and safety?

risk of developing secondary endogenous and exogenous infection, and we believe they should not be reported in the denominator of pediatric ICU infection rates. A total of 1,241 children were enrolled in the study: 520 had infections, with an overall infection rate of 41.9%; viral infections accounted for 14.5% and bacterial/yeast infections for 33.0%. The incidence of blood-stream infection and lower airway infection was 21.0 and 9.1 episodes per 1,000 patient days, respectively; 13.3% of the children were infected with a microorganism acquired in the pediatric ICU; 4.0% of admitted patients developed infections due to resistant microorganisms. The mortality rate was 9.6%.

References

1. Vollaard EJ, Clasener HAL (1994) Colonisation resistance. Antimicrob Agents Chemother 335:409–414
2. Vlaspolder F, de Zeeuw G, Rozenberg-Arska M et al (1987) The influence of flucloxacillin and amoxicillin with clavulanic acid on the aerobic flora of the alimentary tract. Infection 15:241–244
3. Harbarth S, Liassine N, Dharan S et al (2000) Risk factors for persistent carriage of methicillin-resistant *Staphylococcus aureus*. Clin Infect Dis 31:1380–1385
4. Shek FW, Stacey BSF, Rendell J et al (2000) The rise of *Clostridium difficile*: the effect of length of stay, patient age and antibiotic use. J Hosp Infect 45:235–237
5. Donskey CJ, Chowdry TK, Hecker MT et al (2000) Effect of antibiotic therapy on the density of vancomycin-resistant enterococci in the stool of colonised patients. N Engl J Med 343:1925–1932
6. van Saene R, Fairclough S, Petros A (1998) Broad- and narrow-spectrum antibiotics: a different approach. Clin Microbiol Infect 4:56–57
7. Buck AC, Cooke EM (1969) The fate of ingested *Pseudomonas aeruginosa* in normal persons. J Med Microbiol 2:521–525
8. van Saene HKF, Stoutenbeek CP, Geitz JN et al (1988) Effect of amoxycillin on colonisation resistance in human volunteers. Microb Ecol Health Dis 1:169–177

9. Vollaard EJ, Clasener HAL, Janssen AJHM et al (1990) Influence of amoxycillin on microbial colonisation resistance in healthy volunteers. A methodological study. J Antimicrob Chemother 25:861–871
10. Vollaard EJ, Clasener HAL, Janssen AJHM et al (1990) Influence of cefotaxime on microbial colonisation resistance in healthy volunteers. J Antimicrob Chemother 26:117–123
11. Vollaard EJ, Clasener HAL, Janssen AJHM (1992) Influence of cephradine on microbial colonisation resistance in healthy volunteers. Microb Ecol Health Dis 5:147–153
12. Krook A, Danielsson D, Kjellander J, Jarnerot G (1979) Changes in the fecal flora of patients with Crohn's disease during treatment with metronidazole. Scand J Gastroenterol 14:705–710
13. Meijer BC, Kootstra GJ, Geertsma DG, Wilkinson MHE (1991) Effects of ceftriaxone on faecal flora: analysis by micromorphometry. Epidemiol Infect 106:513–521
14. Toltzis P, Yamashita T, Vilt L et al (1998) Antibiotic restriction does not alter endemic colonisation with resistant Gram-negative rods in a pediatric intensive care unit. Crit Care Med 26:1893–1899
15. Samonis G, Gikas A, Toloudis P et al (1994) Prospective study of the impact of broad-spectrum antibiotics on the yeast flora of the human gut. Eur J Clin Microbiol Infect Dis 13:665–667
16. Krcmery V Jr, Oravcova E, Spanik S et al (1998) Nosocomial breakthrough fungaemia during antifungal prophylaxis or empirical anti-fungal therapy in 41 cancer patients receiving anti-neoplastic chemotherapy: analysis of aetiology risk factors and outcome. J Antimicrob Chemother 41:373–380
17. Lode H, von der Höh N, Ziege S et al (2001) Ecological effects of linezolid versus amoxicillin/clavulanic acid on the normal intestinal microflora. Scand J Infect Dis 33:899–903
18. Cunha AC (2001) Effective antibiotic-resistance control strategies. Lancet 357:1307–1308
19. Lee SC, Fung CP, Liu PYF et al (1999) Nosocomial infections with ceftazidime-resistant *Pseudomonas aeruginosa*: risk factors and outcome. Infect Control Hosp Epidemiol 20:205–207
20. Fink MP, Snydman DR, Niederman MS et al (1994) Treatment of severe pneumonia in hospitalised patients: results of a multi-center, randomised, double-blind trial comparing intravenous ciprofloxacin and imipenem-cilastatin. Antimicrob Agents Chemother 38:547–557
21. Carmeli Y, Troillet N, Eliopoulos GM, Samore MH (1999) Emergence of antibiotic-resistant *Pseudomonas aeruginosa*: comparison of risks associated with different anti-pseudomonal agents. Antimicrob Agents Chemother 43:1379–1382
22. Lacey RW, Lord VL, Howson GL et al (1983) Double-blind study to compare the selection of antibiotic resistance by amoxicillin or cephradine in the commensal flora. Lancet 2:529–532
23. de Man P, Verhoeven BAN, Verburgh HA et al (2000) An antibiotic policy to prevent emergence of resistant bacilli. Lancet 355:973–978
24. Cunha BA (2000) Antibiotic resistance. Med Clin North Am 84:1407–1429
25. Mingeot-Leclercq MP, Glupczynski Y, Tulkens PM (1999) Aminoglycosides: activity and resistance. Antimicrob Agents Chemother 43:727–737
26. Gerding DN, Larson TA, Hughes RA et al (1991) Aminoglycoside resistance and aminoglycoside usage: ten years of experience in one hospital. Antimicrob Agents Chemother 35:1284–1290
27. Toltzis P, Dul M, O'Riordan MA et al (2003) Cefepime use in a pediatric intensive care unit reduces colonization with resistant bacilli. Pediatr Infect Dis J 22:109–114
28. Gillespie T, Masterton RG (2002) Investigation into the selection frequency of resistant mutants and the bacterial kill rate by levofloxacin and ciprofloxacin in non-mucoid *Pseudomonas aeruginosa* isolates from cystic fibrosis patients. Int J Antimicrob Agents 19:377–382
29. Livermore DM (2002) Multiple mechanisms of antimicrobial resistance in *Pseudomonas aeruginosa*: our worst nightmare? Clin Infect Dis 34:634–640

30. Dofferhoff AS, Nijland JH, de Vries-Hospers HG et al (1991) Effects of different types and combinations of antimicrobial agents on endotoxin release from Gram-negative bacteria: an in vitro and in vivo study. Scand J Infect Dis 23:745–754
31. Jackson JJ, Kropp H (1992) Beta-lactam antibiotic-induced release of free endotoxin: in vitro comparison of penicillin-binding protein (PBP) 2-specific imipenem and PBP 3-specific ceftazidime. J Infect Dis 165:1033–1041
32. Prins JM, van Deventer SJH, Kuijper EJ, Speelman P (1994) Clinical relevance of antibiotic-induced endotoxin release. Antimicrob Agents Chemother 38:1211–1218
33. Luchi M, Morrison DC, Opal S et al (2000) A comparative trial of imipenem versus ceftazidime in the release of endotoxin and cytokine generation in patients with Gram-negative urosepsis. J Endotoxin Res 6:25–31
34. Prins JM, van Agtmael MA, Kuijper EJ et al (1995) Antibiotic-induced endotoxin release in patients with Gram-negative urosepsis: a double-blind study comparing imipenem and ceftazidime. J Infect Dis 172:888–891
35. Holzheimer RG, Hirte JF, Reith B et al (1996) Different endotoxin release and IL-6 plasma levels after antibiotic administration in surgical intensive care patients. J Endotoxin Res 3:261–267
36. Crosby HA, Bion JF, Penn CW, Elliott TSJ (1994) Antibiotic-induced release of endotoxin from bacteria in vitro. J Med Microbiol 40:23–30
37. Artenstein AW, Cross AS (1989) Inhibition of endotoxin reactivity by aminoglycosides. J Antimicrob Chemother 24:826–828
38. Foca A, Matera G, Berlinghieri MC (1993) Inhibition of endotoxin-induced interleukin 8 release by teicoplanin in human whole blood. Eur J Clin Microbiol Infect Dis 12:940–944
39. Siedlar M, Szczepanik A, Wieckiewicz J et al (1997) Vancomycin down-regulates lipopolysaccharide-induced tumour necrosis factor alpha (TNF alpha) and TNF alpha mRNA accumulation in human blood monocytes. Immunopharmacology 35:265–271
40. Prentice HG, Hann IM, Herbrecht R et al (1997) A randomized comparison of liposomal versus conventional amphotericin B for the treatment of pyrexia of unknown origin in neutropenic patients. Br J Haematol 98:711–718
41. Peters M, Petros A, Dixon G et al (1999) Acquired immuno-paralysis in paediatric intensive care: prospective observational study. BMJ 319:609–610
42. Kaiser AB (1986) Antimicrobial prophylaxis in surgery. N Engl J Med 315:1129–1138
43. Stoutenbeek CP (1989) The role of systemic antibiotic prophylaxis in infection prevention in intensive care by SDD. Infection 17:418–421
44. Lingnau W, Berger J, Javorsky F et al (1997) Selective intestinal decontamination in multiple trauma patients: prospective, controlled trial. J Trauma 42:687–694
45. Verwaest C, Verhaegen J, Ferdinande P et al (1997) Randomised, controlled trial of selective digestive decontamination in 600 mechanically ventilated patients in a multi-disciplinary intensive care unit. Crit Care Med 25:63–71
46. Krueger WA, Lenhart FP, Neeser G et al (2002) Influence of combined intravenous and topical antibiotic prophylaxis on the incidence of infections, organ dysfunctions, and mortality in critically ill patients. Am J Respir Crit Care Med 166:1029–1037
47. Baxby D, van Saene HKF, Stoutenbeek CP, Zandstra DF (1996) Selective decontamination of the digestive tract: 13 years on, what it is and what it is not. Intensive Care Med 22:699–706
48. Damjanovic V, Connolly CM, van Saene HKF et al (1993) Selective decontamination with nystatin for control of a Candida outbreak in a neonatal intensive care unit. J Hosp Infect 24:245–259
49. de la Cal MA, Cerda E, van Saene HKF et al (2004) Effectiveness and safety of enteral vancomycin to control endemicity of methicillin-resistant Staphylococcus aureus in a medical/surgical intensive care unit. J Hosp Infect 56:175–183
50. Desai MH, Rutan RL, Heggers JP, Herndon DN (1992) *Candida* infection with and without nystatin prophylaxis. Arch Surg 127:159–162

51. Morar P, Makura Z, Jones A et al (2000) Topical antibiotics on tracheostoma prevents exogenous colonisation and infection of lower airways in children. Chest 117:513–518
52. Alcock SR (1990) Short-term parenteral antibiotics used as a supplement to SDD regimens. Infection 13(Suppl 1):S14–S18
53. Sirvent JM, Torres A, El-Ebiary M et al (1997) Protective effect of intravenously administered cefuroxime against nosocomial pneumonia in patients with structural coma. Am J Respir Crit Care Med 155:1729–1734
54. (No authors listed) (1996) Hospital-acquired pneumonia in adults: diagnosis, assessment of severity, initial antimicrobial therapy, and preventative strategies. A consensus statement November 1995. Am J Respir Crit Care Med 153:1711–1725
55. Chastre J, Wolff M, Fagon JY et al (2003) Comparison of 8 vs 15 days of antibiotic therapy for ventilator-associated pneumonia in adults. A randomised trial. JAMA 290:2588–2598
56. A'Court CHD, Garrard CS, Crook D et al (1993) Microbiological lung surveillance in mechanically ventilated patients, using non-directed bronchial lavage and quantitative culture. Q J Med 86:635–648
57. Montravers P, Fagon JY, Chastre J et al (1993) Follow-up protected specimen brushes to assess treatment in nosocomial pneumonia. Am Rev Respir Dis 147:38–44
58. Singh N, Rogers P, Atwood CW et al (2000) Short-course empiric antibiotic therapy for patients with pulmonary infiltrates in the intensive care unit. Am J Respir Crit Care Med 162:505–511
59. Dennesen PJW, van der Ven AJAM, Kessels AGH et al (2001) Resolution of infectious parameters after antimicrobial therapy in patients with VAP. Am J Respir Crit Care Med 163:1371–1375
60. Ibrahim EH, Ward S, Sherman G et al (2001) Experience with a clinical guideline for the treatment of ventilator-associated pneumonia. Crit Care Med 29:1109–1115
61. Condon RE (2002) Bacterial resistance to antibiotics. Arch Surg 137:1417–1418
62. Torres A, Ewig S (2004) Diagnosing ventilator-associated pneumonia. N Engl J Med 350:433–435
63. Ledingham I McA, Alcock SR, Eastaway AT et al (1988) Triple regimen of selective decontamination of the digestive tract, systemic cefotaxime, and microbiological surveillance for prevention of acquired infection in intensive care. Lancet 1:785–790
64. Luna CM, Vujacich P, Niederman MS et al (1997) Impact of BAL data on the therapy and outcome of ventilator-associated pneumonia. Chest 111:676–685
65. Alvarez-Lerma F, ICU-acquired Pneumonia Study Group (1996) Modification of empiric antibiotic treatment in patients with pneumonia acquired in the intensive care unit. Intensive Care Med 22:387–394
66. Sarginson RE, Taylor N, Reilly N et al (2004) Infection in prolonged pediatric critical illness: a prospective four year study based on knowledge of the carrier state. Crit Care Med 32:839–847

Outbreaks of Infection in the ICU: What's up at the Beginning of the Twenty-First Century?

12

V. Damjanovic, N. Taylor, T. Williets and H. K. F. van Saene

12.1 Introduction

Two recent sets of publications were taken into consideration when preparing our analysis of infectious outbreaks in the intensive care unit (ICU). The first concerns the emergence of severe acute respiratory syndrome (SARS) and avian flu in 2003, and a spread across the world of a novel influenza caused by SwH1N1 in 2009. These viral infections had a major impact on intensive care and are described in Chap. 20. This chapter is dedicated to describing outbreaks caused by bacteria and fungi, with references to secondary infections associated with flu and SARS [1, 2]. The second publication concerns the "International Study of the Prevalence and Outcomes of Infection in Intensive Care Units" published in December 2009 [3]. Although this is a point-prevalence study, it provides information about the global epidemiology of Infection in ICUs. Unfortunately, it could not give insight into outbreaks of infection in ICUs, so we searched for specific publications describing such outbreaks.

In the second (2005) edition of this book, we analysed the usefulness of molecular techniques in selected outbreaks [4]. The majority of outbreaks occurred in the last decade of the twentieth century. However, reports were usually published several years later. A similar pattern was observed when we analysed outbreaks published in the first decade of the twenty-first century: the actual outbreaks occurred a few years earlier. Indeed, the above-mentioned point-prevalence study was conducted on 8 May 2007 but published in December 2009 [3]. Therefore, for accuracy, this analysis indicates when outbreaks actually happened and when they were subsequently published. *Acinetobacter* outbreaks were selected to illustrate

---

V. Damjanovic (✉)
Institute of Ageing and Chronic Disease, University of Liverpool,
Liverpool, UK
e-mail: damjan.carmel@btinternet.com

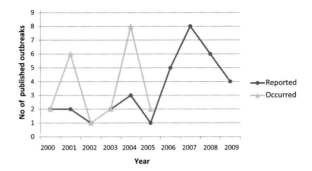

Fig. 12.1 *Acinetobacter* outbreaks published in 2000–2003 actually occurred in 1996–1999

this point (Fig. 12.1). In addition to the reported outbreaks, a number of publications considered many relevant aspects of infection and outbreaks in ICU. Some of these are included in this chapter. We analysed 97 publications, the majority of which met the definition of an outbreak in neonatal (NICU), paediatric (PICU) and adult (AICU) ICUs and reported since 2000. The main objective of this analysis was to find out whether there were any new features in the outbreaks of infection in ICU at the beginning of the new century, including those influenced by new viruses.

12.2 Methods of Analysis

12.2.1 Search Strategy

We searched MEDLINE for outbreaks published between January 2000 and September 2009. The search terms used were intensive care unit, adult ICU, paediatric ICU, neonatal ICU and outbreaks.

12.2.2 Framework of Analysis

We used the same framework as in the second edition of this book; however, outbreaks were not presented separately per ICU type but according to causative organisms, in the following order: methicillin-resistant *Staphylococcus aureus* (MRSA), vancomycin-resistant enterococci (VRE), aerobic Gram-negative bacilli (AGNB), *Pseudomonas* spp., *Acinetobacter* spp. and fungi, together with the selected features searched (Table 12.1). The number of analysed outbreaks is stated, but only selected outbreaks are shown and listed in the references.

Table 12.1 Outbreak microorganisms and features searched

Causative microorganisms	Features				
	Emerging threats	Methods used	Pathogenesis	Prevention and control	Endpoint
MRSA, VRE, AGNB, *Pseudomonas* spp., *Acinetobacter* spp., fungi	New antibiotic resistance, SARS, H1N1	Surveillance cultures, molecular techniques, statistics	Exogenous versus endogenous, endemic infection versus outbreak	Hygiene, anti-sepsis, SDD	Morbidity and mortality associated with outbreak

SDD selective digestive decontamination

12.3 MRSA Outbreaks

We retrieved reports on six outbreaks [5–10] published since 2000; five occurred in AICUs and one in an animal ICU. Reports of two outbreaks were published in 2002 and three in 2004, all occurring between 1997 and 2000. One report published in 2007 did not report the actual time of the outbreak. These outbreaks are summarised briefly according to their countries of origin. A paper from Italy published in 2002 reported a unique experience of controlling a MRSA outbreak of 8 months' duration in a medical/surgical AICU in 1998 using enterally administered vancomycin in mechanically ventilated patients [5]. Another report from Italy, published in 2004, described the identification of a variant of the "Rome clone" of MRSA responsible for an outbreak in a cardiac surgery ICU, which occurred in 1999 in a hospital in Rome. This strain had decreased sensitivity to vancomycin and was resistant to many antibiotics [6]. A study from Germany published in 2002 described the occurrence of MRSA in ICU in terms of endemic and epidemic infections followed from January 1997 to June 2000. This study involved 139 ICUs, 51 of which (37%) had MRSA infections. Outbreaks (three or more MRSA infections within 3 months) were registered in 13 ICUs, clusters (two MRSA infections within 3 months) in further 12 units and single events in 26 [7]. A publication from Spain showed that enterally administered vancomycin can control endemic MRSA in ICUs without promoting VRE. This study was carried out over a 49-month period from July 1996 to 2000 and published in 2004 [8]. In 2007, a report from Canada presented a recent outbreak of MRSA carriage in an animal ICU. This finding appears important, as the strain responsible for the animal outbreak was indistinguishable from a strain in humans commonly isolated in Canada and the USA. Infection control measures, including active surveillance of all animals in the ICU, were used to control the outbreak. As transmission of MRSA within the unit occurred without infections and did not persist for a prolonged period of time, staff screening was surprisingly not initiated [9]. A paper from China published in 2004 described an MRSA outbreak due to an increased acquisition rate in ICU associated with an outbreak of SARS, which occurred in 2003. From 12 March to 31 May, only patients with SARS were admitted to the 22-bed unit. During this period, infection control precautions were upgraded, which included wearing gloves and gowns at all times. However, data suggested that MRSA transmission might be unexpectedly increased if gloves and gowns were worn all the time [10].

12.4 Enterococcal Outbreaks

There have been ten outbreaks in AICUs published since 2000: eight were caused by VRE, one was sensitive to vancomycin and one was sensitive to vancomycin but resistant to linezolid. We selected seven reports and summarised them according to the countries of origin and time of events and publishing.

A paper from Pakistan published in 2002 was the country's first experience with a vancomycin resistant *Enterococcus faecium* outbreak in the ICU and NICU. The outbreak occurred in 2002, lasted 1 month and all but one isolate was of a single clone [11]. All isolates were resistant to gentamicin, ampicillin and tetracycline but sensitive to chloramphenicol. Six patients were colonised and four infected, with positive blood cultures; two of each died before specific therapy could be started (50% mortality rate). In 2005, a report from Italy described an outbreak of VRE colonisation and infection in an ICU that lasted 16 months (2001–2002) [12]. Fifty-six patients were colonised by *E. faecium*, and *E. faecalis* was detected in only two cases. Because of the low pathogenicity of VRE, the authors questioned whether it was worthwhile to have a specific VRE surveillance programme. For the 2004 Lowbury lecture, Pearman reported the Australian experience with VRE, which he described as "from disaster to ongoing control". This was the first outbreak of VRE, which was caused by *E. faecium* in an ICU and hospital wards and lasted 5 months in 2001. A vigilant VRE control programme prevented the epidemic strain from becoming endemic in the hospital [13]. An outbreak due to glycopeptide-resistant enterococci (GRE) in an ICU with simultaneous circulation of two different clones was reported from France in 2008. The outbreak lasted several months in 2003 without infections, but the significant colonisation caused organisational problems in the ICU [14]. An outbreak of VRE in an ICU was reported from China in 2009. The outbreak was caused by *E. faecium* and lasted 11 months (2006–2007). A detailed molecular analysis showed that genetically unrelated isolates had transferred vancomycin resistance by conjugation [15]. A paper from Korea reported an outbreak of VRE in a neurological ICU. VRE was mainly isolated from urine specimens associated with the presence of a Foley catheter. Of 52 patients colonised with VRE, only two had active infection [16]. In 2009, a report from Spain presented an outbreak of linezolid-resistant *E. faecalis* in an ICU and reanimation unit [17]. This was the first report of a clonal outbreak of linezolid-resistant *E. faecalis* in Spain. The strain was sensitive to imipenem, vancomycin, teicoplanin and rifampicin. Most patients were exposed to linezolid within a year (2005–2006). The use of linezolid began in

2002. The increase in its use continued until 2005 when a mutant was identified by molecular analysis.

12.5 AGNB Outbreaks

Fourteen reports on outbreaks were retrieved since 2000. Eight were caused by *Klebsiella pneumoniae*, four by *Serratia marcescens*, one by *Enterobacter cloacae* and one by simultaneous infection of *E. cloacae* and *S. marcescens*. Three *Klebsiella*, three *Serratia* and the remaining two were selected for analysis. We discuss *Pseudomonas* and *Acinetobacter* outbreaks separately.

12.5.1 *Klebsiella* Outbreaks

An outbreak of *Klebsiella* infection in NICU and PICU was published from Spain in 2004; this outbreak occurred in 2002–2003 and lasted 1 year [18]. The outbreak was polyclonal. Two predominant clones of *Klebsiella* harboured a special gene (SHV5) for the beta-lactamase enzyme responsible for multi-drug-resistant *Klebsiella*. According to the authors, this type of *Klebsiella* was not reported previously in Spain. Another clone harbouring two different genes responsible for multidrug resistance but dissimilar from the above was reported. A report from The Netherlands published in 2001 described an outbreak of infections with a multi-drug-resistant *Klebsiella* strain [19] associated with contaminated roll boards in operating rooms. This outbreak in 2000 showed how an unusual source of the outbreak can be revealed by systematic surveillance. In 2008, a polyclonal outbreak of extended spectrum beta-lactamase (ESBL)-producing *K. pneumoniae* in an ICU of a university hospital in Belgium was reported [20]. This was a 2-month outbreak that occurred in 2005 with 18 isolates. There was one predominant clone, two clones with several isolates and four with unique isolates. The cause of the outbreak was not clear but was associated with a dramatic increase in the number of imported carriers during the previous weeks.

12.5.2 *Enterobacter cloacae* Outbreaks

An outbreak caused by ESBL-producing *E. cloacae* in a cardiothoracic ICU was reported from Spain in 2007 [21]. The outbreak occurred in 2005, lasted 3 months, and involved seven patients. Molecular analysis revealed two clones responsible for the outbreak: one carried a single ESBL; the other carried two ESBLs. Both clones showed resistance to quinolones and aminoglycosides. The outbreak was brought under control by the implementation of barrier measures and cephalosporin restrictions.

12.5.3 *Serratia marcescens* Outbreaks

An outbreak was reported from Germany in 2002 [22] in both the NICU and PICU, lasted from September to November 1998 and involved 15 patients. Two epidemic strains were associated with cross-infection in groups of five and ten patients, respectively. Two epidemic clones were detected from the surfaces of an ICU room, but an original source was not identified. The outbreak was stopped by routine infection-control measures. A report from Malaysia in 2004 described an outbreak of *Serratia* infections that lasted 10 days in an AICU [23]. The single outbreak strain was found in insulin and sedative solutions administered to patients. An outbreak of *S. marcescens* colonisation and infection in a neurological ICU that occurred from May 2002 to March 2003 was reported from a Dutch university medical centre in 2006 [24]. The outbreak strain was traced to a healthcare worker (HCW) with long-term carriage on the hands. The skin of the HCW's hands was psoriatic. The epidemic ended after the colonised HCW went on leave, with subsequent eradication treatment. A heterogeneous outbreak of *E. cloacae* and *S. marcescens* infections in a surgical ICU was published by a group of authors from San Francisco, USA [25]. The outbreak lasted from December 1997 through January 1998. Molecular techniques ruled out a point source or significant cross-contamination as modes of transmission. The authors concluded that patient-related factors, such as respiratory tract colonisation and duration of central line placement might have played a role in this outbreak.

12.5.4 *Pseudomonas* Outbreaks

Several reports have been published on infections caused by multi-drug-resistant *Pseudomonas* spp. in ICUs since 2000. We retrieved 19 reports; not all were outbreaks, as some were described as endemic infections. In addition, one outbreak was caused by *Burkholderia cepacia*. We selected a few outbreaks that we believed would represent the main problems occurring in ICUs, such as multidrug resistance, clonality, transmission source and mode and infection severity.

In 2000, a publication from Norway reported an outbreak of multi-drug-resistant *P. aeruginosa* associated with increased risk of death [26]. The outbreak occurred from December 1999 to September 2000, was monoclonal and the strain was introduced into the ICU early in 1998 and was maintained thereafter. All patients were ventilated. The strain was resistant to carbapenems, quinolones and azlocillin. In 13 infected patients, ten of whom died, *Pseudomonas* was found in one or all specimens, such as respiratory secretions, ventilator tubes, connection tubes and the water catcher of the ventilator system. The bacterium was also isolated from water taps. In addition to enhanced control of infection measures, complete elimination of the outbreak was achieved after water taps were pasteurised and sterile water was used when a solvent was needed. In 2003, French authors published a report on the epidemiology of *P. aeruginosa* in an ICU [27]. Although between 1996 and 1997 the prevalence of *P. aeruginosa* infections reached 30% of all hospital-acquired infections, the authors did not call this an outbreak, despite the fact that this was twice the national prevalence of 15% observed in ICUs. However, this high prevalence prompted the authors to conduct a prospective epidemiological study from July 1997 to February 1998. We selected this study as a good example of activities necessary to prevent a major outbreak. The authors described how systematic surveillance was carried out (oropharyngeal and rectal swabs on admission and twice weekly afterwards). This practice revealed that during the study period, the overall incidence of *P. aeruginosa* carriage was 43%: 17% on admission and 26% acquired in the ICU. In addition 16/191 (8%) patients developed the infection. The authors also pointed out that intestinal carriage was a prerequisite for colonisation or infection. Genotyping analysis of 81 isolates indicated that 70% belonged to genotype 1, 4% to genotype 2 and that remaining isolates were not genetically related. It has also been shown that mechanical ventilation was associated with *P. aeruginosa* carriage and ineffective antibiotics significantly increased the risk of colonisation and infection in ICU. The authors concluded that not only do endogenous sources account for the majority of colonisation or infection due to *P. aeruginosa* but that exogenous sources may be involved in some instances. In an epidemic setting, the authors' stance was to reinforce standard barrier precautions. However, the main message of this study is the necessity to adopt and pursue preventive measures.

In 2008, an outbreak of severe *B. cepacia* infections in an ICU was reported from Spain [28]. The outbreak occurred over a period of 18 days in August 2006 when *B. cepacia* were recovered from different clinical samples associated with bacteraemia in three cases, lower respiratory tract infection in one and urinary tract infection in one. Samples of antiseptics, eau de cologne and moisturising milk available on treatment carts were collected and cultured. *B. cepacia* was isolated not only from three samples of the moisturising body milk that had been applied to the patients but also from two new hermetically closed units. All strains recovered from environmental and clinical samples belonged to the same clone. The cream was withdrawn from all hospital units, and no new cases of *B. cepacia* developed. The authors concluded that the presence of bacteria in cosmetic products, even within accepted limits, may lead to severe life-threatening infections in severely ill patients.

12.5.5 *Acinetobacter* Outbreaks

We retrieved 34 publications on *Acinetobacter* outbreaks, 11 of which were not strictly outbreaks, and actually not reported as such, but rather described general epidemiology, antibiotic resistance, infection control or treatment options. Most of these problems are dealt with in relevant chapters of this edition. Following our approach, we summarise only a few outbreaks, which appeared to offer some new findings or insights.

A 2000 report from Italy described an outbreak of infusion-related *A. baumannii* bacteraemia in an eight-bed ICU [29]. From 6 June to 15 July 2000, six cases were identified. All patients received parenterally administered solutions prepared by ICU nurses, which was subsequently proven to be the source of infection. Three patients died from sepsis despite treatment with a combination of meropenem and amikacin, which were shown by laboratory tests to be synergistic. This high mortality rate (50%) was explained by the authors as being due to persistent bacteraemia related to the repeated infusions of contaminated solutions. Once aseptic preparation was carried out in the hospital pharmacy, this outbreak was controlled, and further infusion-related nosocomial bacteraemia was prevented. From the USA, a publication in 2001 reported an outbreak of multiresistant *Acinetobacter* colonisation and infection in an ICU [30]. The strain was sensitive only to polymyxin. The outbreak lasted an entire year between 1996 and 1997 and involved 57 patients, 27 of whom were infected and 25 colonised. The arrival of a colonised burn patient (>50% total body surface area) from an outside hospital was responsible for the outbreak. Although on typing two strains were found, the only identified primary source was the original burn patient. Ten deaths resulted from infections (37% of infected patients). The authors claimed that this outbreak served as a model of eradication of multi-drug-resistant organisms, as the *Acinetobacter* was eliminated from all ICU patients by multidisciplinary measures that included the following: cohort and contact isolation of all colonised and infected patients; introduction of strict aseptic measures such as hand washing, barrier isolation, equipment and room cleaning; sterilisation of ventilator equipment; and individual dedication of medical equipment to each patient. A paper was published from Australia in 2007 regarding carbapenem-resistant *A. baumannii* [31]. We selected this publication as an illustration of an extensive molecular analysis rather than for a critical review of the outbreak, which occurred in an ICU between 1999 and 2000. Based on their findings, the authors claim that antibiotic-resistant genes are readily exchanged between co-circulating strains in epidemics of phenotypically indistinguishable organisms. In conclusion, they recommend that epidemiological investigation of major outbreaks should include whole-genome typing as well as analysis of potentially transmissible genes and their vehicles. Finally, we found a paper in a journal from Kuwait not found by our Internet research [32]. The authors reported three different outbreaks of multi-drug-resistant *A. baumannii* infections involving 24 patients aged 16–75 years that occurred in an ICU in the course of 1 year between 2006 and 2007. The outbreak was polyclonal and successfully controlled with tigecycline, to which two causative clones were sensitive. Three additional distinct clones were isolated from the environment. Due to lack of appropriate surveillance cultures, no explanation was offered for the origin of epidemic clones. Subsequently, in a letter to the editor, our interpretation that "…microbial gut overgrowth increased spontaneous mutation, which led to polyclonality and antibiotic resistance in the critically ill" was accepted by the authors [33, 34].

12.6 Fungal Outbreaks

Thirteen publications were retrieved from MEDLINE, five of which described outbreaks of remarkable findings. The remaining papers reported some important aspects of fungal species, colonisation, infection and treatments, predominantly as surveys, and as such were not included in our analysis.

Outbreaks presented here were caused by uncommon opportunistic fungi. Two reports described ICU outbreaks caused by *Hansenula anomala*, an opportunistic yeast first reported from a Liverpool, UK, NICU in 1986 [35]. In 2001, a report from Croatia described an outbreak in a surgical ICU [36]. *H. anomala* was isolated from blood taken from eight patients between 23 August and 6 December 1993. All patients were treated with antifungal therapy; three died from complications of underlying disease. The introduction of strict hygienic measures stopped the spread of infection, but the outbreak ceased with the introduction of a new batch of cotton from another manufacturer, which was used for venipuncture-site disinfection. However, the authors could not find evidence for infection source and transmission route. The second report, from Brazil (2005), describes an outbreak in a PICU [37]. The authors reported their finding as an outbreak of *Pichia anomala*, a newly introduced name for *H. anomala*. From October 2002 to January 2004, 17 children developed *P. anomala* fungemia. The median age was 1.1 year, and the main underlying conditions were congenital malformations and neoplastic disease. The overall mortality rate was 41.2% despite treatment with amphotericin B. During a 2-week period in April 2003, when new cases occurred, surveillance cultures revealed that 67.9% of patients were colonised with yeasts, but no single patient was found to be colonised with *P. anomala*. Thus, no source was found at that time. The outbreak was not controlled until orally administered prophylaxis with nystatin and topical application of an iodoform to venipuncture sites were started.

An extraordinary outbreak of invasive gastritis caused by *Rhizopus microsporus* in an adult ICU was reported from Spain in 2004 [38]. Over a 14-week period (between November 1995 and March 1996), gastric mucormycosis was diagnosed in five patients, four of whom were admitted to ICU with severe community-acquired pneumonia and one with multiple trauma. The main symptom was upper gastrointestinal haemorrhage. Isolated filamentous fungi were identified as *R. microsporus* var. *rhizopodiformis* and were detected in gastric aspiration samples and traced to wooden tongue depressors used to prepare medication for oral administration (and given to patients through a nasogastric catheter) and in some tongue depressors stored in unopened boxes unexposed to the ICU environment. The outbreak was terminated when contaminated tongue depressors were withdrawn from use. This outbreak was attributable to the 40% mortality rate; wooden material should not be used in the hospital setting.

In 2004, an outbreak of three cases of *Dipodascus capitatus* infection in an ICU was reported from Japan [39]. The index case was pulmonary infection with a fulminant course of fungal infection, which resulted in death, in a patient with acute myelocytic leukaemia who shared a room for at least 1 week with the two other patients, suggesting the possibility of transmission. One of the other two patients died from multiple organ dysfunction. The presence of *D. capitatus* might have been due to contamination in the respiratory ICU. In all cases, *D. capitatus* was identified in sputum, deep tracheal aspiration samples, blood and urine samples. The authors concluded that *D. capitatus* should be added to the lengthening list of opportunistic fungal pathogens that can cause infection in immune-compromised patients, with the danger of transmission and potential outbreak.

An outbreak of *Saccharomyces cerevisiae* fungemia in an ICU was reported from Spain in 2005 [40]. During the period from 15 to 30 April, three patients with *S. cerevisiae* fungemia were identified. The only identified risk factor was treatment with a probiotic containing this yeast. The three patients received the product via nasogastric tube for a mean of 8.5 days before the culture was positive. Surveillance cultures for the control patients admitted at the same time did not reveal any carriers. All three patients died from causes unrelated to *S. cerevisiae*. Discontinuation of use of the product for treatment or prevention of *Clostridium difficile*-associated diarrhoea in the unit stopped the outbreak of infection. In conclusion, the authors warned that the use of *S. cerevisiae* should be carefully reassessed in immune-compromised or critically ill patients.

12.7 Discussion

An outbreak is defined as an event where two or more patients in a defined location are infected by identical, often multi-drug-resistant, microorganisms transmitted via the hands of HCW, usually within an arbitrary time period of 2 weeks. There are two different types of infection involved in outbreaks: secondary endogenous and exogenous. Outbreaks of secondary endogenous infections are invariably preceded by outbreaks of carriage of abnormal flora, whereas outbreaks of exogenous infections are not preceded by outbreaks of abnormal carriage. These two types of outbreaks each require a different type of management: enterally and topically administered antimicrobials for secondary endogenous and exogenous outbreaks, respectively. Ongoing surveillance efforts, i.e. throat and rectal swabs on admission and twice weekly thereafter, to monitor the efficacy of systematic decontamination of the digestive tract (SDD) and to identify the emergence of antimicrobial resistant threats, is an intrinsic component of any decontamination programme. In this sense, a well-designed programme contains an intrinsic degree of protection against antibiotic-resistant organism emergence. Surveillance cultures of throat and rectum are more sensitive in detecting resistance than are diagnostic samples [41]. Additionally, there is a close relationship between surveillance and diagnostic samples. Once a resistant microorganism reaches overgrowth concentrations, i.e. $\geq 10^5$/ml saliva and/or gram of faeces, diagnostic samples become positive [8].

In our review, 28 outbreaks were selected to illustrate the situation at the beginning of this century. As a matter of fact, the majority of the outbreaks was related to the previous decade. However, biased or not, our analysis described 19 outbreaks that occurred after 2000 and nine from last century, although the outbreaks were published in this century (Fig. 12.1). This suggests that some new problems indeed emerged in this century.

It is important to record the number of papers retrieved according the causative organisms: MRSA six, VRE ten, AGNB 14, *Pseudomonas* spp. 19, *Acinetobacter* spp. 23 and fungi 13. Perhaps, against our expectation, AGNB organisms—in

Table 12.2 New and older trends at the beginning of the twenty-first century

New trends	Older trends
Emerging viral infections may increase bacterial and fungal outbreaks	Surveillance cultures mostly used after outbreaks occurred
Extensive use of molecular techniques proved that many outbreaks are polyclonal and detected new genes responsible for antibiotic resistance	Pathogenesis of outbreaks rarely clarified due to lack of surveillance cultures SDD still rarely used for control of outbreaks In general, endemic infections more common than outbreaks
Emergence of new resistant clones	Infection control measures usually enhanced after outbreak occurred
The principle of SDD extended to other antibiotics, e.g. vancomycin to prevent MRSA outbreaks	Mortality primarily attributed to underlying disease, with exception of NICU and direct injection of pathogen

SDD selective decontamination of the digestive tract; *MRSA* methicillin-resistant *Staphylococcus aureus*; *NICU* neonatal intensive care unit

particular, opportunists such as *Pseudomonas* and *Acinetobacter*—prevailed significantly, for which there must be a reason. If we take MRSA as an example, all around the world, this drug-resistant pathogen has been a primary focus for nosocomial infection control and treatment for years. Thus, there are fewer outbreaks. An extensive study from Germany that involved 139 ICUs showed that cluster and single MRSA infections were significantly more common than actual outbreaks (38 ICUs compared with 12, respectively) [7]. To our knowledge, there were no similar studies for VRE and AGNB, but one would anticipate similar findings and interpretation.

On the other hand, opportunistic pathogens such as *Pseudomonas* spp., *Acinetobacter* spp. and fungi often caused unexpected outbreaks, particularly in immunocompromised patients. They originated from external sources and were difficult to treat because of their resistance to multiple antibiotics.

Our search for specific features relevant to published outbreaks revealed some new, and confirmed some older, trends (Table 12.2). Probably the best example of how new viral infections—such as SARS—can change the rate of bacterial and fungal infections in ICUs came from the experience in China [10]. There was a significant increase in the rate of MRSA and *Candida* spp. acquisition in an ICU during the SARS period. It may be anticipated, therefore, that in the future, SARS and influenza viral infections would lead to complex ICU outbreaks.

We pointed out earlier how using molecular techniques revealed that many outbreaks were due to more than one clone [4]. Our analysis confirms this, although the origin of different clones remained obscure in all reports in which polyclonality was detected. However, we recently put forward a hypothesis that microbial gut overgrowth is responsible for increased spontaneous mutation leading to polyclonality and antibiotic resistance [42]. Furthermore, extensive use of molecular techniques not only revealed a number of new genes responsible for antibiotic resistance [18] but showed that genetically unrelated organisms readily exchange antibiotic resistance genes [15, 31]. Yet further, a new trend is related to the SDD concept. Two studies, one from Italy and one from Spain, reported the use of enterally administered vancomycin to control and prevent, respectively, MRSA outbreaks [5, 8]. This is further evidence that the principle of SDD can be used with antimicrobials directed specifically to the causative organism. As early as 1993 we reported how selective decontamination with nystatin successfully controlled a *Candida* outbreak in an NICU [43].

Among older trends, surveillance cultures, or lack of them, are still prominent. Even in 2009 there were authors responsible for infection control in hospitals and ICUs who claimed that "...surveillance cultures of all patients with potential to develop infection are difficult and very costly..." [44]. Some time ago (1994), we expressed an alternative view in response to an identical attitude [45]. Needless to say, lack of surveillance cultures not only delays the recognition of an outbreak and its control but also precludes the understanding of the pathogenesis of the majority of outbreaks. Surveillance cultures are also crucial for detecting outbreaks of exogenous pathogenesis, i.e. without carriage. On the other hand, the source of an exogenous outbreak is readily identified with molecular techniques. Some of these outbreaks are striking, such as one from this analysis in which *Acinetobacter*-contaminated parentally administered solutions were repeatedly infused to patients, leading to a very high mortality rate of 50% [29].

In conclusion, new trends as well as old confirm what we indicated in the previous edition of this book, which is that to control and prevent ICU outbreaks, surveillance cultures and SDD should be integrated in routine infection-control measures.

References

1. El-Masri MM, Williams KM, Fox-Wasylyshyn SM (2004) Severe acute respiratory syndrome: another challenge for critical care nurses. AACN Clin Issues 15:150–159
2. Burns SM (2009) H1N1 influenza is here. J Hosp Infect 73:200–202
3. Vincent JL, Rello J, Marshall J et al (2009) International study of the prevalence and outcome of infection in intensive care units. JAMA 302:2323–2329
4. Damjanovic V, Corbella X, van der Spoel JI, van Saene HKF (2005) Outbreaks of infection in intensive care units—usefulness of molecular techniques for outbreak analysis. In: van Saene HKF, Silvestri L, de la Cal MA (eds) Infection control in the intensive care unit, 2nd edn. Springer, Milan, pp 247–296
5. Silvestri L, Milanese M, Oblach L et al (2002) Enteral vancomycin to control methicillin-resistant *Staphylococcus aureus* outbreak in mechanically ventilated patients. Am J Infect Control 30:391–399
6. Cassone M, Campanile F, Pantosti A et al (2004) Identification of a variant 'Rome clone' of methicillin-resistant *Staphylococcus aureus* with decreased susceptibility to vancomycin, responsible for an outbreak in an intensive care unit. Microb Drug Res 10:43–49
7. Gastmeier P, Sohr D, Geffers C et al (2002) Occurrence of methicillin-resistant *Staphylococcus aureus* infections in German intensive care units. Infection 4:198–202

8. de la Cal MA, Cerda E, van Saene HKF et al (2004) Effectiveness and safety of enteral vancomycin to control endemicity of methicillin-resistant *Staphylococcus aureus* in a medical/surgical intensive care unit. J Hosp Infect 56:175–183
9. Weese JS, Faires M, Rousseau J et al (2007) Cluster of methicillin-resistant *Staphylococcus aureus* colonisation in a small animal intensive care unit. JAMA 231:1361–1364
10. Yap FH, Gomersall CD, Fung KS et al (2004) Increase in methicillin-resistant *Staphylococcus aureus* acquisition rate and change in pathogen pattern associated with an outbreak of severe acute respiratory syndrome. Clin Infect Dis 39:511–516
11. Khan E, Sarwari A, Hasan R et al (2002) Emergence of vancomycin-resistant *Enterococcus faecium* at a tertiary care hospital in Karachi, Pakistan. J Hosp Infect 52:292–296
12. Peta M, Carretto E, Bdbarini D et al (2006) Outbreak of vancomycin-resistant *Enterococcus* spp. on an Italian general intensive care unit. Clin Microbiol Infect 12:163–169
13. Pearman JW (2006) 2004 Lowbury lecture: the Western Australian experience with vancomycin-resistant enterococci—from disaster to ongoing control. J Hosp Infect 63:14–26
14. Delamare C, Lameloise V, Lozniewski A et al (2008) Glycopeptide-resistant *Enterococcus* outbreak in an ICU with simultaneous circulation of two different clones. Pathol Biol 56:454–460
15. Zhu X, Zeng B, Wang S et al (2009) Molecular characterization of outbreak-related strains of vancomycin-resistant *Enterococcus faecium* from an intensive care unit in Beijing, China. J Hosp Infect 72:147–154
16. Se BY, Chun HJ, Yi HJ et al (2009) Incidence and risk factors of infections caused by vancomycin-resistant *Enterococcus* colonization in neurosurgical intensive care unit patients. J Korean Neurosurg Soc 46:123–129
17. Gomez-Gil R, Romero-Gomez MP, Garcia-Arias A et al (2009) Nosocomial outbreak of linezolid-resistant *Enterococcus faecalis* infection in a tertiary care hospital. Diag Microb Infect Dis 65:175–179
18. Brinas L, Lantero M, Zarazaga M et al (2004) Outbreak of SHV-5 beta-lactamase-producing *Klebsiella pneumoniae* in a neonatal–pediatric intensive care unit in Spain. Microb Drug Res 10:354–358
19. van't Veen A, van der Zee A, Nelson J et al (2005) Outbreak of infection with a multiresistant *Klebsiella pneumoniae* strain associated with contaminated roll boards in operating rooms. J Clin Microbiol 43:4961–4967
20. Laurent C, Rodriguez-Villalobos H, Rost F et al (2008) Intensive care unit outbreak of extended-spectrum beta-lactamase-producing *Klebsiella pneumoniae* controlled by cohorting patients and reinforcing infection control measures. Infect Control Hosp Epidemiol 29: 517–524
21. Manzur A, Tubau F, Pujol M et al (2007) Nosocomial outbreak due to extended-spectrum-beta-lactamase-producing *Enterobacter cloacae* in a cardiothoracic intensive care unit. J Clin Microbiol 45:2365–2369
22. Steppberger K, Walter S, Claros MC et al (2002) Nosocomial neonatal outbreak of Serratia marcescens–analysis of pathogens by pulsed field gel electrophoresis and polymerase chain reaction. Infection 30:277–281
23. Alfizah H, Nordiah AJ, Rozaidi WS (2004) Using pulsed-field gel electrophoresis in the molecular investigation of an outbreak of *Serratia marcescens* infection in an intensive care unit. Singap Med J 45:214–218
24. de Vries JJ, Bass WH, van der Ploeg K et al (2006) Outbreak of *Serratia marcescens* colonization and infection traced to a healthcare worker with long-term carriage on the hands. Infect Control Hosp Epidemiol 27:1153–1158
25. Dorsey G, Borneo HT, Sun SJ et al (2000) A heterogeneous outbreak of *Enterobacter cloacae* and *Serratia marcescens* infections in a surgical intensive care unit. Infect Control Hosp Epidemiol 21:465–469
26. Bukholm G, Tannaes T, Kjelsberg AB et al (2002) An outbreak of multidrug-resistant *Pseudomonas aeruginosa* associated with increased risk of patient death in an intensive care unit. Infect Control Hosp Epidemiol 23:441–446

27. Thuong M, Arvaniti K, Ruimy R et al (2003) Epidemiology of *Pseudomonas aeruginosa* and risk factors for carriage acquisition in an intensive care unit. J Hosp Infect 53:274–282
28. Alvarez-Lerma F, Maull E, Terradas R et al (2008) Mosturizing body milk as a reservoir of *Burkholderia cepacia*: outbreak of nosocomial infection in a multidisciplinary intensive care unit. Crit Care 12:R10
29. Menichetti F, Tascini C, Ferranti S et al (2000) Clinical and molecular epidemiology of an outbreak of infusion-related *Acinetobacter baumannii* bacteremia in an intensive care unit. Le Infezioni Medicina 1:24–29
30. Podnos YD, Cinat ME, Wilson SE et al (2001) Eradication of multi-drug resistant *Acinetobacter* from an intensive care unit. Surg Infect 2:297–301
31. Valenzuela JK, Thomas L, Partridge SR et al (2007) Hospital gene transfer in a polyclonal outbreak of carbapenem-resistant *Acinetobacter baumannii*. J Clin Microbiol 45:453–460
32. Jamal W, Salama M, Dehrab N et al (2009) Role of tigecycline in the control of carbapenem-resistant *Acinetobacter baumannii* outbreak in an intensive care unit. J Hosp Infect 72: 234–242
33. Damjanovic V, Taylor N, van Saene HKF (2009) Origin of epidemic clones of *Acinetobacter* in the critically ill. J Hosp Infect 73:285–286
34. Rotimi VO, Jamal W, Salama M (2009) Control of *Acinetobacter* outbreaks in the intensive care unit. J Hosp Infect 73:286–287
35. Murphy N, Damjanovic V, Hart CA et al (1986) Infection and colonisation of neonates by *Hansenula anomala*. Lancet 1:291–293
36. Kalenic S, Jandrlic M, Vegar V et al (2001) *Hansenula anomala* outbreak at a surgical intensive care unit: a search for risk factors. Eur J Epidemiol 17:491–496
37. Pasqualotto AC, Sukiennik TC, Severo LC et al (2005) An outbreak of *Pichia anomala* fungaemia in a Brazilian pediatric intensive care unit. Infect Control Hosp Epidemiol 26:553–558
38. Maravi-Poma E, Rodriguez-Tudela JL, de Jalon JG et al (2004) Outbreak of gastric mucormycosis associated with the use of wooden tongue depressors in critically ill patients. Intensive Care Med 30:724–728
39. Eroz G, Otag F, Erturan Z et al (2004) An outbreak of *Dipodascus capitatus* infection in the ICU: three case reports and review of the literature. Jpn J Infect Dis 57:248–252
40. Munoz P, Bouza E, Cuenca-Estrella M et al (2005) *Saccharomyces cerevisiae* fungemia: an emerging infectious disease. Clin Infect Dis 40:1625–1634
41. D'Agata EMC, Venkataraman L, De Girolami P et al (1999) Colonization with broad-spectrum cephalosporin-resistant Gram-negative bacilli in intensive care units during a nonoutbreak period: prevalence, risk factors, and rate of infection. Crit Care Med 27: 1090–1095
42. van Saene HK, Taylor N, Damjanovic V et al (2008) Microbial gut overgrowth guarantees increased spontaneous mutation leading to polyclonality and antibiotic resistance in the critically ill. Curr Drug Targets 9:419–421
43. Damjanovic V, Connolly CM, van Saene HKF et al (1993) Selective decontamination with nystatin for control of a *Candida* outbreak in a neonatal intensive care unit. J Hosp Infect 24:245–259
44. Miranda LN, van der Heijden IM, Costa SF et al (2009) Candida colonisation as a source of candaemia. J Hosp Infect 72:9–16
45. Damjanovic V, van Saene HKF, Weindling AM et al (1994) The multiple value of surveillance cultures: an alternative view. J Hosp Infect 28:71–75

Preventing Infection Using Selective Decontamination of the Digestive Tract

13

L. Silvestri, H. K. F. van Saene
and D. F. Zandstra

13.1 Introduction

Selective decontamination of the digestive tract (SDD) is an antimicrobial prophylaxis designed to prevent or minimize endogenous and exogenous infections in critically ill patients. The purpose of SDD is to prevent—or eradicate if initially present— the oropharyngeal and intestinal abnormal carrier state of potentially pathogenic microorganisms (PPMs), mainly aerobic Gram-negative microorganisms, but also methicillin-sensitive *Staphylococcus aureus* (MSSA), and yeasts, leaving the indigenous flora predominately undisturbed. The practice of SDD has four fundamental features, termed the classic Stoutenbeek's tetralogy [1, 2] (Fig. 13.1, Table 13.1):
1. parenteral antibiotics given immediately on admission for 4 days to control primary endogenous infections due to PPMs already present in the admission flora;
2. enteral antimicrobials [polymyxin E, tobramycin, and amphotericin B (PTA)] given throughout treatment in the intensive care unit (ICU) to control secondary carriage and subsequent endogenous infections due to PPMs acquired in the unit;
3. health care workers' hand hygiene throughout treatment in the ICU to control exogenous infections due to transmission of ICU-associated microorganisms;
4. surveillance cultures of patients' throat and rectum on admission and twice weekly to monitor the efficacy of the maneuver.

SDD selectively targets the 15 PPMs and the high-level pathogens, such as *Streptococcus pyogenes*. By design, SDD does not cover low-level pathogens, including anaerobes, viridans streptococci, enterococci and coagulase-negative

---

L. Silvestri (✉)
Department of Emergency, Unit of Anesthesia and Intensive Care,
Presidio Ospedaliero di Gorizia, Gorizia, Italy
e-mail: lucianosilvestri@yahoo.it

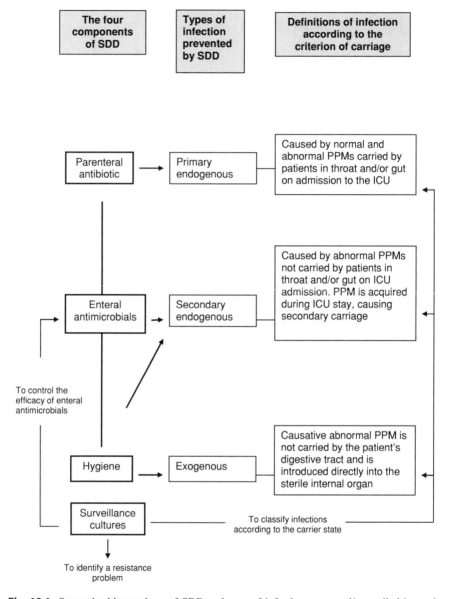

Fig. 13.1 Stoutenbeek's tetralogy of SDD and type of infection prevented/controlled by each component. *SDD* selective decontamination of the digestive tract; *PPM* potentially pathogenic microorganism; *ICU* intensive care unit

Table 13.1 The full four-component protocol of selective decontamination of the digestive tract

Target PPMs and antimicrobials	Total daily dose (divided 4 × daily)		
	<5 years	5–12 years	>12 years
1. Parenteral antimicrobials: normal PPMs: cefotaxime (mg)	150/kg	200/kg	4,000
2. Enteral antimicrobials: abnormal PPMs A. Oropharynx 1. AGNB: polymyxin E with tobramycin 2. Yeasts: amphotericin B or nystatin 3. MRSA: vancomycin	 2 g of 2% paste or gel 2 g of 2% paste or gel 2 g of 4% paste or gel		
B. Gut 1. AGNB: polymyxin E (mg) with tobramycin (mg) 2. Yeasts: amphotericin B (mg) or nystatin units 3. MRSA: vancomycin (mg)	 100 80 500 2×10^6 20–40/kg	 200 160 1,000 4×10^6 20–40/kg	 400 320 2,000 8×10^6 500–2,000
3. Hygiene with topical antimicrobials			
4. Surveillance swabs of throat and rectum on admission, Monday, Thursday			

PPMs potentially pathogenic microorganisms; *AGNB* aerobic Gram-negative bacilli; *MRSA* methicillin-resistant *Staphylococcus aureus*

staphylococci. The most important feature of SDD is the enteral administration of nonabsorbable polymyxin E/tobramycin to eradicate the abnormal aerobic Gram negative bacilli (AGNB). This results in decontamination of the digestive tract. Critically ill patients are unable to clear these pathogens due to their underlying disease. Intestinal overgrowth with AGNB causes systemic immunoparalysis [2]. The reason for the enteral administration of polymyxin E/tobramycin is that it promotes recovery of systemic immunity and because preventing or eradicating abnormal AGNB in throat and gut effectively controls aspiration and translocation of these microorganisms into the lower airways and blood stream, respectively. Enterally administered antimicrobials have been shown to be effective in controlling secondary endogenous infections. However, their use does not affect primary endogenous and exogenous infections. The second component is adequate parenteral administration of an antimicrobial to control primary endogenous infections. Cefotaxime has been used in most trials to cover both normal and abnormal pathogens. In adding enterally to parenterally administered antibiotics, the original pre-1980s antibiotics remain useful, without the development of antimicrobial resistance. Third, high standards of hygiene are indispensable for reducing hand contamination and subsequent transmission from external sources. Finally, surveillance samples of the throat and rectum are an integral component of the SDD protocol. Knowledge of the carrier state allows compliance and efficacy of this prophylactic protocol to be monitored.

13.2 Efficacy

After 25 five years of clinical research, SDD has been assessed in 63 randomized controlled trials (RCTs) [3–65] and ten meta-analyses of RCTs only (Table 13.2) [66–75].

13.2.1 Carriage

SDD significantly reduced oropharyngeal carriage by 87% [odds ratio (OR) 0.13, 95% confidence interval (CI) 0.07–0.2] and rectal carriage due to Gram-negative PPMs by 85% (OR 0.15; 95% CI 0.07–0.31) [72]. Gram-positive carriage was also reduced, but not significantly. Additionally, fungal carriage was significantly reduced by 68% (OR 0.32, 95% CI 0.19–0.53) [70].

13.2.2 Lower Airway Infection

All meta-analyses showed a significant reduction of lower respiratory tract infection. The meta-analysis from the Italian Cochrane Centre demonstrated that enteral and parenteral administration of antimicrobials for SDD reduced lower airway infections by 82% (OR 0.28; 95% CI 0.20–0.38) [74]. Only four patients needed to be treated with SDD to prevent one case of pneumonia. Moreover, lower airway infection due to Gram-negative bacteria was reduced by 89% (OR 0.11, 95% CI (0.05–0.20) and that due to Gram-positives by 48% (OR 0.52 95% CI 0.34–0.78) [72].

13.2.3 Bloodstream Infection

SDD significantly reduced bloodstream infections by 27% (OR 0.73, 95% CI 0.59–0.90), particularly those due to Gram-negative bacteria (OR 0.39; 95% CI 0.24–0.63) [71].

13.2.4 Fungal Infection

SDD including polyene, either amphotericin B or nystatin, significantly reduced fungal infections by 70% (OR 0.30, 95% CI 0.17–0.53). Fungemia was reduced, albeit not significantly, mainly due to the low event rates in test and control groups (OR 0.89, 95% CI 0.16–4.95) [70].

Table 13.2 Efficacy of selective decontamination of the digestive tract assessed in ten meta-analyses of randomized controlled trials only

First author	Year	Lower airway infection: OR (95% CI)	Bloodstream infection: OR (95% CI)	MODS: OR (95% CI)	Mortality: OR (95% CI)
Vandenbroucke-Grauls [66]	1991	0.12 (0.08–0.19)			0.92 (0.45–1.84)
D'Amico [67]	1998	0.35 (0.29–0.41)			0.80 (0.69–0.93)
Liberati [68]	2004	0.35 (0.29–0.41)			0.78 (0.68–0.89)
Safdar [69]	2004				0.82 (0.22–2.45)
Silvestri [70]	2005		0.89 (0.16–4.95)		
Silvestri [71]	2007		0.63 (0.46–0.87)		0.74 (0.61–0.91)
Silvestri [72] Gram negative Gram positive	2008	0.07 (0.04–0.13) 0.52 (0.34–0.78)	0.36 (0.22–0.60) 1.03 (0.75–1.41)		
Silvestri [73]	2009				0.71 (0.61–0.82)
Liberati [74]	2009	0.28 (0.20–0.38)			0.75 (0.65–0.87)
Silvestri [75]	2010			0.50 (0.34–0.74)	0.82 (0.51–1.32)

OR odds ratio; *CI* confidence interval; *MODS* multiple organ dysfunction syndrome

13.2.5 Mortality

Mortality rate was an outcome measure in eight of the ten meta-analyses [66–69, 71, 73–75]. There was a consistent survival benefit in all meta-analyses that assessed the full four-component SDD protocol providing the sample size was large enough [67, 68, 71, 73, 74]. The Italian meta-analysis, which assessed only RCTs in which the full SDD protocol was used, showed a mortality rate reduction of 29% (OR 0.71, 95% CI 0.61–0.82) [73]. This effect achieved a 42% mortality rate reduction in studies where SDD eradicated the carrier state (OR 0.58, 95% CI 0.45–0.77) [73]. Eighteen patients need to be treated with the full SDD protocol to prevent one death [73, 74]. The meta-analyses of Vandenbroucke-Grauls and Vandenbroucke [66], Safdar et al. [69], and Silvestri et al. [75] showed an impact on mortality rate that was not significant due to the small sample size. Two Dutch RCTs with the primary endpoint of mortality have been published. In the first [17], the randomization unit was the ICU and not the patient and included about 1,000 patients. The risk of mortality was significantly reduced by 40% in the unit in which SDD was administered to all patients (OR 0.6; 95% CI 0.4–0.8). The second [19] is the largest study on SDD ever published and included about 6,000 patients. The primary endpoint was mortality, whereas resistance was among the secondary endpoints. The study compared SDD, selective oropharyngeal decontamination (SOD), a modified SDD protocol without the gut component and the parenterally administered antibiotic, and standard care. Both SDD and SOD significantly reduced the odds of death compared with standard care [OR 0.83 ($p = 0.02$), and 0.86 ($p = 0.045$), respectively]. However, mortality rate reduction was higher, albeit not significantly, in the SDD group than in the SOD group. These results regarding SOD have been confirmed by a recent meta-analysis of the nine RCTs using SOD and including 4,733 patients [76]. Although SOD has been shown to significantly reduce the odds of pneumonia, the meta-analysis failed to demonstrate any significant impact on survival (OR 0.93; 95% CI 0.81–1.07). Additionally, SOD has been shown to be associated with a 33% and SDD with a 45% reduction in ICU-acquired Gram-negative bacteremia [77], explaining why SDD, and not SOD, is associated with a significant mortality rate reduction.

13.2.6 Miscellaneous

One meta-analysis explored the efficacy of SDD in preventing multiple organ dysfunction syndrome (MODS) [75]. Seven RCTs involving 1,270 patients reported available information and demonstrated that SDD reduces MODS by 50% (OR 0.50, 95% CI 0.34–0.74). Overall mortality rates for SDD versus control patients were 18.7 and 22.9%, respectively, demonstrating a nonsignificant reduction in the odds of death (OR 0.82, 95% CI 0.51–1.32), due to the small sample size.

Another meta-analysis verified whether SDD reduced ventilator-associated tracheobronchitis (VAT) [78]. Twelve RCTs involving 2,252 patients (1,102 SDD; 1,150 controls) provided useful information on VAT. There were 135 (12.25%) patients with VAT in the SDD group and 234 (20.34%) in controls, indicating a 46% VAT reduction in the group receiving SDD (OR 0.54; 95% CI 0.42–0.69).

The efficacy of SDD in selected patient groups, such as burn patients and patients receiving esophageal surgery, has been explored. The meta-analysis on mortality rates in burn patients assessed three RCTs recruiting 440 patients [79]. There were 48 deaths: 15 (5.2%) in the SDD group and 33 (21.8%) in controls. SDD significantly reduced the odds of death by 78% (OR 0.22; 95% CI 0.12–0.43). Three RCTs investigating gastroesophageal surgery were pooled in a meta-analysis of 410 patients (198 SDD, 212 controls) [80]. Fifty-six patients developed pneumonia: 15 (7.65%) in the SDD group and 41 (19.34%) in controls. SDD significantly reduced the odds for pneumonia by 64% (OR 0.36; 95% CI 0.19–0.69; $p = 0.0018$). Interestingly, anastomotic leakage was significantly reduced by SDD.

13.3 Safety

The use of parenterally administered antibiotics has been shown to lead to the emergence of antimicrobial resistance, which has not been shown in RCTs of SDD [81]. This may be explained by the fact that the addition of enterally administered antibiotics to the parenterally administered antibiotics may have kept the systemic agents useful. An intriguing aspect of 25 years of clinical research in SDD is the experience that the pre-1980s antibiotics, such as cefotaxime, are still active as long they are combined with successful eradication of AGNB from the gut.

Resistance was the endpoint of three RCTs of SDD [13, 17, 19]. A *Klebsiella pneumoniae*—producing extended-spectrum beta-lactamase was endemic in a French hospital [13]: carriage and infection rates were 19.6 and 9%, respectively. Once enterally administered antimicrobials were added to those administered parenterally, there was a significant reduction in both carriage and infection (19.6 vs. 1%; 9 vs. 0%). A Dutch single-center RCT of about 1,000 patients reported that carriage of AGNB resistant to imipenem, ceftazidime, ciprofloxacin, tobramycin, and polymyxins occurred in 16% of patients receiving parenterally and enterally administered antimicrobials compared with 26% of control patients who received antibiotics parenterally only, with a relative risk of 0.6 (95% CI 0.5–0.8) [17]. The largest multicenter RCT to date is also from The Netherlands and comprised about 6,000 patients [19]. The proportion of patients with AGNB shown in rectal swabs that were not susceptible to the marker antibiotics was lower with SDD than with standard care or SOD. For example, carriage of multi-drug-resistant *Pseudomonas aeruginosa* was 0.4% in SDD versus 0.8% in SOD and 1.3% in the group receiving standard care ($p < 0.005$). Moreover, the study authors reported in a separate analysis of the same RCT results on bacteremia and lower respiratory tract colonization due to highly resistant microorganisms (HRMO), namely aerobic Gram-negative bacilli [82]. Bacteremia due to HRMO was significantly reduced by SDD compared with SOD (OR 0.37; 95% CI 0.16–0.85). Lower respiratory tract colonization due to HRMO was less with SDD (OR 0.58; 95% CI 0.43–0.78) than with SOD (OR 0.65; 95% CI 0.49–0.87) compared with standard care. Therefore, SDD was superior to SOD and to standard care in preventing antimicrobial resistance.

In an ecological study [83] conducted during the study periods of the Dutch RCT [19], an increase in resistance after discontinuation of SOD and SDD was observed, which seems to contradict the reduction in resistance. However, that ecological analysis has an important limitation, i.e., the use of a point-prevalence survey in which all patients in the unit (whether enrolled in the SDD or SOD trial) were included. Moreover, the average prevalence of AGNB resistant to ceftazidime, tobramycin, and ciprofloxacin in the respiratory tract was significantly lower during SDD/SOD than the pre- and post-intervention periods, and AGNB resistance to ciprofloxacin and tobramycin in rectal swabs was significantly reduced during SDD compared with standard care/SOD [84, 85].

The target microorganisms of SDD include PPMs belonging to the normal flora, including *S. pneumoniae* and MSSA, as well as the opportunistic aerobic Gram-negative bacilli, including *Klebsiella*, *Acinetobacter*, and *Pseudomonas* spp. Methicillin-resistant *S. aureus* (MRSA), by design, is not covered by the original SDD protocol, and hence, six randomized trials conducted in ICUs in which MRSA was endemic at the time of the study showed a trend toward higher MRSA infection rates in patients receiving SDD. These observations suggest that the parenterally and enterally administered antimicrobials of the SDD protocol, i.e., cefotaxime, polymyxin, tobramycin, and amphotericin B, may select for and promote MRSA. Under these circumstances, SDD requires the addition of oropharyngeally and intestinally administered vancomycin. Two studies showed that adding vancomycin to SDD is an effective and safe maneuver [86, 87].

SDD is not active against vancomycin-resistant enterococci (VRE). All SDD randomized trials were undertaken in ICU and hospital settings without VRE experience. SDD was evaluated in two observational studies undertaken in ICU with a low VRE prevalence [87, 88]. In the Spanish study, VRE was imported into the unit, but no change in policy was required, as extensive spread did not occur [87]. In the American study, SDD was evaluated in a unit with a low incidence of VRE, and the authors reported that SDD did not increase the incidence of VRE carriage and infection [88].

13.4 Conclusions

SDD is the only evidence-based maneuver that prevents infection in the critically ill. It significantly reduces lower respiratory tract infections, bloodstream infections, multiple organ failure, mortality rates, and resistance if the full four-component protocol is used. SOD only significantly reduces pneumonia but not mortality rates. Moreover, the full SDD protocol significantly reduces intestinal carriage of multi-drug-resistant aerobic Gram-negative microorganisms, thus reducing the occurrence of ICU-acquired bacteremia.

References

1. Stoutenbeek CP, van Saene HKF, Miranda DR, Zandstra DF (1984) The effect of selective decontamination of the digestive tract on colonization and infection rate in multiple trauma patients. Intensive Care Med 10:185–192
2. van Saene HKF, Petros AJ, Ramsay G, Baxby D (2003) All great truths are iconoclastic: selective decontamination of the digestive tract moves from heresy to level 1 truth. Intensive Care Med 29:677–690
3. Abdel-Razek SM, Abdel-Khalek AH, Allam AM et al (2000) Impact of selective gastrointestinal decontamination on mortality and morbidity in severely burned patients. Ann Burns Fire Disasters 13:213–215
4. Abele-Horn M, Dauber A, Bauernfeind A et al (1997) Decrease in nosocomial pneumonia in ventilated patients by selective oropharyngeal decontamination (SOD). Intensive Care Med 23:1878–1895

5. Aerdts SJA, van Dalen R, Clasener HAL et al (1991) Antibiotic prophylaxis of respiratory tract infection in mechanically ventilated patients. A prospective, blinded, randomized trial of the effect of a novel regimen. Chest 100:783–791
6. Arnow PA, Caradang GC, Zabner R et al (1996) Randomized controlled trial of selective decontamination for prevention of infections following liver transplantation. Clin Infect Dis 22:997–1003
7. Barret JP, Jeschke MG, Herndon DN (2001) Selective decontamination of the digestive tract on severely burned pediatric patients. Burns 27:439–445
8. Bergmans DCJJ, Bonten MJM, Gaillard CA et al (2001) Prevention of ventilator-associated pneumonia by oral decontamination. A prospective, randomized, double-blind, placebo-controlled study. Am J Respir Crit Care Med 164:382–388
9. Bion JF, Badger I, Crosby HA et al (1994) Selective decontamination of the digestive tract reduces Gram-negative pulmonary colonization but not systemic endotoxemia in patients undergoing elective liver transplantation. Crit Care Med 22:40–49
10. Blair P, Rowlands BJ, Lowry K et al (1991) Selective decontamination of the digestive tract: a stratified, randomized, prospective study in a mixed intensive care unit. Surgery 110:303–310
11. Boland JP, Sadler DL, Stewart W et al (1991) Reduction of nosocomial respiratory tract infections in the multiple trauma patients requiring mechanical ventilation by selective parenteral and enteral antisepsis regimen (SPEAR) in the intensive care [abstract]. 17th congress of chemotherapy, Berlin, N°0465
12. Bouter H, Schippers EF, Luelmo SAG et al (2002) No effect of preoperative selective gut decontamination on endotoxemia and cytokine activation during cardiopulmonary bypass: a randomized, placebo-controlled study. Crit Care Med 30:38–43
13. Brun-Buisson C, Legrand P, Rauss A et al (1989) Intestinal decontamination for control of nosocomial multiresistant gram-negative bacilli. Study of an outbreak in an intensive care unit. Ann Intern Med 110:873–881
14. Camus C, Bellisant E, Sebille V et al (2005) Prevention of acquired infections in intubated patients with the combination of two decontamination regimens. Crit Care Med 33:307–314
15. Cerra FB, Maddaus MA, Dunn DL et al (1992) Selective gut decontamination reduces nosocomial infections and length of stay but not mortality or organ failure in surgical intensive care unit patients. Arch Surg 127:163–169
16. Cockerill FR, Muller SR, Anhalt JP et al (1992) Prevention of infection in critically ill patients by selective decontamination of the digestive tract. Ann Intern Med 117:545–553
17. de Jonge E, Schultz M, Spanjaard L et al (2003) Effects of selective decontamination of the digestive tract on mortality and acquisition of resistant bacteria in intensive care: a randomised controlled trial. Lancet 363:1011–1016
18. de la Cal MA, Cerdà E, Garcia-Hierro P et al (2005) Survival benefit in critically ill burned patients receiving selective decontamination of the digestive tract. A randomized, placebo-controlled, double-blind trial. Ann Surg 241:424–430
19. de Smet AMGA, Kluytmans JA, Cooper BS et al (2009) Decontamination of the digestive tract and oropharynx in ICU patients. N Engl J Med 360:20–31
20. Diepenhorst GMP, van Ruler O, Besselink MGH et al (2011) Influence of prophylactic probiotics and selective decontamination on bacterial translocation in patients undergoing pancreatic surgery. Shock 35:9–16
21. Farran L, Llop J, Sans M et al (2008) Efficacy of enteral decontamination in the prevention of anastomotic dehiscence and pulmonary infection in esophagogastric surgery. Dis Esophagus 21:159–164
22. Ferrer M, Torres A, Gonzalez J et al (1994) Utility of selective decontamination in mechanically ventilated patients. Ann Intern Med 120:389–395
23. Finch RG, Tomlinson P, Holliday M et al (1991) Selective decontamination of the digestive tract (SDD) in the prevention of secondary sepsis in a medical/surgical intensive care unit [abstract]. 17th congress of chemotherapy, Berlin, N°0471

24. Flaherty J, Nathan C, Kabins SA et al (1990) Pilot trial of selective decontamination for prevention of bacterial infection in an intensive care unit. J Infect Dis 162:1393–1397
25. Gastinne H, Wolff M, Delatour F et al (1992) A controlled trial in intensive care units of selective decontamination of the digestive tract with nonabsorbable antibiotics. N Engl J Med 326:594–959
26. Gaussorgues Ph, Salord F, Sirodot M et al (1991) Efficacité de la décontamination digestive sur la survenue des bactériémies nosocomiales chez les patients sous ventilation mécanique et recevant des bêtamimétiques. Réanimation Soins Intensive et Médicine d'Urgence 7:169–174
27. Georges B, Mazerolles M, Decun J-F et al (1994) Decontamination digestive selective: resultats d'une etude chez le polytraumatise. Reanim Urgences 3:621–627
28. Gosney M, Martin MV, Wright AE (2006) The role of selective decontamination of the digestive tract in acute stroke. Age Aging 35:42–47
29. Hammond JMJ, Potgieter PD, Saunders GL et al (1992) Double-blind study of selective decontamination of the digestive tract in intensive care. Lancet 340:5–9
30. Hellinger WC, Yao JD, Alvarez S et al (2002) A randomized, prospective, double blinded evaluation of selective bowel decontamination in liver transplantation. Transplantation 73:1904–1909
31. Jacobs S, Foweraker JE, Roberts SE (1992) Effectiveness of selective decontamination of the digestive tract (SDD) in an ICU with a policy encouraging a low gastric pH. Clin Intensive Care 3:52–58
32. Kerver AJH, Rommes JH, Mevissen-Verhage EAE et al (1988) Prevention of colonization and infection in critically ill patients: a prospective randomized study. Crit Care Med 16:1087–1093
33. Korinek AM, Laisne MJ, Nicolas MH et al (1993) Selective decontamination of the digestive tract in neurosurgical intensive care unit patients: a double-blind, randomized, placebo-controlled study. Crit Care Med 21:1466–1473
34. Krueger WA, Lenhart F-P, Neeser G et al (2002) Influence of combined intravenous and topical antibiotic prophylaxis on the incidence of infections, organ dysfunctions, and mortality in critically ill surgical patients. A prospective, stratified, randomized, double-blind, placebo-controlled clinical trial. Am J Respir Crit Care Med 166:1029–1037
35. Laggner AN, Tryba M, Georgopulos A et al (1994) Oropharyngeal decontamination with gentamicin for long-stay ventilated patients on stress ulcer prophylaxis with sucralfate? Wien Klin Wochenschr 106:15–19
36. Lingnau W, Berger J, Javorsky F et al (1997) Selective intestinal decontamination in multiple trauma patients: prospective, controlled trial. J Trauma 42:687–694
37. Luiten EJT, Hop WCJ, Lange JF et al (1995) Controlled clinical trial of selective decontamination for the treatment of severe acute pancreatitis. Ann Surg 222:57–65
38. Martinez-Pellus AE, Merino P, Bru M et al (1993) Can selective digestive decontamination avoid the endotoxemia and cytokine activation promoted by cardiopulmonary bypass? Crit Care Med 21:1684–1691
39. Martinez-Pellus AE, Merino P, Bru M et al (1997) Endogenous endotoxemia of intestinal origin during cardiopulmonary bypass. Role of type of flow and protective effect of selective digestive decontamination. Intensive Care Med 23:1251–1257
40. Oudhuis GJ, Bergmans DG, Dormans T et al (2011) Probiotics versus antibiotic decontamination of the digestive tract: infection and mortality. Intensive Care Med 37:110–117
41. Palomar M, Alvarez-Lerma F, Jordà R et al (1997) Prevention of nosocomial infection in mechanically ventilated patients: selective digestive decontamination versus sucralfate. Clin Intensive Care 8:228–235
42. Pneumatikos I, Koulouras V, Nathanail C et al (2002) Selective decontamination of subglottic area in mechanically ventilated patients with multiple trauma. Intensive Care Med 28:432–437

43. Pugin J, Auckenthaler R, Lew DP et al (1991) Oropharyngeal decontamination decreases incidence of ventilator-associated pneumonia. A randomized, placebo-controlled, double-blind clinical trial. JAMA 265:2704–2710
44. Quinio B, Albanese J, Bues-Charbit M et al (1996) Selective decontamination of the digestive tract in multiple trauma patients. A prospective double-blind, randomized, placebo-controlled study. Chest 109:765–772
45. Rayes N, Seehofer D, Hansen S et al (2002) Early enteral supply of *Lactobacillus* and fiber versus selective bowel decontamination: a controlled trial in liver transplant recipients. Transplantation 74:123–128
46. Rios F, Maskin B, Saenz Valliente A et al (2005) Prevention of ventilation associated pneumonia (VAP) by oral decontamination (OD). Prospective, randomized, double blind, placebo-controlled study. ATS interventional conference, San Diego, USA, C95, Poster 608 (abstract) available at http://abstracts2view.com/ats05/view.php?nu=ATS5L-3301
47. Rocha LA, Martin MJ, Pita S et al (1993) Prevention of nosocomial infection in critically ill patients by selective decontamination of the digestive tract. A randomized, double-blind, placebo controlled study. Intensive Care Med 18:398–404
48. Rodriguez-Roldan JM, Altuna-Cuesta A, Lopez A et al (1990) Prevention of nosocomial lung infection in ventilated patients: use of an antimicrobial pharyngeal nonabsorbable paste. Crit Care Med 18:1239–1242
49. Rolando N, Gimson A, Wade J et al (1993) Prospective controlled trial of selective parenteral and enteral antimicrobial regimen in fulminant liver failure. Hepatology 17:196–201
50. Rolando N, Wade JJ, Stangou A et al (1996) Prospective study comparing the efficacy of prophylactic parenteral antimicrobials. With or without enteral decontamination, in patients with acute liver failure. Liver Transpl Surg 2:8–13
51. Ruza F, Alvarado F, Herruzo R et al (1998) Prevention of nosocomial infection in a pediatric intensive care unit (PICU) through the use of selective digestive decontamination. Eur J Epidemiol 14:719–727
52. Sanchez Garcia M, Cambronero Galache JA, Lopez Diaz J et al (1998) Effectiveness and cost of selective decontamination of the digestive tract in critically ill intubated patients. A randomized, double-blind, placebo-controlled, multicenter trial. Am J Respir Crit Care Med 158:908–916
53. Schardey HM, Joosten U, Finke U et al (1997) The prevention of anastomotic leakage after total gastrectomy with local decontamination. A prospective, randomized, double-blind, placebo-controlled, multicenter trial. Ann Surg 225:172–180
54. Smith SD, Jackson RJ, Hannakan CJ et al (1993) Selective decontamination in pediatric liver transplants. A randomized prospective study. Transplantation 55:1306–1309
55. Stoutenbeek CP, van Saene HKF, Zandstra DF (1996) Prevention of multiple organ failure by selective decontamination of the digestive tract in multiple trauma patients. In: Faist E, Baue AE, Schildberg FW (eds) The immune consequences of trauma, shock and sepsis–mechanisms and therapeutic approach. Pabst Science Publishers, Lengerich, pp 1055–1066
56. Stoutenbeek CP, van Saene HKF, Little RA et al (2007) The effect of selective decontamination of the digestive tract on mortality in multiple trauma patients: a multicenter randomized controlled trial. Intensive Care Med 33:261–270
57. Tetteroo GWM, Wagenvoort JHT, Castelein A et al (1990) Selective decontamination to reduce gram-negative colonisation and infections after oesophageal resection. Lancet 335:704–707
58. Ulrich C, Harinck-de Weerd JE, Bakker NC et al (1989) Selective decontamination of the digestive tract with norfloxacin in the prevention of ICU-acquired infections: a prospective randomized study. Intensive Care Med 15:424–431
59. Unertl K, Ruckdeschel G, Selbmann HK et al (1987) Prevention of colonization and respiratory infections in long-term ventilated patients by local antimicrobial prophylaxis. Intensive Care Med 13:106–113

60. Verwaest C, Verhaegen J, Ferdinande P et al (1997) Randomized, controlled trial of selective digestive decontamination in 600 mechanically ventilated patients in a multidisciplinary intensive care unit. Crit Care Med 25:63–71
61. Wiener J, Itokazu G, Nathan C et al (1995) Randomized, double-blind, placebo-controlled trial of selective digestive decontamination in a medical-surgical intensive care unit. Clin Infect Dis 20:861–867
62. Winter R, Humphreys H, Pick A et al (1992) A controlled trial of selective decontamination of the digestive tract in intensive care and its effect on nosocomial infection. J Antimicrob Chemother 30:73–77
63. Yu J, Xiao YB, Wang XY (2007) Effects of preoperatively selected gut decontamination on cardiopulmonary bypass-induced endotoxemia. Chin J Traumatol 10:131–137
64. Zobel G, Kutting M, Grubbauer H-M et al (1991) Reduction of colonization and infection rate during pediatric intensive care by selective decontamination of the digestive tract. Crit Care Med 19:1242–1246
65. Zwaveling JH, Maring JK, Klompmaker IJ et al (2002) Selective decontamination of the digestive tract to prevent postoperative infection: a randomized placebo-controlled trial in liver transplant patients. Crit Care Med 30:1204–1209
66. Vandenbroucke-Grauls CMJ, Vandenbroucke JP (1991) Effect of selective decontamination of the digestive tract on respiratory tract infections and mortality in the intensive care unit. Lancet 338:859–862
67. D'Amico R, Pifferi S, Leonetti C et al (1998) Effectiveness of antibiotic prophylaxis in critically ill adult patients: systematic review of randomised controlled trials. BMJ 316:1275–1285
68. Liberati A, D'Amico R, Pifferi S et al (2004) Antibiotic prophylaxis to reduce respiratory tract infections and mortality in adults receiving intensive care. Cochrane Database Syst Rev 1:CD000022
69. Safdar N, Said A, Lucey MR (2004) The role of selective digestive decontamination for reducing infection in patients undergoing liver transplantation: a systematic review and meta-analysis. Liver Transpl 10:817–827
70. Silvestri L, van Saene HKF, Milanese M et al (2005) Impact of selective decontamination of the digestive tract on fungal carriage and infection: systematic review of randomised controlled trials. Intensive Care Med 31:898–910
71. Silvestri L, van Saene HKF, Milanese M et al (2007) Selective decontamination of the digestive tract reduces bacterial bloodstream infections and mortality in critically ill patients. Systematic review of randomised, controlled trials. J Hosp Infect 15:187–203
72. Silvestri L, van Saene HKF, Casarin A et al (2008) Impact of selective decontamination of the digestive tract on carriage and infection due to Gram-negative and Gram-positive bacteria. A systematic review of randomised controlled trials. Anaesth Intensive Care 36:324–338
73. Silvestri L, van Saene HKF, Weir J, Gullo A (2009) Survival benefit of the full selective digestive decontamination regimen. J Crit Care 24:e7–e14
74. Liberati A, D'Amico R, Pifferi S et al (2009) Antibiotic prophylaxis to reduce respiratory tract infections and mortality in adults receiving intensive care. Cochrane Database Syst Rev 4:CD000022
75. Silvestri L, van Saene HKF, Zandstra DF et al (2010) Impact of selective decontamination of the digestive tract on multiple organ dysfunction syndrome: systematic review of randomized controlled trials. Crit Care Med 38:1370–1376
76. Silvestri L, van Saene HKF, Zandstra DF et al (2010) SDD, SOD or oropharyngeal chlorhexidine to prevent pneumonia and to reduce mortality in ventilated patients: which manoeuvre is evidence-based? Intensive Care Med 31:1436–1437
77. Oostdijk EAN, de Smet AMGA, Kesecioglu J, Bonten MJM, on behalf of the Dutch SOD-SDD Trialsts Group (2011) The role of intestinal colonization with Gram negative bacteria as a source for intensive care unit-acquired bacteremia. Crit Care Med 39:961–966
78. Silvestri L, Milanese M, Taylor N et al (2010) Selective digestive decontamination reduces ventilator-associated tracheobronchitis. Respir Med 104:1953–1955

79. Silvestri L, de la Cal MA, Taylor N et al (2010) Selective decontamination of the digestive tract in burn patients: an evidence-based maneuver that reduces mortality. J Burn Care Res 31:372–373
80. Silvestri L, van Saene HKF (2010) Selective digestive decontamination to prevent pneumonia after esophageal surgery. Ann Thor Cardiovasc Surg 16(3):220–221
81. Silvestri L, van Saene HKF (2006) Selective decontamination of the digestive tract does not increase resistance in critically ill patient. Evidence from randomized controlled trials. Crit Care Med 34:2027–2029
82. de Smet AM, Kluytmans J, Blok H et al (2010) Effects of selective digestive and selective oropharyngeal decontamination on bacteraemia and respiratory tract colonization with highly resistant micro-organisms. Clin Microbiol Infect 16(suppl 2):S98
83. Oodstijk EAN, de Smet AMGA, Blok HEM et al (2010) Ecological effects of selective decontamination on resistant Gram-negative bacterial colonization. Am J Respir Crit Care Med 181:452–457
84. Zandstra DF, Petros AJ, Taylor N et al (2010) Withholding selective decontamination of the digestive tract from critically ill patients must now surely be ethically questionable given the vast evidence base. Crit Care 14:443
85. Petros AJ, Taylor N, V Damjanovic et al (2010) Worlds apart; proof that SDD works. Am J Respir Crit Care Med 182:1564
86. Silvestri L, Milanese M, Oblach L et al (2002) Enteral vancomycin to control methicillin-resistant *Staphylococcus aureus* outbreak in mechanically ventilated patients. Am J Infect Control 30:391–399
87. de la Cal MA, Cerdà E, van Saene HKF et al (2004) Effectiveness and safety of enteral vancomycin to control endemicity of methicillin-resistant *Staphylococcus aureus* in a medical/surgical intensive care unit. J Hosp Infect 56:175–183
88. Bhorade SM, Christensen J, Pohlman AS et al (1999) The incidence of and clinical variables associated with vancomycin-resistant enterococcal colonization in mechanically ventilated patients. Chest 115:1085–1091

Part IV
Infections on ICU

Lower Airway Infection

14

J. Almirall, A. Liapikou, M. Ferrer
and A. Torres

14.1 Definition

Lower respiratory tract infections (RTI) in intubated patients include ventilator-associated tracheobronchitis (VAT) and ventilator-associated pneumonia (VAP). Both are hospital-acquired infections that occur within 48 h after intubation [1, 2]. Diagnostic criteria for VAT and VAP overlap in terms of clinical signs and symptoms. In contrast to VAT, VAP requires the presence of new and persistent pulmonary infiltrates on a chest radiograph, which may be difficult to interpret in some critically ill patients, and two or more of the following criteria: fever (>38.3°C) or hypothermia; leukocyte count >10,000/μl; purulent tracheobronchial secretions, or a reduced partial pressure of oxygen in arterial blood (PaO_2)/fraction of inspired oxygen (FiO_2) ratio $\geq 15\%$ according to the US centers for disease control and prevention definitions. patients with a clinical pulmonary infection score >6 are also considered to have pneumonia [3].

The apparent crude incidence of VAT ranges from 3 to 10%, but it is difficult to determine the exact incidence and importance of VAT for several reasons. The major reason is that to confirm the absence of infiltrates on a chest radiograph, a computed tomography (CT) scan is required. VAT is probably an intermediate process between lower respiratory tract colonization and VAP. Postmortem studies show a continuum between bronchitis and pneumonia in mechanically ventilated (MV) ICU patients [4]. VAP that occurs during the first 4 days of MV is defined as early onset in order to differentiate it from late-onset VAP, which develops thereafter.

A. Torres (✉)
Servei de Pneumologia i Al·lèrgia Respiratòria,
Hospital Clínic, Barcelona, Spain
e-mail: atorres@ub.edu

The term ventilator-associated pneumonia, however, is a misnomer, as the MV is not the main risk factor for lung colonization and pneumonia. The endotracheal tube (ETT) seems to play the most important role in the pathogenesis of VAP, as it creates a direct conduit for bacteria to reach the lower airways and greatly impairs host defenses. Interestingly, studies demonstrate that MV could also increase the risk of pneumonia. Indeed, lungs become highly susceptible to bacterial colonization when injurious ventilatory settings are applied, i.e., with high tidal volumes and low positive end expiratory pressures (PEEP).

Therefore, either ETT-associated pneumonia or ventilation-acquired pneumonia are better terms to describe pneumonia in tracheally intubated and MV patients, as they emphasize the role of ETT and MV in the pathogenesis of such pneumonia. The term ventilation-acquired pneumonia would allow physicians and scientists to maintain the current acronym VAP [5].

14.2 Pathogenesis

Tracheally intubated patients can be colonized via exogenous and endogenous bacterial sources. When bacteria gain access to the lower respiratory tract in healthy, nonintubated patients, colonization is prevented by several defense mechanisms, such as cough, cilia, mucous clearance, polymorphonuclear leukocytes, macrophages and their respective cytokines, antibodies [immunoglobulin (Ig)M, IgG, IgA], and complement factors. Critically ill patients are already at high risk of infection because of the illness, comorbidities, and malnutrition. In MV patients, the tracheal tube may encourage aspiration by bypassing normal defenses, allowing secretions to pool in the upper part of the trachea. It also creates a direct conduit for bacteria to reach the airways, impairs cough, compromises mucociliary clearance, and facilitates bacterial adhesion to the airways through cuff-related injury to the tracheal mucosa. When endotracheal tubes are inserted nasally instead of orally, sinusitis is significantly more likely to occur through blockage of the sinus ostia. The occurrence of nosocomial sinusitis has been associated with VAP.

High-volume, low-pressure, endotracheal tube cuffs, commonly used during prolonged MV, are not leakproof, and micro- and macroaspiration of bacteria-laden oropharyngeal secretions often occurs. Patients are colonized from exogenous bacterial sources via the hands and apparel of healthcare personnel, contaminated aerosols, and invasive devices such as tracheal aspiration catheters and fiberoptic bronchoscopes (FOB). Pathogens are also acquired from the patient's endogenous flora, though there is still controversy regarding the primary source of infection (oropharynx, stomach). It is well acknowledged, however, that in critically ill patients, oral flora quickly shifts to a predominance of aerobic Gram-negative pathogens *Pseudomonas aeruginosa* and methicillin-resistant *Staphylococcus aureus* (MRSA). Following bacterial aspiration and colonization of the proximal airways, the occurrence of VAP mainly depends on the size of the inoculum, functional status, exposure to antibiotics, and potential host defenses.

14.3 Epidemiology

Nosocomial pneumonia accounts for 31% of all nosocomial infections, and a large majority (83%) of patients who develop nosocomial pneumonia are mechanically ventilated. The exact incidence of VAP is difficult to obtain due to overlapping lower RTIs and the difficulty in diagnosing VAP correctly. The incidence of VAP ranges from 9 to 67% of patients on MV. The rate of VAP, expressed as the total number of episodes of VAP/1,000 ventilator days, ranges from 5 to 16 [6]. VAP can increase the time on a ventilator by 10 days, length of ICU stay by 6 days, and length of total hospital stay by 11 days.

Disease incidence depends greatly on the type of population studied, the presence or absence of risk factors for colonization by multi-drug-resistant pathogens, and the type and intensity of preventive strategies applied. Tracheal intubation and MV are the main risk factors for VAP during the first week of ventilation (risk assessed at approximately 3% per day in the first week of MV). A one-day point-prevalence study conducted in 1,417 intensive care units (ICUs) in Western Europe reported that VAP was the most common ICU-acquired infection and MV was associated with a threefold increased risk of developing pneumonia [7]. Studies conducted in several countries in the European Union have shown varying incidence density ranging from approximately 9–25 cases/ 1,000 ventilation days [6]. Epidemiological studies on a large United States database with medical, surgical, and trauma patients have shown a VAP incidence of 9.3%.

Hospital mortality rate of patients with VAP is significantly higher than that of patients without VAP. Crude VAP mortality rates range between 20 and 50%, depending on comorbidities, illness severity, pathogens, and quality of antibiotic treatment [1]. Ventilated ICU patients with VAP appear to have a two- to tenfold higher risk of death compared with patients without pneumonia. However, several patients with VAP die and not because of VAP. However, mortality rates vary from one study to another, and the prognostic impact is debated. It is well recognized that one-third to one-half of all VAP deaths are directly attributable to the disease. Mortality rates are higher when VAP associated with bacteremia, especially with *P. aeruginosa* or *Acinetobacter* spp., medical rather than surgical illness, and treatment with ineffective antibiotic therapy [2].

VAP is associated with higher medical care costs. Patients who develop VAP during a hospital stay remain longer in the ICU and the hospital, and the increased level of care and need for additional invasive procedures drastically increases healthcare costs. It has been reported that each case of VAP is associated with additional hospital costs of $20000 to more than US $40000. Infection with MRSA increases hospital costs by an additional $7731 per patient. These data emphasize the need for prevention and better outcomes [8].

14.4 Etiologic Agents

The etiological cause of VAP is usually identified via semiquantitative microbiologic analysis of tracheal aspirates with or without initial microscopic evaluation. When VAP is diagnosed using a microbiologic strategy following clinical suspicion of lung infection, samples from the lower respiratory tract are collected and quantitative cultures performed. Pathology studies clearly show that the sensitivity of microbiological studies is drastically reduced when antibiotics are administered. Therefore, new antibiotics should be administered after sampling. Specimens can be obtained noninvasively via a tracheal suction catheter or invasively through an FOB. When an FOB is used, pathogens from the lower respiratory tract are retrieved mainly through bronchoalveolar lavage (BAL) or protected specimen brush (PSB). Several modifications of these techniques have been developed, such as mini-BAL and blind PSB sampling. During pneumonia, pathogens colonize the lower respiratory tract at concentrations of 10^5–10^6 colony-forming units/milliliter (CFU/ml). With regard to sample size, the commonly accepted diagnostic threshold for PSB, BAL, and tracheal aspirates are 10^3, 10^4–10^5, and 10^5–10^6 CFU/ml, respectively. Most of the current debate regarding VAP diagnosis still concerns invasive versus. noninvasive sampling techniques. Five randomized clinical trials attempted to demonstrate differences in outcome between techniques; only one study showed significant survival benefit using invasive sampling techniques [9].

Studies in the 1990s confirmed the association between oral bacterial colonization and nosocomial pneumonia in MV patients. In addition, patients in the ICU have higher mean plaque scores than patients in non-ICU control groups. Pathogens isolated from plaque of these ICU patients included MRSA. These findings suggest that dental plaque may also provide a reservoir for pathogenic bacteria that contribute to VAP.

The most common microorganisms implicated as causative agents of VAP are *P. aeruginosa* (24%), *S. aureus* (20%), and Enterobacteriaceae (14%) [10–12]. Increasing resistance of *S. aureus* to methicillin/oxacillin has been reported for many years, reaching almost 60% in recent studies [13]. Multiple etiologic agents are often present. All bacteria implicated in the VAP etiology are reported in Table 14.1.

Several differences in the etiology of early- and late-onset pneumonia can be recognized, with the former mainly caused by pathogens with enhanced antibiotic susceptibility and better outcome, such as *Haemophilus influenzae* and *S. pneumonia*. Anaerobic bacteria play a minor role in VAP pathogenesis. Theoretically, patients who develop VAP within 4 days may have aspirated oropharyngeal contents colonized by anaerobic bacteria, but the need to administer antianaerobic drugs has not been clearly established. In general, viruses and fungi are potential causes of VAP only in immunosuppressed patients.

Table 14.1 Causative agents of ventilator-associated pneumonia (VAP)

	Kollef [8] $n = 398$	Agbath [9] $n = 313$	Kollef [10] $n = 93$
Gram-positive			
MSSA	35 (8.8)	68 (21.7)	15 (16.1)
MRSA	59 (14.8)	25 (8.0)	10 (10.7)
Streptococcus pneumoniae		24 (7.7)	6 (6.4)
Streptococcus spp.		13 (4.2)	
Gram-negative			
Pseudomonas aeruginosa	57 (14.3)	43 (13.7)	19 (20.4)
Haemophilus influenzae		52 (16.6)	6 (6.4)
Enterobacteriaceae	38 (9.5)	64 (20.4)	15 (16.1)
Acinetobacter baumannii	8 (2.0)	10 (3.2)	6 (6.4)

MRSA methicillin-resistant *Staphylococcus aureus*; *MSSA* methicillin-sensitive *Staphylococcus aureus*

14.5 Risk Factors

A number of papers using both univariate and multivariate statistical techniques highlight the risk factors associated with VAP. Knowledge of these risk factors is crucial in implementing effective preventive measures. These risk factors can be modifiable or nonmodifiable conditions (Table 14.2). More importantly, several identified risk factors have been modified in studies aiming at reducing VAP incidence. These include enteral feeding, ventilator-circuit manipulation, patient positioning, MV modes, and strategies for stress-ulcer prophylaxis. Recent guidelines classify recommendations for preventative interventions of modifiable risk factors [2]. Presumed relationships between identified risk factors, preventive strategies, and VAP pathogenesis are shown in Fig. 14.1.

14.6 Preventive Strategies

The high morbidity and mortality rates of VAP and the costs of the disease, both in terms of treatment and increasing hospital length of stay, have led to efforts to reach consensus in control measures and prevention. Many hospitals have developed and implemented evidence-based prevention protocols and educational programs for physicians and nurses. These strategies have often improved quality of care and reduced VAP incidence. When North American epidemiological data from the 2008 National Healthcare Safety Network (NHSN) report are compared with data from the 2003 National Nosocomial Infections Surveillance (NNIS), pneumonia incidence densities are slightly lower overall, suggesting that new preventive strategies applied in the meantime have had a positive effect [13].

Table 14.2 Risk factors for ventilator-associated pneumonia (VAP)

Modifiable risk factors	Nonmodifiable risk factors
Supine patient position	Age >60 years
Large-volume gastric aspiration	COPD/ARDS/pulmonary disease
Colonization of the ventilator circuit	Organ failure
Low endotracheal cuff pressure	Coma/impaired consciousness
Staff hand infection	Tracheostomy
Nasotracheal intubation	Reintubation
Oropharyngeal colonization	Intracranial pressure monitor
Histamine type 2 (H_2) antagonists and antacids	Length of stay in the ICU Duration of intubation and mechanical ventilation >2 days Prior antibiotics Enteral nutrition Therapeutic interventions Use of sedative and paralytic agents

COPD chronic obstructive pulmonary disease; *ARDS* acute respiratory distress syndrome; *ICU* intensive care unit

14.6.1 Ventilator and VAP Bundles

Preventive strategies have focused on reducing/avoiding cross-transmission, pulmonary aspiration across the cuff, and bacterial load in the oropharynx. Several strategies with proven efficacy in reducing MV-related morbidity and mortality rates have been grouped as a ventilator bundle and could bring about a 45% reduction in VAP rates [14]. The interventions are recommended by the Institute for Healthcare Improvement (IHI) and include:
1. elevating the head of the bed by 30–45°;
2. daily "sedation vacations" and assessment of readiness for extubation;
3. peptic ulcer disease prophylaxis;
4. deep venous thrombosis prophylaxis.

Although the aforementioned bundle was not specifically designed to prevent VAP, effects of body position, sedation vacation, and assessment of readiness for extubation have generated significant reduction in VAP rates. The bundle was subsequently implemented specifically to address VAP prevention, and two additional strategies were incorporated: (1) daily oral use of chlorhexidine; (2) subglottic secretion drainage.

14.6.2 Endotracheal Intubation

Intubation and MV is undoubtedly associated with increased risk of VAP and therefore should be avoided whenever possible. Noninvasive positive-pressure ventilation (NPPV) is an attractive alternative for patients with acute

14 Lower Airway Infection 225

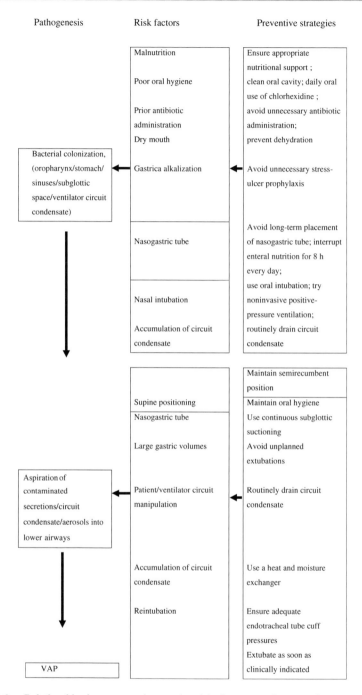

Fig. 14.1 Relationship between pathogenesis, risk factors, and preventive strategies for ventilator-associated pneumonia (VAP)

exacerbations of chronic obstructive pulmonary disease (COPD) or acute hypoxemic respiratory failure and should be used whenever possible in selected (immunosuppressed patients) with pulmonary infiltrates, fever, and respiratory failure and to facilitate difficult weaning. Reintubation should be avoided, if possible, as it increases the risk of VAP [15]. Orotracheal intubation should be preferred over nasotracheal intubation to prevent nosocomial sinusitis and thus reduce the risk of VAP.

Specific strategies, such as improved methods of sedation and the use of protocols to facilitate and accelerate weaning, have been recommended to reduce intubation and MV duration but are dependent on adequate ICU staffing. Daily interruption or lightening of sedation, in particular, can decrease time on MV, as well as avoiding paralytic agents, which is also recommended so as not to depress defence mechanisms.

14.6.3 Tracheal Tube, Ventilatory Circuit, and Gas Conditioning

Most endotracheal tubes used in the ICU have high-volume, low-pressure (HVLP) cuffs. The internal volume of standard HVLP cuffs can exceed the internal diameter of the trachea by up to 40%, so when inflated, HVLP cuffs seal the trachea without being stretched, and their internal pressure closely reflects pressure exerted against the tracheal wall. Nevertheless, longitudinal folds invariably form, and bacteria-laden oropharyngeal secretions easily leak along these folds, increasing risks for airways infection and pneumonia. Cuffs made of new materials such as polyurethane have been developed. During inflation, these cuffs form smaller folds and can prevent or greatly reduce the aspiration of secretions past the cuff. Leakage of oropharyngeal contents past the ETT cuff has also been reduced with a new endotracheal tube that contains a separate dorsal lumen, which opens into the subglottic region and allows continuous aspiration of subglottic secretions (CASS tube) This strategy has significantly reduced the incidence of pneumonia, particularly early-onset VAP, and should be used if available [16]. The internal pressure of the endotracheal tube cuff pressure must also be maintained between 25–30 cm H_2O, particularly when no PEEP is applied, to prevent leakage of contaminated secretions past the cuff into the lower airways and tracheal injury. Patients who require prolonged endotracheal intubation or bedside percutaneous dilation tracheostomy for prolonged MV are also at risk of developing swallowing dysfunctions that may predispose to aspiration and the subsequent development of nosocomial pneumonia [17].

The ventilatory circuit can become colonized and facilitate bacterial inoculation. The frequency of ventilator circuit change does not affect the incidence of VAP, but the condensate fluid collected in the ventilator circuit can increase the risk of exogenous and endogenous bacterial colonization. Therefore, the inadvertent flushing of contaminated condensate into the lower airway should be avoided through careful emptying of ventilator circuits.

There are no consistent data showing reduced VAP incidence [2] and better outcome using either heat and moisture exchangers (HME) or heated humidifiers (HH). Neither humidification strategy can be recommended as a pneumonia prevention tool at this stage; however, inspiratory gases should be delivered at body temperature or slightly below and at the highest relative humidity in order to prevent heat and moisture loss from the airways and, more importantly, change in rheologic properties of secretions and impairment of mucociliary clearance.

14.6.4 Gastric Colonization and Body Position

Gastric sterility is maintained in an acidic environment. In critically ill patients, use of antacids for stress-ulcer prophylaxis, and enterally administered nutrition alkalinizes gastric contents and facilitates bacterial colonization of the stomach. Retrograde colonization of the oropharynx and pulmonary aspiration past the ETT cuff causes bacterial colonization of the lower respiratory tract and pneumonia. Guidelines recommend elevating the head of a patient's bed 30–45°, especially during enteral feeding, to reduce gastroesophageal reflux and incidence of nosocomial pneumonia [2]. Differences between the semirecumbent and supine positions have been reported in one randomized clinical study. Drakulovic et al. [18] showed that the semirecumbent position (45°) lowered the risk for onset of nosocomial pneumonia by 78% in comparison with completely supine position (0°), reducing the gastrooropharyngeal route of pulmonary infection.

14.6.5 Enterally Administered Nutrition

Enterally administered nutrition in supine patients is a risk factor for VAP development through increased risk of aspiration of gastric contents. Residual volume should be carefully monitored and, in the case of consistently large volumes, the use of agents that increase gastrointestinal (GI) motility (e.g., metoclopramide). When necessary, enterally administered nutrition should be withheld to reduce aspiration risk. Enterally administered nutrition acidification and postpyloric tube placement and nutrition suspension 8 h daily (intermittent nutrition) are strategies that should reduce gastric colonization and risk of gastroesophageal reflux, although investigators have reported inconsistent results [19]. However, the effectiveness of such interventions awaits validation in clinical trials. Nevertheless, intubated patients should be kept in a semirecumbent position (30–45°) to prevent aspiration, especially when receiving enterally administered nutrition.

14.6.6 Stress-Ulcer Prophylaxis

As mentioned above, gastric sterility is maintained in an acidic environment within the stomach. A gastric pH >4 facilitates bacterial colonization mostly due to Gram-negative bacteria. However, the majority of critically ill patients are at a higher risk for GI bleeding during MV; hence, stress-ulcer prophylaxis is essential. Antacids, histamine-2-receptor antagonists (H2 blockers), and proton-pump inhibitors (PPI) are usually administered to prevent GI lesions. Sucralfate, an alternative gastroprotective agent, does not change gastric acidity and prevents GI bleeding, protecting gastric mucosa. Several randomized clinical trials and meta-analyses investigated the rates of VAP using sucralfate versus agents that alkalinize gastric juice (antacids, H2 blockers, PPI) with conflicting results. An additional risk for GI bleeding using sucralfate has also been found [20]. Thus, the use of sucralfate as VAP-preventive strategy should only be recommended in patients with low risk of GI bleeding.

14.6.7 Oropharyngeal and Digestive Tract Colonization

Progression from colonization to tracheobronchitis and pneumonia is a dynamic process, and identifying the different entities depends on the specificity of diagnostic tools. Oropharyngeal colonization, either present on admission or acquired during ICU stay, has been identified as an independent risk factor for the development of ICU-acquired pneumonia caused by enteric Gram-negative bacteria and *P. aeruginosa* [21]. In tracheally intubated patients, oral flora rapidly shifts from a predominance of aerobic Gram-positive bacteria and anaerobes to a majority of aerobic Gram-negative pathogens. Oropharyngeal decontamination can be achieved through topical administration of antiseptics, such as chlorhexidine. Using chlorhexidine in cardiac postsurgical patients and patients requiring MV for at least 48 h has been shown to reduce the incidence of VAP. Despite the reduction in nosocomial pneumonia, no survival benefits were demonstrated.

Selective oropharyngeal decontamination (SOD) and subglottic decontamination can be obtained via topical administration of nonabsorbable antibiotics, the most common being polymyxin E, tobramycin/gentamicin, and amphotericin B, all of which provide antimicrobial activity against all aerobic Gram-negative pathogens. An additional short course of systemic third-generation cephalosporins, such as cefotaxime or ceftriaxone, has also been used for selective digestive decontamination (SDD) to prevent early infections caused by *H. influenzae* and *S. pneumonia*. Several randomized clinical trials and meta-analyses have shown reduced bacterial colonization and VAP; however, effects on ICU length of stay and mortality rates are inconsistent. Several concerns have dampened the enthusiasm for the SDD preventive strategy: possible emergence of antibiotic-resistant bacteria; lack of consistent survival benefits demonstrated by randomized clinical trials, and, ultimately, increased healthcare costs. A large randomized clinical trial involving 5,939 patients shows an absolute reduction in mortality of 2.5 and 3.5 percentage points with SOD and SDD, respectively, without evidence of increased emergence of antibiotic resistance [22]. Currently, they are not recommended for routine use, especially in patients who may be colonized with multi-drug-resistant pathogens.

14.6.8 Probiotics

Probiotics are viable microorganisms that colonize the host GI tract by adhering to the intestinal mucosa and compete with the adhesion of pathogens to epithelial binding sites, thus creating an unfavorable local milieu for pathogen colonization. Probiotic products have been shown to be of some benefit in the following diseases: acute infectious diarrhea in children, necrotizing enterocolitis in very-low-birth-weight infants, allergic atopic dermatitis prevention in children, and prevention of relapses of ulcerative colitis. In critically ill patients, studies demonstrate that oral administration of a probiotic *Lactobacillus* preparation delayed respiratory tract colonization with *P. aeruginosa* and resulted in a reduced rate of ventilator-associated pneumonia caused by *P. aeruginosa*. Also, Morrow et al. [23] found that patients treated with *Lactobacillus* were significantly less likely to develop microbiologically confirmed VAP compared with patients treated with placebo (40.0 vs. 19.1%, $p = 0.007$). A meta-analysis of five randomized controlled trials concluded that probiotic administration is associated with lower incidence of VAP [24]. Future studies need to be designed with standardization of the probiotic product and dosing (both daily dose and therapy duration).

14.6.9 Bacterial Biofilm

Bacterial biofilm is a highly structured, matrix-enclosed bacterial community. Sessile bacteria encased within the matrix express genes in a different pattern from their planktonic counterpart to achieve a survival advantage in a hostile environment. Studies show evidence that following tracheal intubation, bacterial biofilm is formed early within the internal surface of the endotracheal tube. These sessile communities develop resistance to antibiotics, to cellular and humoral immune defenses, and are the cause of persistent infection. Certain bacteria, such as *Pseudomonas* spp., appear to be more capable of forming biofilms, especially in the presence of abnormal airway mucosa, such as that which as exists in patients with cystic fibrosis. Bacteria from within the biofilm can be dislodged mechanically through tracheal suction catheters, bronchoscope, or airflow and can ultimately increase the risk for VAP. Coating medical devices, such as intravascular and urinary catheters, with antimicrobial agents such as silver is a widely applied method to reduce the incidence of device-associated infections. In the last decade, several in vitro and in vivo laboratory studies have tested the efficacy and safety of silver-coated ETTs, demonstrating reduced bacterial colonization of the ETT without associated adverse effects. However, results from animal studies have also emphasized that the antibacterial effect may not last beyond 24–48 h, mainly due to mucus accumulation within the ETT. A large randomized clinical trial comparing bactericidal effects of silver-coated tracheal tubes to standard tubes showed a relative VAP risk reduction of 36% and greatest efficacy within the first 10 days of MV [12]. Silver-coated ETT is an attractive approach to decreasing risk of pneumonia, and further studies should be performed to improve antimicrobial efficacy and assess limitations of the strategy.

14.7 Prognostic Factors

Medical conditions predisposing patients to serious infections, such as COPD, immunosuppression, chronic heart failure, chronic hepatopathy, and chronic renal failure can have an impact on the severity of VAP episodes. The presence of specific factors may be associated with poorer outcomes in VAP patients, such as older age, duration of ventilation before enrolment, presence of neurologic disease on admission, failure of the PaO_2/FiO_2 ratio to improve by day 3, acute renal failure, and shock. But the most important prognostic factor associated with mortality is appropriate initial antibiotic treatment. The percentage of inadequate treatment ranges between 22 and 73% in the literature. Multi-drug-resistant microorganisms, such as *P. aeruginosa*, *Acinetobacter* spp., and MRSA, are the more common pathogens that are not susceptible to initial antibiotic therapy. Susceptibility to antibiotics of microorganisms that cause VAP varies between patient populations, hospitals, and ICUs. The most recent American Thoracic Society guidelines [2] list the following risk factors for colonization and infection with multi-drug-resistant bacteria: antibiotic treatment within the last 90 days; current hospitalization or within the last 90 days of >5 days duration; high frequency of multi-drug-resistant organism in the hospital/unit; presence of risk factors for healthcare-associated pneumonia (hospitalization for ≥ 2 days in the preceding 90 days; residence in a nursing home or extended care facility; home infusion therapy; chronic dialysis within the last 30 days; home wound care; family members carriers of multi-drug-resistant bacteria); immunosuppressive disease and/or treatment.

VAP onset is an important issue regarding the associated mortality risk for ICU patients. Late-onset VAP has the worst prognosis in comparison with early-onset pathogens. Typically, late-onset VAP is caused by high-risk microorganisms, and hospital mortality rates can be as high as 65% when VAP is caused by *P. aeruginosa, Acinetobacter* spp. or *Stenotrophomonas maltophilia*. Bacteremia has been associated with increased mortality rates in patients with community-acquired pneumonia, but less information is available for bacteremic episodes of VAP.

Most prognostic factors are included in several scores designed to stratify patients according to disease severity on ICU admission. Some examples are the acute physiology and chronic evaluation (APACHE) score versions I, II, III, and IV; and the simplified acute physiology score (SAPS) versions I, II, and III. When patients are infected, the following scores can be used: sequential organ failure assessment (SOFA), a tool that evaluates six organs and has been recognized as a valuable prognostic scoring system, multiple organ dysfunction score (MODS) and the organ dysfunction and/or infection (ODIN) score. However, no score has been developed to assess severity in VAP patients at the time of diagnosis. In the ICU setting, attending physicians daily have to confront patients in whom a pulmonary infection can complicate their already critical situation.

A predisposition, infection, response, organ failure (PIRO)-based model could be useful for assessing severity and stratifying mortality rate. This four-variable score is based on the patient's predisposition to the disease, gravity of the insult, host's response, and related organ dysfunction [25]. The VAP PIRO score could be useful in daily practice, as it classifies patients according to their mortality risk with only one measurement on the day of the VAP diagnosis. This simple tool has been tested in different situations and has proven efficiency in assessing VAP severity and predicting ICU mortality rate. It has also shown worse outcomes in patients with a score of >2.

References

1. Chastre J, Fagon JY (2002) Ventilator-associated pneumonia. Am J Respir Crit Care Med 165:867–903
2. Niederman MS, Craven DE, Bonten MJ (2005) American Thoracic Society and Infectious Diseases Society of America (ATS/IDSA) Guidelines for the management of adults with hospital-acquired, ventilator-associated, and healthcare-associated pneumonia. Am J Respir Crit Care Med 171:388–416
3. Garner JS, Jarvis WR, Emori TG et al (1998) CDC definitions for nosocomial infections 1998. Am J Infect Control 16:128–140
4. Nseir S, Favory R, Jozefowicz E, VAT Study Group et al (2008) Antimicrobial treatment for ventilator-associated tracheobronchitis: a randomized, controlled, multicenter study. Crit Care 12:R62
5. Torres A, Ewig S, Lode H et al (2009) Defining, treating and preventing hospital acquired pneumonia: European perspective. Intensive Care Med 35:9–29
6. National Nosocomial Infections Surveillance (NNIS) (2004) System Report, data summary from January 1992 through June 2004, issued October 2004. Am J Infect Control 32:470–485
7. Vincent JL, Bihari DJ, Suter PM et al (1995) The prevalence of nosocomial infection in intensive care units in Europe. Results of the European prevalence of infection in intensive care (EPIC) study. EPIC international advisory committee. JAMA 274:639–644
8. Rello J, Ollendorf DA, Oster G et al (2002) Epidemiology and outcomes of ventilator-associated pneumonia in a large US database. Chest 122:2115–2121
9. Fagon JY, Chastre J, Wolff M et al (2000) Invasive and noninvasive strategies for management of suspected ventilator-associated pneumonia. Ann Intern Med 132:621–630
10. Kollef MH, Morrow LE, Niederman MS et al (2006) Clinical characteristics and treatment patterns among patients with ventilator-associated pneumonia. Chest 129:1210–1218
11. Agbaht K, Diaz E, Muñoz E et al (2007) Bacteremia in patients with ventilator-associated pneumonia is associated with increased mortality: a study comparing bacteremic vs nonbacteremic ventilator-associated pneumonia. Crit Care Med 35:2064–2070
12. Kollef MH, Afeas B, Anzuelo A et al (2008) NASCENT investigation group silver-coated endotracheal tubes and incidence of ventilator-associated pneumonia: the NASCENT randomized trial. JAMA 300:805–813
13. Rosenthal VD, Maki DG, Jamulitrat S, INICC members et al (2010) International nosocomial infection control consortium (INICC) report, data summary for 2003–2008, issued June 2009. Am J Infect Control 38(2):95–104.e2
14. Resar R, Pronovost P, Haraden C et al (2005) Using a bundle approach to improve ventilator care processes and reduce ventilator-associated pneumonia. Jt Comm J Qual Patient Saf 31:243–248
15. Torres A, Gatell JM, Aznar E et al (1995) Re-intubation increases the risk of nosocomial pneumonia in patients needing mechanical ventilation. Am J Respir Crit Care Med 152:137–141

16. Valles J, Artigas A, Rello J et al (1995) Continuous aspiration of subglottic secretions in preventing ventilator-associated pneumonia. Ann Intern Med 122:179–186
17. Romero CM, Marambio A, Larrondo J et al (2010) Swallowing dysfunction in nonneurologic critically ill patients who require percutaneous dilatational tracheostomy. Chest 137: 1278–1282
18. Drakulovic MB, Torres A, Bauer TT et al (1999) Supine body position as a risk factor for nosocomial pneumonia in mechanically ventilated patients: a randomised trial. Lancet 354: 1851–1858
19. Heyland DK, Drover JW, Dhaliwal R, Greenwood J (2002) Optimizing the benefits and minimizing the risks of enteral nutrition in the critically ill: role of small bowel feeding. JPEN J Parenter Enteral Nutr 26:S51–S55
20. Cook DJ, Fuller HD, Guyatt GH et al (1994) Risk factors for gastrointestinal bleeding in critically ill patients. N Engl J Med 330:377–381
21. Bonten MJM, Bergmans DCJJ, Ambergen AW et al (1996) Risk factors for pneumonia, and colonization of respiratory tract and stomach in mechanically ventilated ICU patients. Am J Respir Crit Care Med 154:1339–1346
22. de Smet AM, Kluytmans JA, Cooper BS et al (2009) Decontamination of the digestive tract and oropharynx in ICU patients. N Engl J Med 360:20–31
23. Morrow LE, Kollef MH, Casale TB (2010) Probiotic prophylaxis of ventilator-associated pneumonia: a blinded, randomized, controlled trial. Am J Respir Crit Care Med 182(8): 1058–1064
24. Siempos II, Ntaidou TK, Falagas ME (2010) Impact of the administration of probiotics on the incidence of ventilator-associated pneumonia: a meta-analysis of randomized controlled trials. Crit Care Med 38(3):954–962
25. Lisboa T, Diaz E, Sa-Borges M et al (2008) The ventilator-associated pneumonia PIRO score: a tool for predicting ICU mortality and health-care resources use in ventilator-associated pneumonia. Chest 134:1208–1216

Bloodstream Infection in the ICU Patient

15

J. Vallés and R. Ferrer

15.1 Introduction

Hospital-acquired infections (HAI) occur in 5–10% of patients admitted to hospitals in the Unites States and remain a leading cause of morbidity and mortality [1]. The endemic rates of HAI vary markedly between hospitals and between areas of the same hospital. Patients in intensive care units (ICUs), representing 8–15% of hospital admissions, experience a disproportionately high percentage of HAI compared with patients in noncritical care areas [2–8]. Patients admitted to ICUs account for 45% of all HA pneumonias and bloodstream infections (BSIs), although critical care units comprise only 5–10% of all hospital beds [3]. The severity of the underlying disease, invasive diagnostic and therapeutic procedures that breach normal host defenses, contaminated life-support equipment, and the prevalence of resistant microorganisms are critical factors in the high rate of infection in the ICUs [9]. On the other hand, 40% of patients admitted to the ICU present infections acquired in the community, and 17% of them present BSI [10]. The incidence rate of patients with community-acquired (CA) BSI admitted in a general ICU is about nine to ten episodes per 1,000 admissions [11, 12] representing 30–40% of all episodes of BSI in a medical–surgical ICU (Fig. 15.1).

In this chapter, we discuss the characteristics and prognosis of BSI in the ICU, including hospital- and CA episodes.

J. Vallés (✉)
Critical Care Center, Hospital Sabadell,
Sabadell, Barcelona, Spain
e-mail: jvalles@tauli.cat

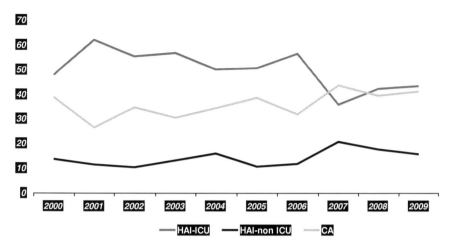

Fig. 15.1 Distribution of bloodstream infections (BSI) in the medical–surgical intensive care unit (ICU) of Hospital Sabadell (2000–2009) *HAI-ICU*, hospital-acquired BSI in ICU; *HAI-non ICU*, hospital-acquired BSI in wards; *CA*, community-acquired BSI

15.2 Hospital-Acquired Bloodstream Infections in the ICU

15.2.1 Epidemiology

HA BSI in the ICU is defined in a patient with a clinically significant blood culture positive for a bacterium or fungus and that is obtained more than 72 h after admission or previously, if it is directly related to a invasive manipulation on admission in the ICU (e.g., urinary catheterization or insertion of intravenous line) [13]. Patients in the ICU not only have higher endemic rates of HAI than patients in general wards, but the distribution of their infections also differs. The two most important HAI in general wards are urinary tract and surgical wound infections, whereas in the ICU, lower respiratory tract infections and BSI are the most frequent [14]. This distribution is related to the widespread use of mechanical ventilation and intravenous catheters. Data compiled through the national nosocomial infections surveillance system (NNIS) of the centers for disease control and prevention (CDC) in the USA revealed that bloodstream infections accounted for almost 20% of HAI in ICU patients, 87% of which were associated with a central line [15]. A recent nationwide surveillance study in 49 US hospitals (SCOPE) reported that 51% of HA BSIs occurred in the ICU [16]. Studies conducted in critically ill patients show that the incidence rate of nosocomial BSI in the ICU ranges from 27 to 68 episodes per 1,000 admissions [17–21] (Table 15.1), depending on the type of ICU (surgical, medical, coronary care unit), severity of patient's illness, use of invasive devices, and the length of ICU stay. These infection rates among ICU patients are as much as five to ten times higher than those recorded for patients admitted to general wards.

Table 15.1 Rates of hospital-acquired bloodstream infections (BSIs) in the intensive care unit (ICU)

Year	Type of ICU	Episodes of nosocomial BSIs per 1,000 admissions	First author
1994	Medical–surgical	67.2	Rello [17]
1994	Surgical	26.7	Pittet [19]
1996	Adult, multicenter study	41	Brun-Buisson [20]
1997	Adult, multicenter study	36	Vallés [18]
2006	Adult, multicenter study	68	Garrouste-Orgas [21]

15.2.2 Risk Factors

Conditions that predispose an individual to BSI include not only the patient's underlying conditions but also therapeutic, microbial, and environmental factors. Illnesses that have been associated with an increased BSI risk include hematologic and nonhematologic malignancies, diabetes mellitus, renal failure requiring dialysis, chronic hepatic failure, immune deficiency syndromes, and conditions associated with the loss of normal skin barriers, such as serious burns and pressure ulcers. In the ICU, therapeutic maneuvers associated with an increased risk of HA BSI include procedures such as placement of intravascular and urinary catheters, endoscopic procedures, and drainage of intra-abdominal infections. Several risk factors have been associated with the acquisition of BSI by specific pathogens. Coagulase-negative staphylococci are mainly associated with central venous line infection and with the use of intravenously administered lipid emulsions. *Candida* spp. infections are related to exposure to multiple antibiotics, hemodialysis, isolation of *Candida* spp. from sites other than the blood, azotemia, and the use of indwelling catheters [22]. In an analysis of risk factors for HA candidemia in our ICU, we found that exposure to more than four antibiotics during the ICU stay [odds ratio (OR) 4.10], parenterally administered nutrition (OR 3.37), previous surgery (OR 2.60), and the presence of solid malignancy (OR 1.57) were the variables that were independently associated with the development of *Candida* spp. infection [23].

15.2.3 Microbiology

The spectrum of microorganisms that invade the bloodstream in patients with HAI during their stay in the ICU has been evaluated in several studies. Although almost any microorganism can produce BSI, staphylococci and Gram-negative bacilli account for the vast majority of cases. However, among the staphylococci, coagulase-negative staphylococci (CNS) have become a clinically significant agent of BSIs in the ICU [17, 18, 24, 25]. The ascendance of this group of staphylococci has increased the interpretative difficulties for clinicians, as a high number of CNS

Table 15.2 Microorganisms causing nosocomial bloodstream infection in adult intensive care units

Reference	Gram-positive microorganisms	Gram-negative microorganisms	Fungi	Polymicrobial episodes (%)
Rello [17]	44.1% CNS S. aureus[a] Enterococcus spp.	40.5% P. aeruginosa[b] E. coli Enterobacter spp.	5.4% Candida spp.	9.9
Pittet [19]	51.0% CNS S. aureus[a] Enterococcus spp.	39.0% Enterobacter spp. Klebsiella spp. S. marcescens[c]	4.8% Candida spp.	21
Vallés [18]	49.8% CNS S. aureus[a] Enterococcus spp.	32.6% P. aeruginosa[b] A. baumannii[d] K. pneumoniae[e]	4.4% Candida spp.	12.7
Jamal [27]	46.8% CNS S. aureus[a] Enterococcus spp.	36.6% Enterobacter spp. S. marcescens[c] K. pneumoniae[e]	17.6% Candida spp.	9.8
Garrouste-Orgas [21]	52.5% ECN S. aureus[a] Enterococcus spp.	29.3% Enterobacter spp. P. aeruginosa[b] Other	6.6% Candida spp.	11.6

CNS coagulase-negative staphylococci
[a] Staphylococcus
[b] Pseudomonas
[c] Serratia
[d] Acinetobacter
[e] Klebsiella

isolations represent contamination rather than true BSI. The increased importance of CNS BSI seems to be related to the high incidence of multiple invasive devices used in critically ill patients and to the multiple antimicrobial therapies used for Gram-negative infections in ICU patients, which results in selection of Gram-positive microorganisms. The change in the spectrum of organisms causing HA BSIs in an adult ICU is confirmed by Edgeworth et al. [26], who analyzed the evolution of HA BSIs over 25 years in the same ICU. Between 1971 and 1990, the frequency of isolation of individual organisms changed little, with *S. aureus*, *P. aeruginosa*, *Escherichia coli*, and *Klebsiella pneumoniae* predominating. However, between 1991 and 1995, the number of BSIs doubled, largely due to the increased isolation of CNS, *Enterococcus* spp., and intrinsically antibiotic-resistant Gram-negative organisms, particularly *P. aeruginosa* and *Candida* spp.

The leading pathogens among cases of HA BSIs in the ICU are Gram-positive microorganisms, representing nearly half of the organisms isolated [17–19, 21, 27] (Table 15.2). CNS, *S. aureus,* and enterococci are the most frequent Gram-positive bacteria in all studies, and CNS is isolated in 20–30% of all episodes of BSI.

Table 15.3 Major sources of hospital-acquired bloodstream infection in the ICUs

Type of infection	Rello [17] (%)	Pittet [19] (%)	Vallés [18] (%)	Edgewort [26] (%)	Garrouste-Orgas [21] (%)
Intravenous catheter	35	18	37.1	62	20.2
Respiratory tract	10	28	17.5	3	16.3
Intra-abdominal	9	NA	6.1	6.9	NA
Genitourinary tract	3.6	5.4	5.9	2.4	2.5
Surgical wound	8	8	2.4	3	9.9
Other	7	14.5	2.9	–	12.9
Unknown origin	27	20	28.1	22.4	32.7

Gram-negative bacilli are responsible for 30–40% of BSI episodes, and the remaining cases are mostly due to *Candida* spp. Polymicrobial episodes are relatively common, representing about 10%. Anaerobic bacteria are isolated in fewer than 5% of cases. Among Gram-positive BSIs, the incidence of pathogens is similar in the different ICUs, with CNS being the most frequently isolated organism and *S. aureus* the second commonest pathogen in all studies. Only the incidence of strains with antibiotic resistance, such as methicillin-resistant *Staphylococcus aureus* (MRSA) or vancomycin-resistant enterococci (VRE), differs substantially according to the characteristics of individual institutions and depending on whether they become established as endemic nosocomial pathogens in the ICU. On the other hand, the Gram-negative species isolated from HA BSIs in ICUs of different institutions show marked variability. The relative contribution of each Gram-negative species to the total number of isolates from blood varies from hospital to hospital and over time. The antibiotic policy of the institution may induce the appearance of highly drug-resistant microorganisms and the emergence of endemic nosocomial pathogens, in particular, *Pseudomonas* spp, *Acinetobacter* spp., and Enterobacteriaceae, with extended-spectrum beta-lactamase (ESBL).

15.2.4 Sources

The vast majority (70%) of nosocomial BSIs in the ICU are secondary bacteremias, including the BSIs related to intravascular catheter infection, and the remaining 30% are bacteremias of unknown origin. Table 15.3 summarizes the sources of nosocomial bacteremias in the ICU reported in several series [17–19, 21, 26]. As shown, intravascular catheter-related infections and respiratory tract infections are the leading sources of secondary episodes. The source of nosocomial BSIs varies according to microorganism. Coagulase-negative staphylococci and *S. aureus* commonly complicate intravenous-related infections, whereas Gram-negative bacilli are the main etiology for secondary BSIs following respiratory tract, intra-abdominal, and urinary tract infections. Among bacteremias of unknown origin, most are caused by Gram-positive microorganisms, mainly CNS, and may originate also in device-related infections not diagnosed at the time of BSI development.

15.2.5 Systemic Response

The host reaction to invading microbes involves a rapidly amplifying polyphony of signals and responses that may spread beyond the invaded tissue. Fever or hypothermia, chills, tachypnea, and tachycardia often herald the onset of the systemic inflammatory response to microbial invasion, also called sepsis. BSI and fungemia have been simply defined as the presence of bacteria or fungi in blood cultures, and four stages of systemic response of increasing severity have been described: the systemic inflammatory response syndrome (SIRS), which is identified by a combination of simple and readily available clinical signs and symptoms (i.e., fever or hypothermia, tachycardia, tachypnea, changes in blood leukocyte count); sepsis, in patients in whom the SIRS is caused by documented infection; severe sepsis, when patients have dysfunction of the major organs; septic shock, which describes patients with hypotension and organ dysfunction in addition to sepsis [28]. The presence of organisms in the blood is one of the most reliable criteria for characterizing a patient presenting with SIRS as having sepsis or one of its more severe presentations, such as severe sepsis or septic shock.

In a multicenter study, Brun-Buisson et al. [20] analyzed the relationship between BSI and severe sepsis in adults ICUs and general wards in 24 hospitals in France. Of the 842 episodes of clinically significant BSI recorded, 162 (19%) occurred in patients hospitalized in ICUs. Three hundred and seventy-seven episodes (45%) of BSIs were HA, and their incidence was 12 times greater in ICUs than in wards. The frequency of severe sepsis during BSI differed markedly between wards and ICUs (17% vs. 65%, $p < 0.001$). HA episodes in the ICU represented an incidence rate of 41/1,000 admissions, and the incidence rate of severe sepsis among patients with HA BSI in the ICU was 24 episodes per 1,000 admissions. A multicenter study reported by our group [18] analyzed 590 HA BSIs in adult ICUs of 30 hospitals in Spain and classified their systemic response as sepsis in 371 episodes (62.8%), severe sepsis in 109 (18.5%), and septic shock in the remaining 110 (18.6%). Episodes of BSI associated with intravascular catheters showed the lowest rate of septic shock (12.8%); episodes of BSI secondary to lower respiratory tract, intra-abdominal, or genitourinary tract infections showed the highest incidence of severe sepsis and septic shock. In the study by Brun-Buisson et al. [20] involving patients hospitalized in ICUs, intravascular catheter-related BSI was also associated with a lower risk of severe sepsis [OR 0.2; 95% confidence interval (CI) 0.1–0.5; $p < 0.01$). Systemic response may differ according to the microorganism causing the episode. Gram-negative and *Candida* spp. have been associated with a higher incidence of severe sepsis and septic shock [18], whereas CNS caused the lowest incidence of septic shock. In the French multicenter study, episodes caused by CNS were also associated with a reduced risk of severe sepsis (OR 0.2; $p = 0.02$) relative to other microorganisms [20].

15.2.6 Prognosis

HA BSIs remain a leading cause of morbidity and mortality in critically ill patients. The crude mortality rate related to HA BSIs in ICU patients ranges from 20 to 60%, and the mortality rate directly attributable to BSI infection ranges from 14 to 38% [17–21]. Although one-third of deaths occur within the first 48 h after symptom onset, death can occur 14 or more days later. Late deaths are often due to poorly controlled infection, complications during ICU stay, or failure of multiple organs. Bueno-Cavanillas et al. [29] analyzed the impact of HAI on the mortality rate in an ICU. Overall crude relative risk (RR) of mortality was 2.48 (95% CI 1.47–4.16) in patients with a HAI compared with noninfected patients, and 4.13 (95% CI 2.11–8.11) in patients with BSI. In a matched, risk-adjusted multicenter study in 12 ICUs, Garrouste-Orgas et al. [21] found that HA BSI was associated with a threefold increase in mortality.

The risk of dying is influenced by the patient's prior clinical condition and the rate at which complications develop. Analysis using prognostic stratification systems (such as Acute Physiology and Chronic Health Evaluation (APACHE) or the Simplified Acute Physiological Score (SAPS) II) indicate that factoring in the patient's age and certain physiologic variables results in more accurate estimates of the risk of dying. Variables associated with the high-care fatality rates include acute respiratory distress syndrome (ARDS), disseminated intravascular coagulation (DIC), renal insufficiency, and multiple organ dysfunction (MOD). Microbial variables are less important, although high-care fatality rates have been observed for patients with BSI due to *P. aeruginosa* and *Candida* spp., and for patients with polymicrobial BSI [21].

15.2.7 Prevention

Indwelling vascular catheters are a leading source of BSIs in critically ill patients. More than 250,000 vascular-catheter-related BSIs (CR-BSI) occur annually in the USA [30–32], resulting in substantial morbidity and mortality rates and costs [33–35]. Despite the publication of clinical practice guidelines [30] on managing and preventing intravascular catheter-related infection, CR-BSI are common. According to the NNIS system of the CDC, the median rate of all types of CR-BSI ranges from 1.8 to 5.2 episodes per 1,000 catheter days. In Spain, the mean rate of CR-BSI in the National Study of Nosocomial Infections Surveillance in the ICU (ENVIN-UCI) in 2006 was five episodes per 1,000 catheter days [36]. In our medical–surgical ICU in 2006, central venous catheters (CVC) were used in 83% of patients, and the incidence of CR-BSI was 5.8 episodes per 1,000 catheter-days.

Pronovost et al. [37] implemented an evidence-based intervention in 108 ICUs to reduce CR-BSI, designating a team leader for each hospital instructed in the different interventions and responsible for disseminating this information among their colleagues. The intervention consisted of five evidence-based procedures recommended by the CDC: hand washing, using full-barrier precautions during CVC insertion, cleaning the skin with chlorhexidine, avoiding the femoral site if possible, and removing unnecessary catheters. A checklist was used to ensure adherence to infection-control practices. Three months after implementing the intervention, their median rate of CR-BSI had decreased from 2.7/1,000 catheter days at baseline to 0/1,000 catheter days ($p < 0.002$), and their mean rate had decreased from 7.7/1,000 catheter days at baseline to 1.4/1,000 catheter days ($p < 0.002$). This improvement was maintained throughout the 18-month study period.

In 2007 in our ICU, we implemented a similar multiple-system intervention applying evidence-based measures and reduced the incidence of catheter-relate BSI from 6.7/1,000 catheter days to 2.4/1,000 catheter days (RR 0.36; 95% CI 0.16–0.80; $p = 0.015$), with a 20% reduction in the incidence of HA BSIs in the ICU [38] (Fig. 15.1).

15.3 Community-Acquired Bloodstream Infections in the ICU

15.3.1 Epidemiology

CA BSI is defined as infection that develops in a patient prior to if the bacteremia develops within the first 48 h of hospital and ICU admission and is not associated with any procedure performed after admission. CAI represent an important reason for ICU admission. Severe CA pneumonia and intra-abdominal infections are the most frequent, and approximately 20% also present bacteremia. A few epidemiologic studies focusing solely on CA BSI on ICU admission are available. Data from a multicenter study reported a CA BSIs rate of 10.2/1,000 ICU admissions [39].

15.3.2 Microbiology

In CA BSIs in patients admitted to the ICU, the incidence of Gram-positive is similar to Gram-negative microorganisms, and almost 10% are polymicrobial episodes. *E. coli, Streptococcus pneumoniae,* and *S. aureus* are the leading pathogens, and the prevalence of these microorganisms is related to the main sources of BSIs found in these patients, such as urinary tract and pulmonary tract infections and those of unknown origin [11, 12, 39] (Table 15.4).

15.3.3 Sources

Among CA BSIs, lower respiratory tract, intra-abdominal, and genitourinary infections represent >80% of episodes of bacteremia admitted in the ICU (Table 15.4). Approximately 20–29% of episodes are of unknown origin, including mainly meningococcal and staphylococcal infections [11, 12, 39].

Table 15.4 Microorganisms and sources of community-acquired bloodstream infections admitted to the intensive care unit

Reference	Sources (%)		Microorganisms (%)	
Forgacs [11]	Pulmonary	38.5	S. pneumoniae[a]	32.3
	Genitourinary	23.0	E. coli[b]	27.2
	Endocarditis	8.0	S. aureus[c]	13.5
	Biliary tract	5.9	Other GNB	14.2
	Other	11.1	Other GPC	8.2
	Unknown origin	20.0	Other	14.2
Vallés [39]	Pulmonary	20.0	E. coli[b]	28.1
	Abdominal	20.1	S. pneumoniae[a]	17.9
	Genitourinary	19.8	S. aureus[c]	14.9
	Other	10.3	Other GNB	18.6
	Unknown origin	29.2	Other GPC	9.5
			Other	11.07

GNB Gram-negative bacilli; *GPC* Gram-positive cocci
[a] *Streptococcus*
[b] *Escherichia*
[c] *Staphylococcus*

15.3.4 Systemic Response

The incidence of severe sepsis and septic shock in patients with CA BSIs is higher than in HA episodes, in part because the severity of the systemic response is the reason for ICU admission. In a multicenter French study, 74% of CA BSI episodes presented severe sepsis or septic shock at admission [20]. In a multicenter Spanish study carried out in 30 ICUs, the incidence of severe sepsis and septic shock was 75%. In that study, Gram-negative microorganisms and urinary tract and intra-abdominal infections were associated more frequently with septic shock [39].

15.3.5 Prognosis

Patients admitted to the ICU with CA BSI present a crude mortality rate close to 40%, compared with 18% in patients admitted to general wards [12, 39, 40]. This is due in part to the severity of systemic response (severe sepsis and septic shock) and associated complications, which is the reason for admission [12, 39]. The appropriateness of empiric antimicrobial treatment is the most important variable influencing the outcome of these patients [12, 39]. The incidence of inappropriate antibiotic treatment in CA BSIs ICU patients ranges between 15% and 20% in two studies, and the mortality rate among patients with inappropriate empiric antibiotic treatment is >70% [12, 39, 41].

15.4 Health-Care-Associated Bloodstream Infections in the ICU

15.4.1 Epidemiology

Patients residing in the community and who are receiving care at home, living in personal-care and rehabilitation centers, receiving chronic dialysis, and receiving chemotherapy in physicians' offices may present BSIs, which have traditionally been categorized as CA infections. However, the difference between community- or HA BSIs has become less clear. Therefore, some investigators propose a new classification—healthcare-associated infections—that are distinct from CAI and HAI [42, 43]. Health-care-associated BSI has been defined when a positive blood culture is obtained from a patient at the time of or within 48 h of hospital admission if the patient fulfilled any of the following criteria:
1. received intravenous therapy at home, received wound care or specialized nursing care, or had self-administered intravenously administered medical therapy;
2. attended a hospital hemodialysis clinic or received chemotherapy intravenously;
3. was hospitalized in an acute-care hospital for ≥ 2 days in the 90 days before the BSI;
4. resided in a personal- or long-term-care facility [43].

According to this new classification, approximately 40–50% of patients admitted with BSI traditionally defined as CA should be classified as having healthcare-associated BSI [42, 43]. In a large US database, healthcare-associated BSI accounted for more than half of all BSIs. If patients with healthcare-associated BSI had been included in the CA BSI category, according to the traditional classification scheme, they would have accounted for approximately 60% of CA BSI patients who needed hospitalization [44].

There are no studies available regarding the importance of healthcare-associated BSI in ICU patients using this new classification. However, recent studies suggest that healthcare-associated BSIs are less frequent than HA- and CA BSI in critically ill patients. In a multicenter study carried out in three hospitals in Spain, 1,157 BSI episodes were studied: 50% were CA, 26% HA, and 24% healthcare-associated BSI [45]. In patients admitted to the ICU, 60% of BSIs were HA, 30% CA, and 10% healthcare associated.

We conducted a multicenter study in 28 ICUs in Spain (unpublished data) analyzing 1,590 BSI episodes and confirmed the low incidence of healthcare-associated BSI in ICU patients compared with patients admitted to conventional wards. The most frequent BSIs were HA (77%), CA (21%), and healthcare associated (8%). Compared with patients with CA episodes, patients with healthcare-associated BSI were older and more likely to have severe comorbidities, such as congestive heart failure, peripheral vascular disease, chronic renal disease, and cancer. This high number of comorbidities and the patient's basal condition may be the reason for a lower ICU admission rate of these patients due

Table 15.5 Pathogens most frequently found in bloodstream infections through epidemiologic type of infection in a Spanish multicenter study [45]

Pathogen	Total $n = 1{,}157$ (%)	CBSI $n = 581$ (%)	HBSI $n = 295$ (%)	HCBSI $n = 281$ (%)	P value
Escherichia coli	472 (40.8)	308 (53)	61 (20.7)	103 (36.7)	<0.001
MSSA	86 (7.4)	25 (4.3)	31 (10.5)	30 (10.6)	<0.001
CN staphylococci	62 (5.3)	4 (0.7)	49 (16.6)	9 (3.2)	<0.001
Streptococcus pneumoniae	80 (6.9)	64 (11)	5 (1.7)	11 (3.9)	<0.001
Pseudomonas aeruginosa	63 (5.4)	9 (1.5)	27 (9.2)	27 (9.6)	<0.001
Klebsiella pneumoniae	41 (3.5)	23 (4)	9 (3.1)	9 (3.2)	NS
Candida spp	12 (1)	0 (0)	11 (3.7)	1 (0.3)	<0.001
Polymicrobial	72 (6.2)	23 (3.9)	26 (8.8)	23 (8.1)	0.01

CBSI community-acquired bloodstream infection; *HBSI* hospital-acquired bloodstream infection; *HCBSI* healthcare-associated bloodstream infection; *MSSA* methicillin-sensitive *Staphylococcus aureus*; *CN* coagulase-negative

to a possible limitation of therapeutic effort by physicians in wards or emergency areas prior to the patient's admission to the ICU. Consequently, the number of patients with healthcare-associated infections admitted in the ICU may be reduced.

15.4.2 Microbiology

The pathogens responsible for healthcare-associated BSI and their susceptibility patterns are similar to HAI. In a prospective observational study of 504 patients with BSIs, Friedman et al. [43] found that *S. aureus* was the most common pathogen in patients with healthcare-associated and HA bacteremia. MRSA was present in 19% of healthcare-associated BSI and 20% in HA episodes. Moreover, ampicillin–sulbactam and ciprofloxacin resistance occurred with similar frequency in Enterobacteriaceae isolated from patients with healthcare-associated and HA BSI. A US multicenter study found similar results in the frequency of *S. aureus* and MRSA in healthcare-associated and HA BSIs [44]. However, the distribution of pathogens in both groups was not identical. Whereas *E. coli* and *Proteus* spp. were identified more frequently in patients with healthcare-associated infections, fungal organisms were more prevalent in patients with HA BSI. In our experience [45], the distribution of pathogens isolated from patients with healthcare-associated BSI shares more similarity with HA than with CA BSIs (Table 15.5). In addition, episodes with healthcare-associated BSI had a higher prevalence of MRSA infections (5%) than CA (0.2%) (OR 30.4; 95% CI 3.9–232.4; $p < 0.001$)

or HA (0.7%) (OR 7.7; 95% CI 1.7–34.1; $p = 0.001$) episodes. A study in Spain found a high MRSA prevalence (16.8; 95% CI 14.9–18.8) among residents in community long-term-care facilities and was isolated from 15.5% of nasal swabs and 59% of decubitus ulcers [46].

15.4.3 Sources

Urinary tract infection, intravascular-device-related BSI, gastrointestinal-related bacteremia, and respiratory tract infections are the most frequent sources of healthcare-associated BSIs [43, 45]. Patients with healthcare-associated and those with HA BSIs have similar frequencies of intravascular-device-related bacteremia.

15.4.4 Systemic Response

In a multicenter study of ICU patients in Spain, 50–60% with healthcare-associated BSI presented septic shock. The frequency of severe sepsis and septic shock was similar to CA and HA BSI (non-ICU-acquired) that originated in conventional wards because they were the main causes for ICU admission (unpublished data).

15.4.5 Prognosis

Friedman et al. [43] found a mortality rate at follow-up greater in patients with healthcare-associated BSI (29% vs. 16%; $p = 0.019$) or HA infection (37% vs. 16%; $p < 0.001$) than in patients with CA infection. Similar results were found by Shorr et al. [44], where the mortality risk was significantly higher if BSI was acquired in the hospital or associated with previous healthcare exposure. Consistent with these reports, we found a significantly higher mortality rate at follow up in groups with HA BSI (27.3%) and healthcare-associated BSI (27.5%) than in those with CA BSI (10.4%) ($p < 0.001$). Among patients with CA and healthcare-associated BSIs, a multivariate analysis, adjusted for age and comorbidities, showed healthcare-associated BSI (OR 2.4; 95% CI 1.5–3.7; $p < 0.001$) as an independent factor associated with mortality [45].

15.5 Treatment

BSIs are among the most serious infections causing severe sepsis or septic shock acquired by hospitalized patients requiring intensive care. The mainstay of therapy for patients with bacteremia remains antimicrobial therapy associated with a optimal management of consequences of bacteremia, such as shock or metastatic suppurative complications and surgical treatment, such as debridement or drainage of abscesses and removing intravascular devices if necessary [47]. Appropriate antimicrobial therapy has been shown to reduce mortality rates among patients with bacteremia and, when initiated early, to have a favorable effect on outcome in critically ill patients [44]. The initial antimicrobial therapy is necessarily empiric based on targeting the most likely etiologic pathogens. However, inappropriate empirical treatment occurs in 30% of cases and is more frequent in the following circumstances: HAI, healthcare-associated infection, prior administration of antibiotics, and presence of multi-drug-resistant pathogens.

The distribution of pathogens associated with CA BSIs is relatively uniform. However, an increase in the incidence of infections due to antibiotic-resistant microorganisms, such as CA MRSA and infections caused by ESBL-producing *E. coli* or *K. pneumoniae* have been reported in most countries, and these circumstances must be considered when empiric antibiotic treatment is initiated. HA and healthcare-associated BSIs are associated with an increased incidence of resistant microorganisms, such as MRSA, ESBL-producing Enterobacteriaceae, *Acinetobacter baumannii*, and *P. aeruginosa*. In these cases, the appropriateness of empirical treatment is more difficult, especially in ICU patients. In these cases, and despite guideline recommendations, identifying the local flora predominant in each area before initiating empirical antibiotic treatment is indispensable.

15.5.1 Treatment of Severe Sepsis and Septic Shock

Patients with BSI who develop severe sepsis or septic shock require additional treatment: early goal-directed therapy (EGDT) [48], corticosteroids for refractory septic shock [49], recombinant human activated protein C or drotrecogin alfa (activated) for multiorgan failure [50], and lung-protective ventilation strategies [51] have all been associated with survival benefits. These and other therapeutic advances led to the development of the surviving sepsis campaign (SSC) guidelines [52]. To improve care for patients with sepsis, the SSC and the Institute for Healthcare Improvement recommend implementing two sepsis bundles: the resuscitation bundle and the management bundle (Table 15.6):
1. The resuscitation bundle includes lactate determination, early cultures and antibiotics, and EGDT. This bundle describes seven tasks that should begin immediately and must be accomplished within the first 6 h of presentation of severe sepsis or septic shock. Some items may not be completed if the clinical conditions described in the bundle do not prevail in a particular case, but clinicians must assess for these elements.
2. The management bundle includes optimization of glycemic control and respiratory inspiratory plateau pressure and determination of the need for corticosteroids or drotrecogin alfa (activated). Efforts to accomplish these goals should begin immediately, and these items must be completed within 24 h of presentation of severe sepsis or septic shock.

Table 15.6 Surviving sepsis campaign bundles

Resuscitation bundle (first 6 h)
1. Measure serum lactate
2. Obtain blood cultures prior to antibiotic within 3 h from time of presentation for emergency department (ED) admissions and 1 h for non-ED intensive care unit (ICU) admission
3. Administer broad-spectrum antibiotics within 3 h from time of presentation for ED admissions and 1 h for non-ED ICU admission
4. In the event of hypotension and/or lactate >36 mg/dl
a. deliver an initial minimum dose of 20 ml/kg crystalloid (or colloid equivalent)
b. apply vasopressors for hypotension not responding to initial fluid resuscitation to maintain mean arterial pressure (MAP) 65 mmHg
5. In the event of persistent hypotension despite fluid resuscitation (septic shock) and/or lactate >36 mg/dl
a. achieve central venous pressure (CVP) of 8 mmHg
b. achieve central venous oxygen saturation ($ScvO_2$) of 70%
Management bundle (first 24 h)
1. Administer low-dose steroids for septic shock in accordance with a standardized ICU policy
2. Administer drotrecogin alfa (activated) in accordance with a standardized ICU policy
3. Maintain glucose control higher than the lower limit of normal but <150 mg/dl
4. Maintain inspiratory plateau pressures >30 cm H_2O for mechanically ventilated patients

Several studies have evaluated bundled care, and in a meta-analyses [53] including all those studies, done by the National Institutes of Health (NIH) in the United States, bundled care was associated with a consistent and significant increase in survival rate (OR 1.91; CI 1.49–2.45; $p < 0.0001$). Moreover, an international effort to implement bundled care improved survival (hospital mortality rates decreased from 37.0 to 30.8% in two years) [54]. According to these results, bundled care is warranted in all patients with BSI and severe sepsis and septic shock.

15.6 Summary

BSIs are among the most serious infections causing severe sepsis or septic shock in hospitalized patients requiring intensive care. Nosocomial BSIs account for almost 20% of HAI in critically ill patients, >80% of which are associated with a central line. These infection rates among ICU patients are as much as five to ten times higher than those recorded for patients admitted to general wards. CA infections represent an important reason for ICU admission: severe pneumonia and urinary tract and intra-abdominal infections are the most frequent CA infections requiring ICU admission, and approximately 20% of these patients will also present bacteremia, which associated with a high incidence of severe sepsis and septic shock. A new classification scheme for BSIs—healthcare-acquired BSIs—has been proposed to distinguish between infections occurring among outpatients having recurrent or recent contact with the healthcare system and patients with true CA infections. According to this classification, approximately 40–50% of patients admitted to general hospital wards classified as having CA BSIs should be classified as having healthcare-associated BSI. However, the rate of healthcare-acquired BSI among critically ill patients in the ICU seems to be lower (<20% of community-acquired infections) than among patients admitted to conventional wards. BSIs in critically ill patients are associated with greater hospital mortality rates. Clinical efforts should therefore be aimed at improving severe sepsis and septic shock management, reducing the incidence of inadequate antimicrobial treatment, and preventing BSI episodes associated with intravascular devices.

References

1. Wenzel RP (1990) Organization for infection control. In: Mandell GL, Douglas RG Jr, Bennett JE (eds) Principles and practice of infectious diseases. Churchill Livingstone, New York, pp 2176–2180
2. Weinstein RA (1991) Epidemiology and control of nosocomial infections in adult intensive care units. Am J Med 91(Suppl 3B):179S–184S
3. Wenzel RP, Thompson RL, Landry SM et al (1983) Hospital-acquired infections in intensive care unit patients: an overview with emphasis on epidemics. Infect Control 4:371–375
4. Maki DG (1989) Risk factors for nosocomial infection in intensive care: "devices vs nature" and goals for the next decade. Arch Intern Med 149:30–35
5. Donowitz LG, Wenzel RP, Hoyt JW (1982) High risk of hospital-acquired infection in the ICU patient. Crit Care Med 10:355–357
6. Brown RB, Hosmer D, Chen HC et al (1985) A comparison of infections in the different ICUs within the same hospital. Crit Care Med 13:472–476
7. Daschner F (1985) Nosocomial infections in intensive care units. Intensive Care Med 11:284–287
8. Trilla A, Gatell JM, Mensa J et al (1991) Risk factors for nosocomial bacteremia in a large Spanish teaching hospital: a case-control study. Infect Control Hosp Epidemiol 12:150–156
9. Massanari RM, Hierholzer WJ Jr (1986) The intensive care unit. In: Bennett JV, Brachman PS (eds) Hospital infections. Little, Brown and Company, Boston, pp 285–298
10. Ponce de León-Rosales S, Molinar-Ramos F, Domínguez-Cherit G et al (2000) Prevalence of infections in intensive care units in Mexico: a multicenter study. Crit Care Med 28:1316–1321
11. Forgacs IC, Eykyn SJ, Bradley RD (1986) Serious infection in the intensive therapy unit: a 15-year study of bacteraemia. Q J Med 60:773–779
12. Vallés J, Ochagavía A, Rué M et al (2000) Critically ill patients with community-acquired bacteremia: characteristics and prognosis. Intensive Care Med 26(Suppl. 3):S222
13. Garner JS, Jarvis WR, Emori TG et al (1988) CDC definitions for nosocomial infections. Am J Infect Control 16:128–140
14. Trilla A (1994) Epidemiology of nosocomial infections in adult intensive care units. Intensive Care Med 20:S1–S4
15. Richards MJ, Edwards JR, Culver DH et al (1999) Nosocomial infections in medical intensive care units in the United States. Crit Care Med 27:887–892
16. Wisplinghoff H, Bischoff T, Tallent SM et al (2004) Nosocomial bloodstream infections in US Hospitals: analysis of 24, 179 cases from a prospective nationwide surveillance study. Clin Infect Dis 39:309–317

17. Rello J, Ricart M, Mirelis B et al (1994) Nosocomial bacteremia in a medical-surgical intensive care unit: epidemiologic characteristics and factors influencing mortality in 111 episodes. Intensive Care Med 20:94–98
18. Vallés J, León C, Alvarez-Lerma F et al (1997) Nosocomial bacteremia in critically ill patients: a multicenter study evaluating epidemiology and prognosis. Clin Infect Dis 24:387–395
19. Pittet D, Tarara D, Wenzel RP (1994) Nosocomial bloodstream infection in critically ill patients. Excess length of stay, extra costs, and attributable mortality. JAMA 271:1598–1601
20. Brun-Buisson C, Doyon F, Carlet J et al (1996) Bacteremia and severe sepsis in adults: a multicenter prospective survey in ICUs and wards of 24 hospitals. Am J Respir Crit Care Med 154:617–624
21. Garrouste-Orgeas M, Timsit JF, Tafflet M et al (2006) Excess risk of death from intensive care unit-acquired nosocomial bloodstream infections: a reappraisal. Clin Infect Dis 42:1118–1126
22. Wenzel RP (1995) Isolation of *Candida* species from sites other than the blood. Clin Infect Dis 20:1531–1534
23. Díaz E, Villagrá A, Martínez M et al (1998) Nosocomial candidemia risk factors. Intensive Care Med 24(Suppl 1):S143
24. Towns ML, Quartey SM, Weinstein MP et al (1993) The clinical significance of positive blood cultures: a prospective, multicenter evaluation, abstr. C-232. In: Abstracts of the 93rd general meeting of the American society for microbiology. American Society for Microbiology, Washington, DC
25. Weinstein MP, Towns ML, Quartey SM et al (1997) The clinical significance of positive blood cultures in the 1990s: a prospective comprehensive evaluation of the microbiology, epidemiology, and outcome of bacteremia and fungemia in adults. Clin Infect Dis 24:584–602
26. Edgeworth JD, Treacher DF, Eykyn SJ (1999) A 25-year study of nosocomial bacteremia in an adult intensive care unit. Crit Care Med 27:1421–1428
27. Jamal WY, El-Din K, Rotimi VO et al (1999) An analysis of hospital-acquired bacteraemia in intensive care unit patients in a university hospital in Kuwait. J Hosp Infect 43:49–56
28. Levy MM, Fink MP, Marshall JC et al (2003) SCCM/ESICM/ACCP/ATS/SIS International sepsis definitions conference. Intensive Care Med 29:530–538
29. Bueno-Cavanillas A, Delgado-Rodríguez M, López-Luque A et al (1994) Influence of nosocomial infection on mortality rate in an intensive care unit. Crit Care Med 22:55–60
30. O'Grady N, Patchen Dellinger A, Gerberding J et al (2002) Guidelines for the prevention of intravascular catheter-related infections. CID 35:1281–1307
31. Mermel LA (2000) Prevention of intravascular catheter-related infections. Ann Intern Med 132:391–402
32. Warren DK, Cosgrove SE, Diekema DJ et al (2006) A multicenter intervention to prevent catheter-associated bloodstream infections. Infect Control Hosp Epidemiol 27:662–669
33. Renaud B, Brun-Buisson C et al (2001) Outcomes of primary and catheter-related bacteremia. Am J Respir Crit Care Med 163:1584–1590
34. Blot SI, Depuydt P, Annemans L et al (2005) Clinical and economic outcomes in critically ill patients with nosocomial catheter-related bloodstream infections. Clin Infect Dis 41:1591–1598
35. Warren DK, Quadir WW, Hollenbeak CS et al (2006) Attributable cost of catheter-associated bloodstream infections among intensive care patients in a nonteaching hospital. Crit Care Med 34:2084–2089
36. Alvarez-Lerma J, Palomar M, Olaechea P et al (2007) National study of control of nosocomial infection in intensive care units. Evolutive report of the years 2003–2005 (Article in Spanish). Med Intensiva 31:6–17
37. Pronovost P, Needham D, Berebholtz S et al (2006) An intervention to decrease catheter-related bloodstream infections in the ICU. NEJM 355:2725–2732

38. Peredo R, Sabatier C, Villagrá A et al (2010) Reduction in catheter-related bloodstream infections in critically ill patients through a multiple system intervention. Eur J Clin Microbiol Infect Dis 29(9):1173–1177
39. Vallés J, Rello J, Ochagavía A et al (2003) Community-acquired bloodstream infection in critically ill adult patients: impact of shock and inappropriate antibiotic therapy on survival. Chest 123:1615–1624
40. Cartón JA, García-Velasco G, Maradona JA (1988) Bacteriemia extrahospitalaria en adultos. Análisis prospectivo de 333 episodios. Med Clin (Barc) 90:525–530
41. Ibrahim EH, Sherman G, Ward S et al (2000) The influence of inadequate antimicrobial treatment of bloodstream infections on patient outcomes in the ICU setting. Chest 118:146–155
42. Siegman-Igra Y, Fourer B, Orni-Wasserkauf R et al (2002) Reappraisal of community-acquired bacteremia: a proposal of a new classification for the spectrum of acquisition of bacteremia. Clin Infect Dis 34:1431–1439
43. Friedman ND, Kaye KS, Stout JE et al (2002) Health care-associated bloodstream infections in adults: a reason to change the accepted definition of community-acquired infections. Ann Intern Med 137:791–797
44. Shorr AF, Tabak YP, Killian AD et al (2006) Healthcare-associated bloodstream infection: a distinct entity? Insights from a large US database. Crit Care Med 34:2588–2595
45. Vallés J, Calbo E, Anoro E et al (2008) Bloodstream infections in adults: importance of healthcare-associated infections. J Infect 56:27–34
46. Manzur A, Gavalda L, Ruiz de Gopegui E et al (2008) Prevalence of methicillin-resistant *Staphylococcus aureus* and factors associated with colonization among residents in community long-term-care facilities in Spain. Clin Microbiol Infect 14:867–872
47. Dellinger RP, Levy MM, Carlet JM et al (2008) Surviving sepsis campaign: international guidelines for management of severe sepsis and septic shock. Crit Care Med 36:296–327
48. Rivers E, Nguyen B, Havstad S et al (2001) Early goal-directed therapy in the treatment of severe sepsis and septic shock. N Engl J Med 345:1368–1377
49. Annane D, Sebille V, Charpentier C et al (2002) Effect of treatment with low doses of hydrocortisone and fludrocortisone on mortality in patients with septic shock. JAMA 288:862–871
50. Bernard GR, Vincent JL, Laterre PF et al (2001) Efficacy and safety of recombinant human activated protein C for severe sepsis. N Engl J Med 344:699–709
51. The Acute Respiratory Distress Syndrome Network (2000) Ventilation with lower tidal volumes as compared with traditional tidal volumes for acute lung injury and the acute respiratory distress syndrome. N Engl J Med 342:1301–1308
52. Dellinger RP, Carlet JM, Masur H et al (2004) Surviving sepsis campaign guidelines for management of severe sepsis and septic shock. Intensive Care Med 30:536–555
53. Barochia AV, Cui X, Vitberg D et al (2010) Bundled care for septic shock: an analysis of clinical trials. Crit Care Med 38:668–678
54. Levy MM, Dellinger RP, Townsend SR et al (2010) The surviving sepsis campaign: results of an international guideline-based performance improvement program targeting severe sepsis. Intensive Care Med 36:222–231

Infections of Peritoneum, Mediastinum, Pleura, Wounds, and Urinary Tract

G. Sganga, G. Brisinda, V. Cozza and M. Castagneto

16.1 Introduction

Intra-abdominal infections (IAIs) are defined as an inflammatory response of the peritoneum to microorganisms and their toxins, which results in purulent exudate in the abdominal cavity [1–5]. They have two major manifestations: generalized peritonitis and IA abscess. Peritonitis remains a potentially fatal disease and still represents a challenge for surgeons [3]. Although a greater understanding of the pathophysiology of IAIs, improvement in critical care, and timely surgical and/or radiological intervention have reduced the mortality rate associated with severe peritonitis, that rate remains unacceptably high, ranging from 3% in localized abscess to 10% in localized peritonitis, 32% in diffuse suppurative peritonitis, and 70–80% in complicated mixed infections [1–5]. In an effort to improve treatment results, especially of IAIs resulting from anastomotic leakage or perforation of the gastrointestinal tract (GIT), new surgical techniques have been introduced.

16.2 Definition and Classification

Many attempts have been made to classify peritonitis in general and secondary peritonitis in particular, which include a large variety of different pathological conditions ranging in severity from a local problem to a devastating disease. A simplified version is reported in Table 16.1. This differentiates the relatively

G. Sganga (✉)
Istituto di Clinica Chirurgica, Università Cattolica del Sacro Cuore,
Rome, Italy
e-mail: gsganga@tiscali.it

Table 16.1 Classification of intra-abdominal infections (IAIs)

Primary peritonitis
- Diffuse bacterial peritonitis in absence of GIT disruption
- Spontaneous peritonitis in children
- Spontaneous peritonitis in adults
- Peritonitis in patients receiving continuous peritoneal dialysis
- Tuberculous and other granulomatous peritonitis

Secondary peritonitis
- Localized or diffuse peritonitis originating from a defect in GIT
- Acute perforation peritonitis (GIT perforation, intestinal ischemia, pelviperitonitis, and other forms)
- Postoperative peritonitis (anastomotic leak, accidental perforation, and devascularization)
- Posttraumatic peritonitis (after either blunt or penetrating abdominal trauma)

Tertiary peritonitis
- Late peritonitis-like syndrome due to disturbance in the immune response
- Peritonitis without evidence of pathogens
- Peritonitis with fungi
- Peritonitis with low-grade pathogenetic bacteria

GIT gastrointestinal tract

rare forms of primary peritonitis, which usually respond to medical treatment, and tertiary peritonitis, which does not respond to any treatment, from the commonly occurring secondary peritonitis that mandates surgical intervention and antibiotic therapy [2]. IAIs include the following pathological conditions:
1. Infections of single organs (cholecystitis, appendicitis, diverticulitis, cholangitis, pancreatitis, salpingitis, etc.), which may or may not be complicated by peritonitis, even in the absence of perforation.
2. Peritonitis, classified as primary, secondary or tertiary.
3. Intra-abdominal abscesses, classified on the basis of their location and anatomic configuration.

The term complicated IAI (C-IAI) is used to indicate infections that, originating in an organ cavity, extend into the peritoneal space and form an abscess or peritonitis. Resolution of this type of infection requires surgical treatment and percutaneous drainage, as well as systemic antibiotic therapy [6]. They are divided into two types: community c-IAIs, which can be mild or serious; and hospital c-IAIs, which usually occur as postoperative infections. The nature of severe IAIs makes it difficult to precisely define the disease, to assess its severity, and to evaluate and compare therapeutic progress. Both the anatomical source of infection and, to a greater degree, the physiological compromise it inflicts, affects the outcome of IAI.

16.3 Microbiology

Primary peritonitis is a monomicrobial, aerobic infection [2] caused by *Streptococcus pneumoniae*. The underlying risk factor most frequently encountered is the presence of cirrhosis and ascites. Bacteriological cultures grow *Escherichia coli*, whereas anaerobes are rare, and their presence, or a mixed flora, suggests secondary peritonitis [2]. The latter represents a polymicrobial infection (average of four isolates per patient, with the most frequent combination being *E. coli* and *Bacteroides fragilis*) after a spontaneous or traumatic breach in a viscous-containing microorganism, or due to postoperative breakdown of GIT anastomosis [7, 8].

The quantity and variety of microorganisms increase progressively the more the lesion is in a distal part of the GIT: the proximal anatomical regions (stomach and duodenum are usually sterile) usually contain aerobic coliform flora with a small anaerobic component ($<10^4$ CFU). In the more distal regions (for example, the colon), the intestine contains a higher concentration of bacteria (10^{12} obligatory anaerobes and 10^8 facultative anaerobes in 1 g of feces). After colon perforation, the peritoneal cavity can be invaded by >400 different bacterial species, but only some of these are directly responsible for infectious processes. Prolonged hospital stay, especially in ICU, repeated surgery, and administration of systemic or intraluminal antibiotic treatment, may drastically modify the patients' flora ecology, resulting in colonization of the proximal GIT with abnormal microorganisms (fungi, Gram-negative bacteria of low pathogenicity), which may be found in tertiary peritonitis [9], in critically ill patients, in ICU infections, and in multiple organ failure (MOF) [2].

16.4 Inflammatory Response in Peritonitis

The outcome of peritonitis depends on the results of a struggle between the patient's systemic and local defenses [systemic inflammatory response syndrome (SIRS)] on one hand, and the nature, volume, and duration of bacterial contamination on the other. The exact events that follow invasion of the peritoneal cavity with bacteria and adjuvants of infection (blood, bile, barium sulfate), and, subsequently, its translymphatic spread, have been clearly defined in recent studies [1–4, 10, 11]. Microorganisms and their products stimulate the host's cellular defenses to activate several inflammatory mediators, which are responsible for sepsis. Bacterial peritonitis appears to induce an intense compartmentalized inflammatory process [10]. A key element is cytokines [proinflammatory: tumor necrosis factor (TNF), interleukin (IL)-1 and -8; anti-inflammatory: IL-6 and -10], and host-produced pleomorphic immunoregulatory peptides [10, 11]. A trigger, such as a microbial toxin, stimulates production of TNF and IL-1, which in turn promote endothelial-cell-leukocyte adhesion, release of proteases and arachidonate metabolites, and clotting activation. IL-1 and TNF are synergistic and share many biological effects, and their inhibition improves organ function and survival. IL-8 may have an especially important role in perpetuating tissue inflammation. IL-6 and -10, which are perhaps counterregulatory, inhibit the generation of TNF, augment the action of acute phase reactants and immunoglobulins, and inhibit T-lymphocyte and macrophage function [11]. Cytokines are measurable in the systemic circulation and in peritoneal exudates, and the magnitude of the phenomena is negatively correlated with outcome [2, 3]. Most peritoneal cytokines probably derive from macrophages exposed to bacterial endotoxin [12]. Recent findings suggest that female sex hormones play a critical role in maintaining the immune response after trauma hemorrhage by suppressing the production of TNF-α and preventing increased mortality rates from subsequent sepsis [12]. Other potential sources are direct translocation of cytokines through the GIT barrier or production by traumatized tissues [13]. Timely therapeutic intervention is crucial to abort the ensuing, self-perpetuating, SIRS, sequential MOF, and death [2, 10–12].

16.5 Diagnosis

16.5.1 Clinical Diagnosis

Clinical diagnosis of intra-abdominal sepsis is usually assisted by the presence of systemic signs of inflammation (such as fever, neutrophil leukocytosis) and by local abdominal symptoms (defense, rigidity and respiratory hypomobility, absence of peristalsis, paralytic ileum), possibly with the assistance of some diagnostic imaging techniques [abdominal X-ray, ultrasonography (US), computed tomography (CT), magnetic resonance imaging (MRI)]. The typical presentation of secondary peritonitis is spontaneous acute abdominal pain, exacerbated by breathing and movement, accompanied by abdominal distension, fever, nausea or vomiting and irregular bowel sounds. Diffused pain is suggestive of generalized peritonitis, whereas localized pain is more indicative of a process involving an organ or its immediate environment. Diagnosis is often difficult, especially in elderly or immunocompromised patients, because the clinical presentation is less precise; or in those with altered conscience state or sedated for mechanical ventilation [14]. Acute abdominal complications are considered infrequent events in the ICU, although they are characterized by serious prognosis when they do appear. The absence of clinical signs and typical symptoms, with consequent delay in diagnosis and treatment, has assigned to IAIs the role of "silent offender" [15, 16]. Occult IAI can also manifest as renal dysfunction or elevated bilirubin and transaminases. Blood culture is often negative, and the absence of bacteremia in a surgery patient with fever increases the probability of IAI. Polymicrobial or anaerobic bacteremia also suggests the presence of an intraperitoneal infection. Differential diagnosis of unexpected difficulty in breathing or supraventricular arrhythmia occurring 3–4 days after abdominal surgery must include suture dehiscence or other intra-abdominal infectious pathology, and their diagnosis should be excluded through appropriate imaging techniques [17]. Biohumoral data are generally not very specific and do not permit diagnosis, but they can contribute to suspected clinical diagnosis of IAI [18]. In trauma or surgery patients who have undergone operations for secondary peritonitis of community origin, the evolution of an IAI following surgery can manifest with general worsening of the patient's clinical condition. This may be due to the appearance of intra- or extra-abdominal complications or to the development of organ (single or multiple) insufficiency as a consequence of early serious damage due to peritonitis [19].

16.5.2 Diagnostic Imaging Techniques

Radiographic imaging is the definitive diagnostic tool for patients with suspected IAI and can usually identify the problem prior to any planned intervention. White abdomen usually indicates the presence of gas in the peritoneum, an intestinal obstruction, or signs of intestinal ischemia. Studies with contrast medium using hydrosoluble agents can reveal a fold break. Contrast fluid in a drain or fistula can help delineate the anatomy of a complex infection and help verify the adequacy of abscess drainage. US, and especially CT, scans play a principal role in the diagnosis and therapeutic strategy. US has the advantage of being easily available, can be carried out on the patient in bed, and repeated as often as necessary because of its innocuous effect on the patient. It permits investigation of the entire abdominal–pelvic cavity, revealing even mild intraperitoneal effusion (<500 ml), detection of the distribution of the peritoneal cavity or part of it (localized effusion), thus assisting in hypothesizing about the nature of the effusion based on its possible homogeneous aspects, and finally help guide fine-needle percutaneous aspiration [20]. Abdominal CT is the reference standard for evaluating the abdomen in critically ill patients [21]. Most causes of secondary peritonitis can be diagnosed promptly with CT using intravenously administered iodinated contrast fluid and opacification of the digestive tube (using hydrosoluble contrast medium injected orally or rectally) Although CT is an invaluable diagnostic instrument, it usually involves moving a potentially unstable patient from one ward to another. Furthermore, iodinated contrast medium can worsen renal function. Renal insufficiency and paralytic ileum are both contraindications for CT, so the risks must be taken into account when deciding whether to carry out this diagnostic technique. One alternative in a very unstable patient is diagnostic peritoneal lavage, which consists of injecting 1 l of normal saline solution or lactated ringers through a catheter into the peritoneum and subsequently observe the characteristics of the fluid returning from the lavage. This can evidence the presence of bacteria, leukocytes, bile, enteral content, or blood in cases of acute intestinal ischemia [22]. Scintigraphy has a very limited role in IAI diagnosis in critically ill patients because it is not specific enough and cannot provide an accurate enough image to guide drainage [23, 24]. MRI has a very high diagnostic accuracy in evaluating acute intra-abdominal abscess [22].

16.6 Management

16.6.1 Standards of Care

Source control is defined as any and all physical measures necessary to eradicate a focus of infection as well as influence factors that maintain infection and thus promote microbial growth or impair host antimicrobial defenses [7, 25]. Primary peritonitis is essentially a disease that is managed with antibiotics and not surgery [26]. There is no reliable evidence that cefotaxime is the treatment of choice for spontaneous bacterial peritonitis, although many authors have suggested this. Furthermore, results indicate that 4 g/day cefotaxime may be as effective as 8 g/day in terms of reducing mortality rates and symptoms resolution, and that treatment for 10 days is no more effective than treatment for 5 days. Goals for managing secondary peritonitis are summarized in Table 16.2. Several studies have identified *E. coli* and *B. fragilis* as the main target organisms for antibiotic therapy [2, 27]. The current practice of early empirical antibiotic administration, targeted to these bacteria, is well established. However, issues concerning drug choice and timing, the need for surgical cultures, and the duration of postoperative administration are controversial. Despite several published options, antibiotic therapy for secondary peritonitis is simple. The emerging concepts suggest that less in terms of number of drugs and treatment duration is better [2]. Furthermore, recent studies suggest that monotherapy with a single broad-spectrum antibiotic that includes full activity against *E. coli* may be equal or superior to polytherapy with multiple drug combinations [27–30]. The surgical strategy depends on the source of the infection [31, 32], the degree of peritoneal contamination, the patient's clinical condition, and concomitant disease. Moreover, early goal-directed therapy provides significant benefits with respect to outcome in patients with severe sepsis and MOF [33]. Ideally, a severe IAI should be cured with a single surgical procedure; unfortunately, infection often persists or recurs. Traditionally, severe peritonitis has been treated by performing a midline laparotomy to identify and eliminate the source of infection. In certain instances, complete control of the infective focus is not feasible during the first operation [2]. Whereas eliminating the focus and reducing contamination are accepted as conditions of successful treatment, surgical procedures differ for treating residual infection. The following major approaches have been developed: (1) continuous peritoneal lavage; (2) planned relaparotomy; and (3) open treatment by laparostomy. Continuous peritoneal lavage takes the whole concept of lavage to an extreme, with the hypothesis being that continual IA irrigation will enhance removal of bacteria and their products and improve the time to resolution [34]. Various forms of peritoneal lavage are routinely used to manage patients with peritonitis. There is little evidence that supports this approach in either the clinical and scientific literature; moreover, it has been documented that lavage damages mesothelial cells, dilutes agents that are involved in peritoneal defense, and may spread previously contained infection.

Table 16.2 Principles for managing peritonitis and indications for staged abdominal repair

1. Supportive measures • Combat hypovolemia and shock and maintain adequate tissue oxygenation • Treat with antibiotics bacteria not eliminated by surgery • Support failing organ systems • Provide adequate nutrition
2. Operative treatment • Repair and/or control infection source • Evacuate bacterial inoculum, pus, and adjuvants • Treat abdominal compartment syndrome • Prevent or treat persistent and recurrent infection or verify both repair and purge
3. Staged abdominal repair • Critical patient condition due to hemodynamic instability, precluding definitive repair • Excessive peritoneal edema (abdominal compartment syndrome, pulmonary, cardiac, renal, or hepatic dysfunction, decreased visceral perfusion) preventing abdominal closure without tension • Intra-abdominal pressure >15 mmHg • Massive abdominal wall loss • Impossible to eliminate or to control the source of infection • Incomplete debridement of necrotic tissue • Uncertainty of viability of remaining bowel • Uncontrolled bleeding (the need for packing)

In cases of IAI, a single operation may not be sufficient to achieve source control, thus necessitating reexploration [5]. The planned relaparotomy approach involves reoperations at fixed intervals, irrespective of the patient's clinical condition, to prevent development of further septic fluid collections, so precluding their systemic effects. Adverse effects of planned relaparotomies are frequent and include damage to abdominal wall structures and IA viscera. Open management facilitates frequent reexploration and, by treating the entire peritoneal cavity as one large infected collection, continuous exposure for maximal drainage. Furthermore, it serves to reduce the high IA pressure caused by peritoneal edema associated with fluid resuscitation and inflammation, thus obviating the deleterious systemic consequences of abdominal compartment syndrome [35]. GIT fistulas and abdominal wall defects have plagued simple open management; these complications should be minimized by introducing temporary abdominal closure devices, such as artificial mesh-zipper techniques. Tertiary peritonitis develops late in the postoperative course, presents clinically as sepsis, and is associated with a sterile peritoneal cavity or particular microbiology. Further antimicrobial administration and surgical interventions may contribute to peritoneal superinfection with yeasts and other low-level pathogens [2]. The low virulence of these organisms, which represent a marker—not the cause—of tertiary peritonitis reflects the global immunodepression of the affected patients.

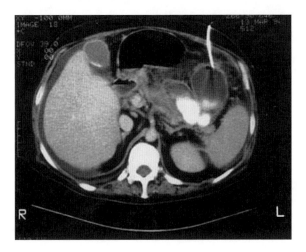

Fig. 16.1 Percutaneous drainage of a pancreatic pseudocyst

16.6.2 Managing Intra-Abdominal Abscess

Abscesses represent a relatively successful outcome of peritonitis. They may be visceral or nonvisceral; extra- or intraperitoneal. Nonvisceral abscesses arise after resolution of diffuse peritonitis in which a localized area of suppuration persists or after a GIT perforation that is effectively localized by peritoneal defenses. Percutaneous US- or CT-guided drainage is the method of choice for single abscess. Although retrospective studies attribute no lesser mortality or morbidity rates to percutaneous drainage versus surgical drainage [36], the former represents a minimally invasive procedure that can spare the patient the unpleasantness of another open abdominal operation (Fig. 16.1). Moreover, a recent study has shown that percutaneous catheter drainage should be considered as the initial therapy for patients with culture-positive peripancreatic fluid collections [37].

16.7 Acute Pancreatitis and Infection of Pancreatic Necrosis

Acute pancreatitis (AP) is an inflammatory process of variable severity (Table 16.3) ranging from a mild self-limiting form with interstitial edema of the pancreas to a severe form with extensive pancreatic and peripancreatic necrosis and hemorrhage [38]. Morbidity and mortality rates associated with AP are substantially higher when necrosis is present (mortality rate 25.8% in severe AP (SAP) and 1.5% in mild disease) [38], especially when the area of necrosis is also infected [39].

Table 16.3 Terminology in pancreatitis

Acute interstitial pancreatitis	A mild, self-limited form of pancreatitis, characterized by interstitial edema and an acute inflammatory response without necrosis, local complications, or systemic manifestations, such as organ failure
Necrotizing pancreatitis	A severe form of pancreatitis characterized by locoregional tissue necrosis and systemic manifestations, such as pulmonary, renal, or cardiac failure; a diffuse or focal area of nonviable pancreas, typically associated with peripancreatic fat necrosis
Sterile necrosis	Acute pancreatitis leading to tissue necrosis without supervening infection
Infected necrosis	Acute pancreatitis with locoregional tissue necrosis complicated by bacterial or fungal infection
Acute fluid collections	Occurring early in the course of acute pancreatitis, located in or near the pancreas, and lacking an epithelial lining or a defined wall of granulation or fibrous tissue
Pancreatic pseudocyst	Pancreatic or peripancreatic fluid collection with a well-defined wall of granulation tissue and fibrosis; absence of epithelial lining. One common complication of pseudocyst is the development of infection
Pancreatic abscess	Circumscribed collection of pus, usually in proximity to the pancreas, containing little or no pancreatic necrosis, arising as a consequence of narcotizing pancreatitis or pancreatic trauma

16.7.1 Pathophysiology

AP pathogenesis remains poorly understood. A number of factors can apparently initiate this process, including obstruction or overdistention of the pancreatic duct, exposure to ethanol and other toxins, hypertriglyceridemia, hypercalcemia, increased permeability of the pancreatic duct, and hyperstimulation of the gland. These diverse factors initiate inappropriate activation of zymogens. Ischemia of the organ appears to transform mild edematous AP into severe hemorrhagic/necrotizing forms [40, 41]. The AP mechanisms and resulting complications are reported in Fig. 16.2. The necrotic pancreas becomes secondarily infected 40–60% of the time, usually with Gram-negative bacteria translocated from the GIT [42, 43]. Enteric organisms predominate, and polymicrobial infection is common. Fungal infection is recognized with increased frequency, and the presence of *Candida* spp. is associated with increased mortality rates [44].

16.7.2 Presentation and Classification

SAP is diagnosed if three or more of Ranson's criteria are present, if the acute physiology and chronic health evaluation (APACHE) II score is ≥ 8, or if one or more of the following are present: shock, renal insufficiency, pulmonary insufficiency. Pancreatic glandular necrosis is usually associated with necrosis of

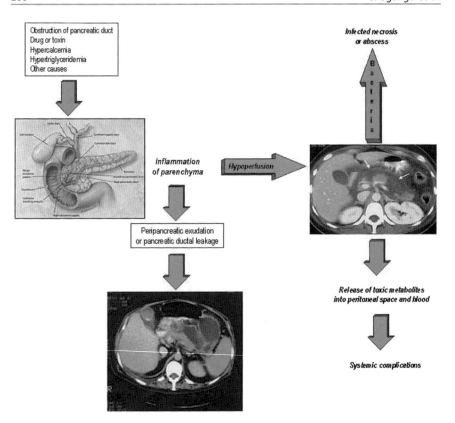

Fig. 16.2 Mechanisms of acute pancreatitis and resulting complications. Acute pancreatitis can be triggered by several events, resulting in inflammation of the parenchyma. Ischemia of the organ appears to transform mild edematous pancreatitis into severe necrotizing forms of the disease. Pseudocysts can form if pancreatic juices and debris leak into the peripancreatic spaces. Necrotic parenchyma becomes secondarily infected 40–60% of the time, usually with Gram-negative bacteria translocated from the GIT. Alternatively, the necrotic pancreas may release toxic factors into the peripancreatic spaces, peritoneal cavity, or systemic circulation, leading to local or systemic complications. Computed tomography scans shown a pancreatic pseudocyst, and lack of enhancement representing necrosis of the head, body, and tail of the pancreas (*arrows*)

peripancreatic fat and, by definition, represents SAP. The risk of infected necrosis increases with the amount of glandular necrosis and the time from AP onset, peaking at 3 weeks. Overall mortality rate in SAP is approximately 30%; as long as necrotizing AP remains sterile, the mortality rate is approximately 10%, and it at least triples if there is infected necrosis. In addition, patients with sterile necrosis and high severity-of-illness scores accompanied by MOF, shock, or renal insufficiency have significantly higher mortality rates. Deaths occur in either of two phases: early deaths (1–2 weeks after AP onset) are due to MOF caused by the release of inflammatory mediators and cytokines; late deaths result from systemic or local infection. Local infections, so-called secondary pancreatic infections, are represented by pancreatic abscess, infected pseudocyst, and infected necrosis. By definition, pancreatic abscess and infected pancreatic pseudocysts are associated with little or no necrosis; in contrast, patients with diffuse or focal areas of nonviable pancreatic parenchyma, often associated with peripancreatic fat necrosis, are categorized as having infected or non-infected pancreatic necrosis.

16.7.3 Recognition

Dynamic intravenous contrast-enhanced abdominal CT diagnoses pancreatic necrosis radiographically. Because the normal pancreatic microcirculation is disrupted during necrotizing AP, affected portions of the pancreas do not show normal contrast enhancement. The lack of normal contrast enhancement may be better detected several days after initial clinical presentation. Contrast-enhanced CT is the gold standard for the noninvasive diagnosis of pancreatic necrosis, with an accuracy of >90% when there is >30% glandular necrosis [45]. Sterile and infected necrosis can be difficult to distinguish clinically, as both may produce fever, leukocytosis, and severe abdominal pain. Distinction is important, because mortality rates among patients with infected necrosis without intervention is nearly 100%. The bacteriologic status of the pancreas may be determined by CT-guided fine-needle aspiration of pancreatic and peripancreatic tissue or fluid [46]. This aspiration method is safe and accurate (sensitivity 96%, specificity 99%) and is recommended for patients with necrotizing AP whose clinical condition deteriorates or fails to improve despite aggressive supportive care. US-guided aspiration may have a lower sensitivity and specificity, but it can be performed at the bedside [47]. Surveillance aspiration may be repeated weekly, as clinically indicated.

16.7.4 Nonsurgical Management of Pancreatic Necrosis

Early studies of antibiotics in patients with AP failed to demonstrate a significant benefit because the studies included both patients with interstitial edematous AP and with pancreatic necrosis. As the development of infected necrosis substantially increases mortality rates among patients with necrotizing AP, preventing infection is critical. Because pancreatic infection occurs primarily as a result of bacterial spread from the colon, studies have shown benefits from both systemic antibiotics and selective gut decontamination [48–54]. Therapy should begin as soon as the diagnosis of necrotizing AP is made and should continue for at least 2–4 weeks. In this respect, intravenous administration of cefuroxime is a reasonable balance between efficacy and cost. Furthermore, imipenem has been recommended on the basis of studies of antibiotic penetration into pancreatic tissue. To meet increased metabolic demands and to "rest" the pancreas, total parenteral nutrition (TPN) is frequently used in patients with pancreatic necrosis [55, 56]. This does not hasten AP resolution, however. In two recent randomized studies, patients with SAP received either TPN or enteral nutrition (EN) within 48 h of illness onset; EN was

Table 16.4 Possible indications for endoscopic retrograde cholangiopancreatography and associated procedures in managing pancreatitis

Acute phase	ERC: diagnosis of biliary pancreatitis in severe cases with an uncertain etiology ES: treatment of severe cases of gallstones, biliary sludge, and other related pathologies, such as ampullary carcinoma
Persisting pancreatitis	ES: for bile duct stones in unresolving mild pancreatitis ERP: disruption of main pancreatic duct or planning surgical intervention
Complications	ERP: assessment of pseudocysts, ascites, and fistulas prior to surgery Stent or NBC: pseudocysts, fistulas, and liquid necrosis in selected cases ERC: endoscopic pseudocystogastrostomy, or endoscopic pseudocystoduodenostomy in selected cases
Convalescent phase	ERCP: establishment of diagnosis in idiopathic cases ERC with bile duct cannulation: CCK-stimulated bile collection for crystal analysis ES: alternative to cholecystectomy in high risk cases
Recurrent pancreatitis	ES: sphincter of Oddi dysfunction or stenosis Stent: trial therapy for pancreas divisum

ERC endoscopic cholangiography; *ERP* endoscopic retrograde pancreatography; *ES* endoscopic sphincterotomy; *NBC* nasobiliary catheter

well tolerated, had no adverse clinical effects, and resulted in significantly fewer total and infectious complications [57, 58]. Acute phase-response scores and disease-severity scores were significantly improved after EN. Studies of endoscopic retrograde cholangiopancreatography (ERCP) and biliary sphincterotomy performed within 72 h of admission in patients with gallstone AP and choledocholithiasis showed an improved outcome in the group of patients who presented with clinically SAP. Improvement was attributed to the relief of pancreatic ductal obstruction and from reduced biliary sepsis. In the presence of pancreatic ductal disruption, a frequent occurrence in pancreatic necrosis, the introduction of infection—transforming sterile to infected pancreatic necrosis—by incidental pancreatography during ERCP may theoretically occur. Therefore, ERCP should be reserved for patients in whom biliary obstruction is suspected (Table 16.4).

16.7.5 Interventions for Pancreatic Necrosis and Secondary Pancreatic Infections

Timing and type of intervention for patients with pancreatic necrosis are controversial. As the mortality rate from sterile necrosis is approximately 10% and surgical intervention has not been shown to lower this figure, most investigators recommend supportive medical therapy [45]. Conversely, infected necrosis is considered uniformly fatal without intervention. Aggressive surgical pancreatic debridement, so-called necrosectomy, remains the standard of care if drainage is

Table 16.5 Results of surgical treatment for secondary pancreatic infections

	Conventional drainage (%)	Open or semiopen procedures (%)	Lesser sac lavage (%)
Small-bowel complications	5	14	4
Large-bowel complications	8	13	2
Bleeding	14	16	8
Pancreatic fistulas	16	17	17
Persistent or recurrent sepsis	44–77	8	16–40
Reoperation	30–55	–	30
Mortality rate	40–76	16–20	25–32

undertaken and may require multiple abdominal explorations. Necrosectomy should be undertaken soon after confirmation of infected necrosis [38]. The benefit of surgery in patients with MOF and sterile necrosis remains unproved, although this scenario is frequently cited as an indication for surgical debridement. In addition, the longer surgical intervention can be delayed after necrosis onset, the better survival is, probably because of improved demarcation between viable and necrotic tissue at the time of operation. The role of delayed, necrosectomy, after MOF resolution, in patients with sterile necrosis also remains controversial.

16.7.6 Surgical Procedures After Debridement

There are three main types of surgical drainage after pancreatic debridement: conventional drainage, open or semiopen procedures, and closed procedures with lesser sac lavage [59–71]. Conventional drainage involves necrosectomy with placement of Penrose/sump drainage. Open or semiopen management involves necrosectomy and either scheduled repeated laparotomies or open packing, which leaves the abdominal wound exposed for frequent dressing changes. Closed management involves necrosectomy with extensive intraoperative lavage of the pancreatic bed; furthermore, the abdomen is closed over large-bore drains for continuous high-volume postoperative lavage of the lesser sac. Results of these procedures are reported in Table 16.5. The principal reason for failure of the conventional surgical approach is the development of recurrent postoperative infection and sepsis. In an extensive review [72] of >1,100 cases of severe pancreatic infections, 76% of postoperative deaths were found to be attributable to persistent or recurrent infection after surgical drainage. A closer examination of the reasons behind the demonstrated failure of Penrose/sump drainage to provide adequate control of postoperative infection unearths the fact that unscheduled re-explorations for recurrent sepsis are necessary in one-third to one half of cases drained in this fashion [73, 74]. Leaving the abdomen open eliminates the need for repeated laparotomy; packing may be changed in ICU. Repeated debridement and manipulation of the abdominal viscera with the open and semiopen techniques results in a high rate of postoperative local complications (pancreatic fistulas, small- and large-bowel complications, bleeding from pancreatic bed). Pancreatic or GIT fistulas occur in up to 40% of patients after surgical necrosectomy and often require additional surgery for closure. The mortality rate from debridement with the open or semiopen technique is approximately 15%. In patients who underwent lesser sac lavage, 16–40% required reoperation for persistent peripancreatic sepsis, and mortality rates varied from 5 to 50%, averaging 30% [72, 75].

16.7.7 Alternative Debridement Methods

Alternative methods for debriding pancreatic necrotic material have recently been described [76–78] but require considerable technical expertise, and the precise role of these techniques in managing pancreatic necrosis will be better defined. One study described the successful treatment of infected necrosis by aggressive irrigation and drainage through large-bore percutaneous catheters in 34 patients. Pancreatic surgery was completely avoided in 47% of patients; in nine patients, sepsis was controlled, and elective surgery was later performed to repair external pancreatic fistulas related to catheter placement. Nine patients required immediate surgery when percutaneous therapy failed, and four (12%) died [78]. Recently, endoscopic drainage of sterile or infected pancreatic necrotic material has been reported [79]. Complete necrosis resolution without the need for surgery was achieved in 25 of 31 patients (81%). Surgical intervention was required more commonly for acute complications of endoscopy than for drainage failure. Laparoscopic approach to SAP treatment has been recently reported [77]. Advantages are the possibility of exploring, irrigating, decompressing, and draining the pancreas, and performing postoperative lavage via the drainage tubes. Pathological disease extent can be determined and appropriate treatment approaches thus planned by laparoscopic exploration. The laparoscopic technique creates less trauma in the early treatment of SAP but, at least theoretically, patients with early severe multiorgan disease without retroperitoneal infection may become victims of a later infection introduced surgically [80, 81].

16.8 Mediastinal Infections

Infection of the mediastinal space is a life-threatening condition with extremely high mortality rates if recognized late or treated improperly. Etiologic factors responsible for the development of mediastinitis include esophageal perforation resulting from instrumentation, foreign bodies, penetrating or blunt trauma, spontaneous disruption, leakage from an esophageal anastomosis, tracheobronchial perforation, and mediastinal extension from an infectious process originating in the pulmonary parenchyma, pleura, chest wall, vertebrae, or great vessels [82–84]. Furthermore, infection may extend from the head and neck downward into the mediastinum: this is described as descending necrotizing mediastinitis because the infection uses the fascial planes in the neck to gain access to the mediastinum [85–87]. It is narcotizing, as the infection is often polymicrobial in etiology and includes gas-producing organisms. The potential spaces that can allow infections from the head or neck to enter the mediastinum include the carotid and prevertebral spaces. Mediastinitis occurs most often after median sternotomy for cardiovascular surgery [88–90]. Risk factors for its development include the use of bilateral internal mammary artery grafts, diabetes mellitus, emergency surgery, external cardiac compression, obesity, postoperative shock (especially when multiple blood transfusions are required) prolonged bypass and operating-room time, reexploration following initial surgery, sternal wound dehiscence, and surgical–technical factors (such as excessive use of electrocautery, bone wax, or paramedian sternotomy). These infections are relatively rare in the era of antibiotic use. In developing countries, mediastinitis still is a common devastating potential complication of head and neck infections. The mortality rate varies from 19–47%, and in the presence of comorbid conditions for patients presenting with established infections, it may be as high as 67% [89].

16.8.1 Microbiology of Mediastinitis

This is often a mixed infection, with facultative and strict anaerobes acting together. *Streptococcus* spp. are the most common facultative organisms (70% of cases), whereas *Bacteroides* spp. are the most common strict anaerobes [91]. Other organisms implicated include *Pseudomonas aeruginosa* and *Fusobacterium*, *Peptostreptococcus*, and *Staphylococcus* spp. Mixed Gram-positive and Gram-negative infections account for about 40% of cases. Isolated Gram-negative infections rarely occur. Mediastinitis not associated with cardiac surgery is usually due to anaerobic organisms. Mixed Gram-negative and Gram-positive infections as well as *Candida* spp. are more common after esophageal perforation or head and neck surgery [82, 92].

16.8.2 Diagnosis

Mediastinitis is manifested clinically by fever, tachycardia, leukocytosis, and pain that may be localized to the chest, back, or neck. Mediastinitis presents within a spectrum that ranges from the subacute patient through the fulminate critically ill who requires immediate intervention in order to prevent death [89]. The typical postoperative patient will present with fever, high pulse rate, and complaints suggestive of a sternal WI. Approximately two-thirds of patients present these symptoms within 14 days following surgery [90]. When mediastinitis is due to esophageal perforation from either trauma or instrumentation, the patient usually presents with neck pain and subcutaneous emphysema because the most common perforation site is at the level of the cricopharyngeal muscle [92]. The diagnosis of mediastinitis is often a clinical one. No single laboratory investigation can confirm the diagnosis. Complete blood count shows leukocytosis, often with a left shift on white blood cell (WBC) differential. Hematocrit decreases if bleeding has occurred. Platelet count increases in early stages of sepsis or decreases as sepsis worsens, or disseminated intravascular coagulation occurs. Bacteremia is found in almost 60% of patients with postoperative mediastinitis. Mediastinal pacing wires should be sent for culture if they are still present and no longer needed. It has been found that pacing-wire culture had a sensitivity of 75%, a specificity of 83%, a positive predictive value (PPV) of 12%, and a negative predictive value (NPV) of 99% [89, 90]. This suggests that sterile cultures argue against a diagnosis of postoperative mediastinitis. Delays in the diagnosis of mediastinitis greatly increase morbidity and mortality rates. The condition is typically recognized through high clinical suspicion in susceptible populations, but radiology studies are often helpful in diagnosis. CT scans are more accurate in identifying air–fluid levels and pneumomediastinum [85]; furthermore, it may demonstrate sternal separation and substernal fluid collections in postoperative mediastinitis. The later the scans are done following surgery, the more accurate the results. If performed after the second postoperative week, CT scans have a sensitivity and specificity of almost 100%. Aspiration of substernal fluid collections under CT guidance may prove helpful in establishing a diagnosis as well as giving practical information from Gram stain and culture [93]. MRI is poorly suited as a diagnostic modality in mediastinitis. Postoperative patients may have sternal wires, vascular clips, metallic valves, and pacing wires that contraindicate MRI. It is also logistically difficult to perform an MRI in an intubated, critically ill patient. Furthermore, esophageal dye studies are the most useful in cases of suspected esophageal perforation.

16.8.3 Treatment

Treating mediastinitis requires correcting the inciting cause and aggressive supportive therapies. Mediastinitis may result in airway compromise, and protecting the airway is often vital. Appropriate, well-directed antibiotic therapy is crucial to successful treatment. In postoperative mediastinitis, because up to 20% of organisms cultured from infected sternotomy sites will be methicillin-resistant *S. aureus* (MRSA), and because another 20% will be Gram-negative organisms, antibiotic coverage must be very broad and deep to include *Pseudomonas* spp. While awaiting results of stains and cultures, a regime of vancomycin, ceftazidime, and a quinolone should provide adequate coverage. If septic shock is present, some would substitute an aminoglycoside for the quinolone, although close watch of drug levels is required to prevent renal damage. Therapy duration is usually prolonged, ranging from weeks to months. Recently, it has suggested that

4–6 weeks of therapy is adequate for most patients. EN should be introduced immediately with a duodenal feeding tube. Recent data suggest that the use of diets formulated with various anti-inflammatory compounds to include omega-3 long-chain fatty acids and arginine provide clinically important benefits for critically ill patients with sepsis [94]. Mediastinitis due to esophageal perforation should be initially treated with broad-spectrum antibiotics that have good anaerobic coverage. Piperacillin–tazobactam and vancomycin provide good empirical coverage while awaiting culture results. Patients with true anaphylaxis to penicillin can be treated with quinolone and clindamycin in place of the piperacillin–tazobactam. The role of antifungal therapy is controversial, although amphotericin B has been used. In patients with mediastinal infections in continuity with empyema, subphrenic abscess or neck abscess, drainage with tube thoracostomy, or percutaneous drainage is frequently successful. In patients who do not respond to the initial measures or in whom mediastinitis occurs from most other causes, thorough debridement of necrotic and infected tissue is necessary in conjunction with surgical drainage [89]. Controversy exists about whether the cervical or transthoracic approach is best. In some case series, the combination of the two has been associated with a lower mortality rate. Surgical treatment is required in severe infections. A simple sternal dehiscence without infection can be effectively treated by rewiring the sternum; this usually yields excellent long-term results. More advanced mediastinitis can be treated with extensive debridement followed by irrigation. Many surgeons prefer to leave the wound open for subsequent debridement efforts. In this case, the wound is packed, and closure via a plastics procedure is delayed until wound cultures have been consistently negative. Ventilator weaning and risk of bleeding from the exposed heart and vessels are disadvantages of the open approach that change thoracic mechanics. However, the most common cause of recurrent mediastinitis is inadequate wound-site debridement and sterilization during the first procedure. Advanced postoperative mediastinitis is best treated with extensive debridement, followed by delayed closure using either muscle or omental flap plastics procedures [95]. Oesophageal perforation was usually fatal; the standard approach has been to operate immediately. In recent years, several case series have addressed medical treatment of esophageal perforation. Shaffer et al. [92] recommend considering nonoperative treatment in absence of crepitus, pneumothorax, pneumoperitoneum, or intraperitoneal extravasation, in esophageal disruptions that are well contained within the mediastinum or a pleural loculus; in instrumental perforations in which the patient was nil per os for the procedure and the perforation was detected early; in patients who are clinically stable; and for perforations with a long delay before diagnosis, such that the patient develops tolerance for the perforation without the need for surgery [92]. Surgery is recommended for Boerhaave syndrome, large perforations with widespread mediastinal contamination, perforations associated with preexisting conditions such as achalasia and cancer, perforation of the IA portion of the esophagus, perforations with pneumothorax, perforations with retained foreign bodies, and unstable patients with shock or other signs of systemic sepsis.

16.9 Pleural Effusion and Empyema

Pleural effusion (PE) is defined as an abnormal accumulation of fluid in the pleural space: approximately 300 ml of fluid is required for the development of costophrenic angle blunting seen on upright chest X-ray; at least 500 ml of effusion is necessary for detection on clinical examination. It is an indicator of a pathologic process that may be of primary pulmonary origin or an origin related to another organ system or to systemic disease. It may occur in the setting of acute or chronic disease (Table 16.6) and is not a diagnosis in and of itself [96–99]. PEs is classified as either transudate or exudate based on fluid protein and lactate dehydrogenase (LDH) concentrations. Normal pleural fluid has the following characteristics: pH 7.60–7.64, protein content <2% (1–2 g/dl), fewer than 1,000 WBCs per cubic millimeter, glucose content similar to that of plasma, and LDH level <50% of plasma. Pleural fluid is exudative if one or more of the following conditions is met and transudative if none are met: ratio of pleural fluid and serum protein levels >0.5, ratio of pleural fluid and serum LDH levels >0.6, and pleural fluid LDH level more than two-thirds of the upper limit for serum LDH levels. Empyema is a pyogenic or suppurative infection of the pleural space. It is exudative in nature, and represents the most common exudative type of PEs [100, 101]. Empyema may be classified into three categories based on the chronicity of the disease process. The acute phase is characterized by PE of low viscosity and cell count. The transitional or fibrinopurulent phase, which can begin after 48 h, is characterized by an increase in WBCs in PE: this begins to loculate and is associated with fibrin deposition on visceral and parietal pleura and progressive lung entrapment. The chronic phase occurs after as little as 1–2 weeks and is associated with an ingrowth of capillaries and fibroblasts into the pleural rind and inexpansible lung. Empyema may occur by direct contamination of the pleural space through wounds of the chest, by hematologic spread, by direct extension from lung parenchymal infections, by rupture of an intrapulmonary abscess or infected cavity, or by extension from the mediastinum. Most often, empyemas are the results of a primary infectious process in the lung.

16.9.1 Frequency and Mortality/Morbidity

In industrialized countries, relative annual incidence of PE is estimated to be 320 per 100,000 people. Approximate PE annual incidences are based on major underlying disease processes, such as congestive heart failure, bacterial pneumonia, malignancy, pulmonary embolus, cirrhosis with ascites, pancreatitis, collagen vascular disease, and tuberculosis. PE morbidity and mortality rates are directly related to cause, disease stage at the time of presentation, and biochemical findings in the pleural fluid. Morbidity and mortality rates of patients with pneumonia and PE are higher than those of patients with pneumonia alone.

Table 16.6 Etiology of pleural effusion (PE)

PE characteristic	Diseases
Transudative	Congestive heart failure (most common transudative PE); hepatic cirrhosis with and without ascites; nephrotic syndrome; peritoneal dialysis/continuous ambulatory peritoneal dialysis; hypoalbuminemia (e.g., severe starvation); glomerulonephritis; superior vena cava obstruction; urinothorax
Exudative	Malignant disorders (metastatic disease to the pleura or lungs, primary lung cancer, mesothelioma, Kaposi sarcoma, lymphoma, leukemia); infectious diseases (bacterial, fungal, parasitic, and viral infections; infection with atypical organisms such as *Mycoplasma, Rickettsiae, Chlamydia, Legionella*); GIT diseases (pancreatic disease, Whipple disease, IA abscess, esophageal perforation, abdominal surgery, diaphragmatic hernia, endoscopic variceal sclerotherapy); collagen vascular diseases (rheumatoid arthritis, systemic lupus erythematosus, drug-induced lupus syndrome, immunoblastic lymphadenopathy, Sjögren syndrome, familial Mediterranean fever, Churg–Strauss syndrome, Wegener granulomatosis); benign asbestos effusion; Meigs syndrome (benign solid ovarian neoplasm associated with ascites and pleural effusion); drug-induced primary pleural disease (nitrofurantoin, dantrolene, methysergide, bromocriptine, amiodarone, procarbazine, methotrexate, ergonovine, ergotamine, oxprenolol, maleate, practolol, minoxidil, bleomycin, interleukin-2, propylthiouracil, isotretinoin, metronidazole, mitomycin); injury after cardiac surgery (Dressler syndrome); uremic pleuritis; yellow nail syndrome; ruptured ectopic pregnancy; electrical burns
Exudative/ transudative	Pulmonary embolism; hypothyroidism; pericardial disease (inflammatory or constrictive); atelectasis; trapped lung (usually a borderline exudate); sarcoidosis (usually an exudate); amyloidosis
Miscellaneous	Hemothorax; following coronary artery bypass graft surgery; after lung or liver transplant; Milk of calcium pleural effusion; ARDS; systemic cholesterol emboli; iatrogenic misplacement of lines or tubes into the mediastinum or the pleural space; radiation pleuritis; necrotizing sarcoid granulomatosis; ovarian hyperstimulation syndrome; postpartum pleural effusion (immediate or delayed); rupture of a silicone bag mammary prosthesis; rupture of a benign germ cell tumor into the pleural space (e.g., benign mediastinal teratoma); syphilis; echinococcosis

GIT gastrointestinal tract; *IA* intra-abdominal; *ARDS* acute respiratory distress syndrome

16.9.2 Symptoms and Physical Findings

Clinical manifestations of PE are variable and often related to the underlying disease process. The most commonly associated symptoms are progressive dyspnea, cough (typically nonproductive), and pleuritic chest pain. Dyspnea is the most common clinical symptom at presentation and usually indicates a large effusion [96, 98]. Chest pain may be mild or severe; it is typically described as sharp or stabbing, is exacerbated with deep inspiration, and is pleuritic. Pain may be localized to the chest wall or referred to the ipsilateral shoulder or upper abdomen, usually because of diaphragmatic involvement. Other signs and symptoms occurring with PEs are associated more closely with the underlying disease process. An acute febrile episode, purulent sputum production, and pleuritic chest pain may occur in patients with PE associated with aerobic bacterial pneumonia [99]. Physical findings are variable and depend on the PE volume. Generally, findings are undetectable for effusions <300 ml. Four main types of fluids in the pleural space are serous fluid (hydrothorax), blood (hemothorax), lipid (chylothorax), and pus (pyothorax or empyema). PE develops in 30–40% of patients with bacterial pneumonia. Those with bacterial pneumonia, especially that caused by *S. pneumoniae*, have a high predilection for complications: these can include bacteremia and multilobar involvement. Moreover, Gram-negative and anaerobic organisms are common cause of empyema [100].

16.9.3 Diagnosis

The initial step in analyzing pleural fluid is to determine whether PE is a transudate or an exudate. Clinical presentation should direct the biochemical and microbiological studies of pleural fluid. The minimal amount of pleural fluid needed for basic diagnostic purposes is 20 ml; if possible, 60 ml should be obtained for potential diagnostic studies. If the clinical presentation is highly suggestive of transudative PE, protein and LDH levels should be determined initially. If the patient has undergone diuretic therapy, the pleural albumin level should be determined simultaneously. Concomitant serum total protein, LDH, and, if indicated, serum albumin levels should be measured. If transudative effusion is diagnosed, no further tests are needed. Exudative PE requires further laboratory investigation. Cytological analysis is strongly recommended for patients with a history of undiagnosed exudative PE, suspected malignancy or *Pneumocystis carinii* infection, or exudative PE with normal fluid glucose and amylase levels [100, 101]. Additional studies should be requested on the basis of the gross appearance of the pleural fluid or when a specific condition is suspected. Gross appearance and results of certain laboratory studies may provide useful diagnostic information (Table 16.7). Laboratory results can aid in narrowing the differential diagnosis of exudative PE (Table 16.8).

16.9.4 Imaging Studies

This step is the most important in the PE evaluation. Common imaging studies used to confirm PE are chest radiography, US, and CT scan [96–101]. Chest radiography is the primary diagnostic tool because of its availability, accuracy, and low cost. It can be used to determine the cause of PE (enlarged cardiac silhouette, underlying lung, parenchymal disease). The most common radiologic appearance is blunting of the costophrenic angle and/or sulci. Upright posteroanterior or anteroposterior radiographs may not show lateral costophrenic angle

Table 16.7 Clinical significance of pleural fluid characteristics

Characteristic	Significance
Bloody	Most likely an indication of malignancy in the absence of trauma; can also indicate pulmonary embolism, infection, pancreatitis, tuberculosis, mesothelioma, or spontaneous pneumothorax
Turbid	Possible increased cellular or lipid content
Yellow or whitish, turbid	Presence of chyle, cholesterol, or empyema
Brown	Rupture of amoebic liver abscess into the pleural space (amebiasis with a hepatopleural fistula)
Black	*Aspergillus* involvement of pleura
Yellow green with debris	Rheumatoid pleurisy
Highly viscous	Malignant mesothelioma (due to increased levels of hyaluronic acid), long-standing pyothorax
Putrid odor	Anaerobic infection of pleural space
Ammonia odor	Urinothorax
Purulent	Empyema
Yellow and thick, with metallic sheen	Effusions rich in cholesterol (longstanding chyliform effusion, e.g., tuberculous or rheumatoid pleuritis)

blunting until 250–500 ml of fluid is present. Lateral radiographs show blunting of the posterior costophrenic angle and the posterior gutter when as little as 175–200 ml of fluid is present. Bilateral decubitus radiographs are recommended, especially with larger effusions. PE location can help in differential diagnosis. Atypical chest radiographic presentations are possible. When an air–fluid level is present in the pleural space, the following must be considered: bronchopleural fistula, pneumothorax, trauma, presence of gas-forming organisms, diaphragmatic hernia, fluid-filled bullae or lung cysts and rupture of the esophagus into the pleural space. Diaphragmatic hernias can be excluded or confirmed with GIT contrast material administration. US can be used to detect as little as 5–50 ml of pleural fluid, with 100% sensitivity for effusions ≥ 100 ml [100]. US helps identify loculated PE and differentiation of pleural fluid from pleural fibrosis, thickening, and parenchymal consolidation. It can help localize the diaphragm if pleural or parenchymal disease obscures it. Unlike CT, US is rapid and available at the bedside. Chest CT scanning permits simultaneous imaging of the entire pleural space, pulmonary parenchyma, and mediastinum. CT scans reveal early-stage pleural abnormalities. Contrast-enhanced scans can depict multiple loculations and localizing PEs; differentiate between lung consolidation versus PE and cystic versus solid lesions; necrotic areas; pleural thickening, nodules, masses, or rounded atelectasis; and peripheral lung abscess versus loculated empyema; and tumoral extent [99, 100].

Table 16.8 Clinical significance of biochemical and cytological pleural fluid characteristics

Characteristic	Significance
Amylase	Can be elevated in acute pancreatitis, pancreatic pseudocyst, esophageal rupture, malignancy, and ruptured ectopic pregnancy. Pancreatic pseudocyst has the highest amylase levels (frequently >100,000 UI). Determination of the amylase isoenzyme level is useful in distinguishing PE caused by pancreatic disease from effusions caused by esophageal rupture or nonpancreatic disease
Glucose	A low PE glucose level is <60 mg/dl. Differential diagnosis includes malignancy, rheumatoid pleurisy, complicated parapneumonic PE, empyema, hemothorax, Churg–Strauss syndrome, and occasionally lupus pleuritis
pH	If <7.20, suggests empyema, complicated parapneumonic PE, esophageal rupture, rheumatoid pleuritis, malignancy, hemothorax, tuberculous pleuritis, lupus pleuritis, or urinothorax. Arterial pH influences pleural fluid pH; therefore, acidemia must be ruled out before any of the above causes are considered. With parapneumonic PE, indications for tube thoracostomy include a pH <7.0, glucose level <40 mg/dl, and positive finding with Gram stains or cultures. To use the pH criteria for chest tube placement in systemic acidosis, the PE pH should be at least 0.3 U less than the arterial pH. A low pleural fluid pH almost always is associated with a high pCO_2
LDH	Indicator of the degree of pleural inflammation. The higher the value, the more inflamed the pleural surface. High concentrations (>1,000 IU/l) occur with complicated parapneumonic PE
RBC and total WBC count	RBC counts >100,000 mm^3 suggest trauma, malignancy, pulmonary embolism, injury after cardiac surgery, asbestos pleurisy, esophageal rupture, pancreatitis, tuberculous pleurisy, and thoracic endometriosis. The total PE leukocyte count is virtually never diagnostic. Neutrophilic predominance indicates an acute inflammatory process near the time of thoracentesis. Significant eosinophilia occurs when the ratio of pleural fluid and total pleural fluid counts is >10%; the most common cause is air or blood in the pleural space. The differential diagnosis of pleural fluid eosinophilia includes pneumothorax, hemothorax, pulmonary infarction, prior thoracentesis, benign asbestos effusion, drug use, parasitic diseases, fungal infections, and Churg–Strauss syndrome; in the absence of these, eosinophilia with pneumonia and pleural effusion is a good prognostic sign, because such effusions rarely become infected. Significant basophilia (counts >10%) is distinctly uncommon; however, if present, it suggests leukemic pleural infiltration
Lymphocyte count	Lymphocytes indicate a long-standing chronic effusion. Pleural fluid lymphocytosis (>50%) suggests malignant disease, particularly lymphoma; however, other conditions (e.g., chronic rheumatoid pleurisy, chronic fungal infection, yellow nail syndrome, chylothorax, trapped lung, benign asbestos PE, sarcoidosis) must be considered. The presence of an undiagnosed exudative effusion with lymphocytosis is an indication for closed pleural biopsy

(continued)

Table 16.8 (continued)

Characteristic	Significance
Mesothelial cell count	These cells line the pleural cavities, and their absence simply indicates diffuse pleural injury or fibrosis. These cells predominate in transudative PE
Plasma cell and macrophage counts	A large number of plasma cells in the pleural fluid suggest multiple myeloma with pleural involvement. A small number of plasma cells are of no particular diagnostic value. The presence of macrophages has no diagnostic value.

PE plural effusion; *LDH* lactose dehydrogenase; *RBC* red blood cells; *WBC* white blood cells

16.9.5 Invasive Diagnostic Procedures

After the presence of PE is established, the cause should be identified. This step can be critical because unnecessary invasive procedures cause morbidity and mortality. When a decision is made to investigate the cause, thoracentesis is the first-line invasive diagnostic procedure [100]. Thoracentesis also can be used as a therapeutic modality. It is the least invasive procedure and it is relatively safe. For stable and asymptomatic patients in whom PE most likely is caused by viral pleurisy, manifestation of a systemic disease, thoracic or abdominal surgery, or childbearing, thoracentesis may not be indicated, or it can be deferred. In this situation, therapy for the specific cause should be initiated, and if no improvement occurs after a few days, diagnostic thoracentesis should be performed. Thoracentesis is also indicated in cases in which the specific cause of PE is unknown or has never been investigated or when the thickness of the free pleural fluid level is >10 mm on the lateral decubitus radiograph. In addition, thoracentesis is indicated if the patient has respiratory compromise, hemodynamic instability, or massive effusion with contralateral mediastinal shift. After thoracentesis, and regardless of its success, chest radiography is recommended to rule out a subsequent pneumothorax. Pneumothorax is the most common complication (incidence 3–20% with unguided thoracentesis, 2–7% with US guidance) and is operator dependent. Other complications include subcutaneous hematoma, infection of the pleural space or soft tissue overlying the thoracentesis site, pain at the site, cough, chest pain, hemothorax, vasovagal reflex, reexpansion pulmonary edema, hypovolemia, hypoxemia, splenic or hepatic laceration, hemoperitoneum, and adverse reactions to local anaesthetics. Definite indications to tube thoracostomy include empyema, hemothorax, large pneumothorax, and parapneumonic PE.

16.9.6 Treatment

Most commonly, PE is an incidental finding in a stable patient. Patients with a toxic condition, respiratory distress, or cardiovascular instability require emergency medical services more frequently. As with any other life-threatening condition, direct initial management is airway stabilization to ensure adequate oxygenation and ventilation [98]. On the basis of presentation, patients with PE may be stable, requiring hospital admission; stable, not requiring hospital admission; or unstable. Stable patients who do not require admission include those in whom the clinical circumstances clearly explain PE and/or prior investigations of the cause were performed, in whom PEs are typical of the disease or are asymptomatic, and in whom diagnostic or therapeutic thoracentesis is not required. Stable patients requiring admission include most patients with PE thicker than 10 mm on the lateral decubitus radiograph. Such patients include those with no prior history of PE, those with parapneumonic PE who do not appear to have a toxic condition, and those with a prior history of PE who have a change in their usual symptoms or effusion. Although these patients are not in acute respiratory distress, diagnostic thoracentesis is imperative. For parapneumonic PE, delay in diagnostic thoracentesis and antibiotic therapy can be detrimental. Simple parapneumonic PE have a great potential to become complicated or empyemas. Antimicrobial therapy alone is not sufficient for complicated parapneumonic PE or empyemas; they require tube thoracostomy and antibiotics [98]. Unstable patients include those with a toxic appearance, respiratory distress, or cardiovascular compromise due to PE. The initial treatment focus should be to stabilize the airway and circulation. Infected pleural fluid with bronchopleural fistula is considered a medical emergency. Bronchopleural fistula should be suspected when a patient with PE produces a larger amount of sputum than that expected from associated pulmonary disease. The presence of an air–fluid level in the pleural space on upright radiographs suggests bronchopleural fistula. These patients require immediate diagnostic thoracentesis and antibiotics [98, 99]. In any patient with chest-penetrating or nonpenetrating trauma, hemothorax should be suspected. Traumatic hemothorax is an indication for the insertion of a large-bore chest tube. Antibiotics and diuretics are commonly used in the initial management of PE. An empiric systemic antibiotic coverage should be initiated in infections or potentially septic conditions (parapneumonic PE, empyemas, esophageal perforation, hemothorax, IA abscesses). Generally, broad-spectrum antibiotics should be used initially for both aerobic and anaerobic microorganisms. Most commonly, two antimicrobial agents are necessary to ensure adequate coverage [97–99]. Various effective combinations exist: one is a third-generation cephalosporin (cefotaxime or ceftriaxone) and clindamycin. If the patient is a nursing home resident, cephalosporin with enhanced antipseudomonas activity is recommended. In children, monotherapy usually is sufficient.

16.10 Wounds Infections

Wound infection (WI) is the most important complication of surgical procedures and continues to be a disconcerting source of mortality in surgical patients [10, 102–104]. Postoperative infections, also, prolong hospitalization and are important causes of postoperative morbidity. Despite antisepsis, surgical site infections (SSI) are the third most frequently reported nosocomial infection, accounting for 14–16%

Table 16.9 Classification of operative wounds

Clean wounds	Infection risk of about 1–5%. Prophylactic antibiotics are not indicated in a clean operation if the patient has no host-risk factors. Factors suggesting the need for prophylaxis are remote infection, diabetes, at least three concomitant medical diagnoses. Additive risk factors are abdominal operations and operations expected to last >2 h. Prostheses implants are clean procedures, some of which requires antibiotic prophylaxis. Inguinal hernia repair with biomaterials does not benefit from antibiotic prophylaxis
Clean-contaminated wounds	≤10% risk of infection. Clean-contaminated surgery usually requires prophylaxis
Contaminated wounds	A 10–20% risk of infection. This type of surgery needs prophylaxis. Biliary, hepatobiliary, and pancreatic operations usually meet criteria of clean-contaminated wounds definitions. In biliary-tract procedures, prophylaxis is required only for cases at high risk of contamination: bile obstruction, jaundice, stones in common duct, reoperation, and cholecystitis. Prophylaxis is always required in hepatobiliary and pancreatic surgery because these operations are long. In gastroduodenal operations, the risk is low if gastric acidity is normal and bleeding, cancer, gastric ulcer and obstruction are absent. Colorectal procedures are usually contaminated cases. The unique goal of prophylaxis includes preoperative reduction of bacterial concentration in feces. In association with mechanical bowel preparation, prophylaxis is used in major elective abdominal procedure (i.e., vascular graft) to prevent bacterial translocation from the gut
Infected wounds	Risk of infection of about 20–50% meeting the following criteria: acute bacterial inflammation, without pus; transection of clean tissue for the purpose of surgical access to a collection of pus; traumatic wound with retained ischemic tissues, foreign bodies, fecal contamination, or delayed treatment. Appropriate treatment is to administer antibiotic therapy, not as prophylaxis, because infection is already present

of all nosocomial infections among hospitalized patients [103]. Among surgical patients, they are the most common nosocomial infection, accounting for 38% of all such infections. Of these, two-thirds were confined to the incision, and one-third involved organs or spaces accessed during the operation. When surgical patients with nosocomial SSI die, 77% of deaths are reported to be related to the infection; the majority (93%) were serious infections involving organs or spaces accessed during the operation [103, 104]. A simple method of evaluating the probability that WI will develop consists of classifying the wound according to the scheme illustrated in Table 16.9.

16.10.1 Risk Factors

Surgical WI occurs whenever the combination of microbial numbers and virulence is sufficiently large to overcome the local host defence mechanisms and establish progressive growth [102–109]. It is immediately evident that different types of surgical procedures, involving a greater or lesser degree of contamination, are then associated with a different probability of developing WI. Several patient factors, besides the type of procedure and operator skill, are important in affecting the probability of incurring a postoperative WI. One is patient age: the higher the age, the higher the incidence. Another factor is the period of hospital stay before surgery: patients hospitalized for >12 days are more susceptible to WI, showing that a relationship is likely to exist between the incidence of infection and the hospital environment and bacterial flora [106, 107].

16.10.2 Factors Involved in WI Development

It is clear that the mechanism whereby a patient develops WI is linked to three critical elements: the closed space; the infectious agent, which must be present in sufficient number and with sufficient virulence; and the susceptible host. Microbial contamination of the surgical site is a necessary precursor of SSI. Quantitatively, it has been shown that if a surgical site is contaminated with $>10^5$ microorganisms per gram of tissue, SSI risk is markedly increased. Injury produces enclosed environments due to pockets of extravasated blood, necrotic tissue, infarcted areas, foreign bodies, and prostheses. The environment in these enclosed spaces soon becomes hypoxic, hypercarbic, and acidic, favoring bacterial growth. In abdominal surgery, GIT represents a huge reservoir of pathogenetic bacteria, and recently it was hypothesized that it could act as an undrained abscess, causing infection and MOF [102, 104, 108]. Any infectious agent can contaminate a closed space, but relatively few cause infection. *Streptococcus* spp. invade even minor breaks in the skin and spread through connective tissue planes and lymphatics. *Staphylococcus* spp. are less invasive but more pathogenic. *Pseudomonas* and *Serratia* spp. are often seen as opportunistic invaders. Many fungi and parasites may cause abscesses or sinus and are typical of the immunocompromised patient. Anaerobes, such as *Bacteroides* spp., and *Peptostreptococcus* spp. are more frequently isolated because of improvements in culture techniques. Postsurgical WI is a multimicrobial disease in which many bacteria act in synergism [108]. Finally, there are host-dependent predisposing factors to the development of postsurgical infections. Among these are diabetes, severe trauma, burns, malnutrition, cancer, hematological disorders, transplantation, and immunosuppressive drugs. In many patients, these factors are believed to be primarily responsible for decreased reactivity to delayed hypersensitivity antigens, creating an anergic state associated with an increased incidence of infectious complications. Considering these three elements, it is easier to understand the cycle: immunosuppression and anergy are highly common in a surgical patient; they lead to infection, and the infection itself can deteriorate the immune system.

16.10.3 Treatment

As infectious complications in surgical patients are responsible for prolonged wound healing, disability, and even death; and as the patient's quality of life can be affected or even permanently altered by them—with huge socioeconomic costs—it is important to prevent them as far as possible. The importance of the nutritional status is emphasized by the higher incidence of infectious and other surgical complications in malnourished patients. Among several nutritional status indices, the prognostic nutritional index (PNI), which explicitly includes serum albumin value, correlates with the probability of infection after surgery: to values of PNI >50%, there corresponds a high risk of postoperative complications; to values between 40 and 49%, an intermediate risk; to values <40% a low risk. Furthermore, perioperative administration of supplemental oxygen is a practical method of reducing the incidence of surgical WIs [110].

16.10.4 Antibiotic Prophylaxis

The first important point about antibiotic prophylaxis is its timing of administration [104, 106]. Administration of antibiotics just before, during, and up to 3 h after surgery effectively prevents WIs. Many studies demonstrate that prophylactic antibiotics are most useful if given to patients before contamination occurs: the most relevant protective effect was observed when antibiotic was given so that good tissue levels were present at the time of the procedure and for the first 3–4 h after surgical incision. A practical approach would then be to contemplate administering a single preoperative dose, followed by an intraoperative dose if the procedure lasts >3 h or twice the half-life of the antibiotic, and massive hemorrhage occurs during surgery [102]. Principles of the proper prophylaxis of WIs include selecting bactericidal antibiotics effective against likely pathogens. Single-agent prophylaxis is almost always effective in the majority of clinical situations, provided that the half-life of the antibiotic is long enough to maintain adequate tissue levels throughout the operation and that the given dose is equal to a full therapeutic i.v. dose. Recommended antibiotics for prophylaxis of WI caused by Gram-positive and Gram-negative aerobic bacteria are cefazolin (1 gm i.v./i.m.) or vancomycin (1 g i.v.) in patients allergic to cephalosporins. First-generation cephalosporins, such as cefazolin, are good choices because they are not expensive, incur a low rate of allergic responses, and have a broad-spectrum of activity against likely aerobic pathogens. Prophylaxis against both Gram-negative aerobes and anaerobes includes clindamycin or metronidazole plus tobramycin, or a single broad-spectrum agent such as cefoxitin or cefotetan, or sulbactam/ampicillin. Gram-negative anaerobes (*Bacteroides* spp.) are of GIT origin and are synergistic with Gram-negative aerobes in causing infections after GIT surgical procedures. Even though the problem is still debated, combination of two antibiotics is in general more powerful than a single broad-spectrum agent active against both bacterial components [102, 106]. A second point concerns the cases for which antibiotic prophylaxis as described is indicated. In general, an approach such as that outlined above is indicated for GIT and anorectal surgery, biliary-tract surgery, vaginal hysterectomy, insertion of artificial devices, or prolonged (>3 h) clean surgery. In contaminated or dirty surgery, appropriate therapy should be started as soon as possible: the right treatment is to administer antibiotic therapy, not as prophylaxis, because infection is already present [102]. In relation to operative contamination and increasing risk of WI, classifying the operative wound includes four categories mentioned above. This is the most widely applied classification of surgical procedures in terms of contamination and probability that a WI will develop; this risk is about 5, 10, 15, and 30% for the four reported classes, respectively [102].

16.11 Urinary Tract Infections

Urinary tract infection (UTI) is defined as significant bacteriuria in the presence of symptoms [111, 112]. This common clinical entity affects an estimated 20% of women at some time during their lifetimes. Successful management includes proper specimen collection, use of immediately available laboratory testing for presumptive diagnosis, appreciation of epidemiological and host factors that may identify patients with clinically unapparent upper UTI, and selection of appropriate antimicrobial therapy with recommendations for follow-up care [113–115].

16.11.1 Pathophysiology

The urinary tract is normally sterile. Uncomplicated UTI involves the urinary bladder in a host without underlying renal or neurological disease. The clinical entity is termed cystitis and represents bladder mucosal invasion, most often by enteric coliform bacteria (*E. coli*), which inhabit the periurethral vaginal introitus and ascend into the bladder via the urethra. Sexual intercourse may promote this migration, and cystitis is common in otherwise healthy young women [114]. Urine is generally a good culture medium; factors unfavorable to bacterial growth include a low pH (≤ 5.5), a high concentration of urea, and the presence of organic acids derived from a diet that includes fruits and protein. Frequent and complete voiding has been associated with a reduced incidence of UTI [115–119]. Normally, a thin film of urine remains in the bladder after emptying, and any bacteria present are removed by the mucosal cell production of organic acids. If lower urinary tract mechanisms fail, upper urinary tract or kidney involvement occurs, which is termed pyelonephritis. Host defences at this level include local leukocyte phagocytosis and renal production of antibodies that kill bacteria in the presence of complement. Complicated UTI occurs in the setting of underlying structural, medical, or neurological disease [115]. Patients with a neurogenic bladder or bladder diverticulum, and postmenopausal women with bladder or uterine prolapse, have an increased frequency of UTI due to incomplete bladder emptying.

This eventually allows residual bacteria to overwhelm local bladder mucosal defences. High urine glucose content and defective host immune factors in patients with diabetes mellitus also predispose to infection.

16.11.2 Frequency and Morbidity/Mortality Rates

An estimated 11% of women in the USA report at least one physician-diagnosed UTI per year, and the lifetime probability that a woman will have a UTI is 60% [120]. Although simple cystitis may resolve spontaneously, effective treatment lessens symptom duration and reduces the incidence of progression to upper UTI. Pyelonephritis is associated with substantial morbidity rate [117–119], including systemic effects such as fever, vomiting, dehydration, and loss of vasomotor tone resulting in hypotension. Complications include acute papillary necrosis with possible development of ureteral obstruction, septic shock, and perinephric abscess. Chronic pyelonephritis may lead to renal scarring with diminished function. Younger patients have the lowest rates of morbidity and mortality. Despite appropriate intervention, 1–3% of patients with acute pyelonephritis die. Factors associated with unfavorable prognosis are general debility and old age, renal calculi or obstruction, recent hospitalization or instrumentation, diabetes mellitus, sickle cell anemia, underlying carcinoma, intercurrent chemotherapy, or chronic nephropathy. The largest group of patients with UTI is adult women. The incidence increases with age and sexual activity. Rates of infection are high in postmenopausal women because of bladder or uterine prolapse, causing incomplete bladder emptying; loss of estrogens, with attendant changes in vaginal flora; loss of lactobacilli, which allows periurethral colonization with Gram-negative aerobes such as *E. coli*; and higher likelihood of concomitant medical illness, such as diabetes. UTI is unusual in men <50 years, and symptoms of dysuria and frequency are usually due to urethral or prostatic infection. In older men, however, the incidence of UTI rises because of prostatic obstruction or subsequent instrumentation.

16.11.3 Symptoms and Physical Findings

Classic symptoms of UTI in the adult are dysuria with accompanying urinary urgency and frequency. A sensation of bladder fullness or lower abdominal discomfort is often present. Bloody urine (hemorrhagic cystitis) is reported in as many as 10% of cases of UTI in otherwise healthy women. Fevers, chills, and malaise may be noted, though these are associated more frequently with pyelonephritis. Most adult women with simple lower UTI have suprapubic tenderness with no evidence of vaginitis, cervicitis, or pelvic tenderness. The patient with pyelonephritis usually appears ill and, in addition to fever, sweating, and prostration, is found to have flank tenderness in the majority of cases.

16.11.4 Diagnosis

If UTI is suspected, the initial test of choice is urinalysis. The midstream-voided technique is as accurate as catheterization if the proper technique is followed. Pyuria, as indicated by a positive result of the leukocyte esterase dip test, is found in the vast majority of patients with UTI. However, low-level pyuria [6–20 WBCs per high power field (HPF) microscopy on a centrifuged specimen] may be associated with an unacceptable level of false-negative results with the leukocyte esterase dip test. In the female patient with appropriate symptoms and examination findings suggestive of UTI, urine microscopy may be indicated despite a negative leukocyte esterase dip test result. Current emphasis in UTI diagnosis rests with pyuria detection. As noted, a positive leukocyte esterase dip test suffices in most instances. According to Stamm and Hooton [119], pyuria levels as low as 2–5 WBCs per HPF in a centrifuged specimen are important in the female patient with appropriate symptoms. The presence of bacteriuria is as significant. A positive result on the nitrate test is highly specific for UTI, typically because of urease-splitting organisms, such as *Proteus* spp. and, occasionally, *E. coli*; however, it is highly insensitive as a screening tool, as only 25% of patients with UTI have a positive nitrite test result. Low-level or, occasionally, frank hematuria may be noted in otherwise typical UTI; its PPV is poor, however. Historically, the definition of UTI was based on the finding of a single organism at culture of 100,000 colonies per millimeter. If the patient has had a UTI within the last month, the same organism probably causes relapse, which represents treatment failure [111]. Reinfection occurs in 1–6 months and is usually due to a different organism (or serotype of the same organism). In the vast majority of patients with UTI, no imaging studies are indicated. If findings are suggestive of nephrolithiasis complicating the presentation, an intravenous pyelogram (IVP) or renal US should be obtained to exclude the possibility of obstruction or hydronephrosis [116–118]. Recent studies with dynamic helical CT scan are proving that this study provides information similar to that yielded by IVP without the need for dye injection. Dynamic CT scans can also serve as a convenient screen for abdominal aortic aneurysm masquerading as UTI or renal colic. Additional testing may be indicated if the diagnosis is in doubt. For example, a pelvic US may be indicated in a young woman with pelvic tenderness, cervical discharge, and unilateral adnexal tenderness; a CT scan may be indicated in the elderly patient whose presentation is not typical for UTI but who has abdominal pain, lower abdominal tenderness, and pyuria. Catheterization is indicated if the patient cannot void spontaneously, is too debilitated or immobilized, or if obesity prevents the patient from obtaining a suitable specimen. Postvoiding residual urine volume, measurable by catheterization, may reveal urinary retention in a host with a defective bladder emptying mechanism.

16.11.5 Treatment

Orally administered therapy with an antibiotic effective against Gram-negative aerobic coliform bacteria, such as *E. coli*, is the principal treatment intervention in patients with UTI. The patient with an uncomplicated, presumed, lower UTI or simple cystitis that has symptom duration <48 h may be treated with one of the following agents for a total of 3 days: (1) cotrimoxazole; (2) ciprofloxacin or similar fluoroquinolone; (3) nitrofurantoin macrocrystals; (4) amoxicillin/clavulanate [115]. Clinical management of UTI is complicated by the increasing incidence of infections caused by strains of *E. coli* that are resistant to commonly used antimicrobial agents [121]. In recent studies, the rate of resistance to trimethoprim–sulfamethoxazole among *E. coli* isolates from women with UTI ranged from 15 to 22% [121]. Pregnant and otherwise healthy women with no evidence of upper UTI may be treated with a 2-week course of a cephalosporin [117, 118]. Pregnant patients should be treated for all episodes of pyuria or bacteriuria, regardless of whether they have symptoms. Ambulatory younger women who present with signs and symptoms of pyelonephritis may be candidates for outpatient therapy. They must be otherwise healthy and must not be pregnant. They must be treated initially with vigorous fluids administered orally or i.v., antipyretic pain medication, and a dose of parenteral antibiotics. Studies show that outpatient therapy for selected patients is as safe as, and much less expensive than, inpatient therapy for a comparable group of patients. The decision regarding admission of a patient with acute pyelonephritis is dependent on age; host factors, such as immunocompromising chemotherapy or chronic diseases; known urinary tract structural abnormalities; renal calculi; recent hospitalization; or urinary tract instrumentation. Initial treatment should include i.v. antibiotic therapy (cotrimoxazole, directed at coliform Gram-negative bacteria; third-generation cephalosporin; or an aminoglycoside), adequate fluid resuscitation to restore effective circulating volume and generous urinary volumes, and antipyretic pain medications [115]. In the patient with a complicated UTI, coverage for unusual or multiple antibiotic-resistant organisms, such as *P. aeruginosa*, must be considered.

16.11.6 Catheter-Associated Urinary Tract Infections

The urinary tract is the most common site of healthcare-associated infection, accounting for >30% of infections reported by acute-care hospitals. Virtually all healthcare- associated UTIs are caused by urinary tract instrumentation. Colonization of urinary catheters is inevitable and expected. Once microorganisms colonize the urine, they rapidly progress, within 72 h, to concentrations >10^5 CFU/ml [122]. The longer the catheter is in place, the more likely colonization will occur. It is believed that extraluminal colonization is the most likely route of entry for microorganisms, particularly via the shorter female urethra. Urinary catheter colonization is perpetuated by microorganism-produced biofilm. Following insertion of a standard urinary catheter, a conditioning film comprising proteins, electrolytes, and other components of urine is deposited on the surface of the catheter [123]. Initially composed of a single species, the biofilm on a long-term indwelling urinary catheter can also contain multiple species. Under unfavorable conditions, organisms can detach from the biofilm and become free-floating. Free-floating organisms in the urine can lead to symptomatic infection. Most microorganisms causing catheter-associated UTIs (CAUTI) derive from the patient's own colonic and perineal flora (such as *E. coli*) or from the hands of healthcare personnel during catheter insertion or manipulation of the collection system. Duration of catheter use is the most important risk factor for infection [124], which increases by an estimated 5–10% each day the catheter remains in place. Patients requiring long-term catheter insertion are almost assured of developing CAUTI. Urinary stasis and bladder overdistention are additional risk factors for bacteriuria and potential infection. Other risk factors are female sex, older age, and failure to maintain a closed drainage system. Catheters coated with nonantibiotic antimicrobial noble metals are now available to help reduce CAUTI, although the main strategy remains avoiding long-term catheter use and unnecessary repositioning.

References

1. Bosscha K, van Vroonhoven JMV, van der Werken C (1999) Surgical management of severe secondary peritonitis. Br J Surg 86:1371–1377
2. Sganga G, Brisinda G, Castagneto M (2001) Peritonitis: priorities and management strategies. In: van Saene HKF, Sganga G, Silvestri L (eds) Infection in the critically ill: an ongoing challenge. Springer, Berlin, pp 23–33
3. Sganga G (2000) Sepsi addominali chirurgiche e insufficienza multiorgano (MOFS). Edizioni Systems Comunicazioni, Milan
4. Bone RG, Balk RA, Cerra FB et al (1992) Definitions for sepsis and organ failure and guidelines for the use of innovative therapies in sepsis. The ACCP/SCCM Consensus Conference Committee. American College of Chest Physicians/Society of Critical Care Medicine. Chest 101:1644–1655
5. Pieracci FM, Barie PS (2007) Intra-abdominal infections. Curr Opin Crit Care 13:440–449
6. Solomkin JS, Mazuski JE, Baron EJ et al (2003) Guidelines for the selection of anti-infective agents for complicated intra-abdominal infections. Clin Infect Dis 37:997–1005
7. Brook I (2008) Microbiology and Management of Abdominal Infections. Dig Dis Sci 53:2585–2591
8. Krepel CJ, Gohr CM, Edmiston CE, Condon RE (1995) Surgical sepsis: constancy of antibiotic susceptibility of causative organisms. Surgery 117:505–509
9. Sganga G, Brisinda G, Castagneto M (2000) Nosocomial fungal infections in surgical patients: risk factors and treatment. Minerva Anestesiol 66(Suppl 1):71–77
10. Wheeler AP, Bernard GR (1999) Treating patients with severe sepsis. N Engl J Med 340:207–214
11. Mannick JA, Rodrick ML, Lederer JA (2001) The immunologic response to injury. J Am Coll Surg 193:237–244
12. Knoferl MW, Angele MK, Diodato MD et al (2002) Female sex hormones regulate macrophage function after trauma-hemorrhage and prevent increased death rate from subsequent sepsis. Ann Surg 235:105–112

13. Sganga G, van Saene HKF, Brisinda G, Castagneto M (2001) Bacterial translocation. In: van Saene HKF, Sganga G, Silvestri L (eds) Infection in the critically ill: an ongoing challenge. Springer, Berlin, pp 35–45
14. Gregor P, Prodger JD (1988) Mead Johnson Critical Care Symposium for the Practic Surgeon. 4. Abdominal crisis in the intensive care unit. Can J Surg 31:331–332
15. Gajic O, Errutia LE, Sewan H et al (2002) Acute abdomen in the medical intensive care unit. Crit Care Med 30:1187–1190
16. Kollef MH, Allen BT (1994) Determinants of outcome for patients in the medical intensive care unit requiring abdominal surgery: a prospective, single-center study. Chest 106:1822–1828
17. Velmahos GC, Kamel E, Berne TV et al (1999) Abdominal computed tomography for the diagnosis of intra-abdominal sepsis in critically injured patients: fishing in murky waters. Arch Surg 134:831–836
18. Mokart D, Merlin M, Sannini A et al (2005) Procalcitonin, interleukin 6 and systemic inflammatory response syndrome (SIRS): early markers of postoperative sepsis after major surgery. Br J Anaesthesiol 94:767–773
19. Wickel DJ, Cheadle WG, Mercer-Jones MA, Garrison RN (1997) Poor outcome from peritonitis is caused by disease acuity and organ failure, not recurrent peritoneal infection. Ann Surg 225:744–756
20. Anbidge AE, Lynch D, Wison SR (2003) US of the peritoneum. Radiographics 23:663–684
21. Go HL, Baarslag HJ, Vermeulen H et al (2005) A comparative study to validate the use of ultrasonography and computed tomography in patients with post-operative intra-abdominal sepsis. Eur J Radiol 54:383–387
22. Whitehouse JS, Weigelt JA (2009) Diagnostic peritoneal lavage: a review of indications, technique, and interpretation. Scandinavian J Trauma Resuscitation Emerg Med 17:13
23. Lin WY, Chao TH, Wang SJ (2002) Clinical features and gallium scan in the detection of post-surgical infection in the elderly. Eur J Nucl Med 29:371–375
24. Shih-Chuan T, Te-Hsin C, Lin WY, Shyh-Jen W (2001) Abdominal abscesses in patients having surgery an application of Ga-67 scintigraphic and computed tomographic scanning. Clin Nucl Med 26:761–776
25. Marshall J, Maier RV, Jimenez M, Dellinger EP (2004) Source control in the management of severe sepsis and septic shock: an evidence-based review. Crit Care Med 32(Suppl 11):S513–S526
26. Soares-Weiser K, Paul M, Brezis M, Leibovici L (2002) Antibiotic treatment for spontaneous bacterial peritonitis. BMJ 324:100–102
27. Solomkin JS, Wilson SE, Christou N et al (2001) Results of a clinical trial of clinafloxacin versus imipenem/cilastatin for intraabdominal infections. Ann Surg 233:79–87
28. Mazuski JE (2007) Antimicrobial treatment for intra-abdominal infections. Expert Opin Pharmacother 8(17):2933–2945
29. Laterre PF (2008) Progress in medical management of intra-abdominal infection. Curr Opin Infect Dis 21(4):393–398
30. Cohen J (2000) Combination antibiotic therapy for severe peritonitis. Lancet 356:1539–1540
31. Holzheimer RG, Dralle H (2001) Paradigm change in 30 years peritonitis treatment. A review on source control. Eur J Med Res 6:161–168
32. Schein M, Marshall J (2004) Source control for surgical infections. World J Surg 28(7):638–645
33. Rivers E, Nguyen B, Havstad S et al (2001) Early goal-directed therapy in the treatment of severe sepsis and septic shock. N Engl J Med 345:1368–1377
34. Platell C, Papadimitriou JM, Hall JC (2000) The influence of lavage on peritonitis. J Am Coll Surg 191:672–680
35. Sganga G, Brisinda G, Castagneto M (2002) Trauma operative procedures: timing of surgery and priorities. In: Gullo A (ed) Critical care medicine. Springer, Berlin, pp 447–467

36. Levison MA, Zeigler D (1991) Correlation of APACHE II score, drainage technique and outcome in postoperative intra-abdominal abscess. Surg Gynecol Obstet 172:89–94
37. Baril NB, Ralls PW, Wren SM et al (2000) Does an infected peripancreatic fluid collection or abscess mandate operation? Ann Surg 231:361–367
38. Brisinda G, Maria G, Ferrante A, Civello IM (1999) Evaluation of prognostic factors in patients with acute pancreatitis. Hepatogastroenterology 46:1990–1997
39. Baron TH, Morgan DE (1999) Acute necrotizing pancreatitis. N Engl J Med 340:1412–1417
40. Beger HG, Rau B, Mayer J, Pralle U (1997) Natural course of acute pancreatitis. World J Surg 21:130–135
41. Bradley EL III (1993) A clinically based classification system for acute pancreatitis. Summary of the international symposium on acute pancreatitis, Atlanta, GA, Sept. 11–13, 1992. Arch Surg 128:586–590
42. Marotta F, Geng TC, Wu CC, Barbi G (1996) Bacterial translocation in the course of acute pancreatitis: beneficial role of nonabsorbable antibiotics and Lactinol enemas. Digestion 57:446–452
43. Foitzik T, Fernandez-del Castillo C, Ferraro MJ et al (1995) Pathogenesis and prevention of early pancreatic infection in experimental acute necrotizing pancreatitis. Ann Surg 222:179–185
44. Isenmann R, Schwarz M, Rau B et al (2002) Characteristics of infection with Candida species in patients with necrotizing pancreatitis. World J Surg 26(3):372–376
45. Bradley EL III (1994) Surgical indications and techniques in necrotizing pancreatitis. In: Bradley EL III (ed) Acute pancreatitis: diagnosis and therapy. Raven Press, New York, pp 105–117
46. Paye F, Rotman N, Radier C et al (1998) Percutaneous aspiration for bacteriological studies in patients with necrotizing pancreatitis. Br J Surg 85:755–759
47. Rau B, Pralle U, Mayer JM, Beger HG (1998) Role of ultrasonographically guided fine-needle aspiration cytology in diagnosis of infected pancreatic necrosis. Br J Surg 85:179–184
48. Mithofer K, Fernandez-del Castillo C, Ferraro MJ et al (1996) Antibiotic treatment improves survival in experimental acute necrotizing pancreatitis. Gastroenterology 110:232–240
49. Sainio V, Kemppainen E, Puolakkainen P et al (1995) Early antibiotic treatment in acute necrotising pancreatitis. Lancet 346:663–667
50. Luiten EJ, Hop WC, Lange JF, Bruining HA (1995) Controlled clinical trial of selective decontamination for the treatment of severe acute pancreatitis. Ann Surg 222:57–65
51. Luiten EJ, Hop WC, Lange JF, Bruining HA (1997) Differential prognosis of gram-negative versus gram-positive infected and sterile pancreatic necrosis: results of a randomized trial in patients with severe acute pancreatitis treated with adjuvant selective decontamination. Clin Infect Dis 25:811–816
52. Pederzoli P, Bassi C, Vesentini S, Campedelli A (1993) A randomized multicenter clinical trial of antibiotic prophylaxis of septic complications in acute necrotizing pancreatitis with imipenem. Surg Gynecol Obstet 176:480–483
53. Ho HS, Frey CF (1997) The role of antibiotic prophylaxis in severe acute pancreatitis. Arch Surg 132:487–493
54. Bassi C, Falconi M, Talamini G et al (1998) Controlled clinical trial of pefloxacin versus imipenem in severe acute pancreatitis. Gastroenterology 115:1513–1517
55. McClave SA, Snider H, Owens N, Sexton LK (1997) Clinical nutrition in pancreatitis. Dig Dis Sci 42:2035–2044
56. Kalfarentzos F, Kehagias J, Mead N et al (1997) Enteral nutrition is superior to parenteral nutrition in severe acute pancreatitis: results of a randomized prospective trial. Br J Surg 84:1665–1669
57. Windsor AC, Kanwar S, Li AG et al (1998) Compared with parenteral nutrition, enteral feeding attenuates the acute phase response and improves disease severity in acute pancreatitis. Gut 42:431–435

58. Bozzetti F, Braga M, Gianotti L et al (2001) Postoperative enteral versus parenteral nutrition in malnourished patients with gastrointestinal cancer: a randomised multicentre trial. Lancet 358:1487–1492
59. Warshaw AL (2000) Pancreatic necrosis. To debride or not to debride–that is the question. Ann Surg 232:627–629
60. Buchler MW, Gloor B, Muller CA et al (2000) Acute necrotizing pancreatitis: treatment strategy according to the status of infection. Ann Surg 232:619–626
61. Farkas G, Marton J, Mandi Y, Szederkenyi E (1996) Surgical strategy and management of infected pancreatic necrosis. Br J Surg 83:930–933
62. Ashley SW, Perez A, Pierce EA et al (2001) Necrotizing pancreatitis. Contemporary analysis of 99 consecutive cases. Ann Surg 234:572–580
63. Gloor B, Muller CA, Worni M et al (2001) Pancreatic infection in severe pancreatitis. The role of fungus and multiresistant organisms. Arch Surg 136:592–596
64. Doglietto GB, Gui D, Pacelli F et al (1994) Open vs closed treatment of secondary pancreatic infection. A review of 42 cases. Arch Surg 129:689–693
65. Kriwanek S, Gschwantler M, Beckerhinn P et al (1999) Complications after surgery for necrotising pancreatitis: risk factors and prognosis. Eur J Surg 165:952–957
66. Dervenis C, Bassi C (2000) Evidence-based assessment of severity and management of acute pancreatitis. Br J Surg 87:257–258
67. Tsiotos GG, Luque-de Leon E, Sarr MG (1998) Long-term outcome of necrotizing pancreatitis treated by necrosectomy. Br J Surg 85:1650–1653
68. del Castillo CF, Rattner DW, Makary MA et al (1998) Debridement and closed packing for treatment of necrotizing pancreatitis. Ann Surg 228:676–684
69. Farkas G (2000) Pancreatic head mass: how can we treat it? Acute pancreatitis: surgical treatment. JOP J Pancreas 1(Suppl 3):138–142
70. Mithofer K, Mueller PR, Warshaw AL (1997) Interventional and surgical treatment of pancreatic abscess. World J Surg 21:162–168
71. Widdison AL, Karanjia ND (1993) Pancreatic infection complicating acute pancreatitis. Br J Surg 80:148–154
72. Lumsden A, Bradley EL III (1990) Secondary pancreatic infections. Surg Gynecol Obstet 170:459–467
73. Aranha GV, Prinz RA, Greenlee HB (1982) Pancreatic abscess: an unresolved surgical problem. Am J Surg 144:534–538
74. Warshaw AL, Jin G (1985) Improved survival in 45 patients with pancreatic abscess. Ann Surg 202:408–417
75. Brisinda G, Mazzari A, Crocco A et al (2011) Open pancreatic necrosectomy in the multidisciplinary management of postinflammatory necrosis. Ann Surg 253(5):1049–1051
76. Ross Carter C, McKay CJ, Imrie CW (2000) Percutaneous necrosectomy and sinus tract endoscopy in the management of infected pancreatic necrosis: an initial experience. Ann Surg 232:175–180
77. Kjossev KT, Losanoff JE (2001) Laparoscopic treatment of severe acute pancreatitis. Surg Endosc 15:1239–1240
78. Freeny PC, Hauptmann E, Althaus SJ et al (1998) Percutaneous CT-guided catheter drainage of infected acute necrotizing pancreatitis: techniques and results. AJR Am J Roentgenol 170:969–975
79. Baron TH, Morgan DE (1997) Organized pancreatic necrosis: definition, diagnosis, and management. Gastroenterol Int 10:167–178
80. Wada K, Takada T, Hirata K et al (2010) Treatment strategy for acute pancreatitis. J Hepatobiliary Pancreat Sci 17:79–86
81. Zhu JF, Fan XH, Zhang XH (2001) Laparoscopic treatment of severe acute pancreatitis. Surg Endosc 15:146–148
82. Clancy CJ, Nguyen MH, Morris AJ (1997) Candidal mediastinitis: an emerging clinical entity. Clin Infect Dis 25:608–613

83. Gamlin F, Caldicott LD, Shah MV (1994) Mediastinitis and sepsis syndrome following intubation. Anaesthesia 49:883–885
84. Isaacs L, Kotton B, Peralta MM Jr et al (1993) Fatal mediastinal abscess from upper respiratory infection. Ear Nose Throat J 72:620–622
85. Becker M, Zbaren P, Hermans R et al (1997) Necrotizing fasciitis of the head and neck: role of CT in diagnosis and management. Radiology 202:471–476
86. Brunelli A, Sabbatini A, Catalini G, Fianchini A (1996) Descending necrotizing mediastinitis. Surgical drainage and tracheostomy. Arch Otolaryngol Head Neck Surg 122:1326–1329
87. Corsten MJ, Shamji FM, Odell PF et al (1997) Optimal treatment of descending necrotising mediastinitis. Thorax 52:702–708
88. Baldwin RT, Radovancevic B, Sweeney MS (1992) Bacterial mediastinitis after heart transplantation. J Heart Lung Transpl 11:545–549
89. El Oakley RM, Wright JE (1996) Postoperative mediastinitis: classification and management. Ann Thorac Surg 61:1030–1036
90. Milano CA, Kesler K, Archibald N (1995) Mediastinitis after coronary artery bypass graft surgery. Risk factors and long-term survival. Circulation 92:2245–2251
91. Brook I, Frazier EH (1996) Microbiology of mediastinitis. Arch Intern Med 156:333–336
92. Shaffer HA Jr, Valenzuela G, Mittal RK (1992) Esophageal perforation. A reassessment of the criteria for choosing medical or surgical therapy. Arch Intern Med 152:757–761
93. Loop FD, Lytle BW, Cosgrove DM (1990) J Maxwell Chamberlain memorial paper. Sternal wound complications after isolated coronary artery bypass grafting: early and late mortality, morbidity, and cost of care. Ann Thorac Surg 49:179–187
94. Gadek JE, DeMichele SJ, Karlstad MD (1999) Effect of enteral feeding with eicosapentaenoic acid, gamma-linolenic acid, and antioxidants in patients with acute respiratory distress syndrome. Enteral nutrition in ARDS study group. Crit Care Med 27:1409–1420
95. Weinzweig N, Yetman R (1995) Transposition of the greater omentum for recalcitrant median sternotomy wound infections. Ann Plast Surg 34:471–477
96. Andrews CO, Gora ML (1994) Pleural effusions: pathophysiology and management. Ann Pharmacother 28:894–903
97. Bartter T, Santarelli R, Akers SM (1994) The evaluation of pleural effusion. Chest 106:1209–1214
98. Fenton KN, Richardson JD (1995) Diagnosis and management of malignant pleural effusions. Am J Surg 170:69–74
99. Kennedy L, Sahn SA (1994) Noninvasive evaluation of the patient with a pleural effusion. Chest Surg Clin N Am 4:451–465
100. Light RW (1995) Pleural diseases, 3rd edn. Williams & Wilkins, New York
101. Sahn SA (1988) State of the art. The pleura. Am Rev Respir Dis 138:184–234
102. Sganga G, Brisinda G, Castagneto M (2001) Practical aspects of antibiotic prophylaxis in high-risk surgical patients. In: van Saene HKF, Sganga G, Silvestri L (eds) Infection in the critically ill: an ongoing challenge. Springer, Berlin, pp 47–58
103. Mangram AJ, Horan TC, Pearson ML et al (1996) The hospital infection control practices advisory committee. Guideline for the prevention of surgical site infection. Infect Control Hosp Epidemiol 20:247–280
104. Sganga G, Cozza V (2009) Intra-abdominal infections: diagnostic and surgical strategies. In: Gullo A, Besso J, Lumb PD, Williams GF (eds) Intensive and critical care medicine. (WFSICCM) World federation of societies of intensive and critical care medicine. Springer, Milan, pp 315–324
105. Kurz A, Sessler DI, Lenhardt R (1996) Perioperative normothermia to reduce the incidende of surgical-wound infection and shorten hospitalization. N Engl J Med 334:1209–1215
106. Classen DC, Evans RS, Pestotnik A (1992) The timing of prophylactic administration of antibiotics and the risk of surgical-wound infection. N Engl J Med 326:281–287

107. Nathens AB, Marshall JC (1999) Selective decontamination of the digestive tract in surgical patients. A systematic review of the evidence. Arch Surg 134:170–176
108. Silvestri L, Mannucci F, van Saene HKF (2000) Selective decontamination of the digestive tract: a life-saver. J Hosp Infect 45:185–190
109. van Saene HKF, Silvestri L, de la Cal M (2000) Prevention of nosocomial infections in the intensive care unit. Curr Opin Crit Care 6:323–329
110. Greif R, Akca O, Horn EP et al (2000) Supplemental perioperative oxygen to reduce the incidence of surgical-wound infection. N Engl J Med 342:161–167
111. Jancel T, Dudas V (2002) Management of uncomplicated urinary tract infections. West J Med 176:51–55
112. Larcombe J (1999) Urinary tract infection in children. BMJ 319:1173–1175
113. Ellis AK, Verma S (2000) Quality of life in women with urinary tract infections: is benign disease a misnomer? J Am Board Fam Pract 13:392–397
114. Hooten TM, Scholes D, Stapleton AE (2000) A prospective study of asymptomatic bacteriuria in sexually active young women. N Engl J Med 343:992–997
115. Howes DS, Young WF (2000) Urinary tract infections. In: Tintinalli A (ed) Emergency medicine. A comprehensive study guide. McGraw-Hill, New York, pp 625–631
116. Leibovici L, Greenshtain S, Cohen O, Wysenbeek AJ (1992) Toward improved empiric management of moderate to severe urinary tract infections. Arch Intern Med 152:2481–2486
117. Millar LK, Wing DA, Paul RH, Grimes DA (1995) Outpatient treatment of pyelonephritis in pregnancy: a randomized controlled trial. Obstet Gynecol 86:560–564
118. Safrin S, Siegel D, Black D (1988) Pyelonephritis in adult women: inpatient versus outpatient therapy. Am J Med 85:793–798
119. Stamm WE, Hooton TM (1993) Management of urinary tract infections in adults. N Engl J Med 329:1328–1334
120. Foxman B, Barlow R, D'Arcy H et al (2000) Urinary tract infection: self-reported incidence and associated costs. Ann Epidemiol 10:509–515
121. Manges AR, Johnson JR, Foxman B et al (2001) Widespread distribution of urinary tract infections caused by a multidrug-resistant Escherichia coli clonal group. N Engl J Med 345:1007–1013
122. Stark RP, Maki DG (1984) Bacteriuria in the catheterized patient. N Engl J Med 311:560–564
123. Trautner BW, Darouiche RO (2004) Catheter-associated infections. Arch Intern Med 164:842–850
124. Lo E, Lindsay N, Classen D et al (2008) Strategies to prevent catheter-associated urinary tract infections in acute care hospitals. Infect Control Hosp Epidemiol 29:S41–S50

Infection in the NICU and PICU

17

A. J. Petros, V. Damjanovic, A. Pigna and J. Farias

17.1 Introduction

In this chapter, we summarise current concepts of infections in neonatal (NICU) and paediatric (PICU) intensive care units and describe the only two proven antibiotic manoeuvres to prevent such infections: surgical prophylaxis, and decontamination of the digestive tract (SDD).

17.2 Current Concepts of Infection

17.2.1 Neonatal Intensive Care Unit

Infections in neonates requiring intensive care are unique in each essential element of the pathogenesis of infection, i.e. the potential pathogen and its source, the mode of transmission and the susceptible host. The pathogen, e.g. hepatitis B virus, or potential pathogen, e.g. *Escherichia coli*, are closely related to source and mode of transmission. Many microorganisms are present in the maternal birth canal (the source). They are most commonly *Streptococcus agalactiae*, *E. coli*, *Herpes simplex* virus, *Listeria monocytogenes* and *Candida albicans*. One or more of these microorganisms can be vertically transmitted from the mother to the neonate. When this type of infection occurs, it will always be present in the first week of the neonate's life (early onset). On the other hand, different microorganisms are acquired in the NICU: in general, these are coagulase-negative staphylococci (CNS),

---

A. J. Petros (✉)
PICU, Great Ormond Street Hospital, London, UK
e-mail: petroa@gosh.nhs.uk

aerobic Gram-negative bacilli (AGNB) (mainly *Klebsiella* spp. and *Pseudomonas aeruginosa*) *S. aureus* and *Candida* spp. The sources of these microorganisms acquired in the NICU are mainly other neonates who carry those microorganisms and/or who are infected with them. NICU staff, mothers, contaminated materials and equipment (environment) are uncommon sources. Although these microorganisms can be transmitted from one neonate to another via equipment, the hands of healthcare workers are the main mode of transmission [1]. Infections due to microorganisms acquired in the unit are usually of late onset following episode period of carriage.

The incidence of infection is higher in the neonatal period than at any time in life. Neonates, particularly preterm, are extremely susceptible to infection, and low birth weight is the single most important risk factor [2]. This increased risk is due primarily to immune system immaturity, poor surface defences, lack of colonisation resistance [3, 4], invasive medical devices and use of broad-spectrum antibiotics. Increased susceptibility to carriage and infection in preterm neonates is the primary contributor to transmission of potential pathogens and subsequent outbreaks of infection on the NICU [1]. Moreover, preterm neonates can be susceptible to new and potential pathogens, usually unknown in an ICU, such as *Hansenula anomala*, a saprophytic yeast known as a contaminant in the brewing industry. This newly recognised potential pathogen caused an outbreak that lasted for 13 months in the Mersey (UK) regional NICU [5].

17.2.2 Paediatric Intensive Care Unit

The three elements—potential pathogen, source and mode of transmission and susceptible host applies to PICU patients. Recent epidemiological studies in children requiring prolonged PICU stay demonstrated that two-thirds of all infections diagnosed were due to microorganisms present in patients' admission flora [6]. These infections practically all manifested within in a week of PICU admission. Infections due to microorganisms acquired in the unit and subsequently carried invariably manifested after 1 week. The three main microorganisms causing infections within the first week are coagulase negative staphylococci, *S. aureus* and *C. albicans*; after one week, the two main microorganisms are *S. aureus* and *P. aeruginosa*. Unlike in the neonate, maternal flora is not the source in a PICU; it is invariably the other patients.

Length of stay in the NICU is substantially longer that in the PICU (median 13 vs. 6.5 days) [4, 7, 8]. An extensive literature search showed that outbreaks are more common in the NICU (Chap. 13). Finally, higher overall mortality rates of 10% versus 5% [9] support the observation that children in the NICU are more susceptible than children in the PICU [4].

17.3 Magnitude of the Problem

17.3.1 Neonatal Intensive Care

The overall infection rates in neonates on intensive care vary between 15 and 20%. This is equal to rates reported for adult medical and surgical units and higher than most paediatric units [10]. The main site of infection is the bloodstream, followed by the lower airways. In a multicenter study of NIUCs in Oakland, New Haven, CT, USA in 1994, Beck-Sague et al. [11] reported that nosocomial bloodstream infection occurred at a rate of 5% when surveillance cultures were performed and was actually half that reported in studies reporting the rate of all infections. Bloodstream infections can account for 50% of all NICU infections. Lower airway infections occur in approximately 3% of neonates during NICU stay [12]. The main organisms are viruses, *S. aureus* and AGNB. The survival benefit of NICU neonates has significantly increased over the last 25 years. In a 2-year study from New York [1977–1978], the mortality rates for early-onset sepsis in neonates <1,000 g was 53.4% and for late-onset sepsis 20.3% [13]. A 5-year study from Oxford, UK (1982–1986) reports mortality rates of 28% and 4% for early- and late-onset sepsis, respectively, in neonates [2]. Data from a 1-year study in a Dutch NICU show a mortality rate <10% (1997) in 436 neonates of about 2,000 g [4].

17.3.2 Paediatric Intensive Care

Nosocomial infection in the PICU is an important cause of morbidity and mortality in ventilated children. Blood stream and lower airways are most common and are almost always due to prolonged use of devices. The incidence of blood stream infection is reported as 10.6–46.9/1,000 catheter days [14] and of lower airways infection 6.5–20.2/1,000 ventilation days.

17.3.2.1 Bloodstream Infections

In a report from a mixed PICU in Birmingham, UK [15], where all children admitted were included, the incidence of blood stream infection was 10.6/1,000 patient days. Consequently, the group as a whole was less ill and stayed for a median of 3 days. The larger denominator of >12,000 patient days also dilutes the real infection rate: 62% of microorganisms causing positive blood cultures were G + bacteria, mainly CNS, *S. aureus* and enterococci; 32% were due to AGNB; the remaining were due to yeasts. In a study from Liverpool, UK, 1,000 children requiring a median of 8 days' ventilation, the overall infection rate was 42.2% [9]. Viral infection accounted for 13.6% and bacterial/yeast infections for 34.6%. The incidence of bloodstream infection was 21/1,000 patient days. The infection rate due to microorganisms acquired in the PICU was 15.8%; 3.7% of admitted children developed infections due to resistant microorganisms. Causative microorganisms were CNS, enterococci, *Pseudomonas* spp., *S. aureus* and yeasts. A study from London, UK, reported an incidence of bloodstream infection of 46.9/1,000 patient days in a subset of 103 children with a line in situ for a median of 6 days [16]. The causative organisms were CNS, *S. aureus, C. albicans* and *Klebsiella* spp.

17.3.2.2 Lower Airway Infections

In a paediatric trauma unit, the rate of lower airway infections was 5.5% [17]. The most common organisms were *S. aureus, Haemophilus influenzae, Enterobacter* and *Pseudomonas* spp. [17]. In the Liverpool study, the overall airway infection rate was 11%, with a rate of 9.3 episodes/1,000 patient days [9]. The three main organisms were *S. aureus, P. aeruginosa* and *H. influenzae*.

17.4 Assessing the Magnitude of the Problem

17.4.1 Carrier State: Endogenous Versus Exogenous

The magnitude of the problem can be assessed in different ways based upon carrier state (Chap. 5). Endogenous must be distinguished from exogenous infection. Endogenous infection is caused by potential pathogens previously carried by the patient; if the potential pathogen was present on that patient's admission, then the infection due to this potential pathogen is called primary endogenous. This type of infection tends to occur early, within the first week. If the infection is due to a potential pathogen acquired in the unit, after the patient goes through the carriage phase, then the infection is termed secondary endogenous. Infections caused by microorganisms not carried by the patient at all are termed exogenous. Obviously, surveillance cultures are indispensable for this classification [6, 9].

17.4.2 Pathogenicity Index

Some microorganisms cause more serious clinical disease than others. This differential pathogenic effect can be used to develop a pathogenicity index for an individual microorganism, in a specific organ system and in a particular homogeneous population for which surveillance cultures are useful [18]. The ratio between the number of ICU patients infected by a particular microorganisms and the number of patients simply carrying that organism in their throat and/or gut is defined as the intrinsic pathogenicity index for a particular microorganism. Indigenous flora, including anaerobes, will rarely cause infections in the lower airways of patients requiring ventilation for more than 3 days despite being carried in high concentrations. This is because they have intrinsic pathogenicity index values of between 0.01 and 0.03. Low-level pathogens, such as viridans streptococci, enterococci and CNS are also carried in high concentrations in the oropharynx by a substantial percentage of ICU patients and are unable to cause lower airway infections. High-level pathogens such as *S. pyogenes* and *Salmonella* spp. have an intrinsic pathogenicity index approaching 1 and diseases manifest in virtually all oropharyngeal and gut carriers. The concept of carriage recognises

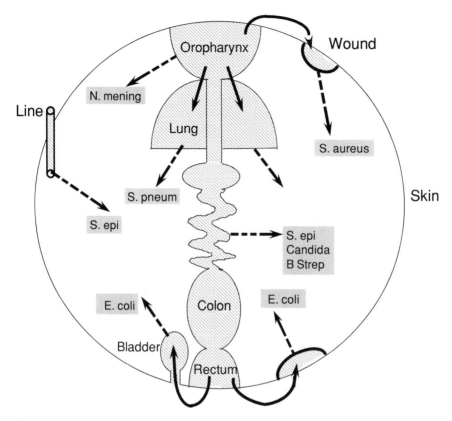

Fig. 17.1 Schematic representation of the digestive tract, illustrating that the throat and gut are the major internal sources of potential pathogens causing endogenous infections of blood, lower airways, bladder and wounds

about 15 potentially pathogenic microorganisms, with intrinsic pathogenicity indices between 0.1 and 0.3. these consist of the six normal microorganisms *S. pneumoniae*, *H. influenzae*, *Moraxella catarrhalis*, *E. coli*, *S. aureus* and *C. albicans* present in previously healthy individuals, and nine abnormal bacteria carried by patients with an underlying chronic or acute condition, namely: *Klebsiella*, *Proteus*, *Morganella*, *Enterobacter*, *Citrobacter*, *Serratia*, *Pseudomonas* and *Acinetobacter* spp. and methicillin-resistant *S. aureus* (MRSA). The overall mortality in our PICU is in the range of 5%, but the mortality rate rises to 10% in the subset of children who require prolonged mechanical ventilation [9].

17.5 Pathogenesis

Figure 17.1 describes the pathogenesis of infection in neonates and children requiring intensive care. Practically all infections in these two groups are endogenous—patients become infected with microorganisms they carry. A recent study in 400 PICU children requiring ventilation demonstrated that 90% of all lower airway infections were endogenous; 80% were primary endogenous, 10% secondary endogenous and the remaining 10% exogenous [6].

Bloodstream infections occur due to translocation. Microorganisms in overgrowth of the terminal ileum ($>10^5$ microorganisms/ml) migrate into the bloodstream [19]. This mechanism applies to *S. agalactiae*, *S. aureus* and *C.* spp. Neonates and children staying longer that 1 week in the NICU or PICU, CNS and AGNB cause septicaemia due to translocation [20].

Lower airway infections are caused by microorganisms carried in the oropharynx, which then migrate into the lower airways. In a previous healthy child *S. pneumoniae*, *H. influenzae* and *S. aureus* cause bacterial lower airway infections. AGNB and MRSA are causative organisms in children who require intensive care >1 week.

Bladder infections are, in general, endogenous due to migrating faecal bacteria. Wound infections of the head, neck and thorax are, in general, caused by oral bacteria, whereas wound infections between the waist and knee are primarily caused by gut bacteria.

Exogenous infections vary between 5% and 25% and are a particular problem in patients with tracheostomies [21]. Children with wounds, particularly burns, are at high risk of exogenous colonisation and infection [9]. Up to 16% of bloodstream infections are of exogenous pathogenesis following contamination of an indwelling intravascular device [19]. Gastrostomies can also be considered as a wound, and recurrent exogenous colonisation/infection is not uncommon in children with such devices [9]. To identify an exogenous infection, surveillance samples of throat and rectum are indispensable. Blood cultures or lower airway secretions are positive for a potential pathogen that is not present in throat and or rectal cultures.

17.5.1 Risk Factors

Risk factor analysis in the pathogenesis of NICU and PICU infections invariably includes low birth weight; administration of total parenteral nutrition; presence of invasive and indwelling devices, including endotracheal tube and mechanical ventilation; length of stay; and prior use of antibiotics [2, 22, 23]. All these factors are reflected in illness severity and are difficult to modify to control infection. Risk factor analysis cannot easily contribute to infection control.

17.6 Diagnosis

17.6.1 Infection

Infection is a microbiologically proven, clinical diagnosis of local and/or general inflammation. The signs of generalised infections in NICU patients, e.g. septicaemia, are often nonspecific and may be clinically indistinguishable from those of noninfectious conditions [2]. For instance, the clinical picture of respiratory distress in early onset sepsis may be identical to hyaline membrane disease. Furthermore, the clinical diagnosis of local infection, such as meningitis, may not differ from that of systemic sepsis without meningeal involvement. On the other hand, infections in the PICU patient are more specific, and the following description of local and general infection is related to paediatric patients.

17.6.2 Pneumonia

17.6.2.1 Microbiologically Proven Pneumonia
1. presence of new or progressive pulmonary infiltrates on a chest X-ray for ≥ 48 h, and
2. purulent tracheal aspirate, and
3. fever $\geq 38.5°C$, and
4. leucocytosis [white blood cells (WBC) > 12,000/ml] or leucopenia (WBC < 4,000/ml), and
5. tracheal aspirate $\geq 10^5$ colony forming units (CFU)/ml of potentially pathogenic microorganism or bronchoalveolar lavage (BAL) yielding $\geq 10^4$ CFU/ml.

17.6.2.2 Clinical Diagnosis
Criteria 1–4 above and sterile BAL or tracheal aspirate.

17.6.3 Tracheitis/Bronchitis

1. purulent tracheal aspirate, and
2. fever $\geq 38.5°C$, and
3. leucocytosis (WBC > 12,000/ml) or leucopenia (WBC < 4,000/ml), and
4. tracheal aspirate yielding $\geq 10^5$ CFU/ml, and, most importantly
5. normal chest X-ray.

17.6.4 Systemic Inflammatory Response Syndrome

Clinical signs of generalised inflammation caused by microorganisms and/or their products, including at least three of the following: fever, temperature instability, lethargy, poor perfusion, hypotension.

17.6.5 Blood Stream Infections

Criteria as for Systemic Inflammatory Response Syndrome (SIRS), with a positive blood culture from either a peripheral vein or an intravascular device.

17.6.6 Intra-Abdominal Infection

Intra-abdominal infection is defined as affecting an abdominal organ and the peritoneal cavity (peritonitis), with local signs such as abdominal tenderness and generalised symptoms including fever and leucocytosis. Peritonitis can be a localised or generalised infection of the peritoneal cavity. Following ultrasound and/or computed tomography scan and/or laparotomy, the diagnosis is confirmed by the isolation of microorganisms of $\geq 3 +$ or $\geq 10^5$ CFU/ml and >++leucocytes in the diagnostic sample [24].

17.6.7 Urinary Tract Infection

Infection of the urinary tract most often involves the bladder. The common features of dysuria, suprapubic pain and urinary frequency and urgency are often not assessable in PICU patients. Therefore, the diagnosis of cystitis is based upon freshly obtained catheter urine containing $\geq 10^5$ CFU/ml and ≥ 5 WBC/ml high power light microscopy field.

17.6.8 Wound Infection

Purulent discharge from wounds, a culture yielding $\geq 3 +$ or $\geq 10^5$ CFU/ml of pus and signs of local inflammation. Isolation of skin flora is considered to be contamination.

17.7 Prevention

Besides the five infection-control interventions (Chap. 10), there is evidence for the effectiveness of only two antibiotic manoeuvres that prevent infection in NICU and PICU patients: surgical prophylaxis [25–27] and selective decontamination of the digestive tract (SDD) (Table 17.1) [28–33].

17.7.1 Cardiac Surgical Prophylaxis

The aim of prophylactic antibiotics in cardiac surgery is to prevent infections of the mediastinal incision and the heart. The main microorganisms causing endocarditis are CNS, viridans streptococci and enterococci; less common are AGNB and yeasts. S. aureus, both sensitive and resistant to methicillin, are the main cause of mediastinal wound infections. A commonly used combination of antimicrobials prior to cardiac surgery is a glycopeptide and an aminoglycoside. A glycopeptide such as teicoplanin covers all streptococci and staphylococci, whereas an aminoglycoside such as netilmicin is active against AGNB that may translocate following gut

17 Infection in the NICU and PICU

Table 17.1 Cardiac and general surgical prophylaxis and prevention protocol for selective decontamination of the digestive tract (SDD)

Surgical prophylaxis	Total daily dose (mg/kg)			
	<7 days	>7 days	1 month–12 years	>12 years
Cardiac				
Teicoplanin	16 then 8		20, then 10, then 6	400 mg then 200 mg
Netilmicin	3 < 2 kg 6 > 2 kg	6	6	200 mg
General				
Cefotaxime	100	150	100–200	6–12 g
Metronidazole	22.5	22.5	22.5	1.5 g
Gentamicin	3 < 2 kg 6 > 2 kg	6 < 2 kg 7.5 > 2 kg	7.5	3–5

SDD	Total daily dose (mg/day)		
	<5 years	5–12 years	>12 years
Oropharynx			
AGNB: polymyxin E with tobramycin	2 g of 2% paste/gel	2 g of 2% paste/gel	2 g of 2% paste/gel
Yeasts: amphotericin B	2 g of 2% paste/gel	2 g of 2% paste/gel	2 g of 2% paste/gel
MRSA: vancomycin	2 g of 2% paste/gel	2 g of 2% paste/gel	2 g of 2% paste/gel
Gut			
AGNB: polymyxin E with tobramycin	100 80	200 160	400 320
Yeasts: amphotericin B	400	1,000	2,000
MRSA: vancomycin	20–40 mg/kg	20–40 mg/kg	500–2,000

Therapy	Total daily dose (mg/kg)			
	<7 days	>7 days	1 month–12 years	>12 years
Neonatal ICU				
Ampicillin: active against *L. monocytogenes* and *S. agalactiae* Gentamicin: AGNB	50	100		
Paediatric ICU				
Cefotaxime: community + hospital microbes excluding *P. aeruginosa*	100	150	100–200	6–12 g
Ceftazidime: *P. aeruginosa*	60	90	100–150	6–9 g
Gentamicin: AGNB	3 < 2 kg 6 > 2 kg	6 < 2 kg 7.5 > 2 kg	7.5	3–5
Cephradine: *S. aureus*	50	50	100	4 g
Vancomycin: MRSA	15 then 20	15 then 30	45	2 g
Amphotericin B: yeasts, fungi (lipophilic)	1–3	1–3	1–3	1–3

ICU intensive care unit; *AGNB* aerobic Gram-negative bacilli; *MRSA* methicillin-resistant *Staphylococcus aureus*; L. monocytogenes, *Listeria monocytogenes*; S. agalactiae, *Streptococcus agalactiae*; P. aeruginosa, *Pseudomonas aeruginosa*

ischaemia. Short-term prophylaxis of three doses is normally administered: one immediately prior to surgery to achieve high tissues concentrations, and two further doses 8-h apart. Under certain circumstances, such as a chest splinted open because of cardiac oedema, these antibiotics may be continued for 5 days, though there is no evidence to support the added efficacy of this practice.

17.7.2 General Surgical Prophylaxis

The type of antimicrobial prescribed depends on the proposed surgery and the associated contamination risk. Clean, sterile procedures do not need antibiotic cover, whereas clean procedures with the likelihood of contamination need cover with one antimicrobial, such as cefotaxime. If there is likely to be faecal contamination, then an aminoglycoside such as gentamicin is also necessary to cover AGNB and enterococci. Finally, if the surgical procedure is likely to be associated with ischaemia and possible necrotic tissue, then metronidazole should be added to the prophylactic regimen. Again, three doses as above will suffice.

17.7.3 Selective Decontamination of the Digestive Tract

SDD is a prophylactic intervention designed to prevent early and late infection and is recommended in the critically ill child requiring >1 week of intensive care (Chap. 14). Four prospective randomised controlled trials [28–32] demonstrate a significant reduction in infectious morbidity using SDD. As the overall mortality rate in this population is approximately 10%, a reduction in that rate is harder to demonstrate than in adults; a huge sample size would be necessary. However, in adults, where the overall mortality rate is approximately 30%, this method demonstrates a significant reduction of 40% [33–35].

There is particular indication for SDD in the NICU, namely, for controlling an infection outbreak. A decade ago, SDD with nystatin was used to control a *C. parapsilosis* outbreak in the Mersey, UK, regional NICU: 76 of 106 neonates who carried the outbreak strain received nystatin in the throat and gut during the 12-month open trial; six neonates developed fungaemia. Once the carriage rate fell from 50 to 5%, no new cases of systemic *Candida* infection were observed. This was the first report of SDD intervention to control an infection outbreak in an NICU [36].

17.8 Meta-Analysis of Randomised Control Trials in Children with Severe Lower Airway and Bloodstream Infections Using SDD

Data was extracted from four randomized controlled trials (RCTs) of selective digestive decontamination in the *paediatric population* (Table 17.2). *The four RCTs* enrolled 335 patients. Pneumonia occurred in five of 170 (2.9%) of patients

Table 17.2 Data extracted from four randomised controlled trials of selective decontamination of the digestive tract in the paediatric population

Author	Patients		Patients with infection		Patients with pneumonia		Mortality	
	SDD	C	SDD	C	SDD	C	SDD	C
Zobel [28]	25	25	2	10	1	6	3	2
Smith [29]	18	18	3	11[a]	0	2	2	3
Ruza [30]	116	110	NA	NA	3	8	6	5
Barret [31]	11	12	5	3	1	0	2	1

SDD selective decontamination of the digestive tract; *C* control; *NA* not available
[a] Patients with Gram-negative infections

Table 17.3 Meta-analysis of the impact of selective decontamination of the digestive tract on secondary endpoints

Outcome	RCTs	No. of patients		No. of patients with outcome		OR[a] (95 CI)	p value	I^2 (%)
		SDD	C	SDD	C			
Infection	3	54	55	10	24	0.34 (0.05–2.18)	0.25	4.7
Mortality	4	170	163	13	11	1.18 (0.50–2.76)	0.70	0

RCTs randomised controlled trials; *OR* odds ratio; *CI* confidence interval; *SDD* selective decontamination of the digestive tract; *C* control
[a] OR less than the unit favours treatment; OR more than the unit favours controls

who received SDD and in 16 of 163 (9.8%) in the control group. This was a significant reduction in the incidence of pneumonia with SDD [odds ratio (OR) 0.31; 95% confidence interval (CI), 0.11–0.87; *P = 0.027*]. A meta-analysis was performed on the impact of SDD on the secondary endpoints of pneumonia and overall infection rates (Table 17.3). In the three eligible RCTs of a total of 109 children, infections of various origins were confirmed in ten of 54 (13%) on SDD and in 24 of 55 (15.9%) in the control group. SDD had no impact on general infection rates, with no significant difference between groups (OR 0.34; 95% CI 0.05–2.18; $P = 0.25$).

Subgroup analyses of type of SDD regimen, randomisation and blinding revealed a significant impact on pneumonia and infection rates when the full protocol of parenteral and enteral antimicrobials was used rather than solely enterally administered antimicrobials. A significant impact on pneumonia and overall infection was demonstrated when randomisation was adequate and in unblinded studies. The subgroup analyses for mortality were consistent with previous pooled results whether the intervention was parenteral/enteral or enteral, whether the design was blinded or not and whether the randomisation process was adequate or not. SDD made no significant impact on mortality rates.

Day one: absence of knowledge of causative microorganism
Empirical treatment: Cefotaxime combined with gentamicin if seriously ill

Day two: presumptive identification of causative microorganism				
Tailored treatment:				
Normal potential patmhogen			Abnormal potential pathogen	
S. pneumoniae	*S. aureus*	*Candida* spp.	Aerobic Gram-negative bacilli	*Pseudomonas* spp.
Stop gentamicin	Stop cefotaxime/ gentamicin	Stop cefotaxime/ gentamicin	Continue cefotaxime/ gentamicin	Replace cefotaxime with ceftazidime
Monotherapy: cefotaxime	Monotherapy: cephradine	Monotherapy: amphotericin B		

Day three: clinical improvement

Day five: stop or change antimicrobial treatment	
Stop	Change
Improved after careful clinical, radiological and microbiological evaluation	Not improved after careful clinical, radiological and microbiological evaluation

Fig. 17.2 Flow diagram for treating an infection

17.9 Treatment

17.9.1 Neonatal Intensive Care Unit

Early-onset infections in the NICU may be due to *L. monocytogenes* and/or *S. agalactiae*. Ampicillin is the most active antibiotic against these two microorganisms, which are acquired from the mother, and is combined with gentamicin to cover AGNB and *S. aureus*. Late-onset infections are treated in the manner described in Fig. 17.2.

17.9.2 Paediatric Intensive Care Unit

When a child is admitted to the PICU with a severe infection, a decision must be made as to which antimicrobial will be used. Antimicrobials are used in combination depending on the severity of the illness; our experience over 20 years led us to choose cefotaxime and gentamicin. This choice is empirical due to the absence of any knowledge regarding the causative microorganism, though reasonable assumptions can be made depending of the child's presentation. For example, a child with meningococcal disease requires cefotaxime only; metronidazole can be added in case of presumed anaerobic involvement. When a presumptive identification of the microorganism can be made, the physician can then tailor therapy. Cefotaxime/gentamicin can be replaced by cephradine for an infection due to *S. pneumoniae*, *S. pyogenes* and *S. aureus*. When *P. aeruginosa* is isolated, ceftazidime should replace cefotaxime and the gentamicin continued. Yeast infections require liposomal amphotericin B in place of cefotaxime/gentamicin (Fig. 17.2). The efficacy of the antimicrobial treatment can be monitored using C-reactive protein (CRP) levels in addition to the clinical, radiographic and microbiological variables. Providing the antimicrobials used are correct, the child will improve within 3 days; in our experience, a short, 5-day course of intravenously administered antibiotics is as effective as a course of 2 weeks or more (Chap. 12). After 5 days, the child is monitored for signs of infection; when there are no signs of infection, antibiotics are discontinued. Should there be no improvement after 5 days, a change in antibiotic regimen is necessary.

Metronidazole is given for 3 days only. The antifungal agent, liposomal amphotericin B, is given for 3 weeks and may be discontinued once the CRP level is normal. Systemic antimicrobials are combined with enterally administered SDD agents to guarantee prevention of potential pathogens becoming resistant to the systemic agents.

References

1. Damjanovic V, van Saene HKF (1998) Outbreaks of infection in a neonatal intensive care unit. In: van Saene HKF, Silvestri L, de la Cal MA (eds) Infection control in the intensive care unit. Springer, Milan, pp 237–248
2. Isaacs D, Moxon ER (1991) Neonatal infections. Butterworth-Heinemann, Oxford
3. van Saene HKF, Leonard EM, Shears P (1989) Ecological impact of antibiotics in neonatal units. Lancet II:509–510
4. de Man P, Verhoeven BAN, Verburgh HA et al (2000) An antibiotic policy to prevent emergence of resistant bacilli. Lancet 355:973–978
5. Murphy N, Damjanovic V, Hart CA et al (1986) Infection and colonisation of neonates by *Hansenula anomala*. Lancet I:291–293

6. Silvestri L, Sargison RE, Hughes J et al (2002) Most nosocomial pneumonias are not due to nosocomial bacteria in ventilated patients: evaluation of the accuracy of the 48 h time cut-off using carriage as the gold standard. Anaesth Intensive Care 30:275–282
7. Petros AJ, O'Connell M, Roberts C et al (2001) Systemic antibiotics fail to clear multidrug-resistant *Klebsiella* from a paediatric ICU. Chest 119:862–866
8. Goldmann DA, Leclair J, Macone A (1978) Bacterial colonization of neonates admitted to an intensive care environment. J Pediatr 2:288–293
9. Sarginson RE, Taylor N, Reilly N et al (2004) Infection in prolonged pediatric critical illness: a prospective three year study based on knowledge of the carrier state. Crit Care Med 32(3):839–847
10. Baltimore RS (1998) Neonatal nosocomial infections. Semin Perinatol 22:25–32
11. Beck-Sague CM, Azimi P, Fonseca SN et al (1994) Bloodstream infections in neonatal intensive care unit patients: results of a multicenter study. Pediatr Infect Dis J 13:1110–1116
12. Gaynes RP, Martone WJ, Culver DH et al (1991) Comparison of rates of nosocomial infections in neonatal intensive care units in the United States. Am J Med 91(suppl 3B):192–196
13. La Gamma EF, Drusin LM, Mackles AW et al (1983) Neonatal infections: an important determinant of late NICU mortality in infants less than 1,000 g at birth. Am J Dis Child 137:838–841
14. Richards MJ, Edwards JR, Culver DH, Gaynes RP, The National Nosocomial Infections Surveillance System (1999) Nosocomial infection in pediatric intensive care units in the United States. Pediatrics 103(4):e39
15. Gray J, Gossain S, Morris K (2001) Three-year survey of bacteraemia and fungemia in a pediatric intensive care unit. Pediatr Infect Dis J 20:416–421
16. Pierce CM, Wade A, Mok Q (2000) Heparin-bonded central venous lines reduce thrombotic and infective complications in critically ill children. Intensive Care Med 26:967–972
17. Patel JC, Mollitt DL, Pieper P, Tepas JJ III (2000) Nosocomial pneumonia in the pediatric trauma patient: a single center's experience. Critical Care Med 28:3530–3533
18. Leonard EM, van Saene HKF, Stoutenbeek CP et al (1990) An intrinsic pathogenicity index for micro-organisms causing infections in a neonatal surgical unit. Microb Ecol Health Dis 2:151–157
19. van Saene HKF, Taylor N, Donnell SC et al (2003) Gut overgrowth with abnormal flora: the missing link in parenteral nutrition-related sepsis in surgical neonates. Eur J Clin Nutrit 57:548–553
20. Donnell SC, Taylor N, van Saene HKF et al (2002) Infection rates in surgical neonates and infants receiving parenteral nutrition: a five year prospective study. J Hosp Infect 52:273–280
21. Morar P, Singh V, Makura Z et al (2002) Differing pathways of lower airway colonization and infection according to mode of ventilation (endotracheal vs. tracheostomy). Arch Otolaryngol Head Neck Surg 128:1061–1066
22. Singh-Naz N, Sprague BM, Patel K et al (2000) Risk assessment and standardized nosocomial infection rate in critically ill children. Crit Care Med 28:2069–2075
23. Mahieu LM, De Muynck AO, De Dooy JJ et al (2000) Prediction of nosocomial sepsis in neonates by means of a computer-weighted bed side scoring system (NOSEP score). Crit Care Med 28:2026–2033
24. A'Court CH, Garrard CS, Crook D et al (1993) Microbiological lung surveillance in mechanically ventilated patients, using non-directed bronchial lavage and quantitative culture. QJM 86:635–638
25. Petros AJ, Marshall JC, van Saene HK (1995) Should morbidity replace mortality as an endpoint for critical trials in intensive care? Lancet 345:369–371
26. Kaiser AB (1986) Antimicrobial prophylaxis in surgery. New Engl J Med 315:1129–1138
27. Infection in Neurosurgery Working Party of the British Society for Antimicrobial Chemotherapy (1994) Antimicrobial prophylaxis in neurosurgery and after head injury. Lancet 344:1547–1551

28. Zobel G, Kuttnig GHM et al (1991) Reduction of colonization and infection rate during pediatric intensive care by selective decontamination of the digestive tract. Crit Care Med 19:1242–1246
29. Smith SD, Jackson RJ, Hannakan CJ et al (1993) Selective decontamination in pediatric liver transplants. Transplantation 55:1306–1309
30. Ruza F, Alvarado F, Herruzo R et al (1998) Prevention of nosocomial infection in a pediatric intensive care unit (PICU) through the use of selective decontamination. Eur J Epidemiol 14:719–727
31. Barret JP, Jeschke MG, Herndon DN (2001) Selective decontamination of the digestive tract in severely burned pediatric patients. Burns 27:439–445
32. Alder Hey Therapeutic Guideline Index.http://www.nppg.scot.nhs.uk/protocols/therapeutic_guidelines_index.htm
33. D'Amico R, Pifferi S, Leonetti C et al (1998) Effectiveness of antibiotic prophylaxis in critically ill adult patients: systematic review of randomized controlled trials. BMJ 316:1275–1285
34. Nathens AB, Marshall JC (1999) Selective decontamination of the digestive tract in surgical patients: a systematic review of the evidence. Arch Surg 134:70–76
35. De Jonge E, Schultz MJ, Spanjaard L et al (2002) Effects of selective decontamination of the digestive tract on mortality and antibiotic resistance. Intensive Care Med 28(Suppl 1):S12
36. Damjanovic V, Connolly CM, van Saene HKF et al (1993) Selective decontamination with nystatin for the control of a Candida outbreak in the neonatal intensive care unit. J Hosp Infect 24:245–259

Early Adequate Antibiotic Therapy

R. Reina and M. A. de la Cal

18.1 Introduction

The most widely accepted definition of inappropriate antibiotic treatment in the intensive care unit (ICU) encompasses the use of an agent to which the pathogen is resistant [1] or delay in prescribing the antibiotic to which the pathogen is sensitive. Some attention has been given to the fact that failure of anti-infective therapy in the ICU might also occur due to inappropriate dosing, potentially leading to suboptimal exposure to the broad-spectrum antimicrobial agent at the infection site, even if it is administered in a timely manner [2].

The pattern of in vitro antibiotic sensitivity/resistance has been universally accepted as the main component of antibiotic therapy appropriateness. The delay between initial symptoms and antimicrobial administration is still a matter of discussion and might vary according to the study and symptom severity of the included patients. Kollef et al. [3] defined inadequate antimicrobial treatment as microbiological documentation of infection that was not effectively treated at the time the causative microorganism and its antibiotic susceptibility were known, without paying attention to the time delay between the first symptoms of sepsis and the microbiological results. Harbarth et al. [4], in a population of septic patients, considered their treatment as inappropriate because the antimicrobial agent was not administered within 24 h of primary microbial isolation from blood or a remote infection site. Kumar et al. [5], in septic shock patients, considered therapy to be effective when antimicrobials with in vitro activity appropriate for the isolated pathogen or pathogens was received after the onset of recurrent or persistent

M. A. de la Cal (✉)
Department of Intensive Care Medicine,
Hospital Universitario de Getafe, Getafe, Spain
e-mail: mcal@ucigetafe.com

hypotension or initiated within 6 h of administration of the first new antimicrobial agent.

18.2 Impact on Morbidity and Mortality

Appropriate antibiotic treatment was consistently associated with reduced mortality rates in infected ICU patients, and this benefit was higher in patients with severe sepsis and septic shock [3, 4]. Garnacho et al. [6] conducted a retrospective case-control study of 87 ICU patients with sepsis adjusted by origin of sepsis, inflammatory response at admission, surgical or medical status, hospital- or community-acquired sepsis, Acute Physiology and Chronic Health Evaluation (APACHE) II score (+2 points) and age (+10 years). Therapy was considered inadequate when no effective drug against the isolated pathogen(s) was included in the empirical antibiotic treatment within the first 24 h of admission to the ICU or the doses and pattern of administration were not in accordance with current medical standards. ICU mortality rates in patients with inadequate treatment were 67.8% [95% confidence interval (CI) 58.0–77.6] versus 28.7% (95% CI 19.2–38.2) in patients receiving appropriate treatment. ICU length of stay in surviving patients was 11 (7–19) and 7 (6–19) days, respectively. Kumar et al. [5], in a retrospective study of 2,731 patients with septic shock, found a strong relationship between delay in effective antimicrobial initiation and in-hospital mortality rates [adjusted odds ratio (OR) 1.12 per hour delay, 95% CI 1.103–1.136]. This increased mortality rate per hour of delay was not associated with the type of infection. A clinical conclusion of the study was that in patients with septic shock, the adequate treatment should be initiated as soon as possible after taking samples for microbiological cultures when indicated. Barochia et al. [7] performed a systematic review of eight unblinded trials, one randomized trial, and seven with historical controls to assess the efficacy of all the recommended practices in treating patients with sepsis [8]. They concluded that for all studies reporting the impact in mortality rates, the only intervention consistently associated to a reduced rate is the appropriateness of antibiotics. Five trials [9–13] provided data of the association between actual mean time from presentation and antibiotic administration. All but one [9] showed a survival benefit of early antibiotic administration.

18.3 Empirical Treatment: Monotherapy Versus Combined Therapy

The rationale for appropriate antibiotic therapy is to increase the likelihood that the infective pathogen will be susceptible in vivo to the prescribed antimicrobial. It implies the in vitro susceptibility to the antibiotic, delay between symptoms and antibiotic administration, dose, and pharmacodynamics (PD) and pharmacokinetics (PK) of antimicrobials. According to these premises, prescription of the adequate antibiotic must taken into account:

- type of infection: community-acquired pneumonia, ventilator-associated pneumonia, abdominal sepsis, catheter-related bloodstream infection, soft-tissue infection, etc;
- antibiotic sensitivity/resistance of ICU flora;
- patient comorbidity: asplenia, renal failure, neutropenia, immunosuppression, allergy, obesity,etc.

Adequate empirical treatment is crucial to reduce mortality risk in severely ill patients. Theoretically, this objective might be better achieved with combined therapy instead of with monotherapy, but this subject is still under discussion [14, 15].

The effect of monotherapy (meropenem) versus combined therapy (meropenem plus ciprofloxacin) has been assessed in a randomized clinical trial of 740 mechanically ventilated patients who developed suspected ventilator-associated pneumonia (VAP) [16] Patients who were known to be previously infected or colonized with *Pseudomonas* spp. or methicillin-resistant *Staphylococcus aureus* (MRSA) were excluded from the trial. The median time from suspicion of VAP to initiation of study antibiotics was 4 h. The proportion of patients who received adequate initial antibiotics was significantly greater in the combination group than in the monotherapy group (93.1 vs. 85.1%, $p = 0.01$). Reasons for inadequate initial therapy were related to the presence of *Pseudomonas* or *Acinetobacter* spp., *Stenotrophomonas maltophilia*, other multi-drug-resistant Gram-negative bacteria, and MRSA. There were no differences between groups in the main outcomes of mortality, time from randomization to discontinuation of mechanical ventilation alive, and discharge from ICU alive. These results support the use of monotherapy as empirical treatment in patients with suspected pneumonia if local resistance patterns or individual patient risk factors do not suggest the possibility of multi-drug-resistant organisms or other difficult-to-treat organisms.

Garnacho et al. [17] retrospectively estimated the association of monotherapy versus combined therapy with mortality in 183 episodes of VAP caused by *Pseudomonas aeruginosa*. When *P. aeruginosa* was susceptible to the antimicrobial used in monotherapy, there was no difference in mortality rates compared with the group treated with combined therapy. Monotherapy versus combined therapy has been also compared in patients with sepsis and septic shock. In a systematic review, Safdar et al. [18] estimated the effect of both types of therapy in Gram-negative bacteremia. Seventeen studies were included (five prospective cohort studies, two prospective randomized trials, and ten retrospective cohort studies). There was no difference in mortality rates between monotherapy and combined therapy (OR 0.96; 95% CI 0.70–1.32). The same conclusion was reached in a subgroup analysis [19] of four studies (three retrospective cohort studies, one prospective cohort study) of patients with *P. aeruginosa* bacteremia (OR 1.31; 95% CI 0.62–2.79), but the low design quality of the studies and the high heterogeneity of their results (42%) preclude any strong conclusion. The addition of aminoglycoside to beta-lactams increases the risk of nephrotoxicity [20].

Kumar et al. [21], in a subgroup analysis of observational studies and randomized clinical trials of bacterial infections potentially associated with sepsis or septic shock, found that when the monotherapy groups have a mortality rate

>25%, there is a potential benefit of combined therapy (OR 0.49; 95% CI 0.35–0.70). The authors did not provide data of the main confounding factor: appropriateness of the initial antimicrobial treatment.

In conclusion, the best evidence supports that in nonneutropenic critically ill patients, combined therapy is only justified as empirical treatment when it is suspected to be caused by highly resistant microorganisms, such as resistant *Pseudomonas* or *Acinetobacter* spp., other multi-drug-resistant Gram-negative bacteria, and MRSA. Most severe patients, i.e., septic shock patients, may benefit from broad coverage with combined therapy to provide a higher likelihood of adequate treatment.

18.4 De-escalation

Initial empiric therapy can be appropriate in 80–90% patients if it is selected following the recommendations provided by guidelines supported by most authoritative scientific societies. Following initial empiric therapy, de-escalation means using microbiologic and clinical data to change from an initial broad-spectrum or multidrug empiric therapy regimen to a regimen with fewer antibiotics and agents of narrower spectrum, reduced therapy duration, and stopping treatment as dictated by results of microbiological cultures and clinical response [22]. The rationale of de-escalation is to reduce the use of antimicrobials to reduce costs, adverse effects, and antibiotic resistance. It is included as a component of the stewardship to optimize antibiotic use in hospitals [23].

De-escalation strategies have been mostly evaluated in VAP. Alvarez-Lerma et al. [24] performed one prospective multicenter study to evaluate the results of implementing a protocol of nosocomial pneumonia therapy that recommended de-escalation. They enrolled 258 patients; appropriate treatment was prescribed in 89% of cases. In 113 of them, microbiological cultures of respiratory samples were negative, and the empirical treatment was continued unmodified. In 108 patients with adequate treatment, at least one pathogen was identified. In only 56 of those patients (24%) was therapy de-escalated. The results emphasize two conclusions: (1) different options to treat patients with suspected nosocomial pneumonia with negative microbiological cultures should be tested in randomized clinical trials; (2) implementation of de-escalation in ICU may be increased. Similar de-escalation percentages have been reported in another observational study [25].

Singh et al. [26] performed a randomized clinical trial in 81 critically ill patients with suspected nosocomial pneumonia and low clinical pulmonary infection score (≤ 6) to evaluate the outcomes of early discontinuation of empirical treatment (ciprofloxacin) when the score remained ≤ 6 versus standard therapy. Results of a comparison between a short course of ciprofloxacin and standard therapy showed mortality rate 0 versus 7% (not significant); length of ICU stay 9 versus 14 days ($p = 0.04$); antimicrobial resistance 14 versus 38% ($p \leq 0.017$) and total costs of the episode UD $6,482 versus $16,004, respectively.

The usefulness of biomarkers to guide treatment has been estimated in clinical trials. Christ-Crain et al. [27] performed a cluster-randomized clinical trial in 243 patients (87 with pneumonia) with suspected lower respiratory tract infections admitted to the emergency department. Patients were randomly assigned either to standard antimicrobial therapy or procalcitonin-guided antimicrobial treatment. On the basis of serum procalcitonin concentrations, use of antibiotics was more or less discouraged (<0.1 µg/L or <0.25 µg/L) or encouraged ($\geq$0.5 µg/L or $\geq$0.25 µg/L), respectively. Duration of antibiotic treatment was shorter in the procalcitonin group (11 vs. 13 days; $p = 0.03$) as well as antibiotic costs of US $96 versus US $202 per patient ($p < 0.0001$). These results were reproduced by the same group in patients with suspected community-acquired pneumonia [28].

Stolz et al. [29], in a multicenter randomized clinical trial, assigned 101 patients with suspected VAP to a therapy according to the American Thoracic Society guidelines or a protocol guided by serum procalcitonin levels during the first 2 days of treatment. Procalcitonin level at day 2:
- <0.25 µg/L discontinuation of antibiotics was strongly encouraged;
- between 0.25 and 0.5 µg/L or a decrease by $\geq$80% compared with day 0 discontinuation of antibiotics was encouraged;
- $\geq$0.5 µg/L or decrease by <80% compared with day 0 discontinuation of antibiotics was discouraged;
- >1 µg/L antibiotic discontinuation was strongly discouraged.

Overall duration of antibiotic therapy was reduced from 15 to 10 days ($p = 0.04$). The number of mechanical ventilation-free days alive, ICU-free days alive, length of hospital stay, and mortality rate on day 28 for the two groups were similar.

Nobre et al. [30] tested the hypothesis that an algorithm based on serial measurements of procalcitonin allows reduction in antibiotic therapy duration in patients with severe sepsis or septic shock. Patients in the procalcitonin-guided group were re-evaluated following a protocol in which: (1) patients with baseline levels $\geq$1 µg/L were re-evaluated at day 5; if procalcitonin dropped >90% from baseline or <0.25 µg/L was reached, investigators encourage to discontinue antibiotics; (2) patients with baseline levels <1 µg/L were re-evaluated at day 3; treating physicians were encouraged to discontinue antibiotics when the procalcitonin level was <0.1 µg/L. Duration was 3.5 days shorter in the procalcitonin group (6 vs. 9.5 days; $p = 0.15$). In summary guiding treatment using biomarkers is safe but only provides marginal benefits.

18.5 Antibiotics Dosage in Critically Ill Patients with Severe Sepsis and Septic Shock: Pharmacokinetics/Pharmacodynamics Parameters

Prescribing antibiotics, including empirical antibiotics, for critically ill patients is a complex process that requires ongoing patient health evaluation to account for the dynamic sepsis disease process. Pathophysiological changes, such as organ dysfunction, fluid shifts, and altered immune status, are common and are able to

Table 18.1 Time- and concentration-dependent antibiotics

Time-dependent killing	Concentration-dependent killing
Penicillins	
Cephalosporins	Aminoglycosides
Macrolides	Fluoroquinolones
Carbapenems	Amphotericin B
Clindamycin	Metronidazole
Linezolid	Colistine
Vancomycin	
Tigecycline	

reduce the efficacy of anti-infective treatment. In recent years, more attention is being paid to how critical illness can influence the PK/PD parameters of antimicrobials by altering their volume of distribution, rate of excretion and elimination, and impairing penetration into tissues [2, 31, 32], and how these changes may modify the efficacy of prescribed antimicrobials.

PK describes absorption, distribution, metabolism, and elimination of drugs in serum and at infection sites. PD describes the relationship that exists between the drug concentration to which the bacteria is exposed at various sites of infection and bacterial killing activity. For antibiotics, PD activity is integrated with PK parameters and pharmacologic effect with the minimum inhibitory concentration (MIC) for a particular pathogen in order to evaluate the ability of the antibiotic to kill the infective organism or inhibit its growth. According to these PK/PD parameters, antimicrobial agents can be categorized based on their mode of bacterial killing and the presence of a postantibiotic effect. Thus, the pattern of bacterial killing can be concentration- or time dependent [33] (Tables 18.1 and 18.2). Antibiotics are considered concentration dependent if higher concentrations result in more extensive elimination of the pathogen. The kill rate for these antibiotics is closely related to peak or maximum concentration above breakpoint MIC (C_{max}/MIC). An antibiotic is considered time dependent if its bacterial killing effectiveness depends upon the duration of pathogen exposure to the agent. The kill rate is better related to how long concentrations are sustained above breakpoint MIC.

Kasiakou et al. [34] performed a systematic review of randomized clinical trials to evaluate the comparative PK/PD properties of continuous versus intermittent intravenous administration of various antimicrobials. They concluded that from a PD point of view, data suggest that continuous intravenous infusion with time-dependent bacteria-killing activity (β-lactams or vancomycin) seems to be superior to the intermittent intravenous administration, without differences in mortality or nephrotoxicity rates.

Few studies have assessed the relationship between PK/PD data and clinical outcome in humans. Roberts et al. [35] performed a systematic review of randomized clinical trials comparing the efficacy of continuous versus bolus

Table 18.2 Antibiotics, their killing activities, and pharmacokinetic and pharmacodynamic (PK/PD) parameters

Antibiotic	Killing activity	PK/PD parameters
Aminoglycosides	Concentration dependent	C_{max}/MIC
Metronidazole	Concentration dependent	AUC_{0-24}/MIC; C_{max}/MIC
Fluoroquinolones	Concentration dependent	AUC_{0-24}/MIC; C_{max}/MIC
Cholistine	Concentration dependent	AUC_{0-24}/MIC; C_{max}/MIC
Penicillins	Time dependent	T > MIC
Cephalosporins	Time dependent	T > MIC
Carbapenems	Time dependent	T > MIC
Monobactams	Time dependent	T > MIC
Clindamycin	Time dependent	T > MIC
Vancomycin	Time dependent	AUC_{0-24}/MIC; C_{max}/MIC
Macrolides	Time dependent	AUC_{0-24}/MIC; C_{max}/MIC
Linezolid	Time dependent	AUC_{0-24}/MIC; C_{max}/MIC
Tigecycline	Time dependent	AUC_{0-24}/MIC; C_{max}/MIC

AUC area under curve, *MIC* minimum inhibitory concentration, C_{max} maximal concentration, *T* time

administration of β-lactams in 846 patients (14 randomized clinical trials), including a large proportion of critically ill patients. Continuous infusion of a β-lactam antibiotic was consistently not associated with an improved clinical cure (OR 1.04; 95% CI 0.74–1.46) or mortality (OR 1.00, 95% CI 0.48–2.06) rates. The rationale for continuous infusion of β-lactams has been documented from a PD point of view, but new studies should be performed—despite the limitation of requiring a large number of patients to achieve significant results—before making a recommendation about using this PK/PD approach.

18.6 Conclusions

Appropriate early antibiotic treatment for ICU patients with infection is associated with strong reduction in mortality and morbidity rates. At present, the challenge is to achieve a level of adequate empirical therapy ≥90%. Combined therapy is only justified as empirical treatment when the infection is suspected to be caused by highly resistant microorganisms or in the most severely ill patients to provide a higher likelihood of adequate treatment. De-escalation of the initial antibiotic therapy must be encouraged because is saves money and reduces costs. The role of biomarkers in helping to discontinue antibiotic therapy is usually marginal. The PK/PD approach to prescribing the correct dose and route of administration is a potential field of outcome research in humans and should be included in the differential diagnosis of treatment failure.

References

1. Davey PG, Marwick C (2008) Appropriate vs. inappropriate antimicrobial therapy. Clin Microbiol Infect 14(Suppl 3):15–21
2. Pea F, Viale P (2009) Bench-to-bedside review: appropriate antibiotic therapy in severe sepsis and septic shock—does the dose matter? Crit Care 13:214
3. Kollef MH, Sherman G, Ward S, Fraser VJ (1999) Inadequate antimicrobial treatment of infections: a risk factor for hospital mortality among critically ill patients. Chest 115:462–474
4. Harbarth S, Garbino J, Pugin J et al (2003) Inappropriate initial antimicrobial therapy and its effect on survival in a clinical trial of immunomodulating therapy for severe sepsis. Am J Med 115:529–535
5. Kumar A, Roberts D, Wood KE et al (2006) Duration of hypotension before initiation of effective antimicrobial therapy is the critical determinant of survival in human septic shock. Crit Care Med 34:1589–1596
6. Garnacho-Montero J, Ortiz-Leyba C, Herrera-Melero I et al (2008) Mortality and morbidity attributable to inadequate empirical antimicrobial therapy in patients admitted to the ICU with sepsis: a matched cohort study. J Antimicrob Chemother 61:436–441
7. Barochia AV, Cui X, Vitberg D et al (2010) Bundled care for septic shock: an analysis of clinical trials. Crit Care Med 38:668–678
8. Dellinger RP, Levy MM, Carlet JM et al for the International Surviving Sepsis Campaign Guidelines Committee; American Association of Critical-Care Nurses; American College of Chest Physicians; American College of Emergency Physicians; Canadian Critical Care Society; European Society of Clinical Microbiology and Infectious Diseases; European Society of Intensive Care Medicine; European Respiratory Society; International Sepsis Forum; Japanese Association for Acute Medicine; Japanese Society of Intensive Care Medicine; Society of Critical Care Medicine; Society of Hospital Medicine; Surgical Infection Society; World Federation of Societies of Intensive and Critical Care Medicine (2008) Surviving sepsis campaign: international guidelines for management of severe sepsis and septic shock: 2008. Crit Care Med 36(1):296–327. Erratum in: Crit Care Med 36:1394–1396
9. Rivers E, Nguyen B, Havstad S, Early Goal-Directed Therapy Collaborative Group et al (2001) Early goal-directed therapy in the treatment of severe sepsis and septic shock. N Engl J Med 345:1368–1377
10. Shapiro NI, Howell MD, Talmor D et al (2006) Implementation and outcomes of the Multiple Urgent Sepsis Therapies (MUST) protocol. Crit Care Med 34:1025–1032
11. Micek ST, Roubinian N, Heuring T et al (2006) Before–after study of a standardized hospital order set for the management of severe septic shock. Crit Care Med 34:2707–2713
12. Nguyen HB, Corbett SW, Steele R et al (2007) Implementation of a bundle of quality indicators for the early management of severe sepsis and septic shock is associated with decreased mortality. Crit Care Med 35:1105–1112
13. El Solh AA, Akinnusi ME, Alsawalha LN, Pineda LA (2008) Outcome of septic shock in older adults after implementation of the sepsis bundle. J Am Geriatr Soc 56:272–278
14. Cunha BA (2008) Sepsis and septic shock: selection of empiric antimicrobial therapy. Crit Care Clin 24:313–334
15. Abad CL, Kumar A, Safdar N (2011) Antimicrobial therapy of sepsis and septic shock—when are two drugs better than one? Crit Care Clin 27:e1–e27
16. Heyland DK, Dodek P, Muscedere J, Canadian Critical Care Trials Group et al (2008) Randomized trial of combination versus monotherapy for the empiric treatment of suspected ventilator-associated pneumonia. Crit Care Med 36:737–744
17. Garnacho-Montero J, Sa-Borges M, Sole-Violan J et al (2007) Optimal management therapy for Pseudomonas aeruginosa ventilator-associated pneumonia: an observational, multicenter study comparing monotherapy with combination antibiotic therapy. Crit Care Med 35:1888–1895

18. Safdar N, Handelsman J, Maki DG (2004) Does combination antimicrobial therapy reduce mortality in Gram-negative bacteraemia? A meta-analysis. Lancet Infect Dis 4:519–527
19. Paul M, Leibovici L (2005) Combination antibiotic therapy for *Pseudomonas aeruginosa* bacteraemia. Lancet Infect Dis 5:192–193
20. Paul M, Benuri-Silbiger I, Soares-Weiser K, Leibovici L (2004) β-lactam monotherapy versus β-lactam-aminoglycoside combination therapy for sepsis in immunocompetent patients: systematic review and meta-analysis of randomised trials. BMJ 328:668. Erratum in BMJ 328:884
21. Kumar A, Safdar N, Kethireddy S, Chateau D (2010) A survival benefit of combination antibiotic therapy for serious infections associated with sepsis and septic shock is contingent only on the risk of death: a meta-analytic/meta-regression study. Crit Care Med 38: 1651–1664
22. Niederman MS (2006) De-escalation therapy in ventilator-associated pneumonia. Curr Opin Crit Care 12:452–457
23. Dellit TH, Owens RC, McGowan JE et al (2007) Infectious Diseases Society of America and the Society for Healthcare Epidemiology of America guidelines for developing an institutional program to enhance antimicrobial stewardship. Clin Infect Dis 44:159–177
24. Alvarez-Lerma F, Alvarez B, Luque P et al (2006) ADANN study group. Empiric broad-spectrum antibiotic therapy of nosocomial pneumonia in the intensive care unit: a prospective observational study. Crit Care 10:R78
25. Kollef MH, Morrow LE, Niederman MS et al (2006) Clinical characteristics and treatment patterns among patients with ventilator-associated pneumonia. Chest 129:1210–1218. Erratum in Chest 130:138
26. Singh N, Rogers P, Atwood CW et al (2000) Short-course empiric antibiotic therapy for patients with pulmonary infiltrates in the intensive care unit. A proposed solution for indiscriminate antibiotic prescription. Am J Respir Crit Care Med 162:505–511
27. Christ-Crain M, Jaccard-Stolz D, Bingisser R et al (2004) Effect of procalcitonin-guided treatment on antibiotic use and outcome in lower respiratory tract infections: cluster-randomised, single-blinded intervention trial. Lancet 363:600–607
28. Christ-Crain M, Stolz D, Bingisser R et al (2006) Procalcitonin guidance of antibiotic therapy in community-acquired pneumonia: a randomized trial. Am J Respir Crit Care Med 174:84–93
29. Stolz D, Smyrnios N, Eggimann P et al (2009) Procalcitonin for reduced antibiotic exposure in ventilator-associated pneumonia: a randomised study. Eur Respir J 34:1364–1375
30. Nobre V, Harbarth S, Graf JD et al (2008) Use of procalcitonin to shorten antibiotic treatment duration in septic patients: a randomized trial. Am J Respir Crit Care Med 177(5):498–505
31. Pea F, Viale P, Furlanut M (2005) Antimicrobial therapy in critically ill patients: a review of pathophysiological conditions responsible for altered disposition and pharmacokinetic variability. Clin Pharmacokinet 44:1009–1034
32. Roberts JA, Lipman J (2009) Dose adjustment and pharmacokinetics of antibiotics in severe sepsis and septic shock. In: Rello J, Kollef M, Diaz E, Rodriguez A (eds) Infectious diseases in critical care, 2nd edn. Springer-Verlag, Berlin-Heidelberg, pp 122–146
33. Petrosillo N, Drapeau CM, Agrafiotis M, Falagas ME (2010) Some current issues in the pharmacokinetics/pharmacodynamics of antimicrobials in intensive care. Minerva Anestesiol 76(7):509–524
34. Kasiakou SK, Lawrence KR, Choulis N, Falagas ME (2005) Continuous versus intermittent intravenous administration of antibacterials with time-dependent action: a systematic review of pharmacokinetic and pharmacodynamic parameters. Drugs 65:2499–2511
35. Roberts JA, Webb S, Paterson D et al (2009) A systematic review on clinical benefits of continuous administration of beta-lactam antibiotics. Crit Care Med 37:2071–2078

ICU Patients Following Transplantation

A. Martinez-Pellus and I. Cortés Puch

19.1 Introduction

Solid organ and bone marrow transplant recipients are at high risk of infection due to long-term immunosuppressant therapy that is necessary to help prevent transplant rejection. Infection prevention and control in this patient population requires a multifactorial approach using general and pharmacologic measures. In this chapter, we discuss selective decontamination of the digestive tract (SDD) (polymyxin, tobramycin, and amphotericin B) as a prophylactic measure during patient admission to the intensive care unit (ICU); the protective effect of fluconazole and topical antifungals drugs; systematic use of trimethoprim/sulfamethoxazole to manage *Pneumocystis jirovecii*; and ganciclovir as a valid strategy to prevent cytomegalovirus (CMV) infection. Another measure considered is shortening postoperative ICU length of stay by setting quick weaning protocols, using noninvasive mechanical ventilation, initiating physiotherapy, and early catheter removal. Long-term maneuvers strongly depend on patient adherence to a prophylactic regimen over long periods, and educational programs and involving patients in their prognosis help achieve this goal.

19.2 Solid Organ Transplantation

Solid organ transplantation is a widespread procedure that has become the therapy of choice for patients with irreversible and progressive end-stage organ disease. Potential severe postoperative complications (related to the inflammatory response

A. Martinez-Pellus (✉)
Intensive Care Unit, University Hospital "Virgen de la Arrixaca",
Murcia, Spain
e-mail: antonioe.martinez@carm.es

due to ischemia/reperfusion injury of the graft) and the risk of acute organ rejection require close postoperative patient monitoring. This surveillance usually takes place in the intensive care unit (ICU). In the early post-transplant period, patients will frequently require mechanical ventilation and invasive devices, putting them at risk for a large variety of infections. Infections at this stage are frequent [1] and have significant consequences on the prognosis, exceeding the surgical complications as a cause of mortality [2]. The primary goal in the transplant recipient is to avoid organ rejection. This requires achieving an adequate state of immunosuppression, known as net state of immunosuppression [3], which refers to all factors that contribute to the patient's risk of infection. Its major determinants are immunosuppressive treatment dose, regimen, and duration. This state can also be affected by the presence of neutropenia, comorbidities, and concomitant infections with immunomodulating viruses, particularly cytomegalovirus (CMV), Epstein-Barr virus (EBV), and hepatitis B and C viruses. When some of these factors occur in a single patient, excessive immunosuppression takes place, affecting humoral and cellular mechanisms and exposing the patient to infection. On the other hand, the environmental exposure of the transplant recipient to a large variety of potentially infectious agents (viruses, fungi, community-acquired pathogens, endogenous flora, etc.) is continuous and takes place in the community as well as in the hospital. Other pathogens that scarcely provoke community-acquired infections in the immunocompetent host can lead to devastating syndromes in the transplant recipient. This is the case with respiratory viruses, fungi, and mycobacteria. Hence, the application of preventive strategies for long periods is necessary. If infection takes places despite these preventive measures, it will represent a serious problem, leading to hospitalization, complex diagnostic procedures, and empirical broad-spectrum antibiotic treatment. Current immunosuppressive regimens have been reached by relative consensus. They always include steroids, together with cyclosporine or tacrolimus, and mycophenolate or azathioprine, in different combinations. There is evidence that links all of these drugs with several opportunistic pathogens, such as *P. jirovecii* and *Aspergillus* (steroids), reactivation and replication of latent viruses (cyclosporine and tacrolimus), and CMV and bacterial infections (mycophenolate). The risk of infection after transplantation changes over time, especially with modifications in immunosuppression. The maximal immunosuppressive effect of these regimens takes place after several months of treatment. Therefore, we can establish a predictable timeline of the specific infections after transplantation according to the level of immunosuppression achieved (Table 19.1). Exceptions to this timeline are so rare that they suggest either a massive environmental exposure or excessive immunosuppression. This predictable pattern in which infections occur allows the establishment of specific prophylactic measures against them. These preventive strategies must start before surgery and continue during prolonged periods or even for life.

Table 19.1 Timing of infectious complications and preventive measures after transplantation

Time	Infectious risk	Screening	Preventive measures
Pre-transplant period	Previous TBC	Tuberculin test	None
	CMV, EBV, HVZ	Serology	**Vaccination (HBV; HVZ)**
	Toxoplasma	Serology	None
	Bacterias	None	**Vaccination (pneumococcus; HI)**
	Aspergillus[a]	Cultures	Amphotericin B aerosol
	Active infection	Cultures	**Eradicate**
Early post-transplant period	Surgical infection	Cultures	Surgical prophylaxis
	VAP	Cultures/RX	SDD (**LT**); NIV
	Multi-drug-resistant pathogens	Cultures	Antibiotic policies
	Fungal infection	Cultures/serology	SDD (**LT**); Fluconazole
	TBC reactivation	RX/Ziehl	**Isoniazid**
	Long ICU stay		Early discharge
Late post-transplant period	CMV	Serology/PCR	**Ganciclovir**
	Fungal infection	Cultivo/serology	Fluconazole; **itraconazole**[b]
	Pneumocystis[b]	BAL	**Trimethropim/sulfamethoxazole**[b]
	pneumococcus/H.I		**vaccination** (12th and 24th months)
	TBC reactivation	RX/Ziehl	Treatment

Bold indicates measures strongly recommended
TBC tuberculosis, *CMV* cytomegalovirus, *EBV* Epstein-Barr virus, *HVZ* Herpes Varicella zoster, *HI* Haemophilus influenzae, *VAP* ventilator-associated pneumonia, *SDD* selective decontamination of the digestive tract, *LT* liver transplant, *NIV* noninvasive ventilation, *RX* chest X-ray, *BAL* bronchoalveolar lavage
[a] Lung transplant
[b] Cardiac transplant

19.2.1 Preoperative Strategies

Candidates for solid organ transplantation must undergo an exhaustive preoperative evaluation in order to define adequate prophylactic measures. Individualized epidemiologic exams can guide preventive strategies and must include unusual pathogen exposition, childhood vaccinations, previous surgeries, antibiotic treatments, recurrent infections, etc. A tuberculin skin test is necessary, as is serologic testing for CMV, EBV, *Toxoplasma gondii*, and syphilis. If the tuberculin skin test is positive, the measures that should be taken are controversial due to the potential hepatotoxicity of the tuberculostatics and their interferences with the pharmacokinetics of tacrolimus and cyclosporine. Periodic negative clinical and radiologic evaluations should rule out the need for prophylaxis. Vaccination against tetanus, diphtheria, mumps, influenza, pneumococcus, *Haemophilus influenza* type B, and hepatitis B virus must be performed during the pretransplant period if they were not previously completed [4]. Live vaccines are generally contraindicated after transplantation, as they may trigger an infection or facilitate organ rejection. Varicella-zoster vaccination should also be performed if the patient is seronegative, although its effectiveness is doubted [5]. The importance of these measures lies in the fact that all of these infections may be latent in the patient and undergo reactivation during immunosuppression. The transplant recipient must not have a proven or suspected infection by the time of surgery. Respiratory carriage of pathogens such as *Aspergillus* or *Burkholderia cepacia* must be ruled out or eradicated before surgery. In the case of *Aspergillus*, some studies demonstrate a significant reduction in the rate of infections in lung or cardiac transplant recipients who received amphotericin B aerosols as prophylaxis [6]. Nevertheless, the detection of this fungus in a respiratory sample may only indicate colonization and, therefore, the interpretation of this microbiological data is difficult. In an attempt to establish the predictive value of *Aspergillus* isolates, a study revealed that cultures with more than two colonies or more than one site of infection were predictive of significant infection and portended a poor prognosis and development of invasive disease [7].

19.2.2 Early Postoperative Period and Preventive Strategies

Surgical complexity and, particularly, the impact of cold ischemia times and consequent graft reperfusion, as well as the risk of systemic complications, leads to a close immediate postoperative management that usually takes place in the ICU. The probability of ICU hospitalization is highest during the first month following transplantation, when infectious complications are similar to those that occur in an immunocompetent host undergoing surgery. They are comparable in site (surgical wound infection, urinary tract infection, catheter-related bloodstream infections, etc.) and etiology (typical nosocomial pathogens such as *Staphylococcus aureus*, coagulase-negative staphylococcus, and Gram-negative bacilli, to which fungi are progressively added). Prophylactic measures must be directed to these "expected" microorganisms. However, we must be aware that patients with previous prolonged hospitalizations while waiting for transplantation may become colonized with hospital-acquired antimicrobial-resistant organisms (*Pseudomonas*, methicillin-resistant *S. aureus* (MRSA), *Aspergillus*, etc.).

19.2.2.1 Topical Antibiotic Prophylaxis
Preventive strategies based on selective decontamination of the digestive tract (SDD), which include pharyngeal and gastric application of polymyxin,

tobramycin, and amphotericin B (PTA), have proved to be useful in preventing respiratory tract infections in critical care patients [8]. The implementation of these strategies in solid organ transplantation has yielded conflicting results. The aim of selective gut decontamination in these patients is to reduce the bacterial burden of the digestive tract, which is the major reservoir of potentially pathogenic endogenous flora. The first open study in this field [9], performed in a cohort of patients waiting for orthotopic liver transplantation, showed a significant decrease of aerobic Gram-negative bacteria and *Candida* colonization following 3 days of oral administration of polymyxin, gentamicin, and nystatin. This prophylactic measure was continued for 21 days, and there was no documented episode of infection caused by aerobic Gram-negative bacilli during the first month following transplantation. Following discontinuation of SDD, recolonization of the gastrointestinal tract with aerobic Gram-negative bacteria and *Candida* occurred in 90 and 35% of the patients, respectively, within 5 days. More recently, four comparative and randomized studies analyzed the effect of a standard SDD regimen (PTA + systemic antibiotics). Smith et al. [10], in a pediatric population, compared patients receiving standard prophylaxis with systemic antibiotics with patients who received SDD added to the standard prophylaxis regimen. They found a reduction of the incidence of infections from 50 to 11% ($p < 0.001$). In a randomized controlled trial, Bion et al. [11] reported a significant reduction in respiratory tract infections in the SDD group but a similar incidence of endotoxemia episodes and the development of organ system failures. Nevertheless, in that study, SDD was started in the immediate postoperative period, and it has been demonstrated that the eradication of aerobic Gram-negative bacilli (as a source of endotoxemia) requires a minimum of 3 days of SDD [12]. Emre et al. [13], in a retrospective cohort study, compared 212 consecutive orthotopic liver transplant recipients receiving perioperative systemic antibiotics and SDD (polymyxin, gentamicin, and nystatin administered through a nasogastric tube) for 21 days with the next 157 consecutive patients, who only received systemic antibiotics. The results yielded a significant reduction of infections in the SDD group, irrespective of site, caused by either aerobic Gram-negative bacilli or by Gram-positive cocci. However, in a cost-effectiveness study comparing SDD with placebo, van Enckevort et al. [14] found no differences in the global number of infections, with a higher cost in SDD group. Nevertheless, that study was performed in a small sample (26/29 patients), and it does not describe the sites of infections or the pathogens isolated. Furthermore, SDD was applied from the time the patients were enrolled on the transplant waiting list (mean 133 days) until the 30th postoperative day, with frequent surveillance samples, justifying the excessive cost found in the SDD group. In another study with a similar approach, which evaluates the work load and the additional costs related to the use of SDD, no difference was found in these items. Actually, a reduction in the number of processed microbiological samples to rule out infection (blood cultures, bronchial aspirates, exudates, and serological tests) was found [15]. In a systematic literature review, Nathens et al. [16] analyzed mortality rates and the most relevant infections (pneumonia, urinary tract infection, surgical wound infection, bloodstream infections) in surgical patients. The results showed that SDD significantly reduced the incidence of infection in transplant organ recipients [odds ratio (OR) 0.44; 95% confidence interval (CI) 0.23–0.87]. Mortality rates were not significantly altered (OR 0.29; 95% CI 0.06–1.47). In a randomized placebo-controlled trial performed in a small group of liver transplant patients, Zwaveling et al. [17] found a similar incidence of infections in both groups but with a significant reduction in those caused by aerobic Gram-negative bacilli ($p < 0.01$) and *Candida spp* ($p < 0.05$) in the SDD group. In a recent meta-analysis [18] that reviewed four randomized trials comparing SDD versus placebo or no treatment at all, the overall incidence of infection was similar despite the use of SDD (OR 0.88; CI 95%: 0.7–1.1). Nevertheless, SDD was able to reduce the incidence of infections caused by aerobic Gram-negative bacilli (OR 0.16; CI 95% 0.07–0.37) and the incidence of postoperative pneumonias. SDD regimens should be adjusted, however, to the most prevalent pathogens found in each ICU, bearing in mind their particular resistance profile.

The use of probiotics during the pretransplant period could represent an alternative to SDD. In a randomized trial, Rayes et al. [19] compared the administration of a fiber-containing formula plus living *Lactobacillus plantarum* 299 versus SDD. They observed a reduction in the incidence of bacterial infections from 48 to 13%, with early enterally provided nutrition with the probiotics. These findings should be validated in further studies, as this is the first study performed in this field, and it is not powered high enough to draw solid conclusions.

19.2.2.2 Systemic Antibiotic Prophylaxis

Surgical prophylaxis is well standardized in the absence of previous colonization or infection with problematic pathogens. A 24-h regimen of second-generation cephalosporins should be adequate to prevent infection subsequent to the surgical intervention. The use of vancomycin in surgical prophylaxis should be restricted due to the risk of selecting vancomycin-resistant enterococcus.

In patients with risk factors for tuberculosis (latent tuberculosis, familiar exposure, malnutrition, etc.), a 9–12-month course of isoniazid can be considered. This course should start early after transplantation and must include close monitoring of liver enzymes levels.

19.2.2.3 Other Measures to Prevent Infection

An additional risk in the transplant recipient for postoperative infections is a prolonged stay in an area with a high environmental exposure to potential pathogens and multiple instrumentation, such as the ICU. A study analyzing factors related to short-term prognosis of liver transplant recipients [20] found that patients who stayed in the ICU >3 days had a higher mortality rate (19.5 vs. 2%; $p < 0.001$) and more infectious episodes (41.5 vs. 11%; $p < 0.001$) than those who stayed for <3 days (given a similar age of recipient and donor, cold ischemia time, intraoperative bleeding, and previous functional state). Another prospective and randomized trial [21] compared noninvasive ventilation with standard treatment (supplemental oxygen administration) in 51 recipients of solid organ transplantation with acute hypoxemic respiratory failure. The use of noninvasive ventilation was associated with improvement in the partial pressure of oxygen in arterial blood/fractional inspiratory oxygen (PaO_2/FiO_2) ratio in a larger number of patients (60 vs. 25%; $p < 0.03$), as well as with a significant reduction in the rate of endotracheal intubation (20 vs. 70%; $p = 0.002$), length of ICU stay of survivors [mean $\pm$ standard deviation (SD) days 5.5 (3) vs. 9 (4); $p = 0.03$], and ICU mortality rate (20 vs. 50%; $p = 0.05$). Finally, simple maneuvers such as early and continuous postural changes, in order to avoid atelectasis and other problems related to prolonged immobilization, have proven to be effective in decreasing the incidence of lower respiratory tract infections in the early post-transplant period [22].

19.2.3 Late Postoperative and Preventive Maneuvers

Fungal infection is frequent in the transplant recipient, with variable incidence according to the type of transplant. Functional disruption of the intestinal barrier and bacterial translocation are involved in this process [23]. The database of the Spanish Network of Infection in Transplantation (RESITRA), which includes 3,500 solid organ transplant recipients during 2003–2005, estimates the incidence of fungal infection in this population, showing an incidence of *Candida* spp. infection of 3–3.6% and *Aspergillus* spp. between 0.15% (renal transplant) and 5.9% (lung and bone marrow transplants) [24]. These data are markedly less than those reported in the literature two decades ago, with incidences varying between 2 and 40%, depending on the transplanted organ [1]. This could be a reflection of a better management of these patients and the standardization of prophylactic measures. The efficacy of this prophylaxis is amply documented. In a randomized, double-blind, placebo-controlled trial comparing fluconazole (400 mg/day) versus placebo until 10 weeks after transplantation, performed in 212 liver transplant recipients, Winston et al. [25] found a significant reduction in fungal infections (43 vs. 9%; $p < 0.001$), both superficial (28 vs. 4%; $p < 0.001$) and invasive (23 vs. 6%; $p < 0.001$). In another study performed in liver transplant recipients, Fortun et al. [26] compared the administration of lipid amphotericin B (AmBisome) formulations with no treatment at all. They found a significant reduction in the rate of invasive fungal infections (0 vs. 32%; $p = 0.03$), with no significant effect in mortality rates. However, in another randomized study performed in 129 consecutive liver transplant recipients divided into three intervention groups (liposomal amphotericin B i.v. plus itraconazole po; fluconazole i.v. plus itraconazole po; placebo), no significant differences were found regarding the incidence of fungal infection, although fungal colonization was higher in the placebo group [27].

With regard to viruses, CMV infection is one of the most frequent in transplantation recipients [28]. The risk of CMV infection and disease following transplantation is highest in CMV-seronegative recipients receiving a CMV-seropositive organ and is associated with an increased predisposition to chronic allograft rejection due to an immune-mediated vascular lesion [29]. This is why prophylactic measures against CMV have been amply investigated. In a controlled, multicenter trial, 155 organ transplant recipients (seropositive donor/seronegative recipient) received ganciclovir i.v. (5 mg/kg per day) for 5–10 days and then either acyclovir po (400 mg t.i.d.) or ganciclovir po (1 g t.i.d.) for an additional 12 weeks. Treatment with ganciclovir po was associated with a significant decrease in the incidence of CMV symptomatic disease when compared with the acyclovir po group (32 vs. 50%; $p < 0.05$) [30]. In another trial comparing the different strategies of cytomegalovirus prophylaxis in liver transplant recipients, ganciclovir po was found to be the most cost-effective strategy [31]. In a recent systematic revision [32], prophylactic treatment with antivirals was found to be associated with a significant decrease in CMV infection [relative risk (RR) 0.62; 95% CI 0.53–0.73; $p < 0.001$) and disease (RR 0.51; 95% CI 0.41–0.64; $p < 0.001$) compared with placebo or no treatment. This revision failed to show significant differences in the incidence of organ rejection or mortality rates. Another meta-analysis [33] of 1,980 patients from 17 controlled trials raises similar conclusions, showing a significant decrease in the incidence of CMV disease (OR 0.20; 95% CI 0.13–0.31) and the rate of allograft rejection. CMV infection is potentially severe but rarely requires ICU hospitalization. Regardless, this disease should be considered with pneumonias presenting with an atypical course, particularly in patients immunosuppressed with mycophenolate.

Beyond the sixth month after transplantation, the organ recipient achieves a stable degree of immunosuppression, and infectious problems at this stage are similar to those that take place in the immunocompetent host. However, patients with chronic rejection who need a strong and maintained state of immunosuppression, are vulnerable to opportunistic infections (*P. jirovecii*, *Listeria monocytogenes*, *Nocardia asteroides*, *Aspergillus*, *Cryptococcus neoformans*, etc.) [3]. This raises the need for prolonged prophylaxis with cotrimoxazole and antifungals. Some of these prophylactic strategies are already well defined. The use of daily single-dose cotrimoxazole, for example, during the 4–12 months following transplantation, has nearly eradicated the incidence of *P. jirovecii* and has decreased the rate of infections caused by *L. monocytogenes*, *N. asteroides*, and *T. gondii* in high-risk patients such as cardiac transplant recipients.

In this late post-transplant period, the risk of tuberculosis (reactivation of a latent infection) is 20–70 times higher than in the general population. In a large series of 4,634 solid organ transplant recipients, García-Goetz et al. [34] found an incidence of 0.45%, but it can reach 6% in endemic areas [35]. Mortality rates of these patients can be as high a 30%. According to this, patients with risk factors for tuberculosis (latent tuberculosis, familiar exposure, or radiologic suspicion) should receive prophylaxis with isoniazid at least for 9–12 months, starting early after transplantation.

19.2.4 Treatment of Confirmed or Suspected Infections

19.2.4.1 Early Postoperative Infection

The rate of infection in the solid organ transplant recipient is thought to be higher than in other diagnostic groups of critical care patients [1]. Despite this data, an analysis of 429 cardiac and liver transplant recipients admitted to our ICU in the

Table 19.2 Infectious episodes during intensive care unit (ICU) stay (transplanted patients vs overall ICU)

	Transplanted	ICU overall
Patients	75/429 (17.5%)	1796/6192 (29%)
Episodes[a]	152 (35.1*)	2131 (33.8*)
Type of infection [n (*)]		
VAP	9 (2.1)	153 (2.4)
LRTI	5 (1.1)	209 (3.3)
UTI	19 (4.4)	451 (7)
PB + CRB	51 (11.7)	690 (10.9)
Peritonitis	**8 (1.8)**	**54 (0.8)**
Surgical wound	13 (3)	130 (2)
Other	8 (1.8)	160 (2.5)
SB	13 (3)	158 (2.5)

VAP ventilator associated pneumonia, *LRTI* lower respiratory tract infection, *UTI* urinary tract infection, *PB* primary bacteremia, *CRB* catheter-related bacteriemia, *SB* secondary bacteremia
[a] Excludes secondary bacteriemias
*Episodes/1,000 ICU days

last 7 years shows a global incidence of early infection of 17.5%, which is similar to the incidence in other severely ill surgical patients and lower than in the rest of the patients admitted with other diagnoses (29%). According to this analysis, there was no difference in the site and incidence of infections between transplant recipients and the rest of the patients, with exception of peritonitis, which was more frequent in liver transplant recipients (1.8 vs. 0.8 per 1,000 days of stay) (Table 19.2). According to etiology, the analysis showed no difference between groups regarding prevailing bacterial infections over fungal and viral ones (Table 19.3). A low incidence of multi-drug-resistant pathogens was found, with the exception of *Acinetobacter baumannii*, which was more frequent in the transplant recipients (9 vs. 4.3%; $p < 0.005$). Aerobic Gram-negative bacilli were more frequent in the group of nontransplant patients (50 vs. 44%; $p < 0.05$), whereas CMV infection rates were higher in transplant recipients (4 vs. 0%; $p < 0.001$). In a univariate analysis, the risk factors of infection were acute liver failure or "code 0" previous to transplantation, Acute Physiology and Chronic Health Evaluation (APACHE) II score at admission, the need for reintervention for any cause, early organ rejection, and pretransplant ICU length of stay. The rates of days with mechanical ventilation and with central venous catheters were also higher in patients with infection. In a regression analysis, the only risk factors for infection found were code 0 as the cause of transplantation (OR 7.5, 95% CI 2.8–19.5), prolonged mechanical ventilation (OR 11.9, 95% CI 6.1–23.2), and

Table 19.3 Microbiology of infectious episodes in patients admitted to the intensive care unit (ICU) after transplantation versus patients admitted for other reason (each infectious episode could involve several microorganisms)

	After transplantation	Other reason	
Microbiology (n)	224	2,700	p value
CNS	56 (25%)	386 (14.3%)	<0.001
Enterococcus faecalis	14 (6.3%)	326 (12.1%)	<0.004
Enterococcus spp.	6 (2.7%)	40 (1.5%)	ns
Staphylococcus aureus	16 (7.2%)	144 (5.3%)	ns
(% MR)	(45)	(45)	
Other GPC	10 (4.5%)	136 (5%)	ns
Total GPC	46.3%	38.2%	ns
Acinetobacter baumannii	20 (9%)	117 (4.3%)	<0.005
Escherichia coli	18 (8.2%)	303 (11.2%)	ns
Klebsiella pneumoniae	15 (6.8%)	165 (6.1%)	ns
Serratia marcescens	3 (1.3%)	106 (3.9%)	ns
Stenotrophomonas maltophilia	9 (4%)	10 (0.37%)	ns
Pseudomonas aeruginosa	15 (6.8%)	267 (9.8%)	ns
Other AGNB	17 (7.6%)	381 (14.1%)	<0.005
Total AGNB	44%	50.3%	<0.05
Candida albicans	6 (2.7%)	144 (5.3%)	<0.02
Candida spp.	10 (4.5%)	134 (4.9%)	ns
Total fungi	7.2%	10.3%	ns
Anaerobes		11 (0.4%)	ns
CMV	9 (4%)	0	<0.001

CNS coagulase-negative staphylococci, *MR* methicillin-resistant *S. aureus*, *GPC* Gram-positive cocci, *AGNB* aerobic Gram-negative bacillus, *CMV* cytomegalovirus

APACHE II score >16 at the admission (OR 2.19, 95% CI 1.1–4.1). Length of ICU stay and mortality rate were highly conditioned by infection (Table 19.4). Managing these infections should not be difficult, always bearing in mind the characteristic pathogens of each center and their resistance profile.

19.2.4.2 Late Infections

Admission to the ICU of an organ transplant recipient with an infectious disease and who requires hemodynamic or respiratory support is a challenging situation for intensivists. The difficulty lies not only in establishing an etiologic diagnosis, but also in choosing an adequate empiric antibiotic therapy, which should be

Table 19.4 Risk factors for infection in 429 solid-organ-transplanted patients

		Infection		
	Total (%)	Yes (%)	No (%)	p value
Number	429	75 (17.5)	354 (82.5)	
Age	52.5 ± 12	51 ± 13	52.7 ± 11.7	ns
Male	308 (71.8)	52 (69)	256 (72.3)	ns
Cirrhosis	364 (84)	54 (72)	310 (87)	ns
Alcohol abuse	132 (31)	19 (25)	113 (32)	ns
Hepatocarcinoma	44 (10)	9 (12)	35 (10)	ns
Code 0	31 (7.2)	19 (13)	12 (3.4)	<0.001
Unscheduled surgery	38 (8.8)	19 (25.3)	19 (5.4)	<0.001
APACHE II (admission)	13.3 ± 4.7	16 ± 5.4	12.7 ± 4	<0.01
Early rejection	77	28 (37.3)	49 (13.8)	<0.001
Retransplant	9	9 (12)	0	<0.001
ICU stay	10.1 ± 13.6	29 ± 24	6 ± 4	<0.001
Ratio MV	0.49	0.76	0.20	<0.001
Ratio CVC	0.86	0.99	0.73	<0.05
ICU mortality	33 (7.7)	24 (32)	9 (2.5)	<0.001

ICU intensive care unit, *APACHE II* acute physiology and chronic health evaluation, *Ratio MV/CVC* total days of mechanical ventilation (central venous catheter)/total ICU days

started immediately. The chronology after transplantation can be helpful in the decision-making process given a predictable timeline (depending on the level of immunosuppression) that correlates with certain pathogens (most of all viruses).

In a medium-term period following transplantation, immunosuppression favors the development of opportunistic infections (*P. jirovecii*, CMV, *Listeria*, *Toxoplasma* and *Nocardia*) and the reactivation of latent infections (tuberculosis). However, the spectrum of infections in the transplant recipient who is ill enough to require admission to the ICU is similar to the general population. When starting an immediate empirical treatment, local resistance profiles must be kept in mind (prevalence of MRSA, extended-spectrum betalactamase-producing *Escherichia coli*, or penicillin-resistant *Streptococcus pneumoniae*).

Beyond the sixth month after transplantation; with an adequate organ function and a minimum degree of immunosuppression, most transplant recipients do relatively well, being at risk from the same infections seen in the general community. However, patients who have had frequent episodes of rejection, requiring augmented immunosuppressive therapy, remain at risk for opportunistic pathogens (*P. jirovecii*, *L. monocytogenes*, *N. asteroides*, *Aspergillus*, *C. neoformans*) [3].

In the rest of the transplant recipients, the most frequent infections during this late period after transplantation are bloodstream and respiratory tract infections. The latter can have an atypical clinical or radiologic pattern, frequently requiring invasive diagnostic procedures and computed tomography (CT) [36]. Acute episodes with a radiologic pulmonary consolidation suggest bacterial infections (including *Legionella*), whereas diffuse edema-like infiltrates usually correspond to a viral processes. Subacute and chronic episodes are mainly caused by fungi, *Nocardia*, tuberculosis, *P. jiroveci*, and viruses. According to our experience with 27 solid organ transplant recipients admitted to our ICU with severe sepsis, most episodes had a bacterial etiology (five *E. coli*, three pneumococcus, three *Pseudomonas*, one *Corynebacterium*, and one MRSA); only three cases of CMV disease where diagnosed. Two patients had influenza H1N1 (during the 2009 pandemic), and in three cases of pneumonia, cultures yielded no results. Baseline characteristics of the patients where similar to those of transplant recipients admitted for any other cause (Table 19.5). The epidemiology of infections was compared between patients with ICU-acquired infections in the immediate post-transplant period and previously transplanted patients who were admitted to the ICU with other diseases. This comparison showed no significant differences in the site and number of infectious episodes between groups (Table 19.6).

During this late post-transplant period, the risk of reactivation of latent tuberculosis is still present. This situation is challenging as a result of drug interactions between tuberculostatics and immunosuppressive agents. Rifampin, for example, decreases tacrolimus and cyclosporine levels. This pharmacokinetic interaction can lead to organ rejection. In these cases, treatment regimens should be based in a combination of other tuberculostatics (isoniazid + ethambutol + pyrazinamide, for example) and may include the possibility of using fluoroquinolones and streptomycin if the course is torpid.

19.3 Bone Marrow Transplants

Unlike solid organ transplant patients, bone marrow transplant recipients are never admitted to the ICU. Nevertheless, they require pretransplant treatment with high-dose radiotherapy, chemotherapy, or both, in order to abolish the patient's immune system. This causes a severe neutropenia as well as damaging the integrity of mucosal barriers, favoring bacterial translocation from the digestive tract. Consequently, infections will be a frequent problem in these patients [37]. Bone marrow recipients need at least 24 months to become immunocompetent. This period may be even longer for allogenic transplants. This fact, as well as the wide etiological spectrum (bacteria, viruses, and fungi) seen in these patients, hinders the establishment of preventive strategies. Even though many infections of the bone marrow recipient have an intestinal origin, prophylactic strategies do not include SDD or systemic antibiotics in the asymptomatic patient due to the lack of evidence of their effectiveness. Some studies in which fluoroquinolones were administered as a prophylactic measure during the period of neutropenia showed a

Table 19.5 Previously transplanted patients with/without infection at ICU admission

	With infection	Without infection	p value
Patients	27	50	
Age	54 ± 16.3	56 ± 13.5	ns
Male	23 (82%)	35 (70)	
Unscheduled surgery	6 (22.2)	10 (20)	ns
APACHE II (admission)	22.4 ± 4.8	21.4 ± 5.9	ns
ICU stay	15.7 ± 13.2	15 ± 18	ns
Ratio MV	0.79	0.79	ns
Ratio CVC	1	1	ns
ICU mortality	10 (37)	21 (42)	ns

APACHE II acute physiology and chronic health evaluation, *ratio MV/CVC* total days of mechanical ventilation (central venous catheter)/total ICU days

Table 19.6 Infectious episodes during ICU stay (admission post-transplant vs. transplant, with admission for other reason)

	Scheduled transplant	Other reason	p value
Patients	75/429 (17.5%)	20/78 (25.6%)	
Episodes[a]	152 (35.1[b])	44 (37.6[b])	ns
Type of infection	n[b]	n[b]	
VAP	9 (2.1)	2 (1.7)	ns
LRTI	5 (1.1)	2 (1.7)	ns
UTI	19 (4.4)	8 (6.8)	ns
PB + CRB	51 (11.7)	15 (12.8)	ns
CVC	39 (8.9)	9 (7.7)	ns
Peritonitis	8 (1.8)	2 (1.7)	ns
Surgical wound	13 (3)	5 (4.2)	ns
Other	8 (1.8)	2 (1.7)	ns
SB	13 (3)	4 (3.4)	ns

VAP ventilator associated pneumonia, *LRTI* lower respiratory tract infection, *UTI* urinary tract infection, *CVC* central venous catheter, *PB* primary bacteremia, *CRB* catheter related bacteriemia, *SB* secondary bacteremia
[a] Excludes secondary bacteriemias
[b] Episodes/1,000 intensive care unit days

reduction in the incidence of bacteremia, with no effect in mortality rates [38]. However, when considering the establishment of a prophylactic protocol, the antibiotics included should be adjusted to the resistance patterns of the most common pathogens present in each center. Moreover, the prevalence of quinolone-resistant staphylococcus, pneumococcus and *E. coli*, as well as the appearance of vancomycin-resistant enterococci, must be borne in mind. Therefore, extensive use of these antibiotics should be avoided. Neutropenic patients are characteristically at risk of fungal infections. Prophylaxis with fluconazole has markedly reduced the incidence of fungal infections (*Candida* spp.), with a favorable impact on mortality rates [39]. However, the emergence of infections caused by non-albicans *Candida* spp. (*C. krusei, C. glabrata*) has been related to this prophylactic strategy [40]. Surveillance cultures could be useful to decide when to administer prophylactic fluconazole in patients with prolonged neutropenia. In a study performed by Guiot et al. [41], patients with low concentrations of *Candida* in the oropharynx (<10 CFU) and fecal samples (<10^3 CFU/g feces) did not develop systemic candidiasis; 19% of those with one high concentration sample and 86% of those with both samples at high concentration had fungemias. There is no consistent evidence so far concerning the use of SDD in this field. However, its use seems justified during the early phase of the transplant regime, considering the expected pathogens at this point (Gram-negative bacilli and fungi). The lack of evidence can be explained by the low number of bone marrow recipients admitted to the ICU and by the fact that SDD is practically limited to the intensive care area. Regarding viruses, the most severe and frequent infectious process (between 30 and 100 days after transplantation) is interstitial pneumonia, which behaves as an acute respiratory distress syndrome and is usually caused by CMV. This has led to the use of prophylactic courses of ganciclovir, aiming to avoid this risk. In a randomized controlled trial [42], bone marrow recipients who had asymptomatic pulmonary CMV infection (positive cultures for CMV in bronchoalveolar lavage while remaining asymptomatic) were randomly assigned to either prophylactic ganciclovir (5 mg/kg twice daily for an initial period of 1–2 weeks, and then five to seven times per week until day 120) or observation alone. The results showed a significant decrease in the incidence of CMV disease and mortality rate, with few side effects. In the late phase after transplantation (>100 days), vaccination against encapsulated bacteria (*S. pneumoniae, H. influenzae*, and *N. meningitidis*) is recommended in allogenic transplant recipients with a chronic form of graft versus host disease requiring treatment with cyclosporine or tacrolimus. Vaccines should be given 12 and 24 months after transplantation.

Regarding infections during the neutropenia phase of bone marrow transplants, the primary site is usually unknown. Therefore, an empirical an immediate antibiotic treatment is necessary [43]. Bacterial and fungal infections are the most frequent.

19.4 Conclusion

Solid-organ and bone marrow transplant recipients are at high risk for infection in the short and medium term. This risk depends on the level of immunosuppression necessary to avoid rejection. Preventive maneuvers aimed at minimizing this problem have gradually increased, and most of them have proven to be effective. The first goal in a global infection prevention plan is to minimize length of ICU stay. This goal can be achieved by implementing quick weaning protocols, removing central lines and drainages as soon as possible, and establishing intensive physiotherapy programs. The fact that in an early phase the epidemiology of infections is comparable in transplant recipients and other surgical patients admitted to the ICU could justify the prophylactic use of SDD. This might be particularly important while the patient is undergoing mechanical ventilation or until a minimum level of immunosuppression can be achieved (cyclosporine monotherapy, for example). The use of SDD could also be supported by the emergence of fungal infections (mainly *Candida* spp.), favored by the use of steroids in immunosuppressive protocols. In the liver transplant recipient, several studies have demonstrated a protective effect of both fluconazole and topical enterally administered nonabsorbable antifungals as part of SDD. The risk of selecting non-albicans *Candida* spp. resistant to azoles, observed with the use of fluconazole, is not likely to exist with topical use of amphotericin B. SDD has been the subject of intense debate given the fact that it has no effect on post-transplant mortality rates. However, this reason should not be enough to refuse treatment with the potential benefit of avoiding infection. To resolve this controversial issue, a study with a complex design and a large sample size is necessary. However, it is unlikely that this kind of study will ever be performed.

In the medium- and long-term periods, the problems concerning prevention rely on the patient's willingness to maintain a long prophylactic regimen, together with the risk of toxicity, interactions with immunosuppressive agents, and selection of resistant pathogens. Reported rates of nonadherence to the medical recommendations after transplantation are unacceptably high in some studies, reaching seven to 36 cases of nonadherence to immunosuppressive treatment per 100 patients/year [44]. Educational programs and greater patient participation in the prognosis are useful tools to achieve this goal.

Regarding the profile of infections in transplant recipients, there are three general time frames to consider: the first month (early postoperative period), the second through the sixth month, and the late post-transplant period (beyond the sixth month or first year). In the early postoperative period, infections are similar in site and etiology to those occurring in general surgical patients. The intermediate period (2–6 months after transplantation), is when the risk of opportunistic infections (*P. jirovecii* and, less frequently, *Listeria* and *Nocardia*), as well as reactivation of latent infections (tuberculosis, CMV, *Toxoplasma*) become manifest. Therefore, these etiologies should be ruled out when a transplant recipient is admitted with an infectious episode. Beyond the first year after transplantation, if the level of immunosuppression is minimal, the recipient has the same risk of infection as the general population, with the exception of the possibility of a reactivation of latent tuberculosis. Although it is unusual that patients with these infections of the late post-transplant period are admitted to the ICU, they can raise a diagnostic challenge. A high index of suspicion is necessary to choose the appropriate diagnostic procedures (serological tests, virus polymerase chain reaction, biopsies, etc.) and to start directed treatment as soon as possible; the patient's prognosis will markedly depend on this.

References

1. Patel R, Paya CV (1997) Infections in solid-organ transplant recipients. Clin Microb Rev 10:86–124
2. Torbenson M, Wang J, Nichols L et al (1998) Causes of death in autopsied liver transplantation patients. Mod Pathol 11:37–46
3. Fishman JA (2007) Infection in solid-organ transplant recipients. N Engl J Med 357:2601–2614
4. Avery RK (2004) Prophylactic strategies before solid-organ transplantation. Curr Opin Infect Dis 17:353–356
5. White CJ (1997) Varicela-zoster virus vaccine. Clin Infect Dis 24:753
6. Reichenspurner H, Gamberg P, Nitschke M et al (1997) Significant reduction in the number of fungal infections after lung, heart-lung, and heart transplantation using aerosolized amphotericin B prophylaxis. Transpl Proc 29:627–628
7. Brown RS, Lake JR, Katzman BA et al (1996) Incidence and significance of Aspergillus cultures following liver and kidney transplantation. Transplantation 61:666–669
8. Liberati A, D'Amico R, Pifferi S, Brazzi L (2007) Antibiotic prophylaxis to reduce respiratory tract infections and mortality in adults receiving intensive care. Cochrane Review. Cochrane Library, Issue 3
9. Wiesner RH, Hermans PE, Rakela J et al (1988) Selective bowel decontamination to decrease gram-negative aerobic bacterial and *Candida* colonization and prevent infection after orthotopic liver transplantation. Transplantation 45:570–574
10. Smith SD, Jackson RJ, Hannakan CJ et al (1993) Selective decontamination in pediatric liver transplants. A randomized prospective study. Transplantation 55:1306–1309
11. Bion JF, Badger I, Crosby HA et al (1994) Selective decontamination of the digestive tract reduces gram-negative pulmonary colonization but not systemic endotoxemia in patients undergoing elective liver transplantation. Crit Care Med 22:40–49
12. van Saene JJM, Stoutenbeek CP, van Saene HKF et al (1996) Reduction of the intestinal endotoxin pool by three different SDD regimens in human volunteers. J Endotoxin Res 3:337–343
13. Emre S, Sebastian A, Chodoff L et al (1999) Selective decontamination of the digestive tract helps prevent bacterial infections in the early postoperativ period after liver transplant. Mt Sinai J Med 66:310–313
14. van Enckevort PJ, Zwaveling JH, Bottema JT et al (2001) Cost effectiveness of selective decontamination of the digestive tract in liver transplant patients. Pharmacoeconomics 19:523–530
15. Garcia-San Vicente B, Canut A, Labora A et al (2010) Descontaminación digestiva selectiva: respercusión en la carga de trabajo y el coste de laboratorio de microbiología y tendencias en la resistencia bacteriana. Enferm Infecc Microbiol Clin 28:75–81
16. Nathens AB, Marshall JC (1999) Selective decontamination of the digestive tract in surgical patients: a systematic review of the evidence. Arch Surg 134:170–176
17. Zwaveling JH, Maring JK, Klompmaker IJ et al (2002) Selective decontamination of the digestive tract to prevent posoperative infection: a randomized placebo-controlled trial in liver transplant patients. Crit Care Med 30:1204–1209
18. Sadfar N, Said A, Lucey MR (2004) The role of selective digestive decontamination for reducing infection in patients undergoing liver transplantation: a systematic review and meta-analysis. Liver Transpl 7:817–827
19. Rayes N, Seehofer D, Hansen S et al (2002) Early enteral supply of lactobacillus and fiber versus selective bowel decontamination: a controlled trial in liver transplant recipients. Transplantation 74:123–127
20. Mor E, Cohen J, Erez E et al (2001) Short intensive care unit stay reduces septic complications and improves outcome after liver transplantation. Transplant Proc 33:2939–2940

21. Antonelli M, Conti G, Bufi M et al (2000) Noninvasive ventilation for treatment of acute respiratory failure in patients undergoing solid organ transplantation: a randomized trial. JAMA 283:235–241
22. Whiteman K, Nachtmann L, Kramer D et al (1995) Effects of continuous lateral rotation therapy on pulmonary complications in liver transplant patients. Am J Crit Care 4:133–139
23. Cole GT, Halawa AA, Anaissie EJ (1996) The role of the gastrointestinal tract in the hematogenous candidiasis: from the laboratory to bedside. Clin Infect Dis 22(Suppl 2): S73–S88
24. Garrido RS, Aguado JM, Diaz-Pedroche C et al (2006) A review of critical periods for opportunistic infection in the new transplantation era. Transplantation 82:1457–1462
25. Winston DJ, Pakrasi A, Busuttil RW (1999) Prophylactic fluconazole in liver transplant recipients. A randomized, double-blind, placebo-controlled trial. Ann Int Med 131:729–737
26. Fortun J, Martin-Davila P, Moreno S et al (2003) Prevention of invasive fungal infections in liver transplant recipients: the role of prophylaxis with lipid formulations of amphotericin B in high risk patients. J Antimicrob Chemother 52:813–819
27. Biancofiore G, Bindi ML, Baldasarri R et al (2002) Antifungal prophylaxis in liver transplant recipients: a randomized placebo-controlled study. Transpl Int 15:341–347
28. Fernandez A, Amezquita Y, Fernandez-Tarrago E et al (2009) Prophylaxis and treatment of cytomegalovirus infection postrenal transplantation in two Madrid units. Transpl Proc 41:2416–2418
29. Arthur SK, Pedersen RA, Kremers WK et al (2009) Delayed-onset primary cytomegalovirus disease and the risk of allograph failure and mortality after kidney transplantation. Clin Infect Dis 46:840–846
30. Rubin RH, Kemmerly SA, Conti D et al (2000) Prevention of primary cytomegalovirus disease in organ transplant recipients with oral ganciclovir or oral acyclovir prophylaxis. Transpl Infect Dis 2:112–117
31. Das A (2000) Cost-effectiveness of different strategies of cytomegalovirus prophylaxis in orthotopic liver transplant recipients. Hepatology 31:311–317
32. Couchoud C (2001) Cytomegalovirus prophylaxis with antiviral agents for solid organ transplantation. Cochrane Database of Systematic Reviews, Issue 4
33. Kalil AC, Levitsky J, Lyden E et al (2005) Meta-analysis: the efficacy of strategies to prevent organ disease by cytomegalovirus in solid organ transplant recipients. Ann Int Med 143: 870–880
34. García-Goetz JF, Linares L, Benito N et al (2009) Tuberculosis in solid organ transplant recipients at a tertiary hospital in the last 20 years in Barcelona, Spain. Transpl Proc 41: 2268–2270
35. Benito N, Sued O, Moreno A et al (2002) Diagnosis and treatment of latent tuberculosis infection in liver transplant recipients in an endemic area. Transplantation 74:1381–1386
36. Torres A, Ewing S, Insausti J et al (2000) Etiology and microbial patterns of pulmonary infiltrates in patients with orthotopic liver transplantation. Chest 117:502–949
37. Kernan NA, Bartsch G, Ash RC et al (1993) Analysis of 462 transplantations from unrelated donors facilitated by the National Marrow Donor Program. N Engl J Med 328(9):593
38. Cruciani M, Rampazzo R, Malena M et al (1996) Prophylaxis with fluoroquinolones for bacterial infection in neutropenic patients: a meta-analysis. Clin Infect Dis 23:795
39. Marr KA, Siedel K, Slavin MA et al (2000) Prolonged fluconazole prophylaxis is associated with persistent protection against candidiasis-related death in allogenic marrow transplant recipients: long-term follow-up of a randomized, placebo-controlled trial. Blood 96:2055
40. Abi-Said D, Anaissie E, Uzun O et al (1997) The epidemiology of hematogenous candidiasis caused by different Candida species. Clin Infect Dis 24:1122
41. Guiot HFL, Fibbe WE, Van't Wout JW (1996) Prevention of invasive candidiasis by fluconazole in patients with malignant hematological disorders and a high grade of candida colonisation. (Abstract LM33) 36th Interscience conference on antimicrobial agents and chemotherapy, New Orleans

42. Schmidt GM, Horak DA, Niland JC et al (1991) A randomized, controlled trial of prophylactic ganciclovir for cytomegalovirus pulmonary infections in recipients of allogenic bone marrow transplants: the City of Hope-Standford-Syntex CMV Study Group. N Engl J Med 324:1005–1011
43. Hughes WT, Armstrong D, Bedey GP et al (1997) 1997 Guidelines for the use of antimicrobials agents in neutropenic patients with unexplained fever. Clin Infect Dis 25(3):551
44. Dew A, Di Martíni AF, De Vito A (2007) Rates and risk factors for nonadherence to the medical regimen after adult solid organ transplantation. Transplantation 83:858–873

Clinical Virology in NICU, PICU and AICU

20

C. Y. W. Tong and S. Schelenz

20.1 Introduction

Viruses are significant causes of nosocomial infections, but their importance has been underappreciated in the past. However, outbreak of severe acute respiratory syndrome (SARS), avian and pandemic influenza with high morbidity and mortality rates increased the awareness of intensivists regarding the devastating effects of nosocomial spread of viral infections in intensive care units (ICU).

Advances in medicine have led to a large number of immunocompromised patients susceptible to severe viral infections. Many such patients are cared for in the ICU and in turn become an infectious hazard for other vulnerable patients. Health care workers can acquire common viral infections from the community and spread them to susceptible patients in the ICU. Patients in neonatal (NICU) and paediatric (PICU) ICUs are most vulnerable because of the lack of prior immunity against many viruses circulating in the community. Recent improvements in diagnostic methods have enabled the rapid diagnosis and monitoring of many viral infections. Rapid and accurate typing of viral strains using a molecular technique can help identify the source of outbreaks. Also, specific postexposure prophylaxis and treatment are now available for many important nosocomial viral infections. In this chapter, we discuss some of the important viruses that could be associated with nosocomial infections in the ICU, according to their usual route of transmission (Table 20.1). Infection control measures recommended for preventing these viral infections are listed in Table 20.2.

C. Y. W. Tong (✉)
Infection, Guy's and St Thomas' NHS Foundation Trust
and King's College London School of Medicine, London, UK
e-mail: William.tong@gstt.nhs.uk

Table 20.1 Mode of viral infection transmission in the intensive care unit

	Respiratory route	Faecal–oral route	Blood and body fluid	Direct contact/fomites
Influenza viruses	+++	–	–	++
Respiratory syncytial virus	+++	–	–	++
Parainfluenza viruses	+++	–	–	++
Adenovirus	+++	++	–	+++
SARS coronavirus	+++	±	–	++
Varicella zoster virus (chickenpox)	+++	–	–	++
Rotavirus	+	+++	–	++
Norovirus	++	+++	–	++
Enterovirus/parechovirus	+	+++	–	++
Hepatitis A virus	–	+++	±	++
Hepatitis B virus	–	–	+++	–
Hepatitis C virus	–	–	++	–
Human immunodeficiency virus	–	–	++	–
Haemorrhagic fever viruses	±	–	++++	+++
Cytomegalovirus	–	–	+	++
Herpes simplex virus	–	–	–	++
Varicella-zoster virus (zoster)	–	–	–	++
Rabies	–	–	±	++

SARS severe respiratory distress syndrome; – Unlikely; ± possible; + common (the number of + is an arbitrary indicator of transmissibility)

20.2 Viruses Transmitted by Droplets and Airborne Route

20.2.1 Influenza Viruses

Influenza viruses (family Orthomyxoviridae) are classified into types A, B and C. Annual seasonal outbreaks of influenza are caused by minor antigenic changes (antigenic drift) seen in influenza A and B viruses. Major changes in antigenic subtypes (antigenic shift) are only found in influenza A virus and typically involve the emergence of novel hemagglutinin (H) and/or neuraminidase (N) proteins on the viral envelope. Pandemic influenza occurs when a new influenza A strain emerges, to which the majority of the world's population has little or no immunity.

Table 20.2 Infection control measures for preventing viral infections

Virus	Isolation or cohorting	Hand washing	Apron/ gown+	Gloves	Masks/ goggles	Incubation	Duration of infectivity
Influenza viruses	✓(negative pressure) IB	✓	✓	✓	✓ IB	1–4 days	Prodromal phase and 7 days after onset
Respiratory syncytial viruses (RSV)	✓ II	✓ IA	✓ IB	✓ IA		2–8 days	48 h before symptoms and 7 days from onset; longer in immunocompromised (up to 30 days)
Parainfluenza viruses	✓	✓	✓	✓		2–4 days	As long as symptoms last
Adenovirus	✓	✓	✓	✓		5–10 days	As long as symptoms last
SARS coronavirus	✓ (negative pressure) IA	✓	✓	✓	✓ (FFP3 or N95) IB	4–6 days (max. reported 14 days)	Peak at day 10 of illness, no reported transmission 10 days beyond resolution of fever
Varicella-zoster virus (chickenpox)	✓(negative pressure) IB	✓	✓	✓		10–21 days	2 days before first vesicle until all lesions are crusted
Rotavirus	✓	✓	✓	✓		2–3 days	2 days before symptoms and up to 4–7 days after onset of illness
Norovirus	✓ IB	✓ IA	✓ IB	✓ IB	±	15–48 h	Up to 48 h after becoming symptom free
Enterovirus/ parechovirus	✓ (young infants often require care in SCBU or NICU)	✓	✓	✓		2–25 days	7–14 days from onset of illness; asymptomatic shedding common
Hepatitis A virus	✓	✓	✓	✓		2–6 weeks	Infectious 1 week before onset of illness, infectivity declines rapidly after onset of illness
Hepatitis B virus		✓		✓		2–3 months	As long as patient is viremic

(continued)

Table 20.2 (continued)

Virus	Isolation or cohorting	Hand washing	Apron/ gown+	Gloves	Masks/ goggles	Incubation	Duration of infectivity
Hepatitis C virus		✓		✓		2–3 months	As long as patient is viremic
Human immunodeficiency virus (HIV)		✓		✓		3–6 weeks	Indefinitely, though viremia can be controlled by therapy
Viral hemorrhagic fever viruses (VHF)	✓ (high security isolation)	✓	✓	✓	✓	3–21 days	High infectivity during illness
Cytomegalovirus (CMV)		✓	(congenital CMV)	(congenital CMV)		3–6 weeks from primary infection.	Congenital infection—from birth. Asymptomatic shedding common
Herpes simplex virus (HSV)		✓		✓		Often due to reactivation	Until lesions have healed
Varicella-zoster virus (shingles)		✓	✓	✓		Due to reactivation	Until vesicles crusted over
Rabies virus	✓	✓	✓	✓	✓	2–8 weeks or longer	Duration of illness

Categorisation of recommendations: *IA* strongly recommended for all hospitals and strongly supported by well-designed experimental or epidemiological studies; *IB* strongly recommended for all hospitals and viewed as effective by experts in the field (these recommendations are based on strong rationale and suggestive evidence, even though scientific studies may not have been performed). *II* suggested for implementation in many hospitals (these recommendations may be supported by suggestive clinical or epidemiological studies, a strong theoretical rationale or definitive studies applicable to some but not all hospitals

FFP3 or N95 high-filtration respirators, *SCBU* special care baby unit, *NICU* neonatal intensive care unit, ✓ recommended and suggested for implementation in most settings, *SARS* severe acute respiratory distress syndrome, *HIV* human immune deficiency virus, *VHF* viral haemorrhagic fevers, *CMV* cytomegalovirus

There were three influenza pandemics in the last century, of which the pandemic in 1918 due to the H1N1 virus was the most severe. The first pandemic of this century occurred in 2009 [1] and was due to another H1N1 variant that emerged through a quadruple reassortment of viral RNAs derived from human, avian, Eurasian and North American swine influenza sources [2]. The presence of animal influenza subtypes, particularly avian influenza viruses such as H5N1, is of continuous concern, as these could be the source of future pandemics. Though with relatively high case-fatality rate, H5N1 avian influenza virus has so far only caused a limited number of human infections in restricted geographical locations with little evidence of human to human spread. However, the 2009 pandemic H1N1 virus proved to be a major burden for ICU staff [3].

Clinically, influenza infection is characterised by abrupt onset of fever, sore throat, myalgia, cough, headache and malaise. Young children may develop croup, pneumonia or middle ear infection. With seasonal influenza, complications are often seen in the elderly, the immunocompromised and those with pre-existing chronic heart or lung disease or diabetes. During the 2009 H1N1 pandemic, children and young adults were more susceptible [4]. Overall fatality rate was <0.5%, but as many as 9–31% of hospitalised patients needed ICU admission [5]. Severe disease and high mortality rates were seen in pregnant women, patients with underlying medical pulmonary, cardiac, metabolic, neuromuscular illness and severe obesity, and those in whom the diagnosis and admission was delayed [6–8]. Respiratory failures could be caused by viral pneumonia and acute respiratory distress syndrome (ARDS). In addition, secondary bacterial infection with *Streptococcus pneumoniae* or *Staphylococcus aureus* (often methicillin resistant) were found in 20–24% of ICU patients and 26–38% of patients who died [3, 5, 9]. Fatal cases were often complicated by multiorgan failure.

Influenza has a short incubation time of 1–4 days. The virus is transmitted via droplets, and patients are infectious during the prodromal phase and up to 7 days after symptom onset. Rapid antigen detection from respiratory secretions is available, but this was found to be insensitive for the 2009 H1N1 pandemic virus [10]. More sensitive and specific real-time polymerase chain reaction (PCR) methods had to be used [11]. Due to the infection-control hazards of taking nasopharyngeal aspirates or bronchoalveolar lavage, the use of throat and nasal swabs were advocated. A complete respiratory diagnostic workup needed to be performed to exclude other viral, bacterial and noninfectious causes. A single negative influenza PCR result on an upper respiratory sample did not definitively exclude the diagnosis [12]. In addition, other concurrent or secondary infections had to be considered. Protocols needed to be in place to ensure satisfactory triage of patients according to severity [13]. Early administration of specific neuraminidase inhibitors, such as oral doses of oseltamivir or inhalation zanamivir, seemed to be beneficial [14]. In more refractory cases, the off-license use of intravenously administered zanamivir or peramivir was tried. Extracorporeal membrane oxygenation (ECMO) was found to be useful in very severe cases [12].

The risk of nosocomial transmission to other hospitalised patients and staff is well documented. Infected patients should ideally be cared for in a single room or cohorted together. Health care workers should be protected through the proper use of personal protective equipments, including respirators or masks, eye protection, gowns/aprons and gloves [15, 16]. High-filtration respirator to FFP3 (Europe) or N95/N99 (USA) standard should be used for staff carrying out aerosol-generating procedures after fit testing and training. Surgical masks should be adequate for nonaerosol contacts [16]. Environmental contamination is an important source of transmission. Good hand hygiene can prevent transmission through this route.

Vaccination is the most specific preventative measure. Annual seasonal influenza vaccination to vulnerable individuals and health care workers has been advocated. A specific vaccine against the H1N1 pandemic strain was developed within months of the onset of the outbreak. However, vaccine uptake rates amongst health care workers are usually poor, and more needs to be done to educate both patients and staff.

20.2.2 Respiratory Syncytial Virus

Respiratory syncytial virus (RSV) (family Paramyxoviridae) is a major cause of lower respiratory tract infections in young children and infants. There are two subtypes, A and B, with varying dominance in different years [17]. The incidence of RSV is seasonal in temperate climates, and hospital admissions usually peak during winter months. Prematurity, bronchopulmonary dysplasia and congenital heart disease are associated with a significant risk for admission to high-dependency units or PICU. In Switzerland, it was estimated that approximately 1–2% of each annual birth cohort required such admission. RSV can also cause significant disease in adults, particularly in immunocompromised individuals such as patients undergoing therapy for haematological malignancies, the elderly and those with chronic pulmonary disease [18].

The most rapid diagnosis of RSV is by direct antigen detection methods such as chromatographic immunoassays. A typical rapid test method is completed within 30 min and can be used as a point of care testing method in emergency rooms and ICUs. However, these rapid tests lack sensitivity [19]. More recently, many laboratories have begun using multiplex real-time nucleic acid amplification techniques (NAAT) to diagnose respiratory tract infections, including RSV [20]. Although NAAT is highly sensitive, it is not a rapid testing method. Hence, it is desirable to have a mixed strategy of diagnostic approaches, such as an initial rapid direct antigen test followed by retesting of negative samples by NAAT.

Nosocomial transmission of RSV in the ICU and haemoncology units has frequently been reported. It is important to identify infected patients and to apply prompt and effective infection control measures (Table 20.2). It is recognised that a combination of cohorting patients using dedicated health care staff, contact isolation of patients, strict adherence to hand hygiene; and screening visitors, family members and health care staff for upper respiratory tract infection symptoms significantly reduce the cross-infection rate of RSV. In haemoncology units, the practice of enhanced seasonal infection control programs for RSV has been shown to be effective [21]. The usefulness of wearing masks and goggles is less clear.

There is no safe and effective vaccine to prevent RSV infection. However, immunoprophylaxis in the form of RSV immunoglobulin (RSV-IG) or humanised monoclonal antibodies (palivizumab) is available as prophylaxis for some high-risk patients to prevent serious RSV disease or to limit further nosocomial spread. Both palivizumab and RSV-IG have been shown to decrease the incidence of RSV hospitalisation and ICU admission, although there was no significant reduction in the risk of mechanical ventilation or mortality rate. When given prophylaxis, infants born <35 weeks gestational age and those with chronic lung and congenital heart disease all had a significant reduction in the risk of RSV hospitalisation [22].

Treating RSV infection is mainly supportive, including oxygen, ventilation and bronchodilatative drugs. Aerosolised ribavirin has often been used in severe cases, with or without gamma globulin i.v. [23]. However, evidence for the clinical efficacy of ribavirin in RSV infection remains inconclusive [24]. The use of aerosolised ribavirin needs to be carefully controlled, as there are potential teratogenic effects on pregnant staff and visitors. Others have tried a combination of palivizumab i.v. with or without ribavirin [25].

Another paramyxovirus, known as human metapneumovirus (hMPV), shares a similar spectrum of clinical illness as RSV. It is likely that general infection control measures against RSV would also be effective against hMPV.

20.2.3 Parainfluenza Viruses

There are four types of human parainfluenza virus (PIV) types: PIV 1–4 (family Paramyxoviridae). Infections with PIV1 and 2 are seasonal, with a peak in autumn affecting mainly children between 6 months and 6 years of age. Clinically, patients often present with croup or a febrile upper respiratory tract infection. In contrast, PIV3 is endemic throughout the year and infects mostly young infants in the first 6 month of life and up to 2 years of age. Clinically, there is no specific presentation in PIV3, but bronchiolitis and pneumonia are not uncommon. In immunocompromised adults, such as stem cell transplant recipients, PIV3 is associated with a high mortality rate. Such patients often present with severe pneumonia and many require admission to the ICU.

The diagnosis of PIV infection can be confirmed by immunofluorescence antigen detection or NAAT [26]. Nosocomial transmission is often due to PIV3 and has been documented in neonatal care and adult haematology units [27]. Infection control precautions are the same as for RSV. Despite several uncontrolled case series of apparent successful use of intravenously, orally or aerosolised administration of ribavirin to treat PIV infections, there is no clear evidence that ribavirin with or without immunoglobulin alters mortality rates from PIV3 pneumonia or decreases the duration of viral shedding from the nasopharynx [28]. Nevertheless, there may be a role for pre-emptive early therapy with ribavirin to prevent progression of upper airway infection to pneumonia.

20.2.4 Adenovirus

Adenovirus (family Adenoviridae) multiplies in the pharynx, conjunctiva or small intestine. Clinically, the infection is localised and typically presents with pharyngitis, conjunctivitis or gastroenteritis depending on serotype. However, in young infants and immunocompromised patients such as organ transplant recipients or AIDS patients, adenovirus can cause severe pneumonia, disseminated infection or haemorrhagic cystitis. The diagnosis can be confirmed by specific antigen detection tests on respiratory or stool samples. Viremia and viruria can be confirmed and quantified using real-time PCR.

In respiratory infections, the virus spreads via droplets or through contaminated hands or fomites. Nosocomial adenovirus infections have been reported and can be a particular problem in neonatal units. It is important to adhere to strict infection control procedures to prevent nosocomial spread (Table 20.2). In vitro, adenovirus is susceptible to antivirals such as cidofovir and ribavirin [29]. Use of cidofovir in selected patients may be successful [30].

20.2.5 Severe Acute Respiratory Syndrome: Coronavirus

A respiratory virus that caused a severe acute respiratory syndrome (SARS) emerged from southern China in 2002. The virus was subsequently identified as a novel virus from the Coronaviridae family and was named SARS coronavirus (SARS CoV) [31]. SARS was associated with a high mortality rate, and of the most concern to the international community was the potential in causing nosocomial infections. From a single index case in a Hong Kong hotel, a series of chains of outbreaks occurred in Vietnam, Singapore and Canada [32]. Subsequently, infections were reported in major cities in Asia, Europe and USA, transmitted through international travel. In total, 8,422 individuals were infected, with 916 deaths around the world. The emergence of SARS was the first wake-up call to the medical community regarding the need for comprehensive infection control policies in hospitals and ICU. This also led to the general provision of personal protective equipment (PPE) with training and fitting programmes for health care workers in many countries.

SARS is infectious from the onset of illness and infectiousness correlates with the degree of viral shedding. Incidences of superspreaders or superspreading events may have accounted for most of the large-scale transmissions. Older age and underlying comorbidity are major risk factors for fatality [33]. Viral loads in various anatomical sites also correlate with the severity of symptoms and mortality. Shedding of SARS CoV peaks at day 10 after the onset of symptoms. The disease pathology is characterized by uncontrolled viral replication, with a major proinflammatory response. The optimal therapy for SARS is still not clear, as there were no randomized controlled trials conducted. Treatment with interferon (IFN)-α, steroid, protease inhibitors (such as lopinavir) together with ribavirin, or convalescent plasma containing neutralising antibody, could all be useful.

Prophylaxis with IFN or hyperimmunoglobulin may also be considered as post-exposure prophylaxis [34].

SARS CoV is identified as a zoonosis with a natural reservoir in Chinese horseshoe bats [35]. Its emergence is associated with local culinary practice in southern China, leading to captured palm civets acting as the amplifying host and passing on infection to human. As long as the reservoirs and amplifying hosts coexist, there is a potential for SARS to re-emerge. Intensivists should always be on the lookout for patients with unexplained severe respiratory infections and consider SARS as a possible differential diagnosis.

20.2.6 Varicella Zoster Virus: Chickenpox

Primary varicella zoster virus (VZV) (family Herpesviridae) infection causes chickenpox. This is a common self-limiting childhood infection characterised by a mild fever and a generalised vesicular rash. Risk factors for severe disease include immunosuppression, smoking and pregnancy. Complications include bacterial sepsis, pneumonia, encephalitis, ataxia, toxic shock, necrotising fasciitis and haemorrhagic chickenpox with disseminated coagulopathy and fatality [36].

Chickenpox is highly infectious and can be transmitted via inhalation of respiratory secretions or by direct contact. Patients are likely to be infective 48 h before the appearance of the rash until the last lesion has crusted over. Outbreaks in the ICU have frequently been reported [37, 38]. Infected patients should be promptly isolated, preferably in negative-pressure rooms.

A rapid diagnosis of chickenpox can be made by electron microscopy or immunofluorescence of scrapings from the vesicle base. A person who has had chickenpox does not develop chickenpox again, but the virus may reactivate as zoster/shingles. Susceptibility to chickenpox can be determined by testing for the presence of VZV immunoglobulin (Ig)G. Infected patients need to be isolated immediately, and exposed patients and staff investigated. Exposed staff who are susceptible to VZV should be excluded from contact with high-risk patients for 8–21 days postexposure. Susceptible individuals at risk of severe disease should receive varicella-zoster immunoglobulin (VZIG) prophylaxis, which could be given up to 10 days after exposure.

Neonates born to mothers who developed chickenpox 7 days before to 7 days after delivery are highly susceptible due to a lack of protective maternal antibodies. In such cases, VZIG prophylaxis to the neonate is recommended. The baby should also be isolated. Intravenously administered acyclovir should be started promptly at the first sign of illness. Most childhood chickenpox does not require treatment. However, in severe cases (e.g. pneumonitis, disseminated disease with visceral involvement and patients requiring hospitalisation), intravenously administered acyclovir (10 mg/kg 8 hourly) is the treatment of choice. Treatment of neonates will require a higher dose (20 mg/kg 8 hourly). A live attenuated vaccine against VZV is available. Susceptible health care workers should be immunised.

20.3 Viruses Transmitted by the Faecal–Oral Route

20.3.1 Rotavirus

Rotavirus (family Reoviridae) is highly infectious and a significant cause of nosocomial gastroenteritis, particularly in children <5 years of age. Patients present with sudden onset of fever, vomiting, abdominal pain and watery diarrhoea. Due to the high viral shedding in the faeces, a diagnosis can be easily obtained using antigen-detection enzyme-linked immunosorbent assay (ELISA) or electron microscopy.

In temperate climates the infection is seasonal with peaks in winter, and hospital outbreaks often coincide with outbreaks in the community. In Europe, it was found that 49–63% of paediatric nosocomial gastroenteritis was positive for rotavirus, with an incidence of 1–2.3 per 1,000 hospital days, leading to prolonged hospitalisation between 1.5 and 4.5 days [39]. Very sick infants with gastroenteritis may require intensive care and could, in turn, be the source of nosocomial infection in ICU. Premature and very low birth weight infants (<1,500 g) are particularly at risk, as severe complications such as necrotising enterocolitis and intestinal perforation are commonly reported. A Dutch study found that amongst all nosocomially acquired viral infections in NICUs, 10% were due to rotavirus, which demonstrates the importance of this infection in the ICU setting [40].

Nosocomial rotavirus infections in adults have also been reported and occasionally cause serious complications in the elderly and immunosuppressed patients. Nosocomial transmission has been previously associated with ungloved nasogastric feeding, contaminated toys, shortage of nurses, overcrowding and high patient turnover. Adherence to effective infection control measures (hand hygiene, enteric precautions; Table 20.3), as well as adequate staffing and patient cohorting/isolation can therefore help prevent or manage an outbreak [41]. The recently developed rotavirus vaccine could substantially reduce the incidence of nosocomial infections [42].

20.3.2 Norovirus

Norovirus (family Caliciviridae) is the most common cause of nosocomial outbreaks of gastroenteritis. Symptoms typically comprise profuse diarrhoea and projectile vomiting. The diagnosis can be confirmed by ELISA, RT-PCR or electron microscopy of stool samples. Noroviruses are highly infectious and are usually transmitted by direct contact via the faecal–oral route or via oropharyngeal exposure to aerosolised vomit. A number of outbreaks have recently been described in NICUs involving mainly premature neonates, some of whom developed necrotising enterocolitis. Neonates and immunocompromised patients can shed the virus for a prolonged time over months, which emphasises the need for rigorous adherence to effective infection control measures (Table 20.3). Additional measures such as increased hand hygiene and wiping of floors and

Table 20.3 General measures to control outbreak of viral gastroenteritis [41]

• Hand washing (liquid soap) or decontamination (aqueous antiseptic/alcohol based-hand rub) (A). However, alcohol-based products are known to be less effective against nonenveloped viruses, for which hand washing with soap and water is preferred (B)
• Wear disposable gloves and aprons when contact with stool or vomitus is likely (B)
• Isolate symptomatic individuals (particularly with uncontrolled diarrhoea, incontinence, and children) (B)
• Avoid unnecessary movement of patients to unaffected areas (B)
• Staff working in affected areas must not work in unaffected areas within 72 h (B)
• Exclude symptomatic staff members from duty until symptom free for 72 h (B)
• If a large number of patients is involved and no further isolation facilities are available, close the unit to new admissions or transfers until 72 h after the last new case (B)
• Terminal cleaning of the environment, using freshly prepared hypochlorite (1,000 ppm) on hard surfaces (B)
• Caution visitors and emphasise hand hygiene (B)

Categorisation of recommendations: *A* strongly recommended for all hospitals and strongly supported by well-designed experimental or epidemiological studies; *B* strongly recommended for all hospitals and viewed as effective by experts in the field

incubators with agents active against caliciviruses have been proven to be particularly useful in controlling outbreaks in NICU wards [43].

20.3.3 Enteroviruses and Parechoviruses

Both enteroviruses and parechoviruses (family Picornaviridae) have numerous subtypes. Enteroviruses include polioviruses, coxsackieviruses, echoviruses and other numbered enteroviruses. There are as many as 14 types of human parechoviruses [44]. Parechovirus type 3, in particular, can cause severe infection in young infants [45].

Both viruses are significant causes of nosocomial infections, particularly in the NICU. Enterovirus outbreaks involving up to 23 neonates have been reported [46], and an attack rate of 29% was reported. Enterovirus infections can present as neonatal sepsis, meningoencephalitis, myocarditis, hepatitis or gastroenteritis. Necrotising enterocolitis with pneumatosis intestinalis is a known complication in neonates. Some enteroviruses, such as *Enterovirus* 71, can cause severe and fatal illness in older children. Parechoviruses can cause meningoencephalitis [47] and a sepsis syndrome in young infants [48]. Enteroviruses and parechoviruses are genetically distinct from each other and require a different RT-PCR for diagnosis. Sequencing of the gene encoding the VP1 region of the virus has been used to identify outbreak strains.

With the global polio eradication programme, poliomyelitis is no longer a common nosocomial infection, although health care workers in the ICU who may be in contact with live vaccine poliovirus shedding infants should ensure that they are immunised.

Rigorous hand washing (Table 20.3) is the most important measure during an outbreak. Cohort nursing, source isolation and screening are other measures frequently used (Table 20.3). Clearance of the virus by the host is antibody-mediated and many have advocated the use of normal human immunoglobulin (NHIG).

20.3.4 Hepatitis A Virus

Hepatitis A virus (family Picornaviridae) belongs to the same family as enteroviruses and is usually transmitted via the faecal–oral route. Nosocomial transmission of hepatitis A virus is well documented. An outbreak in an adult ICU (AICU) occurred as a result of inadequate precautions taken while handling bile of a patient not suspected of incubating hepatitis A [49]. Most other outbreaks occurred in PICUs or NICUs, with attack rates varying between 15 and 25%. Risk factors for outbreaks have been attributed to handling soiled bed pads, nappies or gowns of an index patient, failure to wash hands, and eating in the ICU. In the NICU, vertical transmission and blood transfusion have been implicated as the cause of infection in the index case. The effect of nosocomial hepatitis A infection varies from asymptomatic to classic presentation with acute hepatitis. Diagnosis is by serological detection of hepatitis-A-specific IgM. The use of molecular techniques such as RT-PCR can help identify early infection or in difficult cases, such as those with immunodeficiency. Sequencing of PCR products is useful in establishing epidemiological linkage during outbreaks. NHIG has been successfully used for postexposure prophylaxis to control outbreaks. There is now increasing evidence that hepatitis A vaccine can be used for prophylaxis if the contact occurs within 14 days from onset of illness in the index case [50].

20.4 Viruses Transmitted by Blood and Body Fluid

The most commonly encountered nosocomial blood-borne viruses are hepatitis B virus (HBV), hepatitis C virus (HCV) and human immunodeficiency virus (HIV). The main risks are transmission from patients to health care workers. However, transmissions between patients and from health care workers to patients have been reported. The best way to prevent occupational exposure of blood-borne viruses is to practice universal precautions. Blood and body fluids (Table 20.4) from any patient, whether or not there are identifiable risk factors, should be considered as a potential risk. This encourages good and safe practice and helps prevent unnecessary accidents. Physical isolation of patients with blood-borne virus infection is generally not necessary unless there is profuse uncontrolled bleeding. Infection-control teams and occupational health departments should adopt a proactive approach to educate and prevent sharps injury (Table 20.5). There should also be specific instructions on how to deal with blood and body fluid exposure (Table 20.6).

Table 20.4 Body fluids that may pose a risk for hepatitis B and C virus (HBV, HCV) and human immunodeficiency virus (HIV) after significant exposure

- Amniotic fluid
- Breast milk
- Cerebrospinal fluid
- Exudate from burns or skin lesions
- Pericardial fluid
- Peritoneal fluid
- Pleural fluid
- Saliva after dental treatment
- Synovial fluid
- Unfixed tissues or organs
- Any other fluid if visibly blood stained

Saliva, urine, vomitus or stool that are not blood stained are not considered as high risk for blood borne viruses

20.4.1 Hepatitis B Virus

HBV is the most infectious of the three common blood-borne viruses. The risk of transmission depends on the viral load of the source patient. An HBV-infected individual with hepatitis B "e" antigen (HBeAg) tends to have a high viral load and is therefore more infectious than carriers without HBeAg. Estimate of infectivity ranges from 2% (HBeAg absent) to 40% (HBeAg present). All health care workers should be immunised against HBV. Exposed health care workers who are susceptible (not immunised or vaccine nonresponders) should receive hepatitis B immunoglobulin for postexposure prophylaxis. A booster dose of vaccine should be given to those exposed individual who had previously been successfully immunised.

20.4.2 Hepatitis C Virus

HCV is probably the commonest blood-borne virus encountered in Western countries. In the UK over a 3-year period, 462 incidences of occupational exposure to HCV were reported in comparison with 293 of HIV and 151 of HBV [51]. Follow-up studies of health care workers who sustained a percutaneous exposure to blood from a patient known to have HCV infection have reported an average incidence of seroconversion of 1.8% (range 0–7%). No vaccine or postexposure prophylaxis was available to prevent HCV transmission. Early diagnosis is essential, as early interferon treatment after seroconversion has a high success rate for eradication [52]. Exposed health care workers should be followed up at 6 and

Table 20.5 Example of points for sharps safety education (adapted from the Infection Control Team of Guys and St. Thomas' NHS Foundation Trust, London)

- Never resheath needles
- Dispose all sharps in an approved container
- Dispose sharps at the point of use
- If carried, sharps must be placed in a tray
- Do not overfill sharps bins—dispose of sharps bins when three-fourths full

Table 20.6 Example of actions to be taken immediately after a blood/body fluid exposure (adapted from the Infection Control Team of Guys and St. Thomas' NHS Foundation Trust, London)

- Rinse area thoroughly under running water
- If a wound, wash site with soap, encourage the wound to bleed, and apply a waterproof dressing (if appropriate)
- Report it immediately to:
  - Your supervisor (or line manager)
  - Occupational health or accident and emergency
- Document incident by completing an incident form with source name and details

12 weeks for HCV RNA testing and promptly referred for treatment if found infected.

20.4.3 Human Immunodeficiency Virus

The average risk of HIV transmission after percutaneous exposure to HIV-infected blood is about 0.3%. After mucocutaneous exposure, the risk is estimated to be <0.1%. A case-control study [53] identified four factors with increased risk of transmission:
- deep injury;
- visible blood on the device that caused the injury;
- injury with a needle that has been placed in a source patient's artery or vein;
- terminal HIV-related illness in the source patient.

This study also showed that the use of zidovudine prophylaxis reduce the risk of transmission by 80%. Postexposure prophylaxis (PEP) should therefore be offered to all health care workers who have significant exposure to blood or body fluid from a patient known to be at high risk of or to have HIV infection. Various PEP options are available depending on national recommendations. This should be started as soon as possible after exposure and continued for 4 weeks.

Table 20.7 Viruses responsible for viral haemorrhagic fevers with nosocomial concern in the intensive care unit

Virus	Geographic distribution	Reservoir	Vector
Marburg and Ebola	Sub-Sahara Africa	Bats	None
Rift Valley fever	Mainland Africa	Sheep, cattle	Mosquito
Lassa	West Africa	Rodents	None
Crimean Congo haemorrhagic fever	East, West and South Africa, North and Central Asia, Middle East, India and Pakistan, Balkans, West China	Cows, hares birds, hedgehogs	Ticks

20.4.4 Viral Haemorrhagic Fevers

Viral haemorrhagic fevers (VHFs) are severe and life-threatening diseases caused by a range of viruses. They are either zoonotic or arthropod-borne infections and are often endemic in certain parts of the world. They are often highly infectious through close contact with infected blood and body fluid and therefore pose a significant risk of hospital-acquired infection. As many patients with VHF present with shock and require vigorous supportive treatment, it is a potential problem in the ICU. The major viruses of nosocomial concern in this setting are Marburg, Ebola, Rift Valley fever, Lassa and Crimean Congo haemorrhagic fever (Table 20.7). The incubation period for these VHFs ranges from 3–21 days. Initial symptoms are often nonspecific but may eventually lead to haemorrhage and shock. Any febrile patient who has returned from an endemic area of one of the VHF agents or has a history of contact with cases suspected to have VHF within 3 weeks should be considered as at risk. However, malaria should always be excluded. A risk assessment needs to be performed, and any patient known or strongly suspected to be suffering from VHF should be admitted to a high-security infectious disease unit that is designed to manage these patients. While awaiting transfer to a secure unit, such patients should be placed in a negative-pressure room with strict source isolation. Specimens for patient management should be processed in a high-security laboratory designated for category 4 pathogens, and the aetiological agent established using PCR, serology and virus culture. All areas and materials in contact with infected patients should be autoclaved, incinerated or treated with hypochlorite (10,000 ppm of available chlorine). If the patient dies, the body should be placed in a sealable body bag sprayed or wiped with hypochlorite. Individuals who have been in contact with a case of VHF should be put under surveillance for 3 weeks. The successful i.v. use of ribavirin has been reported in some cases of VHFs (Lassa, Crimean Congo haemorrhagic fever and Hantaan). Apart from yellow fever, no vaccines are available.

20.5 Viruses Transmitted by Direct Contact

20.5.1 Varicella Zoster Virus; Shingles

Shingles or zoster is the result of the reactivation of latent VZV (family Herpesviridae) in the dorsal root or cranial nerve ganglia. The clinical presentation is a painful vesicular eruption covering the affected dermatome. The clinical diagnosis can be confirmed rapidly by immunofluorescence, electron microscopy or PCR of the cellular material obtained from a vesicular scraping. The infection is usually self-limiting but can be more severe in immunocompromised patients, in whom it may present over multiple dermatomes or as a disseminated infection. The latter cases should be managed as if they were chickenpox, and respiratory precautions for infection control have to be enforced.

Patients or health care staff members with classic shingles are contagious from the day the rash appears until the lesions are crusted over. There is some risk of nosocomial transmission if the lesions are on exposed areas of the body or in immunocompromised infected patients. Nonimmune (VZV-IgG negative) patients or health care staff members with no history of chickenpox are susceptible if they have close contact with shingles and should be managed as described for chickenpox contact.

20.5.2 Herpes Simplex Virus

The herpes simplex virus (HSV) (family Herpesviridae) consist of two types: HSV-1 and HSV-2. Clinically, they most commonly manifest with oral (mainly HSV-1) or genital (mainly HSV-2) ulcerations/vesicles, and reactivation is common, particularly in the ICU. Other presentations include keratitis, encephalitis, meningitis, herpetic whitlow or neonatal infection.

The diagnosis can be confirmed rapidly by immunofluorescence, electron microscopy or PCR of vesicle/ulcer scrapings. In the immunocompromised patient, HSV can cause life-threatening disseminated infection and, early treatment with acyclovir i.v. is recommended. It has also been suggested that occult herpes virus reactivation may increase the mortality risk of ICU patients [54].

As the infected lesions contain virus, there is an increased risk of nosocomial transmission until the lesions have crusted over. Standard isolation precautions should be in place to reduce transmission (Table 20.2). Patients with active lesions should be nursed away from high-risk patients (i.e. immunocompromised, severe eczema, burns, or neonates). As patients can be asymptomatic secretors, health care workers should wear gloves when dealing with mucosal secretions (i.e. saliva) to avoid infections such as herpetic whitlow. Infected staff should cover lesions if possible and should not attend those at risk.

Neonatal herpes is usually transmitted from mother to the child at the time of delivery and may not be noticed until the infant develops the disease. Universal precautions, in particularly, hand washing, should always be in place to reduce transmission of infection. To contain or prevent an outbreak, infected cases should be cohorted and nursed by dedicated staff who will not attend noninfected infants.

20.5.3 Rabies Virus

Rabies virus (family Rhabdoviridae) is usually transmitted to humans following exposure to saliva of a rabid animal (e.g. dog, fox, bat) via a bite or scratch, but only 40% of exposed people develop disease. The virus spreads from the wound to the central nervous system causing fatal encephalitis, and the virus may be present in the patient's saliva, skin, eye, and brain tissue. The diagnosis can be confirmed by demonstrating the virus directly in brain tissue or saliva by RT-PCR or by immunofluorescence detection of antigen in skin biopsies from the nape of the neck. Due to the severe and paralysing effect, patients may be admitted to the ICU. To date, no case of nosocomial transmission has been reported apart from two patients who received corneal transplants from infected donors. Suspected or proven cases should be placed in standard isolation and appropriate precautions taken when dealing with potential infectious secretions (e.g. wearing of mask if dealing with oral secretions). Any health care worker with a significant exposure (e.g. splash of secretion onto mucosa or broken skin) should receive rabies vaccine and specific immunoglobulin.

20.6 Summary

Viral infection can cause significant morbidity and mortality and has the potential to result in cross infection, involving patients as well as health care workers. Good infection-control practice is essential to prevent nosocomial infection. Intensivists should be on the alert for important viruses causing infections according to age group of patients and mode of transmission and should never be complacent. Good liaison with the laboratory is essential for determining correct diagnostic tests and timely report of results to help in patient management.

References

1. Fitzgerald DA (2009) Human swine influenza A. Paediatr Respir Rev 10:154–158
2. Trifonov V, Khiabanian H, Rabadan R (2009) Geographic dependence, surveillance, and origins of the 2009 influenza A (H1N1) virus. N Engl J Med 361:115–119
3. Webb SA, Pettila V, Seppelt I et al (2009) Critical care services and 2009 H1N1 influenza in Australia and New Zealand. N Engl J Med 361:1925–1934
4. Itoh Y, Shinya K, Kiso M et al (2009) In vitro and in vivo characterization of new swine-origin H1N1 influenza viruses. Nature 460:1021–1025
5. Writing committee of the WHO consultation on clinical aspects of pandemic (H1N1) 2009 Influenza (2010) Clinical aspects of pandemic 2009 Influenza A (H1N1) virus infection. N Engl J Med 362:1708–1719
6. Siston AM, Rasmussen SA, Honein MA et al (2010) Pandemic 2009 influenza A(H1N1) virus illness among pregnant women in the United States. JAMA 303:1517–1525

7. Campbell A, Rodin R, Kropp R et al (2010) Risk of severe outcomes among patients admitted to hospital with pandemic (H1N1) influenza. CMAJ 182:349–355
8. Hanslik T, Boelle PY, Flahault A (2010) Preliminary estimation of risk factors for admission to intensive care units and for death in patients infected with A(H1N1)2009 influenza virus, France, 2009–2010. PLoS Curr. 2010 March 9; 2:RRN1150
9. Anonymous (2009) Bacterial coinfections in lung tissue specimens from fatal cases of 2009 pandemic influenza A (H1N1)–United States, May–August 2009. MMWR Morb Mortal Wkly Rep 58:1071–1074
10. Anonymous (2009) Evaluation of rapid influenza diagnostic tests for detection of novel influenza A (H1N1) virus–United States, 2009. MMWR Morb Mortal Wkly Rep 58:826–829
11. Ellis J, Iturriza M, Allen R et al (2009) Evaluation of four real-time PCR assays for detection of influenza A (H1N1) viruses. Euro Surveill 14(22): pii: 19230
12. Flagg A, Danziger-Isakov L, Foster C et al (2010) Novel 2009 H1N1 influenza virus infection requiring extracorporeal membrane oxygenation in a pediatric heart transplant recipient. J Heart Lung Transpl 29:582–584
13. Christian MD, Joynt GM, Hick JL et al (2010) Critical care triage. Recommendations and standard operating procedures for intensive care unit and hospital preparations for an influenza epidemic or mass disaster. Intensive Care Med 36(Suppl 1):S55–S64
14. Jain S, Kamimoto L, Bramley AM et al (2009) Hospitalized patients with 2009 H1N1 influenza in the United States, April–June 2009. N Engl J Med 361:1935–1944
15. Taylor BL, Montgomery HE, Rhodes A, Sprung CL (2010) Protection of patients and staff during a pandemic. Recommendations and standard operating procedures for intensive care unit and hospital preparations for an influenza epidemic or mass disaster. Intensive Care Med 36(Suppl 1):S45–S54
16. Cheng VC, Tai JW, Wong LM et al (2010) Prevention of nosocomial transmission of swine-origin pandemic influenza virus A/H1N1 by infection control bundle. J Hosp Infect 74:271–277
17. Reiche J, Schweiger B (2009) Genetic variability of group A human respiratory syncytial virus strains circulating in Germany from 1998 to 2007. J Clin Microbiol 47:1800–1810
18. Berger TM, Aebi C, Duppenthaler A, Stocker M (2009) Prospective population-based study of RSV-related intermediate care and intensive care unit admissions in Switzerland over a 4-year period (2001–2005). Infection 37:109–116
19. Caram LB, Chen J, Taggart EW et al (2009) Respiratory syncytial virus outbreak in a long-term care facility detected using reverse transcriptase polymerase chain reaction: an argument for real-time detection methods. J Am Geriatr Soc 57:482–485
20. Gadsby NJ, Hardie A, Claas EC, Templeton KE (2010) Comparison of the Luminex RVP Fast assay with in-house real-time PCR for respiratory viral diagnosis. J Clin Microbiol 48:2213–2216
21. Lavergne V, Ghannoum M, Weiss K et al (2011) Successful prevention of respiratory syncytial virus nosocomial transmission following an enhanced seasonal infection control program. Bone Marrow Transpl 46(1):137–142
22. Morris SK, Dzolganovski B, Beyene J, Sung L (2009) A meta-analysis of the effect of antibody therapy for the prevention of severe respiratory syncytial virus infection. BMC Infect Dis 9:106
23. Falsey AR, Walsh EE (2000) Respiratory syncytial virus infection in adults. Clin Microbiol Rev 13:371–384
24. Boeckh M, Englund J, Li Y et al (2007) Randomized controlled multicenter trial of aerosolized ribavirin for respiratory syncytial virus upper respiratory tract infection in hematopoietic cell transplant recipients. Clin Infect Dis 44:245–249
25. Chavez-Bueno S, Mejias A, Merryman RA et al (2007) Intravenous palivizumab and ribavirin combination for respiratory syncytial virus disease in high-risk pediatric patients. Pediatr Infect Dis J 26:1089–1093
26. Terlizzi ME, Massimiliano B, Francesca S et al (2009) Quantitative RT real time PCR and indirect immunofluorescence for the detection of human parainfluenza virus 1, 2, 3. J Virol Methods 160:172–177

27. Maziarz RT, Sridharan P, Slater S et al (2010) Control of an outbreak of human parainfluenza virus 3 in hematopoietic stem cell transplant recipients. Biol Blood Marrow Transpl 16:192–198
28. Nichols WG, Corey L, Gooley T et al (2001) Parainfluenza virus infections after hematopoietic stem cell transplantation: risk factors, response to antiviral therapy, and effect on transplant outcome. Blood 98:573–578
29. Lenaerts L, De Clercq E, Naesens L (2008) Clinical features and treatment of adenovirus infections. Rev Med Virol 18:357–374
30. Williams KM, Agwu AL, Dabb AA et al (2009) A clinical algorithm identifies high risk pediatric oncology and bone marrow transplant patients likely to benefit from treatment of adenoviral infection. J Pediatr Hematol Oncol 31:825–831
31. Ksiazek TG, Erdman D, Goldsmith CS et al (2003) A novel coronavirus associated with severe acute respiratory syndrome. N Engl J Med 348:1953–1966
32. Poutanen SM, Low DE, Henry B et al (2003) Identification of severe acute respiratory syndrome in Canada. N Engl J Med 348:1995–2005
33. Lau EH, Hsiung CA, Cowling BJ et al (2010) A comparative epidemiologic analysis of SARS in Hong Kong, Beijing and Taiwan. BMC Infect Dis 10:50
34. Wong SS, Yuen KY (2008) The management of coronavirus infections with particular reference to SARS. J Antimicrob Chemother 62:437–441
35. Cheng VC, Lau SK, Woo PC, Yuen KY (2007) Severe acute respiratory syndrome coronavirus as an agent of emerging and reemerging infection. Clin Microbiol Rev 20:660–694
36. Cameron JC, Allan G, Johnston F et al (2007) Severe complications of chickenpox in hospitalised children in the UK and Ireland. Arch Dis Child 92:1062–1066
37. Aly NY, Al Obaid I, Al-Qulooshi N, Zahed Z (2007) Occupationally related outbreak of chickenpox in an intensive care unit. Med Princ Pract 16:399–401
38. Apisarnthanarak A, Kitphati R, Tawatsupha P et al (2007) Outbreak of varicella-zoster virus infection among Thai healthcare workers. Infect Control Hosp Epidemiol 28:430–434
39. Fruhwirth M, Heininger U, Ehlken B et al (2001) International variation in disease burden of rotavirus gastroenteritis in children with community- and nosocomially acquired infection. Pediatr Infect Dis J 20:784–791
40. Verboon-Maciolek MA, Krediet TG, Gerards LJ et al (2005) Clinical and epidemiologic characteristics of viral infections in a neonatal intensive care unit during a 12-year period. Pediatr Infect Dis J 24:901–904
41. Boyce JM, Pittet D (2002) Guideline for hand hygiene in health-care settings. Recommendations of the healthcare infection control practices Advisory Committee and the HIPAC/SHEA/APIC/IDSA Hand Hygiene Task Force. Am J Infect Control 30:S1–S46
42. Cunliffe NA, Both JA, Lowe SJ et al (2010) Healthcare-associated viral gastroenteritis among children in a large pediatric hospital, United Kingdom. Emerg Infect Dis 16:55–62
43. Armbrust S, Kramer A, Olbertz D et al (2009) Norovirus infections in preterm infants: wide variety of clinical courses. BMC Res Notes 2:96
44. Nix WA, Maher K, Pallansch MA, Oberste MS (2010) Parechovirus typing in clinical specimens by nested or semi-nested PCR coupled with sequencing. J Clin Virol 48:202–207
45. Harvala H, Robertson I, Chieochansin T et al (2009) Specific association of human parechovirus type 3 with sepsis and fever in young infants, as identified by direct typing of cerebrospinal fluid samples. J Infect Dis 199:1753–1760
46. Takami T, Sonodat S, Houjyo H et al (2000) Diagnosis of horizontal enterovirus infections in neonates by nested PCR and direct sequence analysis. J Hosp Infect 45:283–287
47. Gupta S, Fernandez D, Siddiqui A et al (2010) Extensive white matter abnormalities associated with neonatal Parechovirus (HPeV) infection. Eur J Paediatr Neurol 14(6):531–534
48. Benschop KS, Schinkel J, Minnaar RP et al (2006) Human parechovirus infections in Dutch children and the association between serotype and disease severity. Clin Infect Dis 42:204–210
49. Hanna JN, Loewenthal MR, Negel P, Wenck DJ (1996) An outbreak of hepatitis A in an intensive care unit. Anaesth Intensive Care 24:440–444

50. Victor JC, Monto AS, Surdina TY et al (2007) Hepatitis A vaccine versus immune globulin for postexposure prophylaxis. N Engl J Med 357:1685–1694
51. Evans B, Duggan W, Baker J et al (2001) Exposure of healthcare workers in England, Wales, and Northern Ireland to bloodborne viruses between July 1997 and June 2000: analysis of surveillance data. BMJ 322:397–398
52. Maheshwari A, Thuluvath PJ (2010) Management of acute hepatitis C. Clin Liver Dis 14:169–176
53. Cardo DM, Culver DH, Ciesielski CA et al (1997) A case-control study of HIV seroconversion in health care workers after percutaneous exposure. Centers for Disease Control and Prevention Needlestick Surveillance Group. N Engl J Med 337:1485–1490
54. Cook CH, Martin LC, Yenchar JK et al (2003) Occult herpes family viral infections are endemic in critically ill surgical patients. Crit Care Med 31:1923–1929

AIDS Patients in the ICU

F. E. Arancibia and M. A. Aguayo

21.1 Introduction

In the early 1980s in the United States, the first medical reports described outbreaks of Kaposi's sarcoma and *Pneumocystis carinii* (now *P. jiroveci*) pneumonia in homosexual men [1, 2]. These reports rate respiratory infections by opportunistic germs and rare tumors affecting healthy young men. High mortality rates were observed that were most likely caused by acute respiratory failure (ARF). Additionally, each report had abnormal ratios of lymphocyte subgroups. Subsequent reports described an escalating frequency of unusual infections and tumors, suggesting a profound state of immune suppression in many homosexual men, injection-drug users, sexual partners of infected persons, hemophiliacs who had received blood transfusions, and children.

In early 1983, virologists at the Pasteur Institute first isolated the human immunodeficiency virus (HIV) [3], a retrovirus that infects cells of the immune system (subgroup of CD4+ T cells), destroying or impairing their function. The most advanced stage of HIV infection was called AIDS. In the early years, the ICU survival rate of patients with AIDS was low [4]. Based on the belief that ICU care of patients with AIDS was futile, clinical, ethical, and economic issues were raised regarding the benefits and burdens of the critical care of these patients. However, the use of *P. carinii* pneumonia (PCP) prophylaxis, antiretroviral therapy, and corticosteroids for PCP has changed outcomes. Several studies have shown improved survival rates and costs of HIV-infected patients admitted to the ICU [5–8].

F. E. Arancibia (✉)
Unidad de Cuidados Intensivos,
Instituto Nacional Tórax, Santiago, Chile
e-mail: fearancibia@gmail.com

Up to 35–60% of persons with underlying HIV are unaware of their HIV infection at the time of ICU admission [9]. According to other authors, this is due to the fact that the HIV epidemic has two distinct populations of patients. First, there are patients with access to care and to the full armamentarium of HIV-related drugs. In contrast to this patient population is the sizable number of individuals who are either unaware of their HIV status or who lack access to care. These patients continue to appear in emergency rooms and the ICU with the same opportunistic infections that were seen in the 1980s.

HIV is the world's leading infectious killer, with an estimated 2 million AIDS deaths occurring in 2008 alone. The global HIV burden remains enormous. At the end of 2008, an estimated 33.4 million people worldwide were living with HIV. Africa, Asia, and America had the highest incidence. That same year, some 2.7 million people became newly infected with the virus [10].

21.2 Causes for ICU Admission

In the United States and Europe, from 4 to 11% of HIV patients hospitalized require admission to the ICU. All studies show that respiratory failure has remained the most common indication for an ICU admission [5, 8, 11, 12]. Other frequent indications are sepsis and neurological compromise (Table 21.1). Occasionally, patients with severe gastrointestinal symptoms, cardiomyopathies and/or complications such as lactic acidosis and pancreatitis may require intensive care. Finally, these patients may have clinical or surgical conditions requiring ICU admission unrelated to their HIV/AIDS. HIV-infected patients admitted to the ICU following trauma, elective surgery, or gastrointestinal bleeding may have as good a prognosis as patients without HIV infection [9].

However, opportunistic illness rates declined precipitously after the introduction of highly active antiretroviral therapy (HAART) and stabilized at low levels in the subsequent years. Buchacz et al. [13] reported that during 1994–2007, rates of opportunistic infections (per 1,000 person-years) decreased from 89 to 13.3 and rates of opportunistic malignancies were from 23.4 to 3.0 (Fig. 21.1). Due to the dramatic improvement in the prognosis of HIV-infected patients, our notion of HIV as a disease has transformed from a rapidly fatal diagnosis to a treatable chronic condition.

The etiologies of respiratory failure are diverse and include: (1) PCP, initially responsible for a high burden of disease and low survival rates; later studies demonstrated improved survival, even among PCP patients; (2) bacterial pneumonia is more frequent in patients with HIV; (3) cytomegalovirus (CMV) is a minor cause. Also, patients with other associated infections, such as tuberculosis (TB) and fungal infection; or associated malignancy, such as Kaposi's sarcoma and non-Hodgkin's lymphoma; or immune reconstitution syndrome (Fig. 21.2), may develop respiratory failure during disease evolution [9, 14]. The patients with ARF due to *P. jiroveci* and other opportunistic agents can be treated with

Table 21.1 General characteristics, intensive care unit admission diagnosis, mechanical ventilation, and mortality rates of HIV-infected patients

	Nickas 1992–1995 [11] ($n = 394$)	Casalino 1995–1999 [8] ($n = 426$)	Morris 1996–1999 [5] ($n = 354$)	Powell 2000–2004 [12] ($n = 311$)
Age, years, mean (range)	38 (20–64)	38.5	41.7 (23–67)	44 (24–72)
Male, sex	357 (91)	338 (79.3)	285 (80.5)	235 (79.7)
Respiratory failure	203 (46.8)	134 (31.4)	144 (40.7)	131 (42)
Sepsis	54 (12.2)	58 (13.6)	42 (11.9)	62 (20)
Pneumocystis pneumonia	264 (67)	52 (12.2)	36 (10.7)	43 (14)
Neurologic	49 (11.1)	108 (25.4)	44 (12.4)	51 (16)
Cardiac	35 (7.9)	23 (5.4)	35 (9.9)	
Mechanical ventilation	245 (55)	81 (19)	191 (54)	205 (67.7)
HAART use	205 (52)	230 (54)	89 (25)	101 (33)
Mortality	264 (67)	98 (23)	103 (29)	96 (31)

HAART highly active antiretroviral therapy
Values are given as Number (%), unless otherwise indicated

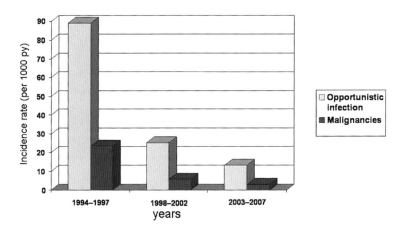

Fig. 21.1 Incidence of AIDS-defining opportunistic infections and malignancies, the HIV infected patient study, 1994–2007 [13]

noninvasive ventilation (NIV). The use of NIV improves gas exchange and avoids intubation and mechanical ventilation. Patients who failed with the use of NIV or present severe ARF still require intubation and mechanical ventilation.

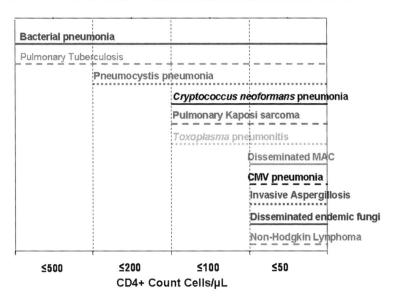

Fig. 21.2 CD4+ cell count ranges for selected HIV-related respiratory illnesses. *CMV* Cytomegalovirus; *MAC Mycobacterium avium* complex [18, 21, 23, 28, 31, 37, 38, 43, 47, 49–51, 54, 57]

The global mortality ratios in hospitalized patients infected with HIV requiring ICU admission went from 23 to 67% [4–8, 11, 12], most frequently due to respiratory failure and septic shock. The death of many HIV-infected patients has been linked directly to late diagnosis and initiation of appropriate antiviral therapy. Several clinical factors are related to the outcome of AIDS patients in the ICU. Predictors of increased mortality risk include the need for mechanical ventilation, and disease severity [high Acute Physiology and Chronic Health Evaluation (APACHE) II score or simplified acute physiological score (SAPS), modified multisystem organ failure (MSOF) score, CD4 count, pneumothorax, presence of cardiovascular instability, and low levels of serum albumin] [14, 15]. Mortality rates of HIV-infected patients and the need for mechanical ventilation early in the epidemic—prior to 1988—reached 82% [16]. However, the use of protective ventilation (lower tidal volume ventilation) is associated with reduced mortality rates in HIV-infected patients with acute lung injury and respiratory failure [17].

21.3 Pneumocystis carinii Pneumonia

PCP remains the most prevalent opportunistic infection in patients infected with the HIV and is often the AIDS-defining illness, occurring most frequently when the T-helper cell count (CD4+) is <200 cells/µl. First identified as a protozoan nearly 100 years ago and reclassified as a fungus in 1988, named *P. carinii* but renamed *P. jiroveci*, has a unique tropism for the lung, where it exists primarily as

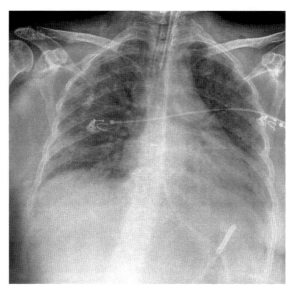

Fig. 21.3 Chest radiograph of a 62-year-old woman who is unaware of her HIV status. Diffuse bilateral reticular pattern with foci of consolidation in the left lower lobe. *Pneumocystis jiroveci* was detected in bronchoalveolar fluid and transbronchial biopsy

an alveolar pathogen without invading the host. In rare cases, pneumocystis disseminates in the setting of severe underlying immunosuppression or overwhelming infection [14, 18].

At the beginning of the AIDS epidemic, around 75% of patients developed at least one episode of PCP, with even higher mortality rates of 35–85% in patients requiring admission to an ICU. With the use of prophylaxis, the incidence of PCP decreased from 47 to 25% [19]. Prophylaxis against *P. jiroveci* pneumonia can be safely discontinued in patients with HIV infection who have had a positive response to HAART (indicated by a CD4 count >200 cells/µl) with minimal risk of recurrent *P. jiroveci* pneumonia [20].

Common symptoms of PCP include the subtle onset of progressive dyspnea, nonproductive cough, and low-grade fever. Physical examination typically reveals tachypnea, tachycardia, and normal findings on lung auscultation. It is typically subacute with a clinical course of days or weeks. Acute dyspnea with pleuritic chest pain may indicate the development of a pneumothorax [14, 18, 21].

Typical radiographic features of PCP are diffuse bilateral interstitial infiltrates involving the entire lung or the lower lung fields [18, 22] (Fig. 21.3). Less common findings include localized infiltrates, upper-lobe infiltrates, solitary or multiple nodules, and pneumatoceles. Pleural effusions and thoracic lymphadenopathy are rare. Approximately 6% of patients can develop spontaneous pneumothoraces during the course of their illness. High-resolution computed tomography, which is more sensitive than chest radiography, may reveal extensive ground-glass

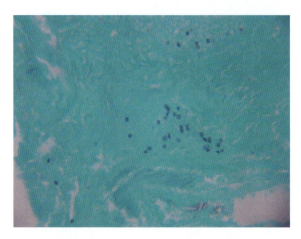

Fig. 21.4 Transbronchial biopsy specimen stained with Grocott's of an adult woman showing typical pneumocystis cyst forms of 5–6 μm (courtesy of Manuel Meneses M.D)

attenuation or cystic lesions. This greater organism burden results in a higher diagnostic yield of induced sputum to confirm PCP in patients with AIDS. If the initial specimen of induced sputum is negative for pneumocystis, then bronchoscopy with bronchoalveolar lavage (BAL) should be performed. Transbronchial or surgical lung biopsy is rarely needed [14, 18, 21] (Fig. 21.4).

PCP may be difficult to diagnose owing to nonspecific symptoms and signs, the use of prophylactic drugs in HIV-infected patients, and simultaneous infection with multiple organisms (such as CMV) in an immunocompromised host. Although an elevated serum lactate dehydrogenase (LDH) level has been noted in patients with PCP, it is likely to be a reflection of the underlying lung inflammation and injury rather than a specific marker for the disease [23].

Since the beginning of the AIDS epidemic, respiratory failure caused by *P. jiroveci* has been the most common indication for ICU admission among patients with HIV infection (Table 21.1). However, the proportion of ICU admissions caused by respiratory failure has declined [16, 18, 24]. Patients with ARF due to *P. jiroveci* can be treated with NIV. In one study, NIV failed only in 13% of HIV-positive patients with severe PCP [25]. Confalonieri et al. [26] compared early NIV in patients with AIDS and PCP with matched controls treated with conventional mechanical ventilation. The mortality rate was 38 versus 100%, respectively. Also, NIV reduced the incidence of pneumothorax.

Patients with HIV infection who also have acute respiratory distress syndrome (ARDS) requiring mechanical ventilation should receive such therapy according to the ARDS Network guidelines with the use of low tidal volumes and plateau pressures [17, 27]. The application of these guidelines is especially crucial in patients with PCP because of the frequent presence of pneumatoceles associated with the infection and the resulting increased risk of pneumothorax during mechanical ventilation. The presence of pneumothorax is an independent risk factor for death in patients with HIV infection and PCP (15).

Trimethoprim/sulfamethoxazole remains the preferred treatment. Other options could be primaquine plus clindamycin, atovaquone, and pentamidine [18, 28]. Early adjunctive corticosteroid therapy to suppress lung inflammation in patients with severe PCP and hypoxemia (partial pressure of arterial oxygen while the patient is breathing room air is <70 mm Hg or the alveolar–arterial gradient is >35) reduces the risks of death in patients with AIDS [29]. In addition, Morris et al. reported an improvement in survival with HAART in HIV-infected patients with severe PCP [30].

In the 1980s and early to mid-1990s, PCP was responsible for a high burden of the disease, and survival rates were low; later studies demonstrated improved survival rates. Among most patients with AIDS and PCP, the mortality rate is 10–20% during the initial infection, but the rate increases substantially with the need for mechanical ventilation [18, 25, 29, 30].

21.4 Bacterial Respiratory Infections

21.4.1 Bacterial Pneumonia

Early in the HIV epidemic, researchers noted that bacterial pneumonia (BP) was a common cause of morbidity. BP is an important cause of morbidity and mortality in patients with HIV infection and is at least five times more frequent in HIV-infected patients compared with healthy individuals. In the precombination ART era, the HIV Infection Study reported the incidence of BP ranged was 3.9–7.3 episodes per 100 person-years. Since the introduction of ART, a reduction in the risk for BP has been observed [21, 31, 32]. BP is still among the most common causes of respiratory failure resulting in ICU admission [32] and might be the first manifestation of underlying HIV infection. BP can occur at any stage during HIV disease and at any CD4+ T-cell count, but it is substantially more frequent among those with <200 CD4+ T-cell counts. Other risk factors include drug use intravenously, previous bacterial infection or PCP, smoking, a low socioeconomic status, alcohol abuse, comorbidities (including cardiovascular disease, renal disease, and hepatic cirrhosis), and malnutrition [31–33].

The microbiologic cause of community-acquired BP identified most frequently in HIV-infected patients, are *Streptococcus pneumoniae* and *Haemophilus* species [21]. *S. pneumoniae* is the most common causative agent and is frequently associated with bacteremic disease [31, 33]. The rate of pneumococcal bacteremia is higher in patients with than without HIV infection [33]. Patients with HIV infection are at increased risk for infection with penicillin and cotrimoxazole-resistant *S. pneumoniae*, and identifying this microorganism could lead to changes in patient management [21, 23, 33].

H. influenzae, both the encapsulated and nonencapsulated types, is also common. *Pseudomonas aeruginosa* pneumonia in some studies has been reported as a common pulmonary complication [33], especially in patients with low leukocyte and CD4+ T-cell counts and ill enough to require ICU admission. Also, there is a growing number of literature reports about the occurrence of pneumonia due to *Staphylococcus aureus*, especially oxacillin-resistant strains, is this population. Atypical pathogens (*Mycoplasma*, *Chlamydia*, and *Legionella*) seem not to play a significant role in HIV-infected patients. Rare causes of pneumonia presenting with cavitation are *Rhodococcus equi* and *Nocardia asteroides* [21, 23, 33].

The clinical and radiographic presentation of BP does not differ substantially for HIV-infected compared with HIV-uninfected patients. Compared with *P. jiroveci* pneumonia and other opportunistic infections of lung, the onset of fever and other symptoms is more abrupt and the patients is more likely to experience a productive cough and pleuritic chest pain. In contrast, patients with low CD4 cell count, who are at an increased risk of BP, often present an atypical clinical picture with milder symptoms and signs, especially when liver cirrhosis is also present. The white blood cell count is usually elevated in persons with BP, and a left shift also might be present. Radiographic features typically include unilateral, focal, segmental, or lobar consolidation. Also, HIV-infected persons might present with multifocal or multilobar involvement and with parapneumonic effusions [31–33]. The American Thoracic Society (ATS) severity criteria developed to assess community-acquired pneumonia (CAP) in patients not infected with HIV have been found to be valid also for HIV-infected patients with bacterial CAP [33].

Prompt and accurate diagnosis is essential, because the outcome of HIV-associated BP appears to be reasonably good with appropriate treatment. Usually, collection of specimens for microbiologic studies should be performed before the initiation of antibiotic therapy. An etiologic diagnosis is obtained in an average of 35% of cases with standard culture methods. In such conditions, urinary antigen test for *S. pneumoniae* identification may help in reaching a rapid and etiologic diagnosis [31]. However, antibiotic therapy should be administered promptly, without waiting for the results of diagnostic testing. Guidelines for managing CAP in persons without HIV infection also apply to HIV-infected persons [34]. Persons with severe pneumonia who require intensive care should be treated with an IV beta-lactam plus either azithromycin intravenously or an IV respiratory fluoroquinolone. If risk factors for *P. aeruginosa* or *S. aureus* infection are present, empiric therapy to cover these pathogens should be contemplated [28].

In all patients presenting with antimicrobial treatment failure, a regular microbial reinvestigation is mandatory in order to find potentially life-threatening etiologies. Given the increased incidence of *Mycobacterium tuberculosis* in HIV-infected persons, the diagnosis of TB should always be suspected in those with pneumonia. Also, noninfectious causes with pulmonary dysfunction should be considered [21, 28, 31].

BP mortality rate is high, and some studies may reach 30%. Factors associated with increased mortality in HIV patients with BP include the presence of septic shock, radiologic progression of infiltrates, and CD4 counts <100 cells/μl.

21.4.2 Nosocomial Pneumonia

Nosocomial pneumonia (NP) appears to be more common in patients with AIDS as a result of the degree of immunosuppression, prior use of antibiotics, and exposure to invasive procedures. Although underestimated, NP is associated with a higher morbidity and mortality rate. NP is most frequently a complication of mechanical ventilation. Improved ART options in developed countries resulted in a decreased hospitalization rate of HIV-infected individuals and the incidence of NP. A study of surveillance of HIV-infected inpatients showed an NP incidence decreasing from 13.9/10,000 patient hospital days between 1994 and 1996 to 5.6/10,000 patient hospital days between 1997 and 1998 [35].

NP in HIV-infected patients is usually caused by Gram-negative bacilli and *S. aureus*, but fungal, viral, and tuberculin infections causes must also be considered. Among atypical agents, *Legionella* pneumonia in HIV-infected patients should be hospital acquired. Clinical and microbiological surveys in HIV-positive patients have found that *P. aeruginosa* is a frequent agent, accounting for 16–67% of nosocomial pneumonias. Empiric antibiotics in HIV-infected patients with suspected hospital-acquired pneumonia should cover potentially multi-drug-resistant organisms such as *P. aeruginosa, Klebsiella pneumonia, Acinetobacter* spp., as well as methicillin-resistant *S. aureus* [21, 23, 35, 36].

21.4.3 Bacteremia Infection

The importance of bacterial infections that complicate the clinical course of patients with HIV infection has been recognized since the beginning of the AIDS epidemic. HIV-infected patients have an increased risk of bacteremia compared with the general population. The presence of bloodstream infection is associated with an increased mortality rate, length of hospital stay, and ICU admission rate. Bacteremia infections are responsible for the immediate cause of death of up to 30% of patients with HIV infection [37].

Several risk factors predispose for bacteremia infections among HIV-infected patients. These include the presence of neutropenia, use of central venous catheters, low CD4+ lymphocyte count, and IV drug use. The common sources of bloodstream infection in patients with HIV infection include the lungs, skin, subcutaneous tissue, and intravascular catheters.

Most bacteremias are community acquired. The most common Gram-positive organism isolated from the bloodstream of patients with HIV is *S. pneumoniae*, followed by *S. aureus*; the most common Gram-negative organisms are *Escherichia coli, Salmonella* spp., and *Pseudomonas* spp. The annual incidence of pneumococcal bacteremia is estimated to be as high as 940/100,000 patients with AIDS [21]. However, similar to other infections, the incidence of bacteremia has been declining since the introduction of HAART. Hospital mortality rates of HIV-positive patients with bloodstream infection range from 9 to 54%, but mortality rates are higher for patients with bacterial sepsis.

21.5 Viral Pneumonias

CMV is the most frequent viral pneumonia seen in persons with HIV infection. Although CMV is often detected in BAL fluid, documented CMV pneumonia is rare and occurs only in severely immunosuppressed patients with CD4 cell counts <50/µl [38]. Some studies suggest that CMV in BAL fluid reflects bronchopulmonary replication of the virus. Although the majority of patients with CMV pneumonia have additional forms of pulmonary pathology, CMV is the only causative agent frequently identified in patients with severe pulmonary disease. Due to the high coinfection rate with *P. jiroveci*, in cases of PCP treatment failure and severe immunosuppression, the main differential diagnosis must be established with CMV. Some authors believe that it represents a preterminal phenomenon in advanced AIDS [21].

Criteria for establishing that CMV is the cause of pneumonitis and pulmonary dysfunction have been difficult to establish. Clinical features are nonproductive cough, fever, progressive dyspnea, hypoxemia, and diffuse interstitial infiltrates [23]. Respiratory symptoms are typically present for 2–4 weeks. Physical examination of the chest may be normal or may reveal crackles or evidence of pleural effusion. The chest radiographic findings of CMV pneumonia vary and include reticular or ground-glass opacities, alveolar infiltrates, and nodules or nodular opacities. Pleural effusions may be seen as well. The latter finding may be helpful in distinguishing CMV pneumonia from *P. jiroveci*, in which pleural effusions are rare. Persons suspected of having CMV pneumonia should undergo a careful dilated retinal examination by an experienced ophthalmologist. Definitive diagnosis of CMV pneumonia requires demonstration of cytopathic inclusions and widespread specific cytopathic changes in the lungs. Confirming the diagnosis is often not easy due to the typically extremely serious condition, making it difficult to perform a lung biopsy. Autopsy studies revealed that patients with AIDS and CMV pneumonia were successfully diagnosed antemortem in only 13–24% of cases. New techniques using in situ DNA hybridization or monoclonal antibodies to detect the virus may improve the diagnostic yield of less invasive procedures, such as bronchoalveolar lavage [39].

When suspected CMV pulmonary disease occurs, therapy must be initiated immediately. Ganciclovir and foscarnet or cidofovir have been used to treat CMV pneumonia [28], although few data establish that such therapy affects outcome. Ganciclovir appears to be less effective against pulmonary infections than against retinitis or gastrointestinal disease, with response rates of 50–60%. Despite the monolithic use of ganciclovir for CMV-related illness, reports of CMV-resistant strains have been mostly limited to long-term usage in patients with HIV infection.

The combination of ganciclovir plus foscarnet may be useful in the setting of ganciclovir-resistant CMV disease [28, 39].

Pneumonitis due to herpes simplex, varicella–zoster, and respiratory syncytial viruses has occasionally been reported in AIDS patients. These viruses are of practical importance due to the availability of effective treatment [9]. Also, data from several studies suggest that Epstein–Barr virus (EBV) has a role in pneumonitis. EBV DNA and proteins have been detected in pulmonary lesions from children with HIV and lymphoid interstitial pneumonitis [40]. The role of influenza and adenoviruses in causing HIV-related pulmonary complications could be important during outbreaks of these infections. Patients with HIV infection frequently developed complications or severe illness with 2009 H1N1 virus infection [41].

21.6 Mycobacteriosis

21.6.1 Tuberculosis

Around the world, TB remains an important public health problem, especially in developing countries. Since the emergence of AIDS, TB and HIV infections have been intimately connected. HIV probably increases susceptibility to infection with *M. tuberculosis* and the risk of progression to TB. Also, TB appears to accelerate the course of HIV disease [21]. By the end of 2000, approximately 11.5 million HIV-infected people worldwide were coinfected with *M. tuberculosis*. Seventy percent of coinfected people were in sub-Saharan Africa and 20% in Southeast Asia [42]. TB is the most common opportunistic disease and the most common cause of death in HIV patients in developing countries [43]. Severe TB requiring ICU care is rare but commonly known to be of markedly bad prognosis (Fig. 21.5). The most common reasons for ICU admission are the development of ARDS and severe organ failure, such as renal failure. ARF caused by TB necessitating mechanical ventilation has been associated with high mortality rates. Several studies also reported a critical course in patients with miliary TB and HIV infection.

The clinical presentation of HIV-infected patients without pronounced immunodeficiency (e.g., CD4+ count >350 cells/µl) with TB is usually similar to that in HIV-negative cases. However, with progressive immunodeficiency, disseminated disease and extrapulmonary involvement occurs more frequently. Weight loss and fever are more common in HIV-positive pulmonary TB patients than in those who are HIV negative. Conversely, cough and hemoptysis are less common in HIV-positive pulmonary TB patients than in those who are HIV negative. This is probably because there is less cavitation, inflammation, and endobronchial irritation in HIV-positive patients. The physical signs in patients with pulmonary TB are nonspecific. The most commonly reported extrapulmonary sites of disease are the lymph nodes, pleura, pericardium, meninges, and genitourinary system. Typical radiographs are seen in only one-third of patients, and they usually have a CD4 count >200 cells/µl [43, 44]. In advanced HIV disease, chest radiographic findings

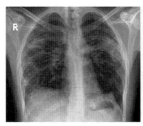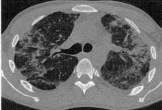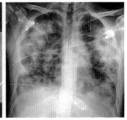

Fig. 21.5 A 27-year-old man with advanced HIV infection and highly active antiretroviral treatment. Chest radiographic (**a**) and high-resolution computed tomography scans (**b**) showing peribronchial thickening, nodularity, and septal lines. Two months later (**c**), progression of lung involvement to multiple nodular infiltrates, confluent lesions, and acute respiratory failure; video thoracoscopic biopsy showed Kaposi's sarcoma

of pulmonary TB commonly include lower lobe, middle lobe, interstitial, and miliary infiltrates; cavitation is less common [28].

The first screening test for suspected pulmonary TB is sputum, bronchial aspirate secretions, or BAL sample for acid-fast bacilli smear and culture. The chances of finding TB bacilli are greater with three respiratory samples than with fewer samples [44]. For patients with signs of extrapulmonary TB, needle aspiration or tissue biopsy of skin lesions, lymph nodes, or pleural or pericardial fluid should be performed. Mycobacterial blood cultures might be helpful for patients with signs of disseminated disease or worsening immunodeficiency [28, 43].

HIV-infected persons who adhere to standard regimens of treatment for TB do not have an increased risk of treatment failure or relapse. Treatment of drug-susceptible TB should include a 6-month regimen with an initial phase of isoniazid, rifampin or rifabutin, pyrazinamide, and ethambutol administered for 2 months, followed by isoniazid and rifampin (or rifabutin) for 4 additional months. However, studies have found that HIV-seropositive patients are more likely to develop acquired drug resistance than are seronegative cases. Patients with TB caused by drug-resistant (especially multi-drug-resistant) organisms should be treated with specialized regimens containing second-line anti-TB drugs. At least four drugs to which the organisms are known or presumed to be susceptible should be used, and treatment should be given for at least 18 months. Delayed clinical suspicion and treatment of active pulmonary TB with ARF may contribute to the persistently high mortality rates in ICU patients with these diseases [28, 43, 44]. The optimal timing for initiating ART in patients with HIV and TB coinfection remains unclear. Despite World Health Organization (WHO) guidelines supporting concomitant treatment of the two diseases (TB/HIV), the initiation of antiretroviral therapy is often deferred until completion of TB therapy because of concern about potential drug interactions between rifampin and some classes of antiretroviral drugs, immune reconstitution inflammatory syndrome, and overlapping side effects. Abdool Karim et al., in a prospective and randomized trial, found that the initiation of ART during TB therapy in patients with confirmed TB and HIV coinfection reduced mortality rates by 56% [45].

21.6.2 Mycobacterium avium

M. avium complex (MAC) infection is common in patients with AIDS. In contrast to the experience in nonimmunocompromised hosts, in whom clinical manifestations are primarily pulmonary, MAC causes disseminated infection, often with documented mycobacteremia in patients with AIDS. In the absence of effective HAART or chemoprophylaxis in those with AIDS-associated immunosuppression, the incidence of disseminated MAC disease is 20–40% [28]. Since early 1980s, MAC infection has been detected at autopsy in >50% of patients dying from AIDS, and in one study, infection due to MAC was detected antemortem in 44%, with blood culture being the most sensitive diagnostic means [46]. In HIV patients, MAC typically occurs among persons with CD4 counts <50 cells/µl, suggesting that specific T-cell products or activities are required for mycobacterial resistance [42]. Natural history studies of persons with AIDS in the pre-ART era showed that almost 40% of patients with <50 CD4+ T cells/µl developed disseminated MAC within 1 year. Other factors associated with increased susceptibility to MAC are high plasma HIV RNA levels (>100,000 copies/ml), previous opportunistic infections, previous colonization of the respiratory or gastrointestinal tract with MAC, and reduced in vitro lymphoproliferative immune responses to *M. avium* antigens, possibly reflecting defects in T-cell repertoire.

Disseminated infection is associated with high mortality rates, especially in those with CD4 counts <100 cells/mm^3. It primarily affects the gastrointestinal tract and lungs and manifests with fever, cough, abdominal pain, diarrhea, and weight loss. A significant proportion of total body burden is on MAC inside macrophages, and this distribution has implications for drug treatment and, therefore, on drug susceptibility testing. A confirmed diagnosis of disseminated MAC disease is based on compatible clinical signs and symptoms coupled with MAC isolation from cultures of blood, lymph node, bone marrow, or other normally sterile tissue or body fluids [28, 42, 46]. Species identification should be performed using specific DNA probes, high-performance liquid chromatography, or biochemical tests.

The treatment is always a combination of three active drugs according to severity. Drugs may include ethambutol, a rifamycin (rifampin or rifabutin), and a macrolide (mainly clarithromycin); other possibilities include aminoglycosides (amikacin) and fluoroquinolones [28, 42].

21.7 Mycoses

21.7.1 Cryptococcosis

Fungal pneumonias—other than PCP—occur in patients with HIV infection but are not common in most geographic areas. The era of effective ART has led to a marked reduction in opportunistic infections in countries where such therapies are available. Opportunistic fungal infections are no exception, and the incidence of such infections is now 20–25% of that seen in the mid-1990s [47]. However, fungal opportunistic infections remain significant causes of morbidity and mortality in persons with HIV in developing countries. After TB and *P. jiroveci* pneumonia, cryptococcosis was the third most common opportunistic infection reported in Thailand [48].

Cryptococcus neoformans is the most common fungal pulmonary infection in patients with AIDS and usually coexists with cryptococcal meningitis. Also, cryptococcal pneumonia may be underdiagnosed and not recognized until dissemination. The majority of cases are observed in patients who have CD4 counts <100 cells/µl. When pulmonary infection is present, symptoms and signs include cough, fever, and dyspnea in association with an abnormal chest radiograph [28]. The radiographic manifestation includes a diffuse reticular or reticulonodular pattern that resembles PCP, lobar or segmental consolidation, or multiple nodules that have a propensity to cavitate. Disseminated disease can occur and manifest as a miliary pattern that may be associated with lymphadenopathy or pleural effusion.

ARF occurring as a complication of cryptococcosis (including pulmonary infection) was initially thought to be uncommon, with only a handful of case reports. Visnegarwala et al. [49] documented ARF as occurring in 29 of 210 cases of AIDS-associated cryptococcosis (13.8%). The clinical presentation was identical to that of PCP. Independent predictors of ARF were black race, LDH level ≥500 IU/L, presence of interstitial infiltrates, and cutaneous lesions. ARF with cryptococcosis in AIDS patients is associated with disseminated disease and high mortality rates.

Diagnosis frequently is not defined before death. Serum cryptococcal antigen testing is a sensitive and rapid screening method in diagnosing cryptococcosis in HIV-infected patients. Also, routine blood cultures are useful [50]. The recommended initial standard treatment is amphotericin B deoxycholate combined with flucytosine or fluconazole [28].

21.7.2 Aspergillosis

Aspergillosis is a life-threatening fungal infection in immunocompromised people, including HIV patients. Invasive pulmonary aspergillosis (IPA) is a relatively uncommon but devastating infection in patients with advanced AIDS [51] and was more common before the advent of HAART. The overall incidence was reported as being 3.5 cases per 1,000 person-years among HIV-infected patients [52]. The infection is most frequently caused by *Aspergillus fumigatus*, although certain cases are caused by *A. flavus, A. niger,* and *A. terreus.* A low CD4 count, generally <100/µl, was present in almost all cases of AIDS-associated aspergillosis. Coexistent neutropenia or use of corticosteroids occurred in about 50% of patients; the remaining cases appear to have no other risk factors other than advanced AIDS [28, 51, 52].

Symptoms of invasive aspergillosis pneumonia are fever, cough, dyspnea, chest pain, hemoptysis, and hypoxemia; chest radiograph might demonstrate a diffuse, focal, or cavitary infiltrate. A halo of low attenuation surrounding a pulmonary nodule or an air crescent on CT scan of the lung is suggestive of disease [53].

Isolation of an *Aspergillus* spp. from respiratory secretions has poor predictive value for invasive disease in AIDS patients. Bronchoscopy with BAL is, however, a safe and useful tool in high-risk patients suspected of having IPA. In addition to obtaining samples for fungal stain and culture, detecting antigens in the BAL fluid may be helpful, as well as excluding other infections. Transbronchial biopsies usually do not add much to the IPA diagnosis and are associated with increased risk of bleeding, so are seldom performed. Histopathological diagnosis, by examining lung tissue obtained by thoracoscopic or open-lung biopsy, remains the gold standard for diagnosing invasive IPA [28, 51, 53]. However, a large proportion of cases of aspergillosis are diagnosed postmortem, suggesting that underdiagnosis antemortem may contribute to poor survival.

Treatment of aspergillosis in the HIV-infected population has not been examined systematically. The recommended treatment for invasive aspergillosis in patients without HIV infection is voriconazole [28]. Amphotericin B deoxycholate, lipid-formulation amphotericin B, and caspofungin and posaconazole are other alternatives; other echinocandins, such as micafungin and anidulafungin, are reasonable alternatives. Response to therapy tends to be particularly poor in this patient population [52]. Other fungi infections, such as *Histoplasma capsulatum* and *Coccidioides immitis*, are less frequent but are present in several regions where the disease is endemic. Their presence in the lung is often indicative of disseminated disease and is associated with significant mortality rates.

21.8 Neoplastic Disease

Kaposi's sarcoma is a well-recognized cause of pulmonary disease in patients with HIV. This was first described in healthy, young, homosexual men, in whom it involved lymph nodes, viscera, mucosa, and skin [2]. Human herpes virus 8 (HHV-8) infection was shown to be the causative viral agent [54]. The variant epidemic, AIDS-associated Kaposi's sarcoma, can progress in weeks or months, and median patient survival is months. However, HAART development has influenced the clinical course and reduced the incidence of Kaposi's sarcoma, but it remains the most common AIDS-associated cancer in the United States [55, 56].

When Kaposi's sarcoma occurs in the lung, imaging features include interstitial or nodular parenchymal opacities. Characteristic peribronchovascular nodule distribution is frequent, and coalescence of nodules is common in late-stage disease (Fig. 21.5). Pleural effusion and lymphadenopathy may also be present [55, 56].

Diagnosis is often anticipated by concurrent skin lesions and the presence of prominent lesions in the tracheobronchial tree, which are easily recognized by bronchoscopy. Definitive diagnosis is not easy to establish. Transbronchial

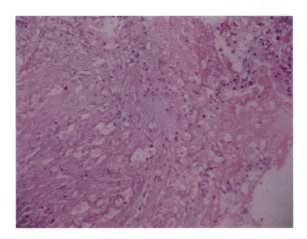

Fig. 21.6 Open lung biopsy specimen shows proliferation of capillaries in a background of spindle-shaped tumor cells in the lung interstitium, which are characteristic histological features of Kaposi's sarcoma (hematoxylin and eosin) (courtesy of Manuel Meneses M.D)

biopsies of the bronchus or lung parenchyma have a high risk of hemorrhage and reveal crush artifacts difficult to distinguish from Kaposi's sarcoma. On cytology, there is no diagnostic feature. Thus, tissue must be obtained on either open lung biopsy or video-assisted thoracoscopy (Fig. 21.6), or a presumptive diagnosis must be made when Kaposi's sarcoma in seen in the tracheobronchial tree and bronchoalveolar lavage reveals no other likely pathogens. Often, there is an associated bloody pleural effusion when thoracentesis is performed [9, 56].

Pulmonary Kaposi's sarcoma can respond well to chemotherapy [57]. HAART and opportunistic infection prophylaxis has contributed to the success rates of management strategies.

Lymphoma continues to be a cause of pulmonary disease. Although primary central nervous system (CNS) lymphomas have greatly diminished in frequency among patients treated with HAART; primary B-cell lymphomas elsewhere continue to occur. Patchy pulmonary infiltrates have been well described. Biopsy or cytology is needed to establish a diagnosis. Combination chemotherapy for HIV-associated lymphoma has become impressively more successful when HAART is continued with opportunistic infection prophylaxis. Stem cell transplantation has also been used successfully.

As patients are now living longer, and experience with large patient populations has increased, other pulmonary neoplastic processes have been recognized that clinicians should be aware of. Primary effusion cell lymphoma can present in the pleural, pericardial, or abdominal cavities as effusions. This HHV-8 and EBV-associated tumor is diagnosed by cytology in many cases. It is not clear how effective chemotherapy is for this tumor.

21.9 Immune Reconstitution Inflammatory Syndrome

During the first few months of HAART, immune reconstitution may be complicated by clinical events in which either previously subclinical infections are found or preexisting partially treated opportunistic infections deteriorate. This condition, termed immune reconstitution inflammatory syndrome (IRIS), is thought to be caused by improvement in the host's immune response to pathogens [58]. The inflammatory response may be such that the patient develops ARF and requires ICU. Abdool Karim et al. [45] reported that the incidence of IRIS was 9.5%. However, the study found the incidence was higher in the integrated-therapy group (anti-TB and ART) than in the sequential-therapy group: 12.4 versus 3.8%, respectively. The term IRIS is most commonly used for mycobacterial infections (TB and disseminated MAC disease) but is also used for other opportunistic infections, including *P. jirovecii* pneumonia, toxoplasmosis, hepatitis B and C viruses, CMV, varicella–zoster virus, cryptococcal infection, and histoplasmosis [28]. The syndrome is manifested as paradoxical worsening of the underlying respiratory disease and occurs days to months after HAART initiation. However, IRIS usually develops within the 4–8 weeks following HAART initiation and is caused by an exuberant inflammatory response to pneumocystis or mycobacterial antigens. On the basis of current knowledge, it is tempting to hypothesize that the immunological basis of IRIS is a HAART-induced rapid clonal expansion and redistribution of *M. tuberculosis*-specific memory T cells, which drives a deregulated immune activation [59] and a cytokine storm [60]. Antigen load could be responsible for the overvigorous inflammatory response of a recovering immune system.

Diagnosing IRIS requires excluding other causes of respiratory decompensation. Clinical presentations are transient worsening or appearance of new symptoms and signs, such as fever, increasing chest radiographic infiltrate, peripheral and mediastinal lymphadenopathy, or changes in radiographic manifestations.

Studies of TB-associated IRIS indicate that this complication is rarely fatal and that severe episodes can be successfully managed with corticosteroids [45]. Patients with severe cases are able to continue ART.

References

1. Centers for Disease Control and Prevention (1981) *Pneumocystis* pneumonia—Los Angeles. MMWR Morb Mortal Wkly Rep 30:250–252
2. Centers for Disease Control and Prevention (1981) Kaposi's sarcoma and *Pneumocystis* pneumonia among homosexual men—New York City and California. MMWR Morb Mortal Wkly Rep 30:305–308
3. Barré-Sinoussi F, Chermann JC, Rey F et al (1983) Isolation of a T-lymphotropic retrovirus from a patient at risk for acquired immune deficiency syndrome (AIDS). Science 220:868–871
4. Schein RMH, Fischl MA, Pitchenik AE et al (1986) ICU survival of patients with acquired immunodeficiency syndrome. Crit Care Med 14:1026–1027

5. Morris A, Creasman J, Turner J et al (2002) Intensive care of human immunodeficiency virus-infected patients during the era of highly active antiretroviral therapy. Am J Respir Crit Care Med 166:262–267
6. Vincent B, Timsit JF, Auburtin M et al (2004) Characteristics and outcomes of HIV-infected patients in the ICU: impact of the highly active antiretroviral treatment era. Intensive Care Med 30:859–866
7. Narasimhan M, Posner AJ, DePalo VA et al (2004) Intensive care in patients with HIV infection in the era of highly active antiretroviral therapy. Chest 125:1800–1804
8. Casalino E, Wolff M, Ravaud P et al (2004) Impact of HAART advent on admission patterns and survival in HIV-infected patients admitted to an intensive care unit. AIDS 18:1429–1433
9. Masur H (2006) Management of patients with HIV in the intensive care unit. Proc Am Thorac Soc 3:96–102
10. Joint United Nations Programme on HIV/AIDS (UNAIDS) and World Health Organization (2009) 2009 AIDS epidemic update. http://data.unaids.org/pub/Report/2009/JC1700_Epi_Update_2009_en.pdf
11. Nickas G, Wachter RM (2000) Outcomes of intensive care for patients with human immunodeficiency virus infection. Arch Intern Med 160:541–547
12. Powell K, Davis JL, Morris AM et al (2009) Survival for patients with HIV ADMITTED to the ICU continues to improve in the current era of combination antiretroviral therapy. Chest 135:11–17
13. Buchacz K, Baker RK, Palella FJ Jr et al (2010) AIDS-defining opportunistic illnesses in US patients, 1994–2007: a cohort study. AIDS 24:1549–1559
14. Huang L, Quartin A, Jones D et al (2006) Intensive care of patients with HIV infection. N Engl J Med 355:173–181
15. Chernilo S, Trujillo S, Kahn M et al (2005) Lung disease among HIV infected patients admitted to the "Instituto Nacional del Tórax" in Santiago, Chile. Rev Med Chile 133:517–524
16. Curtis JR, Yarnold PR, Schwanrtz DN et al (2000) Improvements in outcomes of acute respiratory failure for patients with human immunodeficiency virus related *Pneumocystis carinii* pneumonia. Am J Respir Crit Care Med 162:393–398
17. Davis JL, Morris A, Kallet RH et al (2008) Low tidal volume ventilation is associated with reduced mortality in HIV-infected patients with acute lung injury. Thorax 63:988–993
18. Thomas CF, Limper AH (2004) *Pneumocystis* pneumonia. N Engl J Med 350:2487–2498
19. Muñoz A, Schreger LK, Bacellar H et al (1993) Trends in the incidence of outcomes defining acquired immunodeficiency syndrome (AIDS) in the multicenter AIDS cohort study: 1985–1991. Am J Epidemiol 137:423–427
20. Ledergerber B, Mocroft A, Reiss P et al (2001) Discontinuation of secondary prophylaxis against pneumocystis carinii pneumonia in patients with HIV infection who have a response to antiretroviral therapy. N Engl J Med 344:168–174
21. Speich R (2006) HIV, AIDS, and the lung. In: Torres A, Ewig S, Mandell L, Woodhead M (eds) Respiratory infections. Hodder Arnold, London, pp 719–738
22. DeLorenzo LJ, Huang CT, Maguire GP, Stone DJ (1987) Roentgenographic patterns of *Pneumocystis carinii* pneumonia in 104 patients with AIDS. Chest 91:323–327
23. Erbelding EJ, Chaisson RE (2001) Respiratory infections in persons infected with human immunodeficiency virus. In: Niederman MS, Sarosi GA, Glassroth J (eds) Respiratory infections. Lippincott Williams & Wilkins, Philadelphia, pp 251–264
24. Alves C, Nicolás JM, Miró JM et al (2001) Reappraisal of the aetiology and prognostic factors of severe acute respiratory failure in HIV patients. Eur Respir J 17:87–93
25. Monnet X, Vidal-Petiot E, Osman D et al (2008) Critical care management and outcome of severe *Pneumocystis* pneumonia in patients with and without HIV infection. Critical Care 12:R28. doi:10.1186/cc6806
26. Confalonieri M, Calderini E, Terraciano S et al (2002) Noninvasive ventilation for treating acute respiratory failure in AIDS patients with *Pneumocystis jiroveci* pneumonia. Intensive Care Med 28:1233–1238

27. Acute Respiratory Distress Syndrome Network (2000) Ventilation with lower tidal volumes as compared with traditional tidal volumes for acute lung injury and the acute respiratory distress syndrome. N Engl J Med 342:1301–1308
28. Kaplan JE, Benson C, Holmes KH (2009) Guidelines for prevention and treatment of opportunistic infections in HIV-infected adults and adolescents: recommendations from CDC, the National Institutes of Health, and the HIV medicine association of the infectious diseases society of America. MMWR Recomm Rep 58(RR-4):1–207
29. Bozzette SA, Sattler FR, Chiu J (1990) A controlled trial of early adjunctive treatment with corticosteroids for *Pneumocystis carinii* pneumonia in the acquired immunodeficiency syndrome. N Engl J Med 323(21):1451–1457
30. Morris A, Wachter RM, Luce J et al (2003) Improved survival with highly active antiretroviral therapy in HIV-infected patients with severe *Pneumocystis carinii* pneumonia. AIDS 17:73–80
31. Madeddu G, Fiori ML, Mura MS (2010) Bacterial community-acquired pneumonia in HIV-infected patients. Curr Opin Pulm Med 16:201–207
32. Wolff AJ, O'Donnell AE (2001) Pulmonary manifestations of HIV infection in the era of highly active antiretroviral therapy. Chest 120:1888–1893
33. Cordero E, Pachón J, Rivero A et al (2000) Community-acquired bacterial pneumonia in human immunodeficiency virus-infected patients validation of severity criteria. Am J Respir Crit Care Med 162:2063–2068
34. Mandell LA, Wunderink RG, Anzueto A et al (2007) Infectious diseases society of American/American thoracic society consensus guidelines on the management of community-acquired pneumonia in adults. Clin Infect Dis 44(Suppl 2):S27–S72
35. Tumbarello M, Tacconelli E, de Gaetano Donati K et al (2001) Nosocomial bacterial pneumonia in human immunodeficiency virus infected subjects: incidence, risk factors and outcome. Eur Respir J 17:636–640
36. Petrosillo N, Nicastri E, Viale P (2005) Nosocomial pulmonary infections in HIV-positive patients. Curr Opin Pulm Med 11:231–235
37. Afessa B, Morales I, Weaver B (2001) Bacteremia in hospitalized patients with human immunodeficiency virus: a prospective, cohort study. BMC Infect Dis 1:13
38. Millar AB, Patou G, Miller RF et al (1990) Cytomegalovirus in the lungs of patients with AIDS. Respiratory pathogen or passenger. Am Rev Respir Dis 141(6):1474–1477
39. Drew WL (2007) Laboratory diagnosis of cytomegalovirus infection and disease in immunocompromised patients. Curr Opin Infect Dis 20:408–411
40. Cohen JI (2000) Epstein–Barr virus infection. N Engl J Med 343:481–488
41. Writing Committee of the WHO Consultation on Clinical Aspects of Pandemic (H1N1) 2009 Influenza (2010) Clinical aspects of pandemic 2009 influenza A (H1N1) virus infection. N Engl J Med 362:1708–1719
42. Griffith DE, Aksamit T, Brown-Elliott BA et al (2007) An official ATS/IDSA statement: diagnosis, treatment, and prevention of nontuberculous mycobacterial diseases. Am J Respir Crit Care Med 175:367–416
43. Small PM, Fujiwara PI (2001) Management of tuberculosis in the United States. N Engl J Med 345:189–200
44. Harries A, Maher D, Graham S (2004) TB/HIV: a clinical manual, 2nd edn. Publications of the World Health Organization, Geneva
45. Abdool Karim SS, Naidoo K, Grobler A et al (2010) Timing of initiation of antiretroviral drugs during tuberculosis therapy. N Engl J Med 362:697–706
46. Wallace JM, Hannah JB (1988) Mycobacterium avium complex infection in patients with the acquired immunodeficiency syndrome. A clinicopathologic study. Chest 93:926–932
47. Clark TA, Hajjeh RA (2002) Recent trends in the epidemiology of invasive mycoses. Curr Opin Infect Dis 15:569–574
48. Chariyalertsak S, Supparatpinyo K, Sirisanthana T et al (2002) A controlled trial of itraconazole as primary prophylaxis for systemic fungal infections in patients with advanced human immunodeficiency virus infection in Thailand. Clin Infect Dis 34:277–284

49. Visnegarwala F, Graviss EA, Lacke CE (1998) Acute respiratory failure associated with cryptococcosis in patients with AIDS: analysis of predictive factors. Clin Infect Dis 27: 1231–1237
50. Feldman CH (2003) Cryptococcal pneumonia. Clin Pulm Med 10:67–71
51. Segal BH, Walsh TJ (2006) Current approaches to diagnosis and treatment of invasive aspergillosis. Am J Respir Crit Care Med 173:707–717
52. Holding KJ, Dworkin MS, Wan PC et al (2000) Aspergillosis among people infected with human immunodeficiency virus: incidence and survival. Adult and adolescent spectrum of HIV disease project. Clin Infect Dis 31:1253–1257
53. Zmeili OS, Soubani AO (2007) Pulmonary aspergillosis: a clinical update. Q J Med 100: 317–334
54. Moore PS, Chang Y (1995) Detection of herpesvirus-like DNA sequences in Kaposi's sarcoma in patients with and those without HIV infection. N Engl J Med 332:1181–1185
55. Antman K, Chang Y (2000) Kaposi's sarcoma. N Engl J Med 342:1027–1038
56. Aboulaphia DM (2000) The epidemiologic, pathologic, and clinical features of AIDS-associated pulmonary Kaposi's sarcoma. Chest 117:1128–1145
57. Martin-Carbonero L, Barrios A, Saballs P et al (2004) Pegylated liposomal doxorubicin plus highly active antiretroviral therapy versus highly active antiretroviral therapy alone in HIV patients with Kaposi's sarcoma. AIDS 18:1737–1740
58. Hirsch HH, Kaufmann G, Sendi P et al (2004) Immune reconstitution in HIV infected patients. Clin Infect Dis 38:1159–1166
59. Lawn SD, Bekker LG, Miller RF (2005) Immune reconstitution disease associated with mycobacterial infections in HIV-infected individuals receiving antiretrovirals. Lancet Infect Dis 5:361–373
60. Bourgarit A, Carcelain G, Martinez V et al (2006) Explosion of tuberculin-specific Th1-responses induces immune restoration syndrome in tuberculosis and HIV co-infected patients. AIDS 20:F1–F7

Therapy of Infection in the ICU

22

J. H. Rommes, N. Taylor and L. Silvestri

22.1 Introduction

The 25-year-plus endurance of the selective decontamination of the digestive tract (SDD) strategy as an evidence-based infection prevention maneuver in intensive care medicine has led to fundamental changes in treating infections in intensive care unit (ICU) patients [1]. To appropriately treat such patients, the intensivist must have a thorough knowledge of basic principles, such as carriage, colonization, and infection, normal and abnormal flora, pathogenicity of microorganisms, and infection pathogenesis (Chaps. 1–6). There are six general principles underlying treatment for these patients (Box 22.1):

1. *Obtain surveillance and diagnostic cultures*. Whereas empirical antibiotic treatment needs to be started immediately [2], it is important that diagnostic and surveillance cultures are obtained to identify the causative pathogen(s) as soon as possible so that the initial and empirical treatment can be modified if necessary. Before antibiotic administration, diagnostic blood samples must be collected. Immediately thereafter, parenteral antibiotics should be administered. To obtain diagnostic samples of urine, tracheal aspirate and wounds, together with surveillance samples of the vagina, throat, and rectum takes more time and can be postponed until the antibiotics are initially administered but then must be collected as soon as possible.

2. *Administer immediate and adequate parenteral antibiotic treatment*. Antimicrobial therapy should be administered immediately after obtaining blood samples for culture. Delivery of antibiotics must be reliable, and this may only be realistic using parenterally administered antimicrobial agents. Orally

---

J. H. Rommes (✉)
Gelre Ziekenhuizen Apeldoorn, Intensive Care, Apeldoorn, The Netherlands
e-mail: h.rommes@gmail.com

Box 22.1 Six basic principles for treating infections in ICU patients

1. Obtain both surveillance and diagnostic cultures
2. Administer immediate and adequate parenteral antibiotic treatment
3. Eradicate both internal and external sources of potential pathogens
4. Apply topical antimicrobials
5. Replace or if possible remove all plastic invasive devices
6. Evaluate the efficacy of the treatment

administered drugs in critically ill patients are unpredictable with regard to absorption due to dysfunction of the gastrointestinal tract. The importance of early appropriate antibiotic administration has been shown in numerous studies regardless of infection type and has been confirmed in patients with sepsis, pneumonia, meningitis, and urinary tract infections [3]. The choice between mono- or combination therapy depends on the patient's premorbid health status and infection site. If the patient was previously in reasonably good health, initial empirical monotherapy with cefotaxime is sufficient, as the patient carries normal flora in the oropharynx and gut. Normal flora and highly pathogenic microorganisms such as *Streptococcus pyogenes* or *Neisseria meningitidis* are invariably susceptible to this third-generation cephalosporin. If a previously healthy patient is admitted with a community-acquired pneumonia (CAP), initial empirical combination therapy, i.e., cefotaxime with a macrolide covering the atypical microorganisms must be administered [4]. In the case of an intra-abdominal infection, gentamicin and metronidazole are added to cefotaxime. Yeasts have to be covered as long as the results of the diagnostic cultures of intra-abdominal samples are not available. Carriage of yeasts in the gut is present in 40–50% of patients, and yeast infections are an independent risk factor for mortality [5].

Patients admitted with a chronic underlying condition or who are transferred from another hospital or ward are usually carriers of both normal and abnormal flora [6]. When managing these patients, it is important to be aware that abnormal flora may contain resistant microorganisms. To reduce the likelihood of inappropriate therapy, which is associated with a higher mortality rate, all infections in these patients should be treated by combination therapy with two antibiotics of different mechanisms of action, i.e., aminoglycosides in combination with a beta-lactam antibiotic, e.g., cefotaxime. In patients with septic shock of unknown origin, combination therapy with gentamicin and cefotaxime should be started [7]. On the next day, the microbiologist is able to distinguish normal from abnormal potential pathogens. This information allows the intensivist to adjust the parenteral antimicrobials. There is no evidence to support an antibiotic course exceeding 1 week when treating the majority of infections [8]. Three days' treatment with aminoglycosides is sufficient and should then be discontinued to prevent toxicity (Box 22.2).

3. *Eradicate the source of potential pathogens causing the infection.* The source of potential pathogens causing the infection—whether internal or external—requires elimination to eradicate the original infection and to prevent relapses

Box 22.2 Initial and empirical therapy of infections in critically ill patients

Previously healthy	
Pneumonia	Cefotaxime + erythromycin
Intra-abdominal infection	Gentamicin/cefotaxime/metronidazole/amphotericin B
Urosepsis	Gentamicin/cefotaxime
Sepsis of unknown origin	Gentamicin/cefotaxime
Meningitis	Cefotaxime/ampicillin
Cholangitis	Gentamicin/ceftriaxone/metronidazole
Underlying disease/transferred from another ward or ICU	
Pneumonia	Gentamicin/cefotaxime + erythromycin
Intra-abdominal infection	Gentamicin/cefotaxime/metronidazole/amphotericin B
Urosepsis	Gentamicin/cefotaxime
Sepsis of unknown origin	Gentamicin/cefotaxime
Meningitis	Gentamicin/cefotaxime/ampicillin
Cholangitis	Gentamicin/ceftriaxone/metronidazole

and superinfections. In endogenous infections, the throat and gut of the critically ill are the internal sources of potential pathogens, whereas in exogenous infections, the source of potentially pathogenic microorganisms (PPM) is external, i.e., outside the patient. All patients expected to require ≥ 2 days of mechanical ventilation, immediately receive SDD (Chapter XX). Oropharyngeal, gastrointestinal, and vaginal carriage can be abolished by topical administration of the nonabsorbable polymyxin E, tobramycin, and amphotericin B (PTA), with the aim of eradicating the internal sources. If a patient has a tracheostomy, a paste containing PTA is applied around the tracheostoma [9]. The administration of these nonabsorbable topical antimicrobials is continued until the patient is weaned from the ventilator and extubated. Identifying and eradicating an external source is often more difficult and requires close cooperation between intensivists, nurses, and the infection control team.

4. *Deliver topical antimicrobials to achieve high antibiotic concentrations on the site of infection.* Topical application of antimicrobials is safe and contributes to a more rapid killing of PPMs, resulting in cultures of colonized/infected sites becoming sterile earlier. For example, to increase the antimicrobial activity in the lower airway secretions, topical therapy using aerosolized antibiotics should be considered [10]. Pastes with PTA can be applied topically to tracheostomies, gastrostomies, and pressure sores. These antimicrobial agents mixed with a translucent aquaform gel can also be applied in thin layers over fine mesh gauze to cover, for example, grafted burn wounds [11].

5. *Removal or replacement of invasive devices.* Endotracheal tubes, intravascular lines, and urinary catheters are readily contaminated with microorganisms.

Removal or replacement is thought to contribute to recovery from the original infection by curtailing the supply of potential pathogens [12].
6. *Evaluate efficacy of the therapy*. Generally, if appropriate antimicrobial therapy is administered, diagnostic samples of the infected internal organs are sterile within 3 days [13]. The oropharyngeal and vaginal cavities are free from potential pathogens within 3 days of SDD application. The same applies to topical application of antimicrobial agents to tracheostomies, gastrostomies, and wounds. Decontamination of the gut—in particular, the rectal cavity—depends on peristalsis and passage through the gastrointestinal tract. Liberal use of laxantia and a parasympathomimetic, such as neostigmine, reduce transit time and thus the time to gut decontamination [14].

22.2 Treating Infection on Admission

The majority of patients are admitted to the ICU due to or with an infection. Immediate and adequate therapy based on the six SDD principles should be given to prevent mortality. Details of treatment for the most frequently encountered infections on admission are now described (Box 22.3).

22.2.1 Lower Airway Infection

There are two types of lower airway infections: tracheobronchitis and pneumonia. Tracheobronchitis is an infection of the trachea and/or bronchi with localized (purulent secretion) and generalized clinical signs (fever, leukocytosis, increased C-reactive protein (CRP)). Chest X-ray does not show infiltrates. The tracheal aspirate yields >3+ or >10^5 CFU/ml of a PPM in the presence of >2+ leukocytes. The clinical setting in which this type infection most frequently is encountered is in chronic obstructive pulmonary disease (COPD) patients with acute on chronic respiratory failure or a patient with neuromuscular weakness who develops respiratory failure due to retention of secretions and atelectasis followed by infection. Pneumonia is an infection of the pulmonary tissue. The clinical diagnosis is based on the presence of fever, leukocytosis, and increased CRP and a new or progressive pulmonary infiltrate on chest X-ray. Tracheal aspirate is macroscopically purulent and contains >3+ or >10^5 CFU/ml of a PPM and >2+ leukocytes. Early administration of appropriate antibiotic reduces mortality in patients with a lower respiratory tract infection [15]. Immediately after obtaining diagnostic blood samples, systemic antibiotics should be started. In a previously healthy patient, cefotaxime in combination with a macrolide, e.g., erythromycin, should provide adequate cover of normal and atypical PPMs. Patients with chronic underlying disease and those transferred from the ward or another ICU carry both normal and abnormal PPMs and hence require combination therapy with an aminoglycoside and cefotaxime. Erythromycin is added in case of CAP. Cultures will identify the next day normal or abnormal PPMs so that if necessary, antimicrobial therapy can be adjusted. Infections caused by normal and abnormal

Box 22.3 An effective, rational, and safe antimicrobial drug policy

- Antimicrobials for systemic treatment: gentamicin/tobramycin, cefotaxime, erythromycin, metronidazole, amphotericin B; ceftazidime if *Pseudomonas* spp.; cephradine/cephazolin if *S. aureus*; vancomycin if methicillin resistant *S. aureus*(MRSA); meropenem if extended beta-lactamase (ESBL) producing PPM
- Aminoglycosides; first dose 5 mg/kg, treatment for 3 days under therapeutic drug monitoring (TDM)
- Initial empiric, broad coverage therapy (the first blow is half the battle); after 24 h, tapering down based on culture results
- Therapy duration for infections caused by PPM: 5 days
- Peritonitis: cover yeast with amphotericin B by continuous infusion 30 mg/24 h under TDM

Box 22.4 Dosages of aerosolized antimicrobials

Antimicrobial agent	Dose (mg/5 ml)	Interval (h)
Cefotaxime	500	6
Gentamicin	40	6
Tobramycin	40	6
Ceftazidime	500	6
Cephradine	500	6
Colistin (polymyxin E)	20	6
Amphotericin B	5	6
Vancomycin	250	6

PPM's can be treated with monotherapy, such as cefotaxime for 5 days. If ESBL producing PPMs, *Serratia* or *Morganella* spp are isolated cefotaxim should be replaced by meropenem [16]. If *Pseudomonas* spp. are isolated from throat and/or tracheal aspirate, cefotaxime has to be discontinued and combination therapy with gentamicin (3 days) and ceftazidime should be prescribed. To increase the antimicrobial activity in the lower airway secretions, topical therapy using aerosolized antibiotics should be applied (Box 22.4). Topical application of antimicrobials by nebulization is safe and contributes to a more rapid killing of PPMs, resulting in cultures of the tracheal aspirate becoming sterile earlier [10]. The doses of the different aerosolized antimicrobials are shown in Box 22.4. Tracheal aspirate is obtained daily until cultures are sterile. To prevent recolonization of the lower airways, the tracheal tube should be replaced after 3 days. Gentamicin should be guided by therapeutic drug monitoring (TDM) and generally can be discontinued after 3 days, to prevent toxicity. Systemic antibiotics and nebulized antimicrobials are discontinued when cultures are sterile; usually within 5 days.

22.2.2 Sepsis, Septicemia, Severe Sepsis, and Septic Shock

Sepsis is the clinical picture caused by generalized inflammation due to microorganisms and/or their toxic products. The clinical diagnosis of sepsis (synonymous with the sepsis syndrome) is based on the presence two of more of the following clinical criteria:
- increased heart rate,
- tachypnoe or impaired gas exchange,
- fever or hypothermia,
- leucocytosis or leucopenia plus a documented or suspected infection.

The clinical picture is caused by the release of inflammatory mediators into the circulation, i.e., cytokinemia. Blood cultures are always sterile. Septicemia is defined as sepsis combined with a positive blood culture. Severe sepsis is defined as sepsis plus sepsis-induced organ dysfunction or tissue hypoperfusion. Septic shock is defined as sepsis in combination with the clinical signs of cardiovascular collapse. Once the diagnosis of sepsis, septicemia, or septic shock has been made and blood cultures have been taken, immediate combination therapy should be started to provide an adequate spectrum of antibacterial activity. This is a combination of an aminoglycoside with cefotaxime. If an intra-abdominal focus is suspected, metronidazole and amphotericin B is added to this treatment. Initial empirical therapy is adjusted according to diagnostic culture results. The source of sepsis should be identified and eliminated as soon as possible. SDD using enteral PTA should be commenced immediately to eradicate the internal source.

22.2.3 Intra-Abdominal Infection

Intra-abdominal infection is an infection of an abdominal organ and the peritoneal cavity (peritonitis), with local signs such as abdominal tenderness and generalized symptoms including fever and leukocytosis. Peritonitis can be a localized or generalized. Drainage of the infection site should be performed as soon as possible by the surgeon or interventional radiologist. Again the six basic principles should be applied [17, 18].
1. Cultures taken to identify the organism.
2. Broad-spectrum systemic antimicrobial cover, i.e., an aminoglycoside with cefotaxime, metronidazole and amphotericin B, to empirically cover the likely organisms. This empirical therapy is adjusted when culture results become available after 24 h. Systemic antimicrobials including amphotericin B are given for 5 days.
3. Eradicate the source with SDD. The gut must be considered as an internal abscess that has to be drained [17]. PPM eradication from the gut of patients with peritonitis is often difficult due to the disturbance of both physiology and anatomy. However, decontamination of the gut in that subset of patients is possible but requires commitment and tenacity by the ICU team. Liberal use of laxantia, prokinetics, parasympathetic mimetics such as neostigmine, and enteral feeding

restores digestive tract function. Blind loops are decontaminated with SDD suspension containing 50 mg polymyxin E, 40 mg of tobramycin, and 500 mg of amphotericin B administered via catheters placed in the stoma. In case of rectal overgrowth, i.e., $>10^5$ CFU/ml of PPM, SDD enemas or suppositories are administered twice daily until surveillance cultures are free from PPM.
4. During laparotomy and repeat laparotomy after obtaining cultures, the abdominal cavity is extensively rinsed with a disinfecting agent, 2% Taurolin [19].
5. All potentially contaminated devices may act as a source of infection and should be replaced or, if possible, removed.
6. Treatment is evaluated by ongoing surveillance cultures of throat, stomas and rectum.

22.2.4 Wound Infection

Clinical signs of a wound infection are purulent discharge, redness, swelling, tenderness, and local warmth. The clinical diagnosis is confirmed by isolating $\geq 3+$ or $\geq 10^5$ microorganisms and $\geq 2+$ leukocytes in the purulent discharge [20]. Systemic antimicrobial therapy is seldom indicated, unless symptoms of sepsis, septicemia, or septic shock occur. Local treatment, drainage, debridement, and removal of plastic devices are essential and generally sufficient. Following local treatment, the wounds are rinsed twice daily with a disinfectant, 2% Taurolin, for 3 days. Aquaform gel mixed with 2% PTA and/or vancomycin can be applied to colonized/infected wounds [11].

22.2.5 Urinary Tract Infection

Urinary tract infection is an infection of the *pyelum*, ureter, bladder, or prostate. Severe urinary tract infections and urosepsis occur only if obstruction or lesions in the urinary tract are present. Blood cultures should be taken, followed by antimicrobial therapy. The combination of an aminoglycoside and cefotaxime provides adequate cover. If the Gram stain of the urine reveals yeasts, flucytosine 7,500 mg/day via continuous infusion should be given. Surveillance and additional diagnostic cultures should be taken and an ultrasound of the urinary tract performed as soon as possible. The cornerstone of treatment is drainage: the bladder by catheter, the ureter and kidney by either internal drainage or percutaneous nephrostomy. Following nephrostomy, the patient may deteriorate due to bacteremia induced by insertion of the nephrostomy catheter via the rich vasculature of the kidney into the pus of the *pyelum*.

To prevent new infections, the patient is treated with SDD. Vaginal carriage can be the source of PPM causing bladder infections. After drainage, aminoglycoside can be discontinued, whereas flucytosine and cefotaxime should be continued for a maximum of 5 days.

22.2.6 Acute Bacterial Meningitis

Bacterial meningitis is an infection of the meninges, the membrane lining of the brain, spinal cord, and subarachnoid space. Meningitis is a medical emergency requiring immediate and adequate therapy with antimicrobials and corticosteroids. Clinical diagnosis is often evident, as almost all patients presents with 2 or more of the 4 symptoms: fever, headache, neck stiffness, and altered mental state. Blood cultures must be taken immediately, followed by intravenous infusion of antibiotics. At the same time, dexamethasone 10 mg must be given. A 4-day regimen of dexamethasone 0.6 mg/kg/day divided in four daily doses as additional therapy reduces the risk of mortality and the incidence of cranial nerve impairment, such as hearing loss and other neurological sequelae. Five microorganisms are responsible for the vast majority of community-acquired bacterial meningitis: *Haemophilus influenzae*, *S. pneumoniae*, *Listeria monocytogenes*, and *Streptococcus agalactiae* (in neonates). Empirical treatment with cefotaxime and ampicillin covers these potential causative bacteria. In early-onset meningitis in neonates, an aminoglycoside should be added to cover *E. coli* from the mother's gut. Although rare, patients may develop meningitis during hospital stay. Empirical treatment in this small subset of patients should be guided by clinical history. Recent insertion of an epidural catheter, for instance, is a risk factor for *S. epidermidis* infection requiring vancomycin, whereas meningitis related to a basilar skull fracture or recent neurosurgery must be treated initially with ceftazidime and an aminoglycoside to cover both normal and abnormal PPMs and vancomycin to cover *S. aureus* and *S. epidermidis*.

Only after administration of antimicrobials and dexamethasone does the neurologist have the opportunity to perform lumbar puncture to obtain liquid for clinical chemistry and culture. At the same time, diagnostic and surveillance cultures must be collected. In pneumococcal meningitis, consultation of an otorhinolaryngologist or cardiologist is indicated, as 60% of these patients have contiguous or distant foci of infection, such as sinusitis, otitis, and endocarditis. Antimicrobial treatment should be continued for 5 days.

22.2.7 Biliary Tract Infections

Infections of the gall bladder or biliary-duct system require drainage by the surgeon, radiologist, or endoscopist. While the patient is waiting for definitive therapy, blood cultures should be taken, followed by immediate and adequate antimicrobial treatment. Combination therapy aimed at gastrointestinal flora, including an aminoglycoside, third-generation cephalosporin that provides high levels in the gall (i.e., ceftriaxone and metronidazole) covers the most likely causative microorganisms. Following definitive treatment, aminoglycoside therapy can be discontinued, anaerobic therapy after 3 days, and ceftriaxone after 5 days. *Candida* infections of the gallbladder and biliary tract are rare, and therefore, empirical treatment with antifungals is not indicated.

22.3 Managing Inflammation in a Successfully Decontaminated Patient

Appropriate use of the SDD strategy reduces severe infections of the lower airways and bloodstream by 72 and 37%, respectively [21, 22]. However, although properly decontaminated, some patients may develop signs of inflammation, and the diagnostic process in such a patient is a challenge for the intensive care team. A systematic approach is required (Box 22.5).

If a patient develops symptoms of inflammation such as fever, increased CRP, and leucocytosis, the first step is a thorough clinical reevaluation: Has the tracheal aspirate changed in quantity or quality? Is there deterioration of the pulmonary function? Is the urine cloudy, indicating the presence of leucocytes? How long ago was the central venous catheter inserted and under what conditions? Are there signs of an intra-abdominal problem? Is there a new cardiac murmur? In surgical patients: How are the wounds? Are there signs of an intra-abdominal problem? The next step is to reevaluate the results of the surveillance cultures. If cultures of throat, vagina, and gut are free of PPM, an endogenous infection is very unlikely. Systemic antibiotics should not be prescribed unless vital functions deteriorate progressively and the intensivist is convinced that the patient is suffering from sepsis. Diagnostic samples of lower airways, blood, urine, and wound fluid should be obtained. During decontamination, low-level pathogens such as enterococci and coagulase-negative staphylococci (CNS) may be found in the tracheal aspirate. The clinical impact of isolation of these low-level pathogens in the tracheal aspirate is nil; neither enterococci nor CNS cause lower airway infection. Colonization by *Candida* spp. of the lower respiratory tract on admission is frequently observed and may persist despite decontamination. Fortunately, *Candida pneumonia* is extremely rare and occurs only following hematogenous spread. Changes on X-ray of the thorax require bronchoscopy followed by culture (bacteria, fungi), stains (Gram/Ziehl-Neelsen), and cytology. Cytology of the bronchoalveolar lavage (BAL) should include stains aimed at viral-inclusion bodies suggesting viral infection. Viral pneumonia due to reactivation of herpes or cytomegalovirus (CMV) may occur in critically ill patients. The value of polymerase chain reaction (PCR) on BAL fluid aimed at a virus is unknown but probably limited. In abdominal surgery patients, an abdominal CT scan may provide the diagnosis.

A rather frequent cause of inflammation in a properly decontaminated intensive care patient is an endogenous bloodstream infection with low-level pathogens, i.e. CNS catheter-related bloodstream infection, particularly if the catheter is >7 days in situ [23]. Infections with low-level pathogens are associated with fever and an increase of CRP but do not cause sepsis syndrome or septic shock, as these microorganisms lack endotoxin. Diagnosing catheter-related bloodstream infection is based on one of the following [24]: (1) at least 2 positive blood cultures before catheter removal and persistently negative cultures after removal; (2) isolation of the same microorganism from 2 of the following 3 sites: blood drawn via the suspected line, blood drawn from a peripheral vein, or from the

Box 22.5 Differential diagnostic considerations when confronted with inflammation in a properly decontaminated patient

1. Is the infection present on admission adequately treated?
    i. undrained abscesses/wound infection
    ii. inadequate (too short, decreased susceptibility of PPM) antimicrobial therapy
    iii. source control
2. Is there a new infection?
    i. infection with low pathogens
    • catheter-related bloodstream infection
    • bladder infection
    ii. lower airway
    • exogenous
    • viral infection
    • *Aspergillus*
3. Has the patient an ongoing inflammatory response?
    i. infection excluded but still signs of inflammation
4. Miscellaneous
    i. thromboembolism
    ii. drug fever
    iii. underlying disease such as rheuma, autoimmune disease, malignancy
    iv. pressure sores

catheter tip; (3) quantitative blood cultures drawn via the central venous line and a peripheral vein reveal the same microorganism in a ratio >5:1. However the clinical relevance of this expensive microbiological exercise is limited, as the only effective treatment of a catheter-related bloodstream infection is removal of the contaminated line. If the diagnosis of catheter-related infection is correct, clinical signs of infection, particularly temperature, will normalize within 24 h. The predominant microorganisms involved in this type of infection are the low-level pathogens CNS and enterococci. Systemic treatment with antimicrobials is seldom indicated, even if PPMs such as aerobic Gram-negative bacilli and yeasts are involved. However an *S. aureus* catheter-related bloodstream infection carries the risk of metastatic abscesses and hence requires treatment with a first-generation cephalosporin for 5 days [25].

More complex is the patient with a prosthetic heart valve who develops a catheter-related bloodstream infection. If the signs of infection (fever, increased CRP, leukocytosis) do not resolve within 24 h of removal of the contaminated catheter, an aggressive approach is indicated. Combination therapy with vancomycin and gentamicin should be commenced. If ultrasonography reveals vegetations, antibiotic treatment should be continued for 3 weeks. If after 3 weeks' treatment clinical evaluation reveals signs of persistent infection, surgical replacement of the prosthetic heart valve is indicated [26].

Abscesses and wound infections require drainage. For localized problems, prophylactic systemic antibiotics should be given before drainage; prolonged treatment is not indicated. When the problem is generalized, antibiotics are administered for 5 days.

The incidence of exogenous lower respiratory tract colonization/infection with a potential pathogen, e.g., *Acinetobacter* or *Pseudomonas* spp., depends on the hygiene discipline of ICU workers but should be <15%. Colonization, no signs of infection, and <10^5 PPM/ml requires nebulized antimicrobials. Infection should be treated with both systemic (aminoglycoside and beta-lactam antimicrobial) and nebulized antimicrobials (aminoglycoside or colistine) for 5 days. Replacement of the endotracheal tube or tracheostomy cannula should be performed on the third day. Eradication of the source of the PPM is an important component of effective treatment of respiratory tract infections. Contaminated ventilators, humidifiers, and sinks are potential sources of external PPM. Breaches of hygiene by caregivers, particularly during busy periods, may lead to increased transmission of microorganisms and a higher exogenous infection rate.

Critically ill patients suffer from pronounced immunosuppression, making them vulnerable for all types of respiratory tract infections. If *Aspergillus* spp. are isolated from the tracheal aspirate, immediate antifungal therapy, intravenously and nebulized should always be given. Combination treatment with continuously infused flucytosine (loading dose 2500 mg iv followed by continuous infusion 7500 mg/24 h under TDM) and amphotericin (starting dose 30 mg/24 h) under TDM is safe and effective [27].

The diagnosis of viral pneumonia due to reactivation of herpes or CMV requires the typical inclusion bodies in the cytology of lower airway secretion obtained by BAL and a positive blood PCR.

Streptococcus faecalis or *faecium* bladder infection may occur and is readily diagnosed. Treatment is replacement of the bladder catheter preceded by a single dose of 1,000 mg of vancomycin.

Prolonged inflammation must be considered the moment infection has become unlikely. If the patient's recovery is hampered by this continuing inflammatory response, treatment with a short course of high-dose corticosteroids should be initiated (see below).

22.4 Managing Infections Caused by MRSA

The classic SDD protocol comprising parenteral cefotaxime and enteral PTA is not designed to control MRSA infections. Control requires the addition of enterally administered vancomycin [28–30]. The policy of surveillance cultures of the throat and rectum combined with enterally administered vancomycin in the at-risk patient is analogous to the way in which aerobic Gram-negative bacillary and fungal carriage is managed by the enterally administered antimicrobials PTA. It should be remembered that the principal aim of enterally administered nonabsorbable antimicrobials is the eradication of carriage of potential pathogen

Box 22.6 MRSA eradication protocol

1. Surveillance samples to detect carriers of MRSA
    i. obtain swabs from nose, throat, and rectum

2. Enteral/topical vancomycin to eradicate carriage
    i. treatment of MRSA carrier (5 days)
        • nasal carriage: 2% mupirocin cream 4 times a day or 4% vancomycin cream 4 times a day
        • oropharyngeal carriage: 4% vancomycin paste (0.5 g) 4 times a day, or 4% vancomycin gel (0.5 g) 4 times a day, or 5 mg vancomycin lozenges 4 times a day
        • gastrointestinal carriage: 40 mg of vancomycin/kg per day oral solution in four doses
        • skin carriage: 4% chlorhexidine bath/shower on alternate days
    ii. treatment of colonization/infection (3 days)
        • tracheostomy, gastrostomy: 4% vancomycin paste twice a day; change foreign body
        • lower airways: nebulized vancomycin 4 mg/kg per dose, 4 times a day diluted in normal saline; patient must receive a dose of nebulized salbutamol prior to vancomycin due to the reported risk of bronchoconstriction

3. Limiting the use of flucloxacillin to lift selection pressure on MRSA

4. High level of antistaphylococcal hygiene, including hand washing and device policy

overgrowth, including MRSA. Thus, enterally administered vancomycin not only eliminates a prime source of endogenous MRSA infection in at-risk patients, it also profoundly reduces hand contamination with MRSA and subsequent dissemination within the ICU.

Box 22.6 shows MRSA eradication protocol components. These include surveillance samples to detect the asymptomatic oropharyngeal and gut carrier. These are crucial for controlling antibiotic resistance. Regular surveillance cultures on admission and throughout treatment in the ICU, e.g., Mondays and Thursdays, allow detection of asymptomatic MRSA carriers at an early stage, allowing immediate implementation of isolation, barrier precautions, and enterally administered vancomycin. Relying solely on diagnostic blood, tracheal aspirate, urine, and pus samples results in inherent and substantial delay, permitting MRSA dissemination to other patients and maintaining endemicity. A shift from diagnostic toward preemptive surveillance samples is required to avoid wasting time in controlling MRSA spread. Nasal surveillance must be supplemented with digestive tract surveillance, as gut carriage of MRSA cannot be ignored [31]. Enterally/topically administered vancomycin is used to eradicate MRSA carriage: application of a 4% vancomycin paste or gel has been found to be effective in eradicating oropharyngeal carriage; administration of a vancomycin solution (40 mg/kg/day) through the nasogastric tube readily clears gut carriage; mupirocin or vancomycin intranasally is indicated to eradicate nasal carriage; 4% chlorhexidine liquid soap is used to clear skin carriage.

MRSA has an affinity for both intact and damaged skin, particularly when a plastic device such as a tracheostomy or gastrostomy is present [32, 33]. After device removal and replacement, a 4% vancomycin paste is required to treat colonization and/or infection. In lower airway colonization/infection, aerosolized vancomycin should be delivered via the endotracheal tube. Flucloxacillin should be avoided to lift selection pressure on MRSA. In general, improved antibiotic use to limit selective pressure is not that difficult but unfortunately receives little consideration in therapeutic decision making. Protection of indigenous flora is required to control overgrowth by MRSA. Cephradine is preferred as the first-line antistaphylococcal agent, as flucloxacillin disrupts gut ecology to a greater extent than cephradine [34]. A high level of antistaphylococcal hygiene is important. Improved adherence to infection-control practices—in particular, hand hygiene—cannot be overstated to control MRSA transmission via the hands of carers. It is highly likely that hand washing will be more effective in preventing MRSA transmission in units that implement the new approach. Carriers who receive vancomycin enterally have significantly less MRSA on their skin, so the risk of contaminating carers' hands is less and the level of contamination is lower, making hand washing more effective.

Staphylococci, both coagulase positive and negative, have an affinity for plastic devices. Most patients who require long-term intensive care have indwelling devices, including intubation tubes, intravascular lines, urinary catheters, and tracheostomy and/or gastrostomy tubes. The chance that these devices become contaminated with MRSA is substantial in a patient carrying MRSA in the nose, throat, gut, or skin [32, 33]. A strict device policy is thus required in the ICU. Devices are changed immediately if diagnostic samples are positive for MRSA, e.g., in the case of positive tracheal aspirates, the ventilation tube is replaced; in the case of a positive blood culture taken through an indwelling vascular line or a positive vascular catheter site swab, intravascular lines are removed and replaced.

22.5 Corticosteroids

Severity of infection is related to the extent of the inflammatory response. Excessive and systemic inflammatory response is supposed to play a role in the development of organ dysfunction that occurs during severe sepsis and septic shock. Patients with such an excessive inflammatory response to infection need modulation of this systemic cytokine response. Corticosteroids are potent inhibitors of inflammation by switching off genes that encode proinflammatory cytokines and switching on genes that encode anti-inflammatory cytokines. In a randomized controlled trial (RCT) in patients with typhus, a beneficial effect of high-dose steroids was demonstrated [35]. An RCT done in the 1980s investigated the effect of short courses of high-dose steroids in severe sepsis and septic shock patients [36]. Reversal of shock was significantly earlier in the treatment group, leading to a reduced early mortality rate. However, mortality on day 28 was comparable between controls and study group. The predominant cause of the late mortality was infection related. SDD eradicates the superinfection problem in the ICU patient, thus probably preserving the early beneficial effect of the high doses of corticosteroids.

Based on these considerations, patients with an excessive inflammatory response resulting in sepsis syndrome, severe sepsis, and septic shock should be treated with SDD in combination with a short course of high-dose steroids to block inflammation. Dexamethasone, due to its strong anti-inflammatory action, is preferred at a dose of 5 mg/kg (equivalent to prednisolone 30 mg/kg) for 3 days.

22.6 Conclusion

The old, dogmatic microbiology has been replaced by the sound, evidence-based SDD approach for treating and controlling infection in ICU patients. Recommendations in this chapter, particularly regarding the use of antimicrobial drugs, differ completely from those generated during the numerous consensus meetings and require a renewed mindset from the reader. The reader should keep in mind that evidence showing treatment of infections in critically ill patients using the SDD approach and a limited number of old antimicrobials has reached a grade 1A recommendation for reducing morbidity and mortality rates and preventing the emergence of resistance.

References

1. Zandstra DF, van Saene HKF (2011) Selective decontamination of the digestive tract as infection prevention in the critically ill. A level 1 evidence-based strategy. Minerva Anaesthesiologica 77:212–219
2. Garnacho-Montero J, Garcia-Garmendia JL, Barrero-Almodovar A et al (2003) Impact of adequate empirical antibiotic therapy on the outcome of patients admitted to the intensive care unit with sepsis. Crit Care Med 31:2742–2751
3. Ibraham EH, Sherman G, Ward S et al (2000) The influence of inadequate antimicrobial treatment of bloodstream infections on patient outcomes in the ICU setting. Chest 118:146–155
4. Martin-Loeches I, Lisboa T, Rodriguez A et al (2010) Combination antibiotic therapy with macrolides improves survival in intubated patients with community-acquired pneumonia. Intensive Care Med 36:612–620
5. Montravers P, Dupont H, Gauzit R et al (2006) Candida as a risk factor for mortality in peritonitis. Crit Care Med 34:646–652
6. Viviani M, van Saene HKF, Pisa F et al (2010) The role of admission surveillance cultures in the patients requiring prolonged mechanical ventilation in the intensive care unit. Anaesth Intensive Care 38:325–335
7. Kumar A, Safdar N, Kethireddy S et al (2010) A survival benefit of combination antibiotic therapy for serious infections associated with sepsis and septic shock is contingent only on the risk of death: a meta-analytic/meta-regression study. Crit Care Med 38:1651–1664
8. Chastre J, Wolff M, Fagon JY et al (2003) Comparison of 8 versus 15 days of antibiotic therapy for ventilator associated pneumonia in adults. A randomised trial. JAMA 290:2588–2598
9. Morar P, Makura Z, Jones AS et al (2000) Topical antibiotics on tracheostoma prevents exogenous colonization and infection of lower airways in children. Chest 117:513–518
10. Palmer LB (2009) Aerosolized antibiotics in critically ill ventilated patients. Curr Opinion Crit Care 115:413–418

11. Desai MH, Rutan RL, Heggers JP et al (1992) Candida Infection with and without nystatin prophylaxis. Arch Surg 127:159–162
12. Brown EM (1997) Empirical antimicrobial therapy of mechanically ventilated patients with nosocomial pneumonia. J Antimicrob Chemother 40:463–468
13. Dennesen PJW, van der Ven AJAM, Kessels AGH et al (2001) Resolution of infectious parameters after antimicrobial therapy in patients with ventilator-associated pneumonia. Am J Respir Crit Care Med 163:1371–1375
14. van der Spoel JI, Oudemans-van Straaten HM, Stoutenbeek CP et al (2001) Neostigmine resolves critical illness-related colonic ileus in intensive care patients with multiple organ failure–a prospective, double-blind, placebo-controlled trial. Intensive Care Med 27:822–827
15. Alvarez-Lerma F, Group ICU-Acquired Pneumonia (1996) Modification of empiric antibiotic treatment in patients with pneumonia acquired in the intensive care unit. Intensive Care Med 22:387–394
16. Abecasis F, Sarginson RE, Kerr S, Taylor N, van Saene HK (2011) Is selective digestive decontamination useful in controlling aerobic gram-negative bacilli producing extended spectrum beta-lactamases? Microb Drug Resist 17:17–23
17. Marshall JC, Innes M (2003) Intensive care unit management of intra-abdominal infection. Crit Care Med 31:2228–2237
18. Lamme B, Boermeester MA, Reitsma JB et al (2002) Meta-analysis of relaparatomy for secondary peritonitis. Br J Surg 89:1516–1524
19. Gormans SP, McCafferty DF, Woolfson AD (1987) Reduced adherence of micro-organisms to human mucosal epithelial cells following treatment with taurolin, a novel antimicrobial agent. J Appl Bacteriol 62:315–320
20. Weber JM, Sheridan RL, Pasternack ME et al (1997) Nosocomial infections in pediatric patients with burns. Am J Infect Control 25:195–201
21. Liberati A, D'Amico R, Pifferi S et al (2009) Antibiotic prophylaxis to reduce respiratory tract infections and mortality in adults receiving intensive care. Cochrane Database Syst Rev CD 000022
22. Silvestri L, van Saene HKF, Milanese M et al (2007) Selective decontamination of the digestive tract reduces bacterial bloodstream infections and mortality in critically ill patients. Systematic review of randomised, controlled trials. J Hosp Infect 65:187–203
23. Elliott TSJ, Faroqui MH, Armstrong RF et al (1994) Guidelines for good practice in central venous catheterisation. J Hosp Infect 28:163–176
24. Kurkchubasche AG, Smith MD, Rowe MI (1992) Catheter-sepsis in short bowel syndrome. Arch Surg 127:21–25
25. Naber CK, Baddour LM, Giamarellos-Bourboulis EJ et al (2009) Clinical consensus conference: survey on Gram-positive bloodstream infections with a focus on *Staphylococcus aureus*. Clin Infect Dis 48:S260–S270
26. Brush JL (1998) Infective endocarditis in critical care. In: Cunha BA (ed) Infectious diseases in critical care medicine. Dekker, New York, pp 387–434
27. Grayson ML (ed) (2010) Kucers' The use of antibiotics, 6th edn. Hodder Arnold, London
28. Silvestri L, Milanese M, Oblach L et al (2002) Enteral vancomycin to control methicillin-resistant *Staphylococcus aureus* outbreak in mechanically ventilated patients. Am J Infect Control 30:391–399
29. de la Cal MA, Cerda E, van Saene HKF et al (2004) Effectiveness and safety of enteral vancomycin to control endemicity of methicillin-resistant *Staphylococcus aureus* in a medical/surgical intensive care unit. J Hosp Infect 56:175–183
30. Silvestri L, van Saene HKF, Milanese M et al (2004) Prevention of MRSA pneumonia by oral vancomycin decontamination: a randomised trial. Eur Respir J 23:921–926
31. Coello R, Jimenez J, Garcia M et al (1994) Prospective study of infection, colonization and carriage of methicillin-resistant *Staphylococcus aureus* in an outbreak affecting 990 patients. Eur J Clin Microbiol Infect Dis 13:74–81

32. Steinberg JP, Clark CC, Hackman BO (1996) Nosocomial and community-acquired staphylococcus bacteremias from 1980 to 1993: impact of intravascular devices and methicillin-resistance. Clin Infect Dis 23:255–259
33. Chang FY, Singh N, Gayowski T et al (1998) *Staphylococcus aureus* nasal colonisation in patients with cirrhosis: prospective assessment of association with infection. Infect Control Hosp Epidemiol 19:328–332
34. de Man P, Verhoeven BA, Verbrugh HA et al (2000) An antibiotic policy to prevent emergence of resistant bacilli. Lancet 355:973–978
35. Hoffman SL, Punjabi NH, Kumala S et al (1984) Reduction of mortality in chloramphenicol-treated severe typhoid fever by high-dose dexamethasone. N Engl J Med 310:82–88
36. Sprung CL, Caralis PV, Marcial EH et al (1984) The effects of high-dose corticosteroids in patients with septic shock. New Engl J Med 311:1137–1143

Part V
Special Topics

The Gut in the Critically Ill: Central Organ in Abnormal Microbiological Carriage, Infections, Systemic Inflammation, Microcirculatory Failure, and MODS

23

D. F. Zandstra, H. K. F. van Saene
and R. E. Sarginson

23.1 Introduction

For many years, the gut has been proposed to play a central role in the pathogenesis of infections, multiple organ failure, and other diseases frequently encountered in the critically ill. Also, it is recognized that therapeutic interventions in the critically ill, such as stress ulcer prophylaxis, systemic antibiotics and, vasoconstrictors, can cause inadvertent adverse effects. For example, physiological balances in microbial colonization and microcirculation are impaired, thereby contributing to increased susceptibility to bacterial overgrowth (i.e., abnormal carriage), infections, sepsis, intestinal barrier dysfunction and, ultimately, multiple organ dysfunction syndrome (MODS) [1–4].

The gut consists of different components: microcirculation, mucosa, immune system, enteric nervous system, commensal microflora, and—during critical illness—acquired microorganisms. All these components interact with each other during critical illness, and all elements may become disturbed as a consequence of disease and also its treatment. This may result in alterations in crosstalk between the different elements and yield both beneficial and pathologic responses. The latter responses may induce MODS. Clark and Coopersmith propose that the intestinal epithelium, the intestinal immune system, and the intestines' endogenous bacteria all play vital roles in driving MODS [5]. The complex crosstalk between these three interrelated parts of the gastrointestinal tract cumulatively makes the gut a "motor" of critical illness. The importance of the close relation between

---

D. F. Zandstra (✉)
Department of Intensive Care, Onze Lieve Vrouwe Gasthuis,
Amsterdam, The Netherlands
e-mail: d.f.zandstra@olvg.nl

abnormal microbial carriage, immunity, and intestinal microcirculation in the critically ill is addressed in this chapter. Therapeutic interventions within this context are reviewed.

23.2 Microcirculation

Hippocrates described the clinical triad of cold extremities, fever, and thirst, which implied a bad prognosis. He was probably describing the situation of hypodynamic septic shock. In the first century A.D, Celsus described the classic signs of inflammation: *rubor, tumor, calor, dolor.* Two centuries later, Galen added the *functio laesa* of the affected part as the fifth symptom. These signs can be recognized in systemic inflammatory response syndrome (SIRS), which frequently occurs in patients after trauma, sepsis, and major surgery. *Rubor* is the result of increased blood flow caused by vasodilatation and clinically measured as hypotension. *Tumor* develops as the consequence of the generalized edema associated with increased capillary leak. *Calor* can be recognized systemically as fever caused by substances such as interleukins and other inflammatory mediators that alter the set point of the thermoregulatory center. *Dolor* can be seen as generalized pain, and *functio laesa* as the onset of multiple organ dysfunctions.

23.3 Multiple Organ Failure

The description of multiple organ failure is a rather recent event in the history of medicine. This syndrome was first reported by Tilney et al. in 1973 [6]. They described the onset of sequential organ failure in patients after surgery for ruptured abdominal aneurysm and in whom acute renal failure had developed. Sequential failure of circulation, respiration, liver, and intestines occurred despite intensive therapy. All patients died. All showed gastric mucosal lesions on postmortem investigation, and most patients showed renal tubular necrosis. These findings indicated impaired perfusion of the stomach and kidneys. Postmortem examinations revealed Gram-negative microorganisms in lung slices of all patients. The relationship between shock, impaired gut perfusion, and the ultimate failure of organs was evident. However, the role of Gram-negative infections in the pathogenesis of the syndrome became evident much later [7]. Moreover, the relationship between sepsis and (gut) mucosal ischemia became apparent. Le Gall et al. reported in 1976 extensive gastric mucosal erosions seen on endoscopy in patients with sepsis, whereas patients without sepsis showed normal mucosal surfaces in the stomach [8].

The acid hypothesis as the major factor in the pathogenesis of gut mucosal stress ulceration held sway for many years. Impaired microcirculation, as a consequence of sepsis and shock, was subsequently proposed as a major step in the pathogenesis of gastric mucosal ulceration and bleeding. In a group of high-risk critically ill patients on prolonged mechanical ventilation, a clinical strategy of optimizing microcirculation of the intestinal mucosa, together with preventing abnormal carriage of microorganisms by using selective decontamination of the digestive tract (SDD), resulted in a surprisingly low incidence of stress-ulcer-related bleeding (SURB) without the use of specific SURB prophylaxis [9]. Similar studies 10 years later showed identical results [10, 11]. In patients admitted to the ICU with sepsis, sepsis syndrome, and septic shock, a SURB incidence <1% was shown by focusing on infection prevention using SDD and optimizing microcirculation with aggressive fluid resuscitation, the use of vasodilators, and anti-inflammatory agents without using prophylactic antacids, proton pump inhibitors (PPI), or H_2 antagonists [12].

These findings support the hypothesis that the combination of therapeutic interventions focused on optimizing gut perfusion (fluid resuscitation, vasodilators) and preventing and treating abnormal microbial carriage and organ-site infections (using SDD) are able to prevent some of the universally reported problems in the critically ill. In addition to stress ulcerations of the upper intestinal canal, these problems include loss of colonization resistance, pneumonia, sepsis, and progression from sepsis to multiple organ failure.

SDD significantly reduces the incidence of pneumonia and bloodstream infections, the onset of MODS, and mortality rates in the critically ill [7, 13, 14]. Impaired gastrointestinal motility resulting in delayed or absent gastric emptying and passage of stools are recognized entities in the critically ill [15–17]. Compromised caloric intake leads to impaired mucosal integrity and immune deficiencies. The development of critical-illness-related colonic ileus (CIRCI) may lead to intestinal ischemia by increasing intra-abdominal pressure and subsequently impairing mucosal perfusion. This results in disrupted barrier function of the mucosa, endotoxemia, and finally SIRS. Untreated gut motility disorders contribute to stasis, bacterial overgrowth, and carriage of abnormal microorganisms. Timely intervention with neostigmine may prevent this sequence of events [17].

Commonly used pharmacological agents, such as PPIs, may further contribute to carriage of abnormal microorganisms. PPIs are designed to shut down the gastric proton pump of parietal cells, thereby raising the pH of the stomach and affecting the pH of the colonic content. Although effective in reducing gastric acid production, a number of side effects have been associated with PPI use.

Naturally occurring bacteria, some of which are acid-producing and contain adenosine triphosphatase (ATPase) enzymes, have also been found within the oral cavity, stomach, upper gastrointestinal tract, and colon. Literature reports have suggested that PPIs may affect these bacteria and fungi in two different ways: by directly targeting the proton pumps of bacteria and fungi and by indirectly affecting flora microenvironment via changes in pH. Vesper et al. summarize what is known about the interactions between PPIs and natural human microbiota [18]. Raising colonic pH > 6 may inhibit the growth of indigenous anaerobic flora in the large intestine, contributing to a loss of colonization resistance [19], which in turn may result in overgrowth by potentially pathogenic microorganisms and subsequent infections. An increased susceptibility for infectious complications, such as pneumonia and *Clostridium* infections, has been reported [20–22]. The use of PPIs should be carefully considered in the critically ill, as inadvertent effects may cause harm.

23.4 Microcirculation and the Gut

Regulating microcirculatory perfusion in the gut is complex. Gut functional and structural integrity is maintained under the influence of substances such as catecholamines; hormones; locally released substances, including serotonin, vasopressin, and endothelial vasoactive substances; and food absorption, with the exclusion of bacteria and their products to prevent them from entering the bloodstream [4]. It is increasingly recognized that the normalization of blood pressure during the treatment of septic shock does not automatically result mucosal microcirculation restoration [23–28]. Measuring systemic hemodynamic parameters does not reflect microcirculatory behavior of the intestinal canal [23, 26, 27]. Impairment of effective microcirculation perfusion is the essential step in the pathogenesis of septic shock [29], and persistently impaired microcirculation in septic shock is associated with increased risk of mortality [24].

Early studies from Dietzman and coworkers showed that the pillars for treating (septic) shock were fluid infusion, glucocorticoids, beta agonists, and alpha blockers [30]. Clinical studies show no benefit from adrenergic infusion alone on organ perfusion [31, 32]. Breslow et al. found that norepinephrine (NE) did not prevent reduced renal perfusion in an endotoxin-induced shock model, whereas Johannes et al. demonstrated that dexamethasone improved renal perfusion and prevented the onset of acute renal failure [33, 34]. Reduced perfusion in the pancreas in a septic ovine model could also not be prevented, regardless the agents used (dobutamine, norepinephrine, dopamine, dopexamine, salbutamol) [35]. Dopamine, however, increased liver and intestinal perfusion [36]. Besides vasoconstriction, NE causes thrombocyte hyperaggregation. This may result in impaired microcirculatory flow and subsequently organ dysfunction [37]. NE levels achieved in humans during moderate exercise can result in hyperaggregation [38]. However, infusion of the nitric oxide (NO) donor nitroprusside can prevent NE-induced hyper-aggregation [39]. NE is increasingly used to treat hypotension associated with septic shock, albeit no clinical study shows a survival benefit [40]. Also, low-dose vasopressin infusion increased mortality rates in an ischemia–reperfusion model in mice [41]. Experimental studies further suggest that NE in septic shock also leads to MODS activation via the following:

1. Apoptosis—NE induces apoptosis of alveolar cells and cardiomyocytes within 24 h [42, 43]; epinephrine had a harmful effect on survival that was significantly related to drug dose but not bacterial dose [44].
2. NE impairment of circulating volume—Weil et al. showed in 1975 a sharp decrease in plasma volume after starting NE infusion [31]. In patients with increased lactic acidosis as the consequence of septic shock, impaired peripheral circulation, clinically assessed, identifies these patients [45].

Early goal-directed therapy in patients with septic shock, as proposed by Rivers et al., reduced mortality rates due to acute hemodynamic collapse. This result was achieved by the infusion of more volume and blood rather than an increased administration of catecholamines [46]. Subsequent studies with similar design confirmed these effects [47].

23.5 Immunology of the Gut

The luminal surface of the gut is continually exposed to dense populations of bacteria and their products. The intestinal immune system evolved to facilitate selective absorption of food particles and selective exclusion of bacteria and their products. The intestinal mucosa is the main interface between the immune system and the external environment. The role of the mucosal immune system therefore is to prevent uptake of potentially harmful compounds. A complex system of immunocompetent cells is organized in and around the gut [gut-associated lymphoid tissue (GALT) and mucosa-associated lymphoid tissue (MALT)]. The innate system is the primary barrier against microorganisms, coordinating a targeted response to eradicate invading pathogens. An essential component of the innate system is the presence of T and B-cell receptors and recognition of processed antigens or presenting antigens. In the intestinal tissues, two main immune systems can be identified: (1) the initiation compartment (the GALT), and (2) the effector compartment (consisting of the lamina propria where T-cells reside, migrating after stimulation in the first compartment) [48]. Despite the redundant design with several lines of defense of the immune system, bacterial translocation (BT) may occur and contribute to the development of SIRS and, eventually, MODS. BT has been related to three main conditions: (1) intestinal bacterial overgrowth, (2) disruption of the intestinal barrier, and (3) host immune deficiency [1–3]. These circumstances are usually encountered in the critically ill patient. BT may occur via the hematologic and lymphatic routes; it activates GALT and the mesenteric lymphatic network and seems to be the natural route for immune cells and inflammatory mediators to reach the bloodstream via portal circulation [49, 50].

Interactions between the enteric nervous system and the immune system occur via enteric peptides. Many of these peptides originate from the mucosa. However, they are also produced in the immunocompetent GALT cells, such as macrophages and mast cells. These peptides may instigate different responses, including lymph proliferation, cytokine production, and immunoglobulin (Ig) production. Overgrowth of newly acquired, predominantly Gram-negative, microorganisms may lead to inappropriate activation of immunocompetent cells in the vicinity of the gut. This may result in cytokine release, which further enhances permeability change.

It has been suggested that lymphocyte recruitment to microvessels is affected by the presence of enterobacteria [51, 52]. Increased expression of adhesion molecules leads to increased adherence of lymphocytes to the endothelium of the intestinal microcirculation. This occurs locally in the gut, where enterobacteria are present within the lumen and enter the lymph system, activating the GALT immune response.

A relationship between BT and microcirculation injury has been reported in an experimental setting. Lymph deviated from entering the systemic circulation prevented the onset of mesenteric microcirculation injury; in non-lymph-deviated animals, important and long-lasting injury to the mesenteric microcirculation was observed [50, 53]. It is hypothesized by these authors that the lymphatic route of BT up to the mesenteric lymph nodes (MLN) is the relevant route for the induction of immune response, whereas the portal hematologic route might be the major route for bacteria dissemination from the intestines into systemic organs [49].

23.6 Low Cardiac Output

These events also occur under clinical conditions of low cardiac output, such as chronic heart failure. Sandek et al. reviewed the impact of chronic heart failure on gut functions [54, 55]. Chronic heart failure (CHF) results in increased sympathetic tone, hormonal derangements, anabolic/catabolic imbalance, endothelial dysfunction, and systemic low-grade inflammation affecting various organ systems. Proinflammatory cytokines appear to play important roles in that context. There is increasing evidence that the gut has a pathophysiological role for both chronic inflammation and malnutrition in CHF. Indeed, disturbed intestinal microcirculation and barrier function in CHF seem to trigger cytokine generation, thereby contributing to further impairment in cardiac function. On the other hand, myocardial dysfunction can induce microcirculatory injuries, leading to disruption in the intestinal barrier. This amplifies the inflammatory response. The increased number of adherent bacteria on the intestinal mucosa seen in patients with CHF and elevated systemic levels of antilipopolysaccharide IgA emphasizes this fact. Therefore, the gut is an interesting target for therapeutic interventions in patients with CHF, in many of whom attempts to eliminate Gram-negative bacteria and endotoxins from the gut by using nonabsorbable antibiotics (SDD) improved vascular reactivity and peripheral circulation. Reducing the intestinal endotoxin pool in the gastrointestinal tract by SDD led to decreased monocyte CD14 expression and intracellular cytokine production in patients with severe CHF. The improved peripheral endothelial function could be a marker of the anti-inflammatory effect of SDD [56].

23.7 Probiotics

Immune suppression and bacterial translocation caused by withholding enteral nutrition in the presence of parenteral nutrition in an animal experiment was also reversed and prevented by SDD [57]. In critically ill patients with MODS, the intestinal application of probiotics resulted in an improved immune response as shown by systemic IgA and IgM response and reduced intestinal permeability.

The clinical value of these observations is still debatable [58]. However, these observations emphasize the important interaction between intestinal bacterial content and immune responses.

Probiotic treatment to improve clinical outcome in critically ill patients with pancreatitis resulted in increased mortality rates [59]. The beneficial role of probiotics in the critically ill to prevent infections is still under debate [60, 61]. Eliminating aerobic Gram-negative bacilli (AGNB) from the intestinal canal using SDD with nonabsorbable antibiotics has been shown to reduce the severity and incidence of MODS [7, 62].

23.8 Conclusion

In the critically ill patient, overgrowth with acquired Gram-negative bacteria, disruption of the intestinal barrier, and immune deficiency are often problematic. Therapeutic efforts may be directed at preventing abnormal microbial colonization by SDD; aggressive shock management using early goal-directed therapy and vasodilators to maintain mucosal barrier (i.e., reducing translocation and preserving mucosal integrity); quick restoration of intestinal motility with early feeding; and, if needed, prokinetics. The combination of these interventions contributes to fewer infections, fewer MODS, and a lower mortality rate. The role of probiotics in preventing infections is still under debate.

References

1. Deitch EA (1990) Bacterial translocation of the gut flora. J Trauma 30:S184–S189
2. MacFie J, O'Boyle C, Mitchell CJ et al (1999) Gut origin of sepsis: a prospective study investigating associations between bacterial translocation, gastric micro flora, and septic morbidity. Gut 45:223–228
3. Berg RD (1992) Bacterial translocation from the gastrointestinal tract. J Med 23:217–244
4. Marston A, Bulkley GB, Fiddian Green RC (eds) (1989) Splanchnic ischaemia and multiple organ failure. Edward Arnold, London
5. Clark JA, Coopersmith CM (2007) Intestinal crosstalk: a new paradigm for understanding the gut as the "motor" of critical illness. Shock 28:384–393
6. Tilney NL, Bailey GL, Morgan AP (1973) Sequential system failure after rupture of abdominal aortic aneurysms: an unsolved problem in the postoperative care. Ann Surg 178:117–122
7. Stoutenbeek ChP, van Saene HKF, Zandstra DF (1996) Prevention of multiple organ failure by selective decontamination of the digestive tract in multiple trauma patients. In: Faist E, Baue AE, Schildberg FW (eds) The immune consequences of trauma shock and sepsis. Mechanisms and therapeutic approaches, vols 1, 2. Pabst Science, Berlin, pp 1055–1066
8. Le Gall JR, Mignon FC, Rapin M et al (1976) Acute gastroduodenal lesions related to severe sepsis. Surg Gynecol Obstet 142:377–380
9. Zandstra DF, Stoutenbeek CP (1994) The virtual absence of stress-ulceration related bleeding in ICU patients receiving prolonged mechanical ventilation without any prophylaxis. A prospective cohort study. Intensive Care Med 20:335–340
10. Zandstra DF, van der Voort PH (2004) A more appropriate critical appraisal of the available evidence? Crit Care Med 32:2166–2167

11. Zandstra DF, van der Voort PH (2004) Comment on surviving sepsis campaign guidelines for the management of severe sepsis and septic shock by dellinger et al. Intensive Care Med 30:1984
12. Van Spreuwel-Verheijen M, Bosman RJ, Oudemans-Van Straaten HM et al (2006) Is the surviving sepsis campaign for stress ulcer prophylaxis justified? Intensive Care Med 32(Suppl 1):S23
13. Silvestri L, van Saene HK, Milanese M et al (2007) Selective decontamination of the digestive tract reduces bacterial bloodstream infection and mortality in critically ill patients. Systematic review of randomized, controlled trials. J Hosp Infect 65:187–203
14. de Smet AM, Kluytmans JA, Cooper BS et al (2009) Decontamination of the digestive tract and oropharynx in ICU patients. N Engl J Med 360:20–31
15. Herbert MK, Holzer P (2008) Standardized concept for the treatment of gastrointestinal dysmotility in critically ill patients–current status and future options. Clin Nutr 27:25–41
16. van der Spoel JI, Oudemans-van Straaten HM, Kuiper MA et al (2007) Laxation of critically ill patients with lactulose or polyethylene glycol: a two-centre randomized, double-blind, placebo-controlled trial. Crit Care Med 35:2726–2731
17. van der Spoel JI, Oudemans-van Straaten HM, Stoutenbeek CP et al (2001) Neostigmine resolves critical illness-related colonic ileus in intensive care patients with multiple organ failure–a prospective, double-blind, placebo-controlled trial. Intensive Care Med 27:822–827
18. Vesper BJ, Jawdi A, Altman KW et al (2009) The effect of proton pump inhibitors on the human microbiota. Curr Drug Metab 10:84–89
19. Louis P, Flint H (2009) Diversity, metabolism and microbial ecology of butyrate-producing bacteria from the human large intestine. FEMS Microbiol Lett 294:1–8
20. Dalton BR, Lye-Maccannell T, Henderson EA et al (2009) Proton pump inhibitors increase significantly the risk of clostridium difficile infection in a low-endemicity, non-outbreak hospital setting. Aliment Pharmacol Ther 29(6):626–634
21. Sultan N, Nazareno J, Gregor J (2008) Association between proton pump inhibitors and respiratory infections: a systematic review and meta-analysis of clinical trials. Can J Gastroenterol 22:761–766
22. Vakil N (2009) Acid inhibition and infections outside the gastrointestinal tract. Am J Gastroenterol 104(Suppl 2):S17–S20
23. Spronk PE, Ince C, Gardien MJ et al (2002) Nitroglycerin in septic shock after intravascular volume resuscitation. Lancet 360(9343):1395–1396
24. Spronk PE, Zandstra DF, Ince C (2004) Bench to bedside review: Sepsis is a disease of the microcirculation. Crit Care 8:462–468
25. Sakr Y, Dubois MJ, De Backer D et al (2004) Persistent microcirculatory alterations are associated with organ failure and death in patients with septic shock. Crit Care Med 32:1825–1831
26. De Backer D, Creteur J, Preiser JC et al (2002) Microvascular blood flow is altered in patients with sepsis. Am J Respir Crit Care Med 166:98–104
27. Boerma EC, van der Voort PH, Spronk PE et al (2007) Relationship between sublingual and intestinal microcirculatory perfusion in patients with abdominal sepsis. Crit Care Med 35:1055–1060
28. Boerma EC, Kuiper MA, Kingma WP et al (2008) Disparity between skin perfusion and sublingual microcirculatory alterations in severe sepsis and septic shock: a prospective observational study. Intensive Care Med 34:1294–1298
29. Lush CW, Kvietys PR (2000) Micro vascular dysfunction in sepsis. Microcirculation 7:83–101
30. Dietzman RH, Manax WG, Lillehei RC (1967) Shock: mechanisms and therapy. Can Anaesth Soc J 14:276–286
31. Weil MH, Shubin H, Carlson R (1975) The treatment of circulatory shock. Use of sympathomimetic and related vasoactive agents. JAMA 231:1280–1286
32. Dubin A, Oposo M, Casabella CA et al (2009) Increasing arterial blood pressure with norepinephrine does not improve microcirculatory blood flow: a prospective study. Crit Care 13:r92

33. Breslow MJ, Miller CF, Parker SD et al (1987) Effect of vasopressors on organ blood flow during endotoxin shock in pigs. Am J Physiol 252:H291–H300
34. Johannes T, Mik EG, Klingel K et al (2009) Low-dose dexamethasone-supplemented fluid resuscitation reverses endotoxin-induced acute renal failure and prevents cortical microvascular hypoxia. Shock 31(5):521–528
35. Bersten AD, Hersch M, Cheung H et al (1992) The effects of various sympathomimetics on the regional circulations in hyperdynamic sepsis. Surgery 112:549–561
36. Priebe HJ, Noldge GF, Ambruster K et al (1995) Differential effects of dobutamine, dopamine and noradrenaline on splanchnic hemodynamics and oxygenation in the pig. Acta Anesthesiol Scand 39:1088–1096
37. Marsunaga T, Fujisaki Y, Yamamoto K et al (1985) Norepinephrine in cochlear microcirculation of guinea pigs. Am J Otolaryngol 6:226–230
38. Ikaruga H, Taka T, Nakajima S et al (1999) Norepinephrine, but not epinephrine enhances platelet reactivity and coagulation after exercise in humans. J Appl Physiol 86:133–138
39. Dietrich GV, Heesen M, Boldt J et al (1996) Platelet function and adrenoceptors during and after induced hypotension using nitroprusside. Anesthesiology 85:1334–1340
40. Muellner M, Urbanek B, Havel C et al (2004) Vasopressors for shock (Cochrane review). Cochrane Library, issue 4. Wiley, Chichester
41. Indrambarya T, Boyd JH, Wang Y et al (2009) Low-dose vasopressin infusion results in increased mortality and cardiac dysfunction following ischemia-reperfusion injury in mice. Crit Care 13:98
42. Communal C, Singh K, Pimentell DR et al (1998) Norepinephrine stimulates apoptosis in adult rat ventricular myocytes by activation of the B-adrenergic pathway. Circulation 98:1329–1334
43. Dincer HE, Gangopadhyay N, Wang R et al (2001) Norepinephrine induces alveolar epithelial apoptosis mediated by alfa-, beta-, and angiotensin receptor activation. Am J Physiol Lung Cell Mol Physiol 281:L624–L630
44. Minneci PC, Deans KJ, Banks SM et al (2004) Different effects of epinephrine, norepinephrine, and vasopressin on survival in a canine model of septic shock. Am J Physiol Heart Circ Physiol 287:H2545–H2554
45. Lima A, Jansen TC, van Bommel J et al (2008) The prognostic value of the subjective assessment of peripheral perfusion in critically ill patients. Crit Care Med 34:1294–1298
46. Rivers E, Nguyen B, Havstad S et al (2001) Early goal-directed therapy collaborative group. Early goal-directed therapy in the treatment of severe sepsis and septic shock. N Engl J Med 345:1368–1377
47. Rivers EP, Coba V, Whitmill M (2008) Early goal-directed therapy in severe sepsis and septic shock: a contemporary review of the literature. Curr Opin Anaesthesiol 21:128–140
48. Cheroutre H, Madakamutil L (2004) Acquired and natural memory T cells join forces at the mucosal front line. Nat Rev Immunol 4:290–300
49. Koh IHJ, Liberatore AMA, Menchaca-Diaz JL et al (2006) Bacterial translocation, microcirculation injury and sepsis. Endocr Metab Immune Disord Drug Targets 6:143–150
50. Koh IH, Menchaca-Diaz JL, Farsky SH (2002) Injuries to the mesenteric microcirculation due to bacterial translocation. Transplant Proc 34:1003–1004
51. Rath HC (2003) The role of endogenous bacterial flora: bystander or the necessary prerequisite? Eur J Gastroenterol Hepatol 15:615–620
52. Takebayashi K, Hokari R, Kurihara C et al (2009) Oral tolerance induced by enterobacteria altered the process of lymphocyte recruitment to intestinal microvessels: roles of endothelial cell adhesion molecules, TGF-beta and negative regulators of TLR signaling. Microcirculation 16:251–264
53. Ruiz-Silva M, Silva RM (2006) Can bacterial translocation be a beneficial event? Transplant Proc 38:1836–1837
54. Sandek A, Anker SD, von Haehling S (2009) The gut and intestinal bacteria in chronic heart failure. Curr Drug Metab 10:22–28

55. Sandek A, Rauchhaus M, Anker SD et al (2008) The emerging role of the gut in chronic heart failure. Curr Opin Clin Nutr Metab Care 11:632–639
56. Conraads VM, Jorens PG, De Clerck LS et al (2004) Selective intestinal decontamination in advanced chronic heart failure: a pilot trial. Eur J Heart Fail 6:483–491
57. Späth G, Hirner A (1998) Microbial translocation and impairment of mucosal immunity induced by an elemental diet in rats is prevented by selective decontamination of the digestive tract. Eur J Surg 164:223–228
58. Alberda C, Gramlich L, Meddings J et al (2007) Effects of probiotic therapy in critically ill patients: a randomized, double-blind, placebo-controlled trial. Am J Clin Nutr 85:816–823
59. Besselink MG, van Santvoort HC, Buskens E et al (2008) Probiotic prophylaxis in predicted severe acute pancreatitis: a randomised, double-blind, placebo-controlled trial. Lancet 371:651–659
60. van Silvestri L, van Saene HK, Gregori D et al (2010) Probiotics to prevent ventilator-associated pneumonia: no robust evidence from randomized controlled trials. Crit Care Med 38:1616–1617
61. Morrow LE (2009) Probiotics in the intensive care unit. Curr Opin Crit Care 15:144–148
62. Silvestri L, van Saene HKF, Zandstra DF et al (2010) Impact of selective decontamination of the digestive tract on multiple organ dysfunction syndrome: systematic review of randomized controlled trials. Crit Care Med 38:1–8

Nonantibiotic Measures to Control Ventilator-Associated Pneumonia

24

A. Gullo, A. Paratore and C. M. Celestre

24.1 Introduction

Ventilator-associated pneumonia (VAP) is associated with increased intensive care unit (ICU) stay, higher rates of morbidity and mortality, pressure on critical care capacity and increased costs [1]. Preventing hospital-acquired pneumonia (HAP) and implementing cost-effective strategies to reduce risk and improve patient outcomes should be a priority [2]. Multiple risk factors for VAP involve complex host factors and ubiquitous pathogens, which require several different types of prevention strategies [3]. Risk factors for VAP can be differentiated into modifiable and nonmodifiable conditions, and their identification allows the development of strategies for prevention and the design of treatment protocols. Nonmodifiable risk factors may be patient related (such as male sex, preexisting pulmonary disease, or multiorgan system failure). Prevention efforts should focus on modifiable conditions [4], which are crucial targets that can reduce patient mortality and morbidity rates and promote the cost-effective use of health care resources. There is a growing number of evidence-based strategies for VAP prevention that, if applied in practice, may reduce the incidence of this serious nosocomial infection.

A variety of measures has been suggested for HAP prevention, depending on the setting and the individual risk profile [5]. Effective strategies include the use of strict infection control, hand hygiene, microbiological surveillance with availability of data on local drug-resistant pathogens, monitoring and early removal of invasive devices, and programs to reduce or alter antibiotic prescribing practices. The nonantibiotic prevention strategies include conventional infection control

A. Gullo (✉)
Department of Anesthesia and Intensive Care, School of Medicine,
University Hospital Catania, Catania, Italy
e-mail: a.gullo@policlinico.unict.it

Table 24.1 Recommended nonantibiotic strategies to prevent nosocomial pneumonia in mechanically ventilated patients

Strategy	Recommendation
Conventional infection control measures	Handwashing and use of protective gowns and gloves and chlorhexidine oral rinse
Strategies related to the artificial airway	Respiratory airway care; design of endotracheal tubes; continuous subglottic aspiration
Strategies related to mechanical ventilation	Maintenance of ventilator equipment; heat and moisture exchangers; sedation adjustment; noninvasive mechanical ventilation
Strategies related to the gastrointestinal tract	Stress-ulcer prophylaxis; gastric overdistension: nasogastric tubes, enteral nutrition
Strategies related to patient placement	Semirecumbent position; rotational bed therapy

measures, related to correct care of the artificial airway, and strategies related to the position of intubated patients, the maintenance of mechanical ventilators and equipment, and the gastrointestinal tract (Table 24.1). The Canadian Critical Care trials group's report comprises three classes of evidence: (1) recommended strategies are based on strong rationale and suggestive evidence, (2) strategies may be supported by suggestive clinical or epidemiologic studies, and (3) no recommendations are given for practices for which insufficient evidence or consensus regarding efficacy exists. The report asks three questions related to HAP prevention of HAP: What is not controversial? What is still controversial? What should be investigated? [6].

24.2 Nonantibiotic Management

Table 24.2 shows the preventive measures for VAP with insufficient evidence or consensus regarding efficacy.

24.2.1 Conventional Infection Prevention and Control Measures

24.2.1.1 Multidisciplinary Team Approach
Use of proper infection control practices is the cornerstone for preventing nosocomial pneumonia. Prevention efforts must be part of an evidence-based, multidisciplinary prevention program, with a team that sets benchmarks, establishes goals and time lines, and provides staff education and training. Colonization of carers' hands is always a concern, as it increases the risk of nosocomial infection by cross-colonization during procedures such as tracheal suctioning, manipulation of ventilatory circuits, and bronchoscopy. Cross-contamination via the inoculation of bacteria into upper and lower airways (contamination of

24 Nonantibiotic Measures to Control Ventilator-Associated Pneumonia

Table 24.2 Nonantibiotic measures to prevent ventilator-associated pneumonia still under debate

Preventive strategies	
Infrastructure	
Multidisciplinary team	Programs developed by team consensus are more effective. Input by critical care staff and respiratory therapists is crucial
Target staff education	Staff education/awareness programs reduce VAP. Such programs are adaptable to local needs and are cost effective
Adequate staffing	Critical for maintaining patient safety and adherence to protocols. Particularly important in critical care units; current nursing shortages exist
Patient	
Do not routinely change the breathing circuit more frequently than every week	Not controversial
Humidification system: heat and moisture exchangers versus heated humidification	Still controversial
Handwashing and protective gowns and gloves	Recommended
Chlorhexidine oral rinse	Should be considered
Stress-ulcer prophylaxis	Still controversial, should be investigated
Avoid gastric overdistension	Recommended
Semirecumbent body position and head of bed elevation to 30–45°	Recommended
Postural changes by rotating beds	Should be considered
Enteral nutrition	Should be investigated
Avoid deep sedation	Still controversial, should be investigated
Closed-system suction catheter versus open-system catheter	Still controversial, should be investigated
Orotracheal instead of nasotracheal intubation	Not controversial
Cuff-pressure optimization	Not controversial
Subglottic secretion drainage	Recommended
Noninvasive mechanical ventilation	Still controversial, should be investigated
Early tracheostomy	Still controversial, should be investigated

respiratory equipment, condensed water in ventilator-circuit tubing, excessive manipulation of ventilator circuits) is an exogenous mechanism in VAP pathogenesis. Cross-infection is an important source of acquiring antibiotic resistant organisms (AROs), and hands or gloves of hospital personnel are potential reservoirs for spread [7].

24.2.1.2 Handwashing

Infection control programs, such as hand disinfection; handwashing; and use of protective gowns and gloves, aprons, and masks, to avoid contact with patient secretions have repeatedly demonstrated efficacy in reducing infection rates. Hand washing is widely accepted as the cornerstone of infection control in the ICU. Literature reports show that handwashing and using protective gowns and gloves during patient contact do not significantly reduce the rate of acquired nosocomial infections, especially when handling respiratory secretions or during patient contact when the patient carries an antibiotic-resistant pathogen. However, poor staff compliance is not the only reason for this failure. Although handwashing alone reduces transmission, it does not eliminate it, as transmission is dependent on the bacterial load on health care workers' hands [8]. The lack of easily reachable appropriate physical facilities (sinks, bathrooms) has led many institutions to alcohol-based gels, and clinical data indicate that rates of all nosocomial infection may be significantly reduced by their use. A randomized clinical trial of ICUs is required to support handwashing as the cornerstone of infection control.

24.2.1.3 Modulating Bacterial Colonization

Colonization of the oropharynx with pathogenic organisms is an important risk factor leading to subsequent HAP/VAP. Host-related factors reported in the literature that predispose to oropharyngeal colonization include renal dysfunction, diabetes, coma, shock, advanced age, underlying lung disease, and thoracic or upper abdominal surgery [9]. Oral care has been recommended in several studies, and adequate daily oral hygiene using topical antiseptic agents yielded mixed results.

Topical oral application of antiseptics such as chlorhexidine, an antiseptic solution for controlling dental plaque, or povidone–iodine to the oral mucosa to prevent VAP was studied in randomized controlled trials (RCTs) with conflicting results [10]. Several RCTs examined the influence of chlorhexidine in preventing nosocomial lower respiratory tract infection. Bacteria accumulated in dental plaque have been implicated as VAP pathogens when aspirated to lower airways. Preventive oral washes with chlorhexidine therefore seem reasonable in selected high-risk patients given its easy administration and reasonable cost. The prophylactic use of chlorhexidine prevention strategies is still controversial and is suggested in selected risk patients [11, 12]. The majority of meta-analyses concluded that oral antiseptic rinses seem to be effective in reducing VAP. However, RCTs and meta-analyses should be interpreted with caution, as it seems that these antiseptics may be effective for preventing lower respiratory tract infection only in patients who receive mechanical ventilation no longer than 48 h [13]; their use did not significantly reduce mortality rates. It seems that chemical decontamination with chlorhexidine as a solitary intervention may be insufficient to significantly decrease the risk of pneumonia and that thorough mechanical cleaning is still necessary. Oral decontamination with chlorhexidine did not result in significant reduction in the incidence of nosocomial pneumonia or mortality rates in patients receiving mechanical ventilation.

24.2.1.4 Probiotics

Previous reviews showed no benefit of probiotic administration in critically ill patients, but they did not focus on VAP. Probiotics normally function as colonizers and contribute to the overall health of their hosts by multiple mechanisms, including immune and antibacterial effects. Enteral administration of probiotics may modify the gastrointestinal environment in a manner that preferentially favors growth of minimally virulent species. No adverse events related to probiotic administration were identified [14]. There is no clinical evidence to support the use of probiotics to restore normal human flora in critically ill patients and reduce HAP rates [15]. Literature reports suggest that probiotics (e.g., *Lactobacillus rhamnosus* GG) are safe and recommended in a select, high-risk ICU populations, but administration is not associated with lower incidence of VAP [16, 17].

24.3 Strategies Related to the Artificial Airway and Mechanical Ventilation

24.3.1 Airway, Ventilator Circuit, and Secretion Care

24.3.1.1 Subglottic Secretions Drainage

Accumulation of oropharyngeal secretions above the cuff of the endotracheal tube is thought to increase the risk of secretion aspiration and thus pneumonia. Two meta-analyses of RCTs showed that removing these pooled secretions through suctioning of the subglottic region may reduce the risk of VAP and mortality rates [18, 19]. Not only gross aspiration but also microaspiration to lower airways can facilitate the development of VAP despite the presence of an artificial airway. It is therefore important to maintain adequate tube-cuff pressure to reduce microaspiration. Stagnant oropharyngeal secretions pooled above the cuff can easily gain access to lower airways when the pressure decreases spontaneously or there is a temporal deflation of the cuff, providing a direct route for tracheal colonization and bolus aspiration. Oropharyngeal secretions may descend into the trachea, accumulate above the endotracheal cuff, and later progress to the lower respiratory tract, causing VAP. Investigators have attempted to preemptively remove these secretions to reduce microaspiration and VAP risk and found that continuous aspiration of subglottic secretion reduced the incidence of VAP by half and shortened ICU stay, and thus it is recommended [20]. Continuous aspiration using a specially designed endotracheal tube significantly reduced the incidence of early-onset VAP in several studies but may be a less effective strategy for preventing late-onset disease, which carries a greater risk of ARO infection and higher mortality and morbidity rates. Subglottic secretion drainage is recommended in patients expected to require >72 h of mechanical ventilation, and its regular use should be encouraged in intubated patients. In the meta-analysis by Dezfulian et al., which involved five RCTs, secretion drainage appeared effective in preventing early-onset VAP; no impact on mortality was demonstrated [21, 22]. Subglottic secretion drainage appears effective in preventing early-onset pneumonia due to normal flora with no significant impact on survival. More studies are needed to assess its impact on late-onset VAP, although exogenous infections are an inherent limitation of the maneuver.

24.3.1.2 Silver-Coated Tubes

Preventing biofilm formation in endotracheal tubes is necessary in VAP prophylaxis. Altered surface characteristics of silver-coated endotracheal tubes interfere with the ability of bacteria to adhere to the tubes. Silver-coated tubes can prevent the bacterial colonization requisite for biofilm formation [23, 24], but further investigations are needed. The silver-coated tube showed its greatest effect during the first 10 days of mechanical ventilation, thus primarily affecting microorganisms present in the patient's admission flora, i.e., controls primary endogenous VAP. Inactivation of silver ions by proteins, saliva, mucosal cells, and leukocytes may explain why the silver-coated tubes failed to control secondary endogenous VAP that occurred late during ICU stay. Additionally, exogenous VAP, in which microorganisms are introduced directly into the lower airways due to poor hygiene, bypassing the oropharynx, may be an inherent limitation of the silver-coated tubes. Finally, there was no impact of silver-coated endotracheal tubes on survival. Neither subglottic drainage nor silver-coated tubes have been associated with a survival benefit [25].

24.4 Strategies Related to Patient Placement

Implementing a ventilator care bundle can significantly reduce the incidence of VAP. The original high-impact intervention ventilation care bundle, updated in 2007, consisted of elevating the head of the patient's bed to 30–45° and daily sedation hold [26].

24.4.1 Semirecumbent Position

Aspiration of upper-airway secretions is common, even in healthy adults, in the supine position. Supine patient positioning facilitates aspiration; semirecumbent positioning decreases it. Infection in patients in the supine position was associated with simultaneous administration of enteral nutrition and an increased risk of aspiration of gastric contents. Gastroesophageal reflux occurs less frequently in the semirecumbent position. Thus, it is recommended that intubated patients be managed in a semirecumbent position (>30°), particularly during feeding. Some studies found this position to be associated with lower levels of aspiration into the lower airways but not lower VAP incidence, especially in patients receiving enterally administered nutrition. Several authors and influential scientific societies claim the semirecumbent position prevents VAP [27]. Results were based on experimental studies with radioactive-labeled enteral feeding, which suggested that endotracheal aspiration of gastric content occurred more frequently in supine patients than in patients at a 45° angle. However, clinical data supporting the statement are not robust. Three RCTs and three meta-analyses demonstrated that semirecumbency did not significantly reduce the odds of either microbiological or clinically suspected VAP, and mortality rates were not statistically reduced [28]. The semirecumbent position is a low-cost, easily accessible intervention and may be a more practical and tolerable approach than rotational beds (30–45°, particularly during enteral feeding, continues to be recommended). Patients should thus be nursed in a semirecumbent position [29].

24.5 Conclusion

Despite an increased understanding of HAP/VAP pathogenesis and advances in diagnosis and treatment, risk, cost, morbidity and mortality remain unacceptably high [30]. Implementing preventive measures and cost-effective strategies to reduce patient risk and improve outcomes should be a priority. A variety of measures has been suggested [31], depending on the setting and the individual risk profile; here we focused on nonantibiotic strategies. The gold standard is based on a multidisciplinary team approach. To prevent VAP, authors recommend the orotracheal route of intubation for intubation; a new ventilator circuit for each patient; circuit changes if the circuit becomes soiled or damaged, but no scheduled changes; changing heat and moisture exchangers every 5–7 days or as clinically indicated; using a new closed endotracheal suctioning system for each patient and as clinically indicated; subglottic secretion drainage in patients expected to be mechanically ventilated >72 h; elevating the bed head to 45° when impossible, or as near to 45° as possible. Rotating beds and oral antiseptic rinses should be considered. Bacterial filters and antimicrobial agents such as iseganan are not recommended. We make no recommendations regarding a systematic search for sinusitis, airway humidification type, tracheostomy timing, prone positioning, aerosolized antibiotics, mupirocin intranasally, topically and/or intravenously applied antibiotics, because they are still under debate in medical literature and not universally recommended. In conclusion, prevention is the most important step toward improve standard of care and cost-effectiveness related to HAP/VAP [32].

References

1. Restrepo MI, Anzueto A, Arroliga AC et al (2010) Economic burden of ventilator-associated pneumonia based on total resource utilization. Infect Control Hosp Epidemiol 31:509–515
2. Diaz E, Lorente L, Valles J, Rello J (2010) Mechanical ventilation associated pneumonia. Med Intensiva 34(5):318–324

3. Torres A, Ewig S, Lode H, Carlet J, European HAP Working Group (2009) Defining, treating and preventing hospital acquired pneumonia: European perspective. Intensive Care Med 35:9–29
4. Omrane R, Eid J, Perreault MM et al (2007) Impact of a protocol for prevention of ventilator-associated pneumonia. Ann Pharmacother 41:1390–1396
5. Lorente L, Blot S, Rello J (2010) New issue and controversies in the prevention of ventilator-associated pneumonia. Am J Respir Crit Care Med 182(7):870–876
6. Muscedere J, Dodek P, Keenan S et al, VAP Guidelines Committee and the Canadian Critical Care Trials Group (2008) Comprehensive evidence-based clinical practice guidelines for ventilator-associated pneumonia: prevention. J Crit Care 23:126–137
7. Rotstein C, Evans G, Born A et al (2008) Clinical practice guidelines for hospital-acquired pneumonia and ventilator-associated pneumonia in adults. Can J Infect Dis Med Microbiol 19(1):19–53
8. Silvestri L, Petros AJ, Sarginson RE et al (2005) Handwashing in the intensive care unit: a big measure with modest effects. J Hosp Infect 59(3):172–179
9. Feider LL, Mitchell P, Bridges E (2010) Oral care practices for orally intubated critically ill adults. Am J Crit Care 19:175–183
10. Panchabhai TS, Dangayach NS, Krishnan A, Karnad DR (2009) Effect of oropharyngeal cleansing with 0.2% chlorhexidine in critically ill patients: an open label randomized controlled trial. Chest 135:1150–1156
11. Chan EY, Ruest A, Meade MO, Cook DJ (2007) Oral decontamination for prevention of pneumonia in mechanically ventilated adults: systematic review and meta-analysis. BMJ 334(7599):889
12. Tantipong H, Morkchareonpong C, Jaiyindee S, Thamlikitkul V (2009) Randomized controlled trial and meta-analysis of oral decontamination with 2% chlorhexidine solution for the prevention of ventilator-associated pneumonia. Infect Control Hosp Epidemiol 30: 101–102
13. Kola A, Gastmaier P (2007) Efficacy of oral chlorhexidine in preventing lower respiratory tract infections. Meta-analysis of randomized controlled trials. J Hosp Infect 66:207–216
14. Morrow LE, Kollef MH, Casale TB (2010) Probiotic prophylaxis of ventilator-associated pneumonia: a blinded, randomized, controlled trial. Am J Respir Crit Care Med 182(8):1058–1064
15. Isakow W, Morrow LE, Kollef MH (2007) Probiotics for preventing and treating nosocomial infections: review of current evidence and recommendations. Chest 132:286–294
16. Silvestri L, van Saene HK, Gregori D et al (2010) Probiotics to prevent ventilator-associated pneumonia: no robust evidence from randomized controlled trials. Crit Care Med 38(7): 1616–1617
17. Siempos II, Ntaidou TK, Falagas ME (2010) Impact of the administration of probiotics on the incidence of ventilator-associated pneumonia: a meta-analysis of randomized controlled trials. Crit Care Med 38(3):954–962
18. Dezfulian C, Shojania K, Collard HR et al (2005) Subglottic secretion drainage for preventing ventilator associated pneumonia: a meta-analysis. Am J Med 118:11–18
19. Silvestri L, Milanese M, Piacente N et al (2008) Impact of subglottic secretion drainage on ventilator-associated pneumonia and mortality. Systematic review of randomized controlled trials. In: Proceedings of the 21st anesthesia and ICU symposium Alpe Adria, pp 26–29
20. Lorente L, Lecuona M, Jiménez A et al (2007) Influence of an endotracheal tube with polyurethane cuff and subglottic secretion drainage on pneumonia. Am J Respir Crit Care Med 176:1079–1083
21. Overend TJ, Anderson CM, Brooks D et al (2009) Updating the evidence-base for suctioning adult patients: a systematic review. Can Respir J 16(3):e6–e17
22. Van Saene HKF, Zandstra DF, Petros AJ et al (2009) Infections in ICU: an ongoing challenge. In: Gullo A, Besso J, Lumb PD, Williams GF (eds) Intensive and critical care medicine. Springer, Milan, pp 261–272

23. Niederman MS (2010) Fighting vampires and ventilator-associated pneumonia: is silver the magic bullet? Chest 135:1007–1009
24. Kollef MH, Afessa B, Anzueto A et al, NASCENT Investigation Group (2008) Silver-coated endotracheal tubes and incidence of ventilator-associated pneumonia: the NASCENT randomized trial. JAMA 300:805–813
25. Silvestri L, van Saene HKF, de la Cal MA, de Gaudio AR (2009) Carriage classification of pneumonia rather than time improves survival. Chest 136(4):1188–1189
26. Westwell S (2008) Implementing a ventilator care bundle in an adult intensive care unit. Nurs Crit Care 13:203–207
27. Alexiou VG, Ierodiakonou V, Dimopoulos G, Falagas ME (2009) Impact of patient position on the incidence of ventilator-associated pneumonia: a meta-analysis of randomized controlled trials. J Crit Care 24(4):515–522
28. Silvestri L, Gregori D, van Saene HK et al (2010) Semirecumbent position to prevent ventilator-associated pneumonia is not evidence based. J Crit Care 25(1):152–153
29. Niel-Weise BS, van den Broek PJ (2009) Semi-recumbent position or not? In: Dutch working party for infection prevention (WIP). http://www.wip.nl/systrev.asp?nr=12
30. Rosenthal VD, Maki DG, Jamulitrat S et al, for the INICC Members (2010) International Nosocomial Infection Control Consortium (INICC) report, data summary for 2003–2008, issued June 2009. Am J Infect Control 38:95–104
31. Efrati S, Deutsch I, Antonelli M et al (2010) Ventilator-associated pneumonia: current status and future recommendations. J Clin Monit Comput 24(2):161–168
32. van Saene HKF, Silvestri L, de la Cal MA, Baines PB (2009) The emperor's new clothes; the fairy tale continues. J Crit Care 24:149–152

Impact of Nutritional Route on Infections: Parenteral Versus Enteral

25

A. Gullo, C. M. Celestre and A. Paratore

25.1 Introduction

The significance of nutrition in the intensive care unit (ICU) cannot be overstated [1]. Malnutrition is a marker of poor outcomes and is correlated with longer hospital stays, nutrition-related complications during and after hospitalization, and other adverse outcomes. There is a clear association between malnutrition and postoperative complications. Nutritional status also worsens during hospitalization in surgical patients and during critical illness; malnutrition rates were higher at discharge than at admission. Among seriously ill patients, malnutrition is associated with increased infectious morbidity and prolonged hospital stay. Critical illness is typically associated with a catabolic stress state in which patients commonly demonstrate a systemic inflammatory response. This response is coupled with complications of increased infectious morbidity, multiorgan dysfunction, prolonged hospitalization, and disproportionate mortality rates.

Nosocomial infection in critically ill patients is associated with higher morbidity and mortality rates, prolonged ICU and hospital stay, and consequent higher health care cost [2]. Providing nutritional support has become a standard of care for critically ill patients. A post hoc analysis suggested preoperative administration as the most important period. Preoperative supplementation is as effective as perioperative supplementation in improving outcome [3]. Early nutritional

A. Gullo (✉) · C. M. Celestre (✉) · A. Paratore (✉)
Department of Anesthesia and Intensive Care,
School of Medicine, University Hospital Catania, Catania, Italy
e-mail: a.gullo@policlinico.unict.it

C. M. Celestre
e-mail: chiaracelestre@gmail.com

A. Paratore
e-mail: annalaura79@inwind.it

support, defined as initiation within the first 24–48 h of ICU care, is recommended by clinical practice guidelines as the first-line nutritional therapy in the ICU.

Nutrition administered enterally (EN) and parenterally (PN) should be initiated if the caloric goal will be difficult to attain. The most important goal is to continuously supply the enteric mucosa with useful immunonutrients such as glutamine and fiber to preserve the barrier effect, the mucus layer, and immunological status of the mucosa, with consequent reduced infection rates [4].

25.2 Critical Illness and the Immune System

Critically ill patients are at high risk for nosocomial infections, which can lead to organ dysfunction and death. Thus, the benefits and risks of nutritional therapies in preventing and managing infectious diseases are highly relevant [5, 6]. A major methodological problem is related to the term critically ill, as it does not refer to homogenous populations. The prevalence of malnutrition among critically ill patients, especially those with a protracted clinical course, has remained largely unchanged over several years and has implications on hospital length of stay, illness course, and morbidity rates. The profound and stereotypic metabolic response to critical illness and failure of carers to provide optimal nutritional support therapy during a patient's ICU stay are the principal factors contributing to malnutrition.

Critically ill patients should not be allowed to remain in a state of unopposed starvation, because this increases morbidity and mortality, particularly in the setting of multi-organ-system failure [7]. Immunosuppression occurs as a result of malnutrition, and protein-energy malnutrition has been cited as the major cause of immunodeficiency worldwide. Critical illness results in derangements of all components of the acute immune response, which is organized and executed by innate immunity influenced by the neuroendocrine system. This response starts with sensing danger by pattern-recognition receptors on immunocompetent cells and endothelium [8]. The sensed danger signals, through specific signalling pathways, activate nuclear transcription factor kappa-B and other transcription factors and gene regulatory systems, which up-regulate proinflammatory mediator expression. Plasma cascades are also activated, which together with proinflammatory mediators further stimulate inflammatory biomarker production. The acute inflammatory response underlies the pathophysiological mechanisms involved in the development of multiorgan dysfunction syndrome (MODS). The inflammatory mediators directly affect organ function mediating the production of nitric oxide (NO), leading to mitochondrial anergy and cytopathic hypoxia, a condition of cellular inability to use oxygen.

Understanding the mechanisms of acute immune responses in critical illness is necessary for the development of therapeutic strategies, understanding molecular and biological effects of nutrients in maintaining homeostasis has made exponential advances. Perioperative immune modulation using specialized enteral diets containing specific immunonutrients may improve postoperative outcomes [9]. Some studies investigated the role of nutrition as a modifier of the immune response in specific clinical settings, especially the use of preoperative oral supplementation with immunonutrients in comparison with standard nutrition in surgical and critically ill patients [10]. Several specific nutrients have been shown in laboratory and clinical studies to influence nutritional, immunological, and inflammatory parameters. Immunonutrients are defined as nutrients that provide specific benefits to the immune system and include glutamine, arginine, long-chain n-3 polyunsaturated fatty acids, and nucleotides, either alone or in combination. Usually provided in combination, these nutrients, when added to a standard enteral formula, seem to improve outcomes by reducing infection rates.

The influence of malnutrition on immunity is complex. Studies investigated the effects of immunonutrition on morbidity and mortality rates in critical ill patients, but results are conflicting in terms of study design, population heterogeneity, treatment timing, and suboptimal delivery of nutrients. In selected patient groups, the immunonutrition, can be efficacious to reduce infection and mortality rates, and hospital length of stay. However whether these immunonutrients are beneficial, or should even be used, in critically ill patients remains controversial [11].

Immunonutrition formulae are indicated in specific subgroups of critically ill patients (e.g. patients with trauma, mild sepsis, surgical patients); this conclusion is supported by meta-analyses and recent guidelines.

25.3 Infection, Bacterial Translocation, and Sepsis

Nutritional support for ICU patients is important, as adverse effects of malnutrition are multiple and common and infection is a serious complication [13]. Malnutrition is accompanied by progressive atrophy and disruption of the intestinal mucosa, resulting in a protein-losing enteropathy. Loss of protein promotes an edematous state, complicating patient care, particularly regarding drug administration. Furthermore, lack of nutrition allows translocation of enteric pathogens across the bowel mucosa and into the circulation, leading to sepsis [14]. Adequate EN or PN nutritional support not only improves clinical outcomes but is essential for recovery from critical illness. EN also may be important in maintaining normal gut structure and function, thereby decreasing bacterial translocation (BT) and the risk of systemic infection. EN is particularly beneficial for promoting gut-barrier integrity and reducing infection and mortality rates. Failure of gastrointestinal tract (GIT) barrier function may fuel systemic inflammatory response syndrome (SIRS), sepsis, and organ failure. In these conditions, BT due to gut-barrier failure has been targeted as the trigger of a self-sustaining process for systemic infection and MODS.

In critically ill patients with severe homeostasis disorders, many different factors are involved in the pathophysiology of bacteria and endotoxin translocation, either in conditions of anatomically intact bowel barrier or in conditions of altered intestinal mucosa. Preventing BT can be attained both by improving intestinal function and the host defense mechanism. Therapies against translocation include nutrition, EN, and selective decontamination of the digestive tract (SDD) to increase oxygen delivery and avoid hypoperfusion.

A retrospective study demonstrated no significant decrease in the incidence of fungal infections in critically ill patients receiving SDD between those receiving EN and total PN (TPN). SDD significantly reduced overall bloodstream infections (BSI), Gram-negative BSI [15, 16] and overall mortality, without affecting Gram-positive BSI [17]. The full protocol of systemic SDD reduces mortality rates in critically ill patients, particularly when successful decontamination is achieved [18].

EN is indicated in postoperative patients (GI surgery), reducing the complication rate and hospital stay, and in severe pancreatitis promotes resolution of inflammation and reduces the incidence of infection. Nutrition via the enteral route is often preferred over central venous or TPN due to its relative ease of administration and lower cost. As demonstrated in the literature, it is not only safer and less expensive than PN but modulates an exaggerated cytokine response related to surgical trauma that leads to increased intestinal permeability, BT, and infection. Nutrients administered enterally can reach the bowel lumen where enterocytes draw upon their fuel, preserving the barrier effect and modulating the cytokine response. Parenteral supply does not achieve this target, as the blood supply of nutrients is not as important as the luminal supply. It is only via the enteral route that the barrier effect can be preserved.

Experimental studies show that TPN (enteric starvation) results in rapid and severe atrophy of gut-associated lymphoid tissue (GALT) and increases BT. In patients with an intact GIT, early EN is the preferred route of nutritional support [19]. PN is immunosuppressive and proinflammatory and may be deleterious in patients with pancreatitis. GALT is the source of most mucosal immunity in humans. In addition, TPN is associated with impaired B- and T-cell lymphocyte function, altered leucocyte chemotaxis, and impaired bacterial and fungal killing. Lack of enteral feeding results in atrophy of the GI mucosa, bacterial overgrowth, increased intestinal permeability, and translocation of bacteria or bacterial products into the circulation. TPN may therefore promote BT [20].

Two vital components of critical care are the use of central venous catheters and TPN. The most severely ill patients often require both for survival and recovery. In the ICU, GI dysfunction associated with multiorgan failure and shock or with abdominal surgery is not uncommon. Nutrition therefore must not be compromised. When TPN is suggested for a patient, the risk of infectious complications, especially infection related to central venous catheters, is often thought greater than potential benefits. Of all the potentially devastating infectious complications, catheter-related infection remains the major concern associated with TPN. However, because early provision of nutritional support improves outcomes in critically ill patients, avoiding or delaying TPN administration of solutions is potentially harmful [21].

25.4 Assessing Nutritional Status and Score Index

Many tools are used to assess patients' nutritional status. Traditional nutrition assessment tools (albumin, prealbumin, and anthropometry) are not valid in critical care. Most nutritional assessment techniques are based on their ability to predict clinical outcomes [22]. However, none of these techniques to accurately measure nutritional risk has been validated. Using nutritional assessment to predict clinical outcome can be problematic, because the interaction between malnutrition and other factors that influence outcomes makes it difficult to isolate any putative contribution from malnutrition alone. Recognizing specific prognostic factors might lead to interventions or increased postoperative surveillance, which could improve outcome. However, the validity of these techniques has also not been proven.

Two methods can be applied for nutritional assessment: (1) Subjective Global Assessment (SGA) is used to classify patients into one of three categories of nutritional status: (a) well nourished, (b) moderately malnourished, or (c) severely malnourished (2) Nutritional Risk Index (NRI) is a simple equation that uses serum albumin levels and recent weight loss. An NRI >100 indicates no malnourishment, 97.5–100 mild malnourishment, 83.5–<97.5 moderate malnourishment, and <83.5 severe malnourishment. Whereas the NRI uses serum albumin concentrations, which are influenced by nutritional status in the presence of inflammatory stress due to a disease, the SGA is not influenced by serum proteins. On the other hand, NRI uses some laboratory examination, which requires laboratory costs, but SGA uses only clinical examination, which can easily be done in several minutes. One might say SGA is the more cost-effective means of assessing nutritional risk. Both these nutrition tests are, however, predictive for malnutrition and postoperative complications (infectious-complications-included pneumonia, intra-abdominal abscess, sepsis, wound infection, urinary tract infection, pneumonia, atelectasis, pulmonary complications, anemia, cardiac arrhythmia), length of hospital and ICU stay, and mechanical ventilation duration [23].

Malnutrition is also associated with a delayed recovery from illness and an increased rate of complications. Heart failure, respiratory diseases, impaired immune function, and postoperative wound healing are all influenced by nutritional status. Nutritional assessment includes patient history, physical examination, anthropometric measurements, laboratory data, and changes in immunocompetence. The validity and sensitivity of the parameters, i.e. serum proteins, albumin, transferrin, and retinol-binding protein, to assess nutritional status are diminished for the individual patient. Albumin is commonly thought of as a good indicator of nutritional status and visceral proteins [24]. Although a variety of nutritional indices have been found to be valuable in predicting patient outcome when used alone, there is no consensus on the best method for assessing the nutritional status of hospitalized patients. There are no sensitive markers available to assess the influence of malnutrition on the immunocompetence of an individual patient for clinical purposes. Traditionally, nutritional support in the critically ill population has been regarded as adjunctive care designed to provide exogenous fuels to support the patient during the stress response.

25.5 Enteral Versus Parenteral Administration Route

Nutritional support had three main objectives: to preserve lean body mass, to maintain immune function, and to avert metabolic complications. Nutrition therapy therefore specifically aims at attenuating the metabolic response to stress, preventing oxidative cellular injury, and favorably modulating the immune response. Because EN and PN carry both risks and benefits, in the average patient in the ICU who has no contraindications, the choice of route for nutritional support may be influenced by several factors.

Enteral tube feeding was first employed in the 1600s and was made popular in the medical profession by the famous British surgeon John Hunter at the end of the eighteenth century. The indication for early EN is supported by guidelines published by the European Society for Clinical Nutrition and Metabolism and American and Canadian guidelines, which recommend starting administration within the first 24–48 h of admission to the ICU [25]. Short-term access is usually achieved using nasogastric (NG) or nasojejunal (NJ) tubes; percutaneous endoscopic gastrotomy (PEG) or jejunostomy should be considered if feeding is planned for longer than 1 month. Early EN is recommended for critically ill patients, with special formulas indicated in specific patient subgroups. Early EN enhances immunocompetence, reduced clinical infection rates, and maintained gut structure and function by preserving gut structure/function integrity, balancing intestinal microflora, maintaining effective local and systemic immunocompetence, and potentially attenuating catabolic stress responses in patients after surgery. There is strong evidence that early enteral feeding prevents infections in a variety of traumatic and surgical illnesses [26]. There is, however, little support for similar early feeding in medical illnesses.

Recommendations are to initiate EN as soon as possible whenever the GIT is functioning. The disadvantage of enteral support is that insufficient energy and protein coverage can occur. Evidence shows that EN can result in underfeeding and that nutritional goals are frequently reached only after 1 week. Several observational studies in long-term ICU patients note that cumulative energy deficit is related to increased infectious morbidity (infection rate, wound healing, mechanical ventilation, length of stay, duration of recovery), and costs [27]. Morbidity and mortality rates seem to be linked to such an energy deficit, which often occurs during the first week of stay. Supplemental PN combined with EN can be considered to cover energy and protein targets when EN alone fails to achieve the caloric goal [28]. EN is believed be safer and less expensive than PN. However, total enteral feeding (TEN) is associated with complications such as diarrhea, abdominal distention and cramps, and contamination and infection of an enteral feeding system. In fact EN provides an ideal environment for the development of bacteria, and the ICU team thus plays a vital role in implementing and maintaining appropriate standards of care and minimizing risks of bacterial contamination. Again, if EN is insufficient or fails, PN should be instituted, respecting the often reduced demand for exogenous substrates in critically ill patients [29].

PN therapy is primarily initiated in patients with a contraindication to use of the GIT and when infection is one of its frequent and severe complications. PN is indicated in patients who are unable to obtain adequate nutrients by oral or enteral routes (EN is not feasible). Other indications are short-gut syndrome, high-output fistula, prolonged ileus, or bowel obstruction. Indications for TPN are patients without a functioning GIT or who have disorders requiring complete bowel rest, such as some stages of Crohn's disease or ulcerative colitis, bowel obstruction, certain pediatric GI disorders (congenital GI anomalies, prolonged diarrhea regardless of cause, short-bowel syndrome due to surgery). Short-term PN may be used if a person's digestive system has shut down (peritonitis) and their weight is low enough to cause concerns about nutrition during an extended hospital stay. Long-term PN is occasionally used to treat people suffering the extended consequences of an accident, surgery, or digestive disorder. The nutrient solution consists of water and electrolytes (glucose, amino acids, lipids); essential vitamins, minerals, and trace elements are added or given separately. Previously, lipid emulsions were given separately. In critical patients in perioperative care, PN increases the risk of infection when compared with EN or delayed nutrition [30].

A European meta-analysis showed that PN is superior to delayed EN in critically ill patients. Additional PN thus seems to be the way to avoid cumulative energy deficit associated with insufficient or no EN. Guidelines issued by the American Society for Parenteral and Enteral Nutrition (ASPEN) and the European Society for Clinical Nutrition and Metabolism (ESPEN) are mainly based on observational studies showing a strong correlation between negative energy balance and morbidity–mortality rates. ASPEN guidelines recommend administration of PN to nonmalnourished ICU patients receiving some but not adequate EN during the first 7–10 days after admission [31]; ESPEN guidelines recommend compensating the deficit by adding PN after 24–48 h [32].

The energy deficit accumulated by underfed ICU patients during the first days of stay may play an important role in ICU and hospital outcomes for long-term patients. To reach caloric requirements by artificial nutritional support without harming the patient is still a subject of debate. Frequent questions related to artificial nutrition are: Is there significant benefit or risk associated with the route chosen for nutrition delivery? Would TPN increase the bacteremia rate? Some studies showed that the nutritional support route in severely ill patients in an ICU does not affect the rate of infectious complications [33]; however, comorbid medical conditions and the need of ICU support are more important parameters for determining the risk of infectious complications. Although many studies have reported that catheter-associated infective complications are more frequently elicited by TPN, some studies report that TPN-associated infections can be attributed to hyperglycemia and caloric overload and that insulin therapy can alleviate these infections. Others consider PN to be an independent risk factor for central–venous catheter-related infection [34]. Studies evaluating the impact of feeding route and intestinal permeability on BSI and systemic immune responses concluded that systemic proinflammatory response decreases with increasing EN and PN weaning [35]. In the majority of critically ill patients, it is practical and

Table 25.1 European Society for Clinical Nutrition and Metabolism (ESPEN) guidelines modified. Enteral nutrition (EN): intensive care

Recommendations	
Indications for EN	All patients who are not expected to be on a full oral diet within 3 days should receive EN
Application of early EN	The ESPEN committee recommends that hemodynamically stable critically ill patients who have a functioning gastrointestinal tract should be fed early (<24 h) using an appropriate amount of feed. Exogenous energy supply: • During the acute and initial phase of critical illness: in excess of 20–25 kcal/kg body weight/day may be associated with a less favorable outcome • During the anabolic recovery phase, the aim should be to provide 25–30 kcal/kg body weight/day • Patient with severe undernutrition should receive EN up 25–30 total Kcal/kg body weight/day. If these target values are not reached, supplementary parenteral nutrition (PN) should be given. Consider i.v. administration of metoclopramide or erythromycin in patients with intolerance to enteral feeding (e.g., with high gastric residuals)
Route	Use EN in patients who can be fed via the enteral route There is no significant difference in the efficacy of jejunal versus gastric feeding in critically ill patients Use supplemental PN in patients who cannot be fed sufficiently via the enteral route

safe to use EN instead of PN. The beneficial effects of EN when compared with PN are well documented in numerous prospective randomized controlled trials involving a variety of patient populations in critical illness, including trauma, burns, head injury, major surgery, and acute pancreatitis. Whereas few studies show a differential effect on mortality rates, the most consistent outcome effect from EN is reduced infectious morbidity. When TPN is recommended, the risk of infectious complications, especially infection related to central venous catheters, is often thought greater than potential benefits. However, because early provision of nutritional support improves outcomes in critically ill patients, avoiding or delaying TPN administration is potentially harmful (Table 25.1).

When selecting the appropriate enteral formulation for the critically ill patient, the clinician must first decide if the patient is a candidate for a specialty immunomodulating formulation, which are those supplemented with agents such as arginine, glutamine, nucleic acid, Omega-3 fatty acids, and antioxidants, and which should be used for the appropriate patient population (major elective surgery, trauma, burns, head and neck cancer, critically ill patients on mechanical ventilation) [36]. Results strengthen the indication for a special formula in acute respiratory distress syndrome (ARDS) and acute lung injury [37]. Administration of probiotic, a combination of antioxidant vitamins, and trace minerals in specific critically ill patient populations is still being debated (Table 25.2).

Table 25.2 European Society for Clinical Nutrition and Metabolism (ESPEN) guidelines modified. Special enteral nutrition (EN) formulations for the appropriate patient population

EN formulae and patient population	
Type of formula	Whole-protein formulae are appropriate in most patients because no clinical advantage of peptide-based formulae could be shown
	Immune-modulating formulae (formulae enriched with arginine, nucleotides, and ω-3 fatty acids) are superior to standard enteral formulae
	• In elective upper GI surgical patients (see guidelines surgery)
	• In patients with a mild sepsis (APACHE II <15)
	• In patients with severe sepsis, however, immune-modulating formulae may be harmful and are therefore not recommended
	• In patients with trauma (see guidelines surgery)
	• In patients with ARDS (formulae containing ω-3 fatty acids and antioxidants)
	No recommendation for immunomodulating formulae can be given for burn patients due to insufficient data. In burn patients, trace elements (Cu, Se, Zn) should be supplemented in a higher-than-standard dose
	ICU patients with very severe illness who do not tolerate >700 ml enteral formulae per day should not receive an immunomodulating formula enriched with arginine, nucleotides and ω-3 fatty acids
	Glutamine should be added to standard enteral formula in:
	• Burn patients
	• Trauma patients
	There are not sufficient data to support glutamine supplementation in surgical or heterogenous critically ill patients

GI gastrointestinal tract, *APACHE* Acute Physiology and Chronic Health Evaluation II, *ARDS* acute respiratory distress syndrome, *Cu* copper, *Se* selenium, *Zn* zinc

EN via tube feeding is the preferred method of feeding the critically ill patient, particularly on those who develop a severe inflammatory response, (i.e. patients who have failure of at least one organ during ICU stay) and an important means of counteracting the catabolic state induced by severe diseases. Evidence from primarily low-quality trials shows that EN reduces infections, septic complications, and length of hospital stay, resulting in a better outcome compared with total PN, but not does affect noninfectious complication or hospital mortality rates. That combined nutritional support provides additional benefit on overall outcomes has yet to be proven in further studies, including outcomes of physical and cognitive functioning, quality of life, cost-effectiveness, and cost utility. Meta-analyses of ICU studies showed that PN is not related to a greater mortality rate and may even be associated with improved survival [38].

25.6 Conclusion

The significance of nutritional support in the hospital setting cannot be overstated and is part of the standard of care for the critically ill adult patient. Nutrition is a cornerstone for improved outcomes [39]. Nutritional modulation of the stress response to critical illness includes early EN using the enteral route, which is seen as a proactive therapeutic strategy that may reduce disease severity, diminish complications, decrease length of ICU stay, and favorably impact patient outcome. Guidelines and studies confirm that EN versus PN, early EN initiation, enteral and parenteral glutamine administration, and intensive insulin therapy are all associated with reduced infectious morbidity in critically ill patients [40, 41]. EN compared with PN results in an important decrease in the incidence of infectious complications in the critically ill and may be less costly, and thus should be the first choice for nutritional support in the critically ill. EN reduces infections, septic complications and length of hospital stay, resulting in a better outcome compared with total PN, but it not does affect noninfectious complication or hospital mortality rates.

Guidelines for using TPN while avoiding catheter-related infection may markedly improve its outcome. Appropriately training personnel to care for central venous catheters is imperative and is an effective method of reducing devastating complications of infection [42]. Catheters impregnated with antiseptics and coated with antibiotics are now available. Conceivably, as our understanding of interventions such as central venous catheters and TPN continues to improve, these catheters can be used in situations in which the risk of catheter-related infection is high, such as TPN administration. Evidence-based critical care nutrition clinical practice guidelines recommend EN over PN; time to initiate EN; use of formulas enriched with fish oils; glutamine supplementation; glycemic control; arginine-enriched formulas; motility agents; timing of supplemental PN when appropriate; delivery of hypocaloric PN when appropriate; and adoption of a feeding protocol [43, 44].

Nutritional assessment of the critically ill patient is crucial, as the deterioration of nutritional status is a key factor in surgical and critically ill patient outcomes. Perioperative nutrition with specialized enteral diets improves outcome when compared with standard formulas. One meta-analysis suggests that antioxidant supplementation is associated with no improvement in infectious complications but is associated with increased survival rates. New prospects may be possible in the fight against surgical infections by adding probiotics to EN in order to improve the microenvironment of the colon. Many unanswered questions remain, however, the last but not the least of which is the advocated proactive posture for metabolic support in the ICU [45, 46].

References

1. Cahill NE, Dhaliwal R, Day AG, Jiang X, Heyland DK (2010) Nutrition therapy in the critical care setting: what is "best achievable" practice? An international multicenter observational study. Crit Care Med 38(2):395–401
2. Farber MS, Moses J, Korn M (2005) Reducing costs and patient morbidity in the enterally fed intensive care unit patient. JPEN J Parenter Enteral Nutr 29:S62–S69
3. Martindale RG, Maerz LL (2006) Management of perioperative nutrition support. Curr Opin Crit Care 12:290–294
4. Gianotti L (2006) Nutrition and infections. Surg Infect (Larchmt) 7(Suppl 2):S29–S32

5. Elia M, Engfer M, Green C, Silk DB (2010) Letter to the editor on the new guidelines for adult critically ill patients. JPEN J Parenter Enteral Nutr 34(1):105
6. Taylor B, Krenitsky J (2010) Nutrition in the intensive care unit: year in review 2008–2009. JPEN J Parenter Enteral Nutr 34(1):21–31
7. Saka B, Kaya O, Ozturk GB et al (2010) Malnutrition in the elderly and its relationship with other geriatric syndromes. Clin Nutr74 29(6):745–748
8. Marshall JC, Charbonney E, Gonzalez PD (2008) The immune system in critical illness. Clin Chest Med 29(4):605–616
9. Mizock BA (2010) Immunonutrition and critical illness: an update. Nutrition 26(7–8):701–707
10. Helminem H, Raitanen M, Kellosalo J (2007) Immunonutrition in elective gastrointestinal surgery patients. Scand J Surg 96:46–50
11. Calder PC (2007) Immunonutrition in surgical and critically ill patients. Br J Nutr 98 (Suppl 1):S133–9
12. Klek S, Kulig J, Sierzega M et al (2008) The impact of immunostimulating nutrition on infectious complications after upper gastrointestinal surgery: a prospective, randomized, clinical trial. Ann Surg 248(2):212–220
13. Dhaliwal R, Heyland DK (2005) Nutrition and infection in the intensive care unit: what does the evidence show? Curr Opin Crit Care 11(5):461–467
14. Kang W, Kudsk KA (2007) Is there evidence that the gut contributes to mucosal immunity in humans? JPEN J Parenter Enteral Nutr 31(3):246–258
15. Silvestri L, van Saene HK, Milanese M, Gregori D (2005) Impact of selective decontamination of the digestive tract on fungal carriage and infection: systematic review of randomized controlled trials. Intensive Care Med 31(7):898–910
16. Silvestri L, Zandstra DF, van Saene HK, Petros AJ et al (2008) Antifungal prophylaxis in critically ill patients. Crit Care 12(3):420
17. Silvestri L, van Saene HK, Milanese M et al (2007) Selective decontamination of the digestive tract reduces bacterial bloodstream infection and mortality in critically ill patients. Systematic review of randomized, controlled trials. J Hosp Infect 65(3):187–203
18. Silvestri L, van Saene HK, Weir I, Gullo A (2009) Survival benefit of the full selective digestive decontamination regimen. J Crit Care 24(3):474.e7–474.e14
19. Doig GS, Heighes PT, Simpson F, Sweetman EA (2010) Early enteral nutrition reduces mortality in trauma patients requiring intensive care: a meta-analysis of randomised controlled trials. Injury 42(1):50–56
20. Hanna N, Bialowas C, Fernandez C (2010) Septicemia secondary to ileus in trauma patients: a human model for bacterial translocation. South Med J 103(5):461–463
21. Ziegler TR (2009) Parenteral nutrition in the critically ill patient. N Engl J Med 361(11):1088–1097; comment: N Engl J Med 362(1):83; author reply 83–84
22. Kuzu MA, Terzioğlu H, Genç V et al (2006) Preoperative nutritional risk assessment in predicting postoperative outcome in patients undergoing major surgery. World J Surg 30(3):378–390
23. Paillaud E, Herbaud S, Caillet P et al (2005) Relations between undernutrition and nosocomial infections in elderly patients. Age Ageing 34(6):619–625
24. Lohsiriwat V, Lohsiriwat D, Boonnuch W et al (2008) Pre-operative hypoalbuminemia is a major risk factor for postoperative complications following rectal cancer surgery. World J Gastroenterol 14(8):1248–1251
25. Kreymann KG (2008) Early nutrition support in critical care: a European perspective. Curr Opin Clin Nutr Metab Care 11(2):156–159
26. Artinian V, Krayem H, DiGiovine B (2006) Effects of early enteral feeding on the outcome of critically ill mechanically ventilated medical patients. Chest 129:960–967
27. Singer P, Pichard C, Heidegger CP, Wernerman J (2010) Considering energy deficit in the intensive care unit. Curr Opin Clin Nutr Metab Care 13(2):170–176
28. Wernerman J (2008) Paradigm of early parenteral nutrition support in combination with insufficient enteral nutrition. Curr Opin Clin Nutr Metab Care 11(2):160–163

29. Nagata S, Fukuzawa K, Iwashita Y et al (2009) Comparison of enteral nutrition with combined enteral and parenteral nutrition in post-pancreaticoduodenectomy patients: a pilot study. Nutr J 8:24
30. Tennenberg D, Peris A, di Valvasone S et al (2010) Parenteral nutrition in the critically ill patient. N Engl J Med 362(1):81–82
31. Huhmann MB, August DA (2008) Review of American Society for Parenteral and Enteral Nutrition (A.S.P.E.N.) clinical guidelines for nutrition support in cancer patients: nutrition screening and assessment. Nutr Clin Pract 23(2):182–188
32. Plauth M, Cabré E, Campillo B for ESPEN (2009) Guidelines on parenteral nutrition. Clin Nutr 28(4):436–444
33. Selcuk H, Kanbay M, Korkmaz M et al (2006) Route of nutrition has no effect on the development of infectious complications. J Natl Med Assoc 98(12):1963–1966
34. Hartl WH, Jauch KW, Parhofer K, Rittler P for the Working Group for Developing the Guidelines for Parenteral Nutrition of the German Association for Nutritional Medicine (2009) Complications and monitoring–Guidelines on parenteral nutrition, Ger Med Sci 18;7:Doc17
35. Cole CR, Frem JC, Schmotzer B et al (2010) The rate of bloodstream infection is high in infants with short bowel syndrome: relationship with small bowel bacterial overgrowth, enteral feeding, and inflammatory and immune responses. J Pediatr 156(6):941–947
36. Aiko S, Yoshizumi Y, Tsuwano S et al (2005) The effects of immediate enteral feeding with a formula containing high levels of ω-3 fatty acids in patients after surgery for esophageal cancer. JPEN J Parenter Enteral Nutr 29(3):141–147
37. Singer P, Theilla M, Fisher H et al (2006) Benefit of an enteral diet enriched with eicosapentaenoic acid and gamma-linolenic acid in ventilated patients with acute lung injury. Crit Care Med 34:1033–1038
38. Heidegger CP, Darmon P, Pichard C (2008) Enteral vs. parenteral nutrition for the critically ill patient: a combined support should be preferred. Curr Opin Crit Care 14(4):408–414
39. Hise ME, Halterman K, Gajewski BJ et al (2007) Feeding practices of severely ill intensive care unit patients: an evaluation of energy sources and clinical outcomes. J Am Diet Assoc 107(3):458–465
40. Martindale RG, McClave SA, Vanek VW et al (2009) Guidelines for the provision and assessment of nutrition support therapy in the adult critically ill patient: Society of Critical Care Medicine and American Society for Parenteral and Enteral Nutrition: executive summary. Crit Care Med 37(5):1757–1761
41. Btaiche IF, Chan L-N, Pleva M, Kraft MD (2010) Critical illness, gastrointestinal complications, and medication therapy during enteral feeding in critically ill adult patients. Nutr Clin Pract 25(1):32–49
42. Sriram K, Cyriac T, Fogg LF (2010) Effect of nutritional support team restructuring on the use of parenteral nutrition. Nutrition 26(7–8):735–739
43. Zhou M, Martindale RG (2007) Arginine in the critical care setting. J Nutr 137(6 Suppl 2):1687S–1692S
44. Dos Santos RG, Viana ML, Generoso SV et al (2010) Glutamine supplementation decreases intestinal permeability and preserves gut mucosa integrity in an experimental mouse model. JPEN J Parenter Enteral Nutr 34(4):408–413
45. Scurlock C, Mechanick JI (2008) Early nutrition support in the intensive care unit: a US perspective. Curr Opin Clin Nutr Metab Care 11(2):152–155
46. Bistrian BR (2010) Comment on guidelines for the provision and assessment of nutrition support therapy in the adult critically ill patient. JPEN J Parenter Enteral Nutr 34(3):348–349; author reply 350–352

Gut Mucosal Protection in the Critically Ill Patient: Toward an Integrated Clinical Strategy

D. F. Zandstra, P. H. J. van der Voort, K. Thorburn and H. K. F. van Saene

26.1 Introduction

Traditionally, the critically ill patient is considered at risk for the development of stress-ulcer-related bleeding (SURB) from the intestinal canal. Back-diffusion of H^+ is considered the most important mechanism in the etiology of SURB [1]. In the intensive care unit (ICU), routine administration of specific prophylaxis using antacids, histamine-2 (H_2) receptor antagonists, and cytoprotective agents has been practiced for the past 40 years. Several meta-analyses have shown a reduction from 15 to 5% in SURB after administration of antacids and H_2 receptor antagonists [2–5]. Despite this reduced incidence, overt SURB contributes to both morbidity and mortality [6]. The risk of death is increased only when the bleeding occurs for >4 weeks after ICU admission, which suggests a different pathophysiology for early- and late-onset bleeding [7]. Early bleeding is associated with acute hemodynamic disturbances, such as shock and incomplete resuscitation, whereas late bleeding is due to sepsis and multiple organ dysfunction syndrome (MODS).

26.2 Magnitude of the Problem

The reported incidence of SURB in adult patients who do not receive prophylaxis has also fallen, from 60% in 1978 to 0.65% in 1994 [8]. Since 1994, the incidence of SURB has remained constant (1–5%), irrespective of whether the patient

---

D. F. Zandstra (✉)
Department of Intensive Care Medicine,
Onze Lieve Vrouwe Gasthuis, Amsterdam,
The Netherlands
e-mail: postbus@dfzandstra.demon.nl

received prophylaxis or not [8]. Reduction in mortality rates has never been demonstrated using a prophylactic regimen [9, 10].

26.3 SURB Pathogenesis in the Critically Ill

SURB pathogenesis is complex. Under normal conditions, the mucosa is protected against potentially aggressive factors (e.g., gastric acid, pepsin, and bile) by a mucus layer. The most important mechanisms involved mucosal damage are vascular injury, gastric acid, ischemia, sepsis, endotoxin and inflammation in serious infection, *Helicobacter pylori* gastritis, and parenteral feeding.

26.3.1 Vascular Injury

Time-sequence studies in animal experiments have shown that vascular injury due to various substances is the rate-limiting step in the pathogenesis of mucosal injury. Vascular injury of the superficial mucosal capillaries may lead to reduced or even absent blood flow, with subsequent edema and congestion of the mucosal layer. Whereas the blood supply remains intact, the self-restoring capacity of the mucosal layer is enormous. When the vascular injury is minimal or absent, the lesions of the epithelial surface are covered by migrating cuboidal cells within 60 min [11].

26.3.2 Gastric Acid

Back-diffusion of H^+ ions was considered to be of the utmost importance in SURB development [1]. Recent work questions the pivotal role of gastric acid, however. A meta-analysis showed that ranitidine is no better than placebo in reducing the incidence of SURB [12]. H_2 receptor antagonists are contraindicated in the critically ill, as they contribute to infection [13]. The H_2 receptors are not located on the acid-producing cells of the stomach but on the surface of the immunocompetent cells in the mucosal lining [14]. These cells orchestrate the local immune system in the gut (enteric minibrain). H_2 receptor antagonists downregulate the gut immune system, explaining the higher incidence of infections [13]. Critically ill patients often have gastric exocrine failure, with a subsequent gastric pH >4 [15]. SURB is frequently observed in this particular condition where the critically ill are unable to produce gastric acid; therefore gastric acid can be considered as a secondary factor in SURB pathogenesis. The primary step is impairment of mucosal barrier functions due to ischemia.

26.3.3 Ischemia

Mucosal ischemia plays a key role in SURB pathogenesis [16, 17] and occurs during shock, sepsis, and endotoxemia. The fundus and corpus of the stomach are particularly sensitive to ischemia. Mucosal cells do not have the ability to store glycogen as an energy substrate. During ischemia, these cells cannot maintain cellular function by anaerobic glycolysis [18]. The reduced splanchnic blood flow leads to decreased oxygen delivery and an energy deficit that causes impairment of the barrier function of the mucosa. Back-diffusion of acid may occur, with subsequent mucosal damage and erosions or ulcers.

Hypovolemia, low cardiac output, and vasoconstrictive medication may all reduce splanchnic perfusion. Hypovolemia, particularly in surgical patients, is associated with an increased risk of gastrointestinal complications [19, 20]. There is a relationship between endotoxemia and the central venous pressure [21]. Mechanical ventilation on its own is associated with impaired intestinal perfusion in a high percentage of patients and may lead to impaired oxygenation [20]. Circulation therapy aimed at adequate microcirculation (flow) rather than blood pressure remains crucial in SURB prevention. Ischemia of the mucosa may persist due to arteriovenous shunting in the submucosa. Consequently, reperfusion injury may occur. Several experimental studies have shown that radical oxygen scavengers attenuate mucosal damage [22, 23].

26.3.4 Sepsis

The link between SURB and infection becomes increasingly clear in clinical practice. The incidence of SURB was 20% in patients with ineffectively treated pneumonias, whereas it was <10% in adequately treated patients [24]. Therefore, pneumonia can be considered a major factor in SURB pathogenesis. Ventilator-associated pneumonia in the critically ill patient can effectively be prevented by selective decontamination of the digestive tract (SDD) [25]. The potential role of sepsis in the pathogenesis of coagulation disorders that impact on SURB should be emphasized [10]. Experimental studies that focused on the role of sepsis in SURB pathogenesis are scarce. However, clinical experience shows that sepsis is the most important risk factor of SURB [7]. Various mechanisms are involved: (1) release of vasoactive substances, including serotonin, histamine, adrenaline, and noradrenaline, promotes vasoconstriction following endotoxin release; (2) hemodynamic changes may cause hypotension during the early phase of sepsis and may lead to a redistribution of blood flow between and within organs [26]. During sepsis, a substantial deficit in nutrient flow to the mucosa has been observed despite fluid resuscitation [27]. Increased arteriovenous shunting may cause tissue hypoxemia irrespective of increased blood flow [28].

26.3.5 Endotoxin and Inflammation in Serious Infections

Many clinical conditions are associated with increased intestinal permeability and may lead to endotoxemia, which is related to the degree of permeability [21]. Increased permeability can be prevented by vasodilators and adequate intravascular volume [21]. This inflammatory insult involves activation of leukocytes, which may then adhere to the endothelium of the venular side of the microcirculation. This may block microcirculation by means of subsequent stasis and ulceration [29]. Serious infections such as pneumonia have been shown to result in high levels of interleukin (IL)-6 and tumor necrosis factor (TNF). These inflammatory mediators increase the expression of adhesion molecules on endothelium and leukocytes [30]. Expression of the adhesion molecules can be prevented with steroids. Several anti-inflammatory agents reduce mucosal damage by preventing leukocyte adherence to the venular endothelium [31, 32]. There is good evidence for the role of activated leukocytes in SURB development. Steroids prevent adhesion of leukocytes and thereby mucosal damage. Although steroids were believed to promote SURB, risk analysis failed to substantiate this [10].

26.3.6 Gastritis by *Helicobacter pylori*

H. pylori infection is the most important factor in gastric and duodenal ulceration pathogenesis in the non-ICU patient. In this population, the prevalence of *H. pylori* infection is about 30%. Its potential role in SURB pathogenesis in critically ill patients was investigated in detail in our unit [33, 35–37]. The following endpoints were studied:
1. a new method for detecting *H. pylori* in mechanically ventilated patients using a urea breath test;
2. the incidence of *H. pylori* infection in patients requiring acute admission to the ICU using the urea breath test and serology;
3. the impact of parenterally and enterally administered antibiotics in SDD on *H. pylori* eradication;
4. the incidence and risk factors of mucosal damage by direct endoscopy at ICU admission;
5. *H. pylori* infection as an ICU occupational hazard.

Serological tests are unreliable for identifying *H. pylori* infections ventilated ICU patients; the laser-assisted ratio analyzer (LARA) 13C-urea breath test (Alimenterics, NJ, USA) is more reliable [34]. The incidence of *H. pylori* infections in acute patients admitted to the ICU is 40% [33]. A relationship was found between the degree of gastric mucosal lesions on admission and the presence of active infection [35]. *H. pylori* infection of the stomach causes extensive microvascular leucocyte adhesion and migration into the tissue parenchyma, and significant inflammatory cell infiltration is found [36]. Antimicrobials may be effective in treating *H. pylori* infection of the gastric mucosa, e.g., enterally administered nonabsorbable antibiotics [37]. SDD reduces SURB, in part by eliminating *H. pylori*. Transmission of *H. pylori* from infected patients to nursing staff was shown in our study [38].

26.3.7 Feeding

Enteral feeding can cause infectious morbidity [39]. Delay in initiating enteral feeding promotes mucosal vasoconstriction due to reduced prostaglandin synthesis. Stressful conditions combined with food deprivation increases the incidence of ulceration. Enteral feeding protects the mucosa by: (1) neutralizing acid, (2) stimulating perfusion, and (3) providing intraluminal substrate as fuel for the colonic mucosal cell. Three studies show that enteral feeding has a beneficial effect on the incidence of stress ulceration [40–42]. As the critically ill patient is deprived of adequate swallowing abilities, impaired salivary flow into the stomach results in extreme low gastric levels of nitric oxide (NO). Nitrate-rich saliva enhances bactericidal effects of gastric juices [43, 44]. Dietary nitrate increases gastric mucosal blood flow and mucosal bactericidal defence [45]. Future studies are needed to demonstrate whether NO donors applied topically or systemically prevent SURB.

26.4 Clinical Approach to Controlling SURB

The decreased incidence of SURB in ICU patients without prophylaxis is due to improved treatment in recent decades. The main factors are: optimizing the microcirculation, effective infection control, early enteral feeding, and controlling inflammation/infection due to *H. pylori* (Table 26.1). Aggressive correction of hypovolemia is achieved by adequate fluid replacement and preventing vasoconstriction using vasodilators. Vasoconstricting agents should be administered cautiously. Treating low-cardiac-output syndrome is based inodilator administration following diagnosis. Steroids prevent the release of adhesion molecules, so leukocytes do not adhere to the endothelium.

H_2 receptor antagonists are contraindicated in the critically ill, as they are risk factors for infection. The risk of ventilator-associated pneumonia increases with increased severity of critical illness [46, 47], and the subsequent hyperinflammatory status predisposes the patient to SURB. Effective prevention of serious infection using SDD reduces the incidence of SURB [48] and significantly reduces infectious morbidity and mortality rates.

Enteral feeding protects the gut mucosa and contributes to infection control. SDD using enterally and parenterally administered antibiotics controls *H. pylori* infections, and SDD clears fecal endotoxin, thus preventing endotoxin absorption and subsequent inflammation. Prokinetic use can also promote rapid elimination of the fecal endotoxin pool [49].

Clinical measures are important to optimize microcirculation, prevent nosocomial infections, and reduce hyperinflammation, which in turn reduces the incidence of SURB. This strategy, comprising continuous vasodilators to prevent mucosal ischemia, SDD to control infection and reduce intestinal endotoxin, and steroids to reduce leukocyte adherence, was associated with a SURB incidence of

Table 26.1 Protocol for preventing stress-ulcer-related bleeding (SURB)

Circulation
- Prevent microcirculatory stasis by aggressive correction of hypovolemia and of low cardiac output
- Prevent arteriovenous shunting using vasodilators
- Preven corpuscular endothelial adhesion using steroids
- Prevent infection
- Prevent serious infections, including pneumonia and septicemia, by selective decontamination of the digestive tract and immunonutrition

Intestinal contents
- Remove fecal endotoxins using selective decontamination of the digestive tract
- Prevent stasis of intestinal contents using enema and neostigmine
- Enteral feeding to ensure mucosal energy supply
- Control gastritis due to *Helicobacter pylori*
- Eliminate *H. pylori* using enterally and parenterally administered antimicrobials in selective decontamination of the digestive tract protocol
- Provide nitric oxide donors enterally or systemically
- Consider side effects of proton-pump inhibitors on gut ecology

0.6% in a 7-year cohort of critically ill ICU patients needing mechanical ventilation >48 h [35, 48]. These data, in combination with the lack of efficacy of specific prophylaxis in most recent studies, support the concept that SURB prevention is not only a matter of intragastric-acid control. The proposed guidelines in the Surviving Sepsis Campaign for preventing stress ulceration therefore can be challenged [50, 51]. Also, the potential role of NO donors via saliva into the stomach or systemically administered contributes to improved gastric mucosal microcirculation and increased intragastric microbial killing of potentially pathogenic microorganisms [43]. This challenges the perceived pivotal role of gastric acid in the pathogenesis of SURB in the critically ill. Enhancement of endogenous cytoprotective mechanisms by NO donors as a strategy for SURB prevention, however, needs further evaluation.

Increased susceptibility of potentially the hazardous side effect of increased transmucosal gastric leak caused by of proton-pump inhibitors (PPIs) and the effects on the human (protective) microbiota may further contribute to a reconsideration of PPIs being used to prevent SURB [52, 53]. PPIs impair intestinal colonization resistance and increase susceptibility for *Clostridium difficile* infection [53].

26.5 Pediatric Experience

There is a paucity of information concerning the incidence of clinically significant SURB in pediatric practice, with the reported incidence ranging from 0.4 to 1.6% [54, 55]. The basic pathophysiology is similar in children and adults [56]. There is no clear evidence of improvement with prophylaxis [5]. In a large pediatric ICU in Liverpool, UK, there were only three cases of clinically important SURB in 3,238 admissions (>85% ventilated), including 772 postcardiopulmonary bypass (personal communication). No prophylaxis is used other than infection prevention by SDD in combination with a policy of early enteral feeding. A meta-analysis suggests a weak benefit from PPIs, but high-quality evidence to guide clinical practice is still limited [57].

26.6 Conclusions

During the past 40 years, clinical strategies controlling SURB have shifted from interventions to neutralize intragastric acid (antacids) and inhibit acid synthesis (H_2 receptor antagonists, PPIs) toward maneuvers aimed at maintaining and improving microcirculatory perfusion (aggressive circulatory support, including vasodilators). The use of anti-inflammatory drugs to prevent microcirculatory sludging is important to maintain adequate microcirculation. Infections are a pivotal pathogenetic step in SURB and MODS development [58]. These infections, however, can be prevented by SDD (25). This therapy also suppresses *H. pylori* gastritis, which plays a role in SURB pathogenesis. Implementing SDD guarantees a consistently low incidence (<1%) of SURB in patients requiring a minimum of 2 days of mechanical ventilation. Dietary nitrate is considered important to maintain gastric mucosal blood flow and mucosal defence, including antimicrobial defence. A better understanding of the side effects of PPIs and H_2 antagonists should lead to a more restrictive use of these classes of drugs in the critically ill, as overuse is acknowledged [59, 60].

References

1. Skillman JJ, Gould SA, Chung W et al (1970) The gastric mucosal barrier: clinical and experimental studies in critically ill and normal man, and in the rabbit. Ann Surg 172: 564–582
2. Cook DJ, Witt LJ, Cook RJ (1991) Stress ulcer prophylaxis in the critically ill: a meta-analysis. Am J Med 91:519–527
3. Shuman RB, Schuster DP, Zuckerman GR (1987) Prophylactic therapy for stress bleeding: a reappraisal. Ann Intern Med 106:562–567
4. Lacroix J, Infante-Rivard C, Jecinek M et al (1989) Prophylaxis of upper gastrointestinal bleeding in intensive care units. Crit Care Med 17:862–869
5. Tryba M (1991) Der Einfluss praeventiver Massnahmen auf Morbitaet und Mortalitaet von Intensivpatienten. Anaesthesiol Intensivmed Notfallmed Schmerzther (Suppl)1:42–53
6. Cook DJ, Griffith LE, Walter S et al (2001) Canadian Critical Care Trials Group. The attributable mortality and length of intensive care unit stay of clinically important gastrointestinal bleeding in critically ill patients. Crit Care 5:368–375
7. Zandstra DF, Stoutenbeek CP, Oudemans-van Straaten HM (1989) Pathogenesis of stress ulcer bleeding. In: van Saene HKF et al (eds) Update in intensive and emergency medicine. Springer, Berlin, pp 166–172
8. Zandstra DF (1995) Stress ulceration in the critically ill. No longer a problem? Proceedings SMART. Springer, Milan, pp 30–32
9. Tryba M (1991) Stress bleeding prophylaxis 1990—a meta-analysis. Clin J Gastroenterol 13(Suppl 2):44–55

10. Cook DJ, Fuller HD, Guyatt GH et al (1994) Risk factors for gastrointestinal bleeding in critically ill patients. N Engl J Med 330:377–381
11. Lacey ER, Ito S (1984) Rapid epithelial restitution of the rat gastric mucosa after ethanol injury. Lab Invest 51:573–583
12. Messori A, Trippoli S, Vaiani M et al (2000) Bleeding and pneumonia in intensive care patients given ranitidine and sucralfate for prevention of stress ulcer: metaanalysis of randomized controlled trials. BMJ 321:1103–1106
13. O'Keefe GE, Gentilello LM, Maier RV (1998) Incidence of infectious complications associated with the use of histamine2-receptor antagonists in critically ill trauma patients. Ann Surg 227:120–112
14. Mezey E, Palkovits M (1992) Localisation of targets for anti-ulcer drugs in cells of the immune system. Science 258:1662–1665
15. Stannard VA, Hutchinson A, Morris DL et al (1988) Gastric exocrine failure in critically ill patients: incidence and associated features. BMJ 296:155–156
16. Fiddian-Green RG, McCough E, Pittenger G et al (1983) Predictive value of intramural pH and other risk factors for massive bleeding from stress ulceration. Gastroenterology 85:613–620
17. Hottenrott C, Seufert RM, Becker H (1978) The role of ischaemia in the pathogenesis of stress induced gastric lesions in piglets. Surg Gynecol Obstet 146:217–220
18. Menguy R, Desbaillets L, Masters YF (1974) Mechanisms of stress: influence of hypovolaemic shock on energy metabolism in the gastric mucosa. Gastroenterology 66:46–55
19. Christenson JT, Schmuziger M, Maurice J et al (1994) Gastrointestinal complications after coronary artery bypass grafting. J Thorac Cardiovasc Surg 108:899–906
20. Love R, Choe E, Lipton H et al (1995) Positive end-expiratory pressure decreased mesenteric blood flow despite normalization of cardiac output. J Trauma 39:195–199
21. Oudemans-van Straaten HM, Jansen PG, Velthuis H et al (1996) Endotoxaemia and postoperative hypermetabolism in coronary artery bypass surgery: the role of ketanserin. Br J Anaesth 77:473–479
22. Bhattacharjee M, Bhattacharjee S, Gupta A et al (2002) Critical role of an endogenous gastric peroxidase in controlling oxidative damage in $H.\ pylori$-mediated and nonmediated gastric ulcer. Free Radic Biol Med 32:731–743
23. Biswas K, Bandyopadhyay U, Chattopadhyay I et al (2003) A novel antioxidant and antiapoptotic role of omeprazole to block gastric ulcer through scavenging of hydroxyl radical. J Biol Chem 278:1099–1001
24. Alvarez Lerma F, ICU Acquired Infection Group (1996) Modification of empiric antibiotic treatment in patients with acquired pneumonia in the ICU. Intensive Care Med 22:387–394
25. Liberati A, D'Amico R, Pifferi S et al. (2009) Antibiotic prophylaxis to reduce respiratory tract infections and mortality in adults receiving intensive care. Cochrane Database Syst Rev 4:CD000022
26. Lang CH, Bagby GJ, Ferguson JL et al (1984) Cardiac output and redistribution of organ blood flow in hypermetabolic sepsis. Am J Physiol 246:331
27. Kreimeier U, Yang ZH, Messmer K (1988) The role of fluid replacement in acute endotoxin shock. In: Kox W, Bihari D (eds) Shock and the adult respiratory distress syndrome. Springer, Berlin
28. Bowen JC, LeDoux JC, Harkin GV (1979) Evidence for pathophysiologic arteriovenous shunting in the pathogenesis of acute gastric mucosal ulceration. Adv Shock Res 1:35–42
29. McCafferty DM, Granger DN, Wallace JL (1995) Indomethacin induced gastric injury and leucocyte adherence in arthritic versus healthy rats. Gastroenterology 109:1173–1180
30. Cush JJ, Rothlein R, Lindley HB et al (1993) Increased levels of circulating intercellular adhesion molecules in the sera of patients with rheumatoid arthritis. Arthritis Rheum 36:1098–1102
31. Low J, Grabow D, Sommers C et al (1995) Cytoprotective effects of CI-959 in the rat gastric mucosa; modulation of leukocyte adhesion. Gastroenterology 109:1224–1223

32. Santucci L, Firucci S, Giansanti M et al (1994) Pentoxifylline prevents indomethacin induced acute mucosal damage in rats: role of TNF. Gut 35:909–915
33. van der Voort PHJ, van der Hulst RWM, Zandstra DF et al (1999) Detection of *Helicobacter pylori* in mechanically ventilated patients: the LARA-13C-Urea breath test and serology. Clin Intensive Care 10:91–95
34. van der Voort PH, van der Hulst RW, Zandstra DF et al (2001) Prevalence of *Helicobacter pylori* infection in stress-induced gastric mucosal injury. Intensive Care Med 27:68–73
35. van der Voort PHJ, van der Hulst RW, Zandstra DF et al (2001) Suppression of *Helicobacter pylori* infection during intensive care stay: related to stress ulcer bleeding incidence? J Crit Care 16:182–187
36. van der Voort PH, van der Hulst RW, Zandstra DF et al (2000) In vitro susceptibility of *Helicobacter pylori* to, and in vivo suppression by antimicrobials used in selective decontamination of the digestive tract. J Antimicrob Chemother 46:803–805
37. Suzuki H, Suzuki M, Imeada H et al (2009) *Helicobacter pylori* and microcirculation. Microcirculation 16:547–558
38. van der Voort PH, van der Hulst RW, Zandstra DF et al (2001) Gut decontamination of critically ill patients reduces *Helicobacter pylori* acquisition by intensive care nurses. J Hosp Infect 47:41–45
39. Beale RJ, Bryg DJ, Bihari DJ (1999) Immunonutrition in the critically ill: a systematic review of clinical outcome. Crit Care Med 27:2799–2805
40. Ephgrave KS, Scott DL, Ong A et al (2000) Are gastric, jejunal, or both forms of enteral feeding gastroprotective during stress? J Surg Res 88:1–7
41. Ephgrave KS, Kleiman-Wexler RL, Adair CG (1990) Enteral nutrients prevent stress ulceration and increase intragastric volume. Crit Care Med 18:621–624
42. Raff T, Germann G, Hartmann B (1997) The value of early enteral nutrition in the prophylaxis of stress ulceration in the severely burned patient. Burns 23:313–318
43. Bjorne H, Petersson J, Phillipson H et al (2004) Nitrite in saliva increases gastric mucosal bloodflow. J Clin Invest 113:106–114
44. Bjorne H, Weitzberg E, Lundberg JO (2006) Intraqastric generation of antimicrobial nitrogen oxides from saliva. Physiological and therapeutic considerations. Free Radic Biol Med 41:1404–1412
45. Petersson J, Phillipson M, Jansson EA (2007) Dietary nitrate increases gastric mucosal bloodflow and mucosal defence. Am J Physiol Gastrointest Liver Physiol 292:g718–g724
46. Vincent JL, Rello J, Marshall J et al (2009) International study of the prevalence and outcomes of infection in intensive care units. JAMA 302:2323–2329
47. Zandstra DF, Petros AJ, van Saene HK (2009) The final gasp from the European experts. Intensive Care Med 35:1816
48. Zandstra DF, Stoutenbeek CP (1994) The virtual absence of stress-ulcer related bleeding in ICU patients receiving prolonged mechanical ventilation without any prophylaxis: a prospective cohort study. Intensive Care Med 20:335–340
49. van der Spoel JI, Oudemans-van Straaten HM, Stoutenbeek CP et al (2001) Neostigmine resolves critical illness-related colonic ileus in intensive care patients with multiple organ failure—a prospective, double-blind, placebo-controlled trial. Intensive Care Med 27: 822–827
50. Van Spreuwel–Verheijen M, Bosman RJ, Oudemans–van Straaten HM et al (2006) Is the surviving sepsis campaign for stress ulcer prophylaxis justified? Intensive Care Med 32(Suppl 1):s23
51. Zandstra DF, van der Voort PH (2004) A more appropriate critical appraisal of the available evidence? Crit Care Med 32:2166–2167
52. Vesper BJ, Jawdi A, Altman KW et al (2009) The effect of proton pump inhibitors on the human microbiota. Curr Drug Metab 10:84–89
53. Murray LJ, Gabello M, Rudolph DS et al (2009) Transmucosal gastric leak induced by proton pump inhibitors. Dig Dis Sci 54:1408–1417

54. Lacroix J, Nadeau D, Laberge S et al (1992) Frequency of upper gastrointestinal bleeding in a pediatric intensive care unit. Crit Care Med 20:35–42
55. Chaibou M, Tucci M, Dugas M-A et al (1998) Clinically significant upper gastrointestinal bleeding in a pediatric intensive care unit: a prospective study. Pediatrics 102:933–938
56. Crill CM, Hak EB (1999) Upper gastrointestinal bleeding in critically ill pediatric patients. Pharmacotherapy 19:162–180
57. Reveiz L, Guerrero-Lozano R, Camacho A et al (2010) Stress ulcer, gastritis, and gastrointestinal bleeding prophylaxis in critically ill pediatric patients: a systematic review. Pediatr Crit Care Med 11:124–132
58. Silvestri L, van Saene HK, Zandstra DF et al (2010) Impact of selective decontamination of the digestive tract on multiple organ dysfunction syndrome: systematic review of randomized controlled trials. Crit Care Med 38:1370–1376
59. Heidelbaugh JJ, Goldberg KL, Inadomi JM (2009) Overutilization op protonpump inhibitors: a review of cost-effectiveness and risk in PPI. Am J Gastroenterol 104:527–532
60. Farrel CP, Mercogliano G, Kuntz CL (2009) Overuse of stress ulcer prophylaxis in the critical care setting and beyond. J Crit Care 25(2):214–220

Selective Decontamination of the Digestive Tract: Role of the Pharmacist

27

N. J. Reilly, A. J. Nunn and K. Pollock

27.1 Introduction

Selective decontamination of the digestive tract (SDD) is an antimicrobial prophylactic strategy aimed at preventing both endogenous and exogenous infections of the lower airways and bloodstream in patients requiring treatment in the intensive care unit (ICU) [1]. SDD therapy is based on the concept of microbial carriage and is directed at limiting infections in ICU patients caused by the carriage of 15 potentially pathogenic microorganisms (PPMs) (Table 27.1).

The SDD concept was introduced in 1984 by Stoutenbeek et al. [2] with the aim of controlling primary endogenous, secondary endogenous and exogenous infections, caused by both normal and abnormal PPMs, by means of a parenterally administered antibiotic, topical nonabsorbable antimicrobials, high levels of hygiene and surveillance cultures [3]. To date, there have been 60 randomised controlled trials (RCTs) evaluating SDD [4–17] and ten meta-analyses assessing its efficacy [18–24], providing evidence that SDD significantly reduces infection in patients in the ICU and improves patient survival. Based on the available evidence, the British Society for Antimicrobial Chemotherapy recently recommended that SDD be considered for ICU patients expected to require mechanical ventilation ≥48 h in order to prevent ventilator-associated pneumonia (VAP) [25].

Due to the lack of commercially available topical formulations, application of the SDD concept to hospital practice has required substantial input from pharmacists in both the development and extemporaneous preparation of SDD formulations. This chapter aims to provide the reader with comprehensive information on the pharmaceutical technology involved in implementing SDD and how

---

N. J. Reilly (✉)
Pharmacy Department, Alder Hey Children's NHS Foundation Trust,
Liverpool, Merseyside, UK
e-mail: Nicola.Reilly@alderhey.nhs.uk

Table 27.1 Potentially pathogenic microorganisms (PPMs) causing infection in intensive care unit (ICU) patients

Previously healthy host (normal PPM)	Host with severe underlying disease (abnormal PPM)
1. *Streptococcus pneumoniae*	7. *Klebsiella* spp.
2. *Haemophilus influenzae*	8. *Proteus* spp.
3. *Moraxella catarrhalis*	9. *Morganella* spp.
4. *Escherichia coli*	10. *Enterobacter* spp.
5. *Staphylococcus aureus*	11. *Citrobacter* spp.
6. *Candida albicans*	12. *Serratia* spp.
	13. *Acinetobacter* spp.
	14. *Pseudomonas* spp.
	15. Methicillin-resistant *Staphylococcus aureus* (MRSA)

the role of the pharmacist is essential if this concept is to be successfully applied to reduce carriage, colonisation and infection rates in ICU patients.

27.2 Nonabsorbable Antimicrobials: The PTA Regimen

SDD aims to convert the abnormal carrier state into normal carriage using nonabsorbable antimicrobials. A paste or gel is applied into the inside of the lower cheeks to prevent or eradicate pre-existing oral carriage of abnormal PPMs, i.e., to decontaminate the oropharynx. Suspensions are administered via the nasogastric tube to decontaminate the stomach and gut and control abnormal carriage of aerobic Gram-negative bacilli (AGNB), particularly *Pseudomonas aeruginosa*. Nonabsorbable antimicrobials are given throughout ICU treatment to control morbidity and mortality associated with late secondary endogenous infection, which is caused by abnormal bacteria not present in admission flora but acquired during ICU treatment. It generally occurs after 1 week in the ICU and accounts for 30% of infections.

Topical antimicrobials are also used to control exogenous infections, e.g., by applying paste to a tracheostomy site to control lower airway infections. Grafted burn wounds may also be targeted by mixing topical antimicrobial agents with a translucent hydrogel (Aquaform®) and applying it in thin layers over fine mesh gauze to the wound site [26]. Exogenous infection is caused by abnormal potential pathogens never carried in the patient's digestive tract but introduced directly into the patient. Exogenous infection may occur at any time during ICU treatment and accounts for 15% of infections.

The ideal SDD regimen should use antimicrobials that are nontoxic, inexpensive, palatable and microbiologically active in the presence of faeces, saliva or antacids. The most widely used SDD regimen is that of the Groningen group [2], who devised a protocol using polymyxin E, tobramycin and amphotericin B

(PTA), which is applied as an oral paste and suspension to treat both the throat and gut, respectively. In the UK, polymyxin E is known as colistin.

The combination of polymyxin E and tobramycin is synergistic against *Proteus* and *Pseudomonas* spp. It is the most potent antipseudomonal combination associated with an effective clearance of *Pseudomonas* from the gut. Emergence of resistance to polymyxin is rare. Although there are bacteria-producing tobramycin-inactivating enzymes, polymyxin is thought to protect tobramycin from being destroyed by these enzymes [27]. Tobramycin is the preferred aminoglycoside because it is intrinsically most active against *Pseudomonas* and is minimally inactivated by saliva and faeces. It also has useful activity against *Staphylococcus aureus* [27]. Both agents absorb endotoxins released by AGNB in the gut. This feature is important because endotoxin can be absorbed from the gut of seriously ill patients, producing fever, release of inflammatory mediators and shock. In order to control yeast overgrowth, amphotericin B is also included in the regime. It is intrinsically the most potent antifungal, but there is a high rate of inactivation in the gut requiring the use of high doses [27]. By design, the PTA regimen is inactive against indigenous flora, such as streptococci viridans, enterococci, coagulase-negative staphylococci (CNS) and anaerobes [27], each of which is necessary for normal physiological gut function. Modifications to the PTA regime may need to be made. For example, SDD was not designed to cover methicillin-resistant *Staphylococcus aureus* (MRSA), as MRSA was not a significant problem in the early 1980s. Therefore, in cases of MRSA endemicity, enterally administered vancomycin should be added to the PTA regime [28, 29]. In the case of endemicity of AGNB producing extended-spectrum beta lactamases (ESBL) resistant to tobramycin, tobramycin may have to be replaced by paromomycin, and if *Serratia* endemicity is present, both polymyxin and tobramycin should be replaced by paromomycin [29].

27.3 Indications

In the paediatric ICU (PICU) setting, SDD is indicated to [30]:
1. control infection: in patients expected to require ventilation for >48 h, SDD reduces the risk of endogenous infections;
2. control inflammation: following cardiac surgery (and particularly cardiopulmonary bypass), patients develop the systemic inflammation response syndrome (SIRS) characterized by high levels of cytokines, leucocytes and increased C-reactive protein (CRP); polymyxin E and tobramycin may neutralize endotoxin and therefore reduce gut overgrowth;
3. prevent resistance: SDD eradicates multi-drug-resistant microorganisms detected from surveillance swabs of throat and rectum.
    Once initiated, SDD therapy should be continued until the patient has been extubated.

27.4 Application Method

27.4.1 SDD of the Oropharynx

SDD gel containing 2% PTA is used. A pea-sized application is evenly smeared inside the lower cheeks four times a day(a 5-g tube lasts approximately 5 days).

27.4.2 SDD of the Gastrointestinal Tract

1. The antimicrobials are given orally or through the nasogastric tube. When the patient requires gastric suction, the nasogastric tube is clamped and the suction is discontinued for 1 h.
2. When the normal anatomy of the gastrointestinal tract is disrupted (gastro- or intestinal-fistulae or colostomy), each (blind) loop should be separately treated with approximately one half of the oral PTA dose in an adequate volume [30].

27.4.3 SDD of Tracheostomy and Gastrostomy Sites

When being ventilated in the PICU, patients with tracheostomies or gastrostomies should have SDD paste containing 2% PTA applied four times a day to these sites, in addition to oropharyngeal and gastrointestinal SDD treatments. Preparation dosages used are shown in Table 27.2 [30].

27.5 Pharmaceutical Technology

The development of SDD medication has depended upon close collaboration between pharmacists and microbiologists. For decontamination of the gut in the unconscious adult and in children, liquid preparations for administration via a nasogastric tube are required. For decontamination of the oropharynx, formulations of oral gels, pastes, pastilles and lozenges have been developed and prepared by hospital and academic pharmacists [31]. Solutions or suspensions of the three antimicrobials are used for oral and nasogastric administration [30]. Coated tablets of colistin have also been prepared for positioned release into the colon [32]. No commercial company has yet shown more than a passing interest in the further development, licensing or marketing of these preparations, and this may have influenced the rate of development of the SDD concept.

As all preparations are made extemporaneously in the hospital pharmacy or manufacturing units, they are classed as "hospital specials" and as such are unlicensed. In using these unlicensed products in clinical practice, responsibility for safety and efficacy lies with the prescriber, and responsibility for quality lies with the pharmacist. Ideally, to reduce risks to the patient, it would be preferable to

Table 27.2 Selective decontamination of the digestive tract (SDD): doses [30]

Age	Medication	Dosage
Over 12 years	Polymyxin E/Colistin	100 mg ≡ 3,000,000 units four times daily
	Tobramycin base	80 mg four times daily
	Amphotericin B	500 mg four times daily
	SDD gel	A pea-sized application four times daily
5–12 years	Polymyxin E/Colistin	50 mg ≡ 1,500,000 units four times daily
	Tobramycin base	40 mg four times daily
	Amphotericin B	250 mg four times daily
	SDD gel	A pea-sized application four times daily
<5 years	Polymyxin E/Colistin	25 mg ≡ 750,000 units four times daily
	Tobramycin base	20 mg four times daily
	Amphotericin B	100 mg four times daily
	SDD gel	A pea-sized application four times daily

The dose administered is dependent on gut volume. To be administered 30 min before feeds and not with feeds. Sucralfate significantly reduces concentrations of colistin, tobramycin and amphotericin B; therefore, separate administration by 2–4 h [34]

NB Colistin doses in milligrams are specified as colistin base, where 1 mg = 30,000 units, 1 mg tobramycin base is equivalent to 1.5 mg tobramycin sulphate, 1 mg colistin base is equivalent to 1.5 mg colistin sulphate

use medicines that have been appropriately researched and subjected to the scrutiny of the medicines licensing process. One other problem with extemporaneous production in the UK is that pharmacy departments are limited in the quantities of products that they can prepare, unless they have a manufacturer's licence (specials) issued by the medicines and healthcare products regulatory agency (MHRA).

Because SDD medication is not commercially available or supported by the usual manufacturers' marketing activity, scientific background to the formulations (assay, rheology) is limited. To date, little work has been undertaken to develop assays for PTA ingredients when combined in mixtures or formulations for local and oral application. Assays should indicate activity of the constituent antimicrobials, and therefore, a microbiological assay is preferred to techniques such as high performance liquid chromatography. Suitable microorganisms must be selected for their resistance to the other PTA components, lack of reversion to sensitivity must be demonstrated and diffusion from the gel to agar plate must be matched to that from standard antimicrobial solutions.

Despite commercial apathy, hospital-based research is continuing into areas such as modifications to the gel, development of colonic-positioned release products and production of placebo products for trial work. It should be noted, however, that extemporaneous production of SDD formulations does lead to an increase in a hospital pharmacy department's workload and that involvement in research programmes requires a considerable amount of research and development, which would ideally be best met by commercial support.

27.6 Choice of Formulation

27.6.1 Oropharynx

To abolish PPM carriage in the oropharynx, a contact time of at least 20 min is required for effective decontamination [31]. Pastes, gels, pastilles and lozenges therefore offer advantages over suspensions, aerosols and oral rinses, as they have a longer contact time [33]. The ideal formulation for use in the oropharynx should therefore have a prolonged contact time with the oral mucosa, should release the antimicrobials into the oropharynx throughout the contact period, should be pharmaceutically stable and should be acceptable to the patient [31].

There are four suitable formulations recommended for use in the oropharynx: paste, gel, lozenge and pastille. It should be noted that the shelf life for these products has been assigned on the basis of in vivo microbiological experience and not by traditional pharmaceutical methodology. For use in our PICU, the majority of these preparations are formulated and supplied to us by specialist hospital pharmacy manufacturing units at the Western Infirmary in Glasgow, Scotland, and Stepping Hill Hospital (Stockport Pharmaceuticals), Manchester, UK; however, products may be available from other manufacturing units. La Botica de Argensola is a manufacturing unit in Madrid, Spain, that can supply SDD products to all countries in the European Union and to South America (www.famaciamagistral.com).

27.6.1.1 Paste
Paste has advantages in that it is easy to produce, has good adhesion to the mucosa, has a prolonged release of medicament, is sugar free, is stable and has a well-proven formula [33] (Table 27.3). Although paste effectively eliminates AGNB, it has several drawbacks. It has an unpleasant taste and appearance, can cause considerable drying of the oral mucosa and can be difficult to remove, occasionally causing trauma to the mucosa. Because of this, it has poor acceptability with patients, staff and relatives. We restrict use of the paste to applications around tracheostomy and gastrostomy sites, where the adherence and barrier properties of the paste are particularly useful.

Table 27.3 Formula for selective decontamination of the digestive tract (SDD) paste [33]

Ingredients	g
Amphotericin B powder Ph. Eur	2 (adjusted for potency)
Tobramycin sulphate USP	2
Colistin sulphate Ph. Eur	2
Liquid paraffin Ph. Eur	10
Orabase® paste (ConvaTec)	to 100

Shelf life 1 month; store at room temperature
SDD paste is prepared by mixing each of the antimicrobial powders with 10% w/w liquid paraffin and gradually incorporating Orabase®. Vigorous mixing causes the Orabase® to crack
Ph. Eur = European Pharmacopoeia
USP = United States Pharmacopoeia

Table 27.4 Formula selective decontamination of the digestive tract (SDD): pastilles [33]

Ingredients	
Gelatine Ph. Eur	500 g
Glycerol Ph. Eur	700 g
Sucrose Ph. Eur	100 g
Sodium benzoate Ph. Eur	4 g
Distilled water	600 ml
Lemon oil Ph. Eur	2 ml
Blackcurrant powder	10 g
Amphotericin B powder Ph. Eur	15.88 g (adjusted for potency)
Colistin Sulphate Ph. Eur	12.95 g
Tobramycin sulphate USP	12.95 g

To prepare SDD pastilles, soak the gelatine and water and heat to melt. Add most of the glycerol and the other ingredients, except the antibiotics, and mix well. Heat for 30 min and then add the antibiotics, wetting the amphotericin with glycerine
Shelf life 6 months; store at room temperature
A 1.5 g pastille contains 12 mg amphotericin and 10 mg tobramycin and colistin
Ph. Eur = European Pharmacopoeia
USP = United States Pharmacopoeia

27.6.1.2 Pastille

The advantages of the pastille are that it can be flavoured easily, it has good release characteristics, it is easy to use and it is acceptable to the conscious patient (Table 27.4). Studies in cancer patients have demonstrated that SDD pastilles are effective in eradicating the carriage of AGNB and yeasts, reducing the incidence of radiation mucositis and yeast stomatitis [34]. The pastille, however, has limited, use as it cannot be used in comatose patients, it has high sugar content and therefore cannot be used in diabetics and it is unsuitable for young children. It is

Table 27.5 Formula for selective decontamination of the digestive tract (SDD): lozenge [36]

Ingredients	mg
Antibiotic mixture	
Amphotericin B powder Ph. Eur	10
Colistin Sulphate Ph. Eur	2
Tobramycin sulphate USP	1.6
Basic mixture	
Citric acid	40
Calcium diphosphate	150
Saccharine	795

Shelf life 3 months; store at room temperature
To prepare SDD lozenges, two powder mixtures are prepared. After sieving of the powders, the total mixture is mixed in a Turbula mixer (90 rpm) for 15 min. The total powder mixture is then moistened with 25 ml water, and thereafter, 25 ml sodium carboxymethylcellulose (low viscosity) is added. Further mixing then takes place for 10 min, after which the moistened powder is dried for a minimum of 4 h at 40°C. The dried mixture is then mashed through a 0.75-mm sieve, and the resulting granulate is sieved further through a 0.4 mm sieve to eliminate the fine powder. Prior to the final tableting stage, the granulate is mixed with 0.5% magnesium stearate and 2.5% talc in the Turbula mixer for 2 min
Ph. Eur = European Pharmacopoeia
USP = United States Pharmacopoeia

difficult to produce, as many hospital pharmacy departments do not have appropriate facilities, and therefore this preparation needs to be made in a specialised manufacturing unit.

27.6.1.3 Lozenge

The advantages and disadvantages of the lozenge are very similar to that of the pastille (Table 27.5). In cancer patients, eradication of AGNB and yeasts by SDD lozenges has been shown by Spijkervet et al. [35] to take up to 3 weeks, therefore comparing poorly with eradication rates of 3–4 days that have been achieved in ICU patients with paste. One explanation for these differing eradication rates would be that patients in the ICU are usually unconscious, permitting proper application of sticky paste, whereas patients with head and neck cancer suck their lozenges four times daily and eat normal, unsterilised food. Poor compliance within this group of patients, a lower standard of personal hygiene and an altered oropharyngeal anatomy may also contribute to the longer eradication times. Lozenges, when sucked, will take approximately 15 min to dissolve in vivo. Hence, they do not achieve the same length of contact time with the buccal mucosa as the paste or gel, and this is therefore another factor contributing to poorer eradication rates. These results would suggest a need for new formulations to be developed to allow a more protracted and hence more effective delivery of the antimicrobials to the buccal mucosa of ambulant patients [36].

Table 27.6 Formula for selective decontamination of the digestive tract (SDD): 2% gel [33]

Ingredients	
Sodium carboxymethylcellulose Ph. Eur	10 g
Glycerol Ph. Eur	60 ml
Nipasept®	600 mg
Concentrated peppermint water BP	10 ml
Distilled water	200 ml
Amphotericin B powder Ph. Eur	6 g (adjusted for potency)
Colistin sulphate Ph. Eur	6 g
Tobramycin sulphate USP	6 g

Shelf life one month; store at 2–8°C
A gel base is prepared from sodium carboxymethylcellulose, propylene glycol or glycerol and Nipasept® solution. Peppermint water is added for flavour; 2% by weight each of amphotericin B, colistin sulphate and tobramycin sulphate are stirred into the cold gel base, and the resulting SDD gel is packed into aluminium tubes using a syringe and tube to aid filling. Colistin sulphomethate sodium has been used in the gel in some centres, where a "stringy" texture has been noted when using the sulphate. This method involves using the commercial powder for injection (Colomycin® injection, manufactured by Pharmax)
Ph. Eur = European Pharmacopoeia
USP = United States Pharmacopoeia
BP = British Pharmacopoeia

27.6.1.4 Gel

Gel, as with paste, is sugar free, but it is an improvement on paste in that it is more palatable, much easier to remove and does not dry the oropharyngeal mucosa [33] (Table 27.6). The efficacy of this formulation appears to be equal to that of paste, but patient acceptability with the gel is higher and therefore compliance is better. The gel presents problems in that it is difficult to produce and at present its long-term stability is unknown.

27.6.2 Gastrointestinal Tract

Decontamination of the gut is not difficult. Most ICU patients have gut stasis, there is good contact time between antimicrobials and organisms and it can be demonstrated by surveillance culture that decontamination of the oesophagus, stomach and small intestine occurs within 3 days. However, to clear PPMs from the large intestine, there must be functioning gut motility. Due to this controlling factor, decontamination of the colon and rectum may be longer and may take up to 7 days. A formulation for use in the gastrointestinal tract should ideally release the antimicrobials in the terminal ileum and provide high concentrations of these antimicrobials in the colon and rectum. The product should also be easy to use, acceptable to patients and have good pharmaceutical stability [30]. To date, only oral suspensions and solutions have been used (Tables 27.6, 27.7, 27.8 and 27.9).

Table 27.7 Formula for amphotericin suspension 100 mg/ml [33]

Ingredients	
Amphotericin B Ph. Eur	500 g (adjusted for potency)
Sodium Citrate Ph. Eur	25 g
Sodium carboxymethylcellulose Ph. Eur	12.5 g
VEEGUM K®	25 g
Citric acid monohydrate Ph. Eur	5.95 g to adjust pH to 5.5
Saccharin powder Ph. Eur	470 mg
Lycasin®	750 ml
Nipasept®	6.5 g
Concentrated peppermint water BP	125 ml
Distilled water	to 5330 g

Shelf life 6 months; store at 2–8°C
A suspension is prepared with sodium carboxymethylcellulose as suspending and thickening agent, distilled water, and Lycasin® as the sweetener. VEEGUM K® (hydrated magnesium aluminium silicate) is then added as the anticaking agent. Amphotericin B powder is added gradually to this mixture, stirring after each addition. Nipasept® used as a preservative is dissolved in the concentrated peppermint water and then added to the suspension. Peppermint water is added to mask the metallic taste of amphotericin. Finally, saccharin powder is added to improve palatability and citric acid monohydrate to adjust the pH of the suspension to 5.5. The remaining water is then added to make up to the final weight
Ph. Eur = European Pharmacopoeia
BP = British Pharmacopoeia

Although Crome [31], in 1988, suggested that research was progressing into the development of colon-positioned release tablets/capsules for use in conscious patients, this research does not appear to have lead to the availability or widespread use of these preparations [37]. We used coated colonic colistin capsules only once [32] in conscious, immunocompromised patients who had functioning guts. The aim of coated colonic preparations is that they should allow release of the capsule contents at a pH of approximately 7–7.2, resulting in disintegration in the ascending colon. The resultant local delivery of antibacterial agents into the colon is thought to achieve faecal flora suppression and that, by bypassing the oesophagus and stomach, gastrointestinal side effects such as nausea and vomiting should be reduced.

The widespread use of the orally administered solutions and suspensions in PICU therefore continues. The advantages of these products is that they are stable [33], easy to produce and can be given via a nasogastric tube and are therefore suitable to give to an unconscious patient [31]. Problems with poor taste, however, particularly of colistin, may decrease compliance in conscious patients. Diarrhoea reportedly may be a problem with SDD treatment [5], but a recent publication [38] observed that, in fact, patients receiving SDD had more days with normal stools than days with diarrhoea.

Table 27.8 Constituents of colistin oral solution 100 mg base (3 megaunits) in 1 ml (formula intellectual property of Stockport Pharmaceuticals, Manchester, UK) [42]

Ingredients
Colistin sulphate powder Ph. Eur
Polysorbate 80 Ph. Eur
Sodium methyl hydroxybenzoate (Nipagin® M Sodium) REG. SPEC
Sodium propyl hydroxybenzoate (Nipasol® M Sodium) REG. SPEC
Orange syrup BP
Dilute hydrochloric acid 10%
Purified water
100 mg colistin base ≡ 150 mg colistin sulphate *Shelf life* 12 months Colistin for SDD is prescribed as base; use within 4 weeks of opening; store <25°C A solution is prepared by adding polysorbate 80, followed by colistin powder, to purified water; dissolution is achieved by gentle mixing with an SL2T mixer at 1,100 rpm. Sodium hydroxybenzoate and sodium propyl hydroxybenzoate are dissolved separately in heated purified water, and then these two solutions are mixed together and filtered. The filtrate is added very slowly to the gently mixing colistin solution. Orange syrup is then added to flavour, and hydrochloric acid is added to adjust the pH to 4.5–5.5. (A commercial preparation of colistin is available (Colomycin®) from Forest. It contains 250,000 units of colistin in 5 ml and is stable for 2 weeks when reconstituted) Ph. Eur = European Pharmacopoeia BP = British Pharmacopoeia REG SPEC = Regional Specification

There have been isolated reports of accumulation of enterally administered antibiotics as an adverse effect of SDD resulting in obstructive masses developing in either the oesophagus or jejunum of affected patients [39]. Accumulation of residual buccally applied SDD paste may be the reason for oesophageal obstruction, whereas residual SDD paste and/or suspension could be the cause of jejunal masses. The incidence of clinically relevant obstructive accumulation is probably very low, but to avoid this adverse effect, it is recommended that there be thorough removal of residual SDD paste before each new application. The likelihood of accumulation may also be reduced by using an SDD gel rather than paste and liquids.

In neonates, vomiting and other gastrointestinal problems have been seen, particularly if concentrated solutions are administered to an empty stomach [40]. The osmolality of amphotericin suspension is high, approximately 2,000 mOsm/l compared with an osmolality of approximately 430 mOsm/l with a colistin 25 mg/ml solution and 60 mOsm/l with a 20 mg/ml solution of tobramycin sulphate. Because hyperosmolar medications have been associated with an increased

Table 27.9 Constituents of tobramycin sulphate oral solution 122 mg in 1 ml (equivalent to tobramycin base 80 mg in 1 ml) [42]. (Formula intellectual property of Stockport Pharmaceuticals, Manchester, UK)

Ingredients
Tobramycin sulphate powder USP
Sodium methyl hydroxybenzoate (Nipagin® M sodium) REG. SPEC
Sodium propyl hydroxybenzoate (Nipasol® M sodium) REG. SPEC
Orange syrup BP
Dilute hydrochloric acid 10%
Purified water
Tobramycin for selective decontamination of the digestive tract (SDD) is prescribed as base. *Shelf life* 2 years; store at 2–8°C; use within 4 weeks of opening Sodium methyl hydroxybenzoate and sodium propyl hydroxybenzoate are dissolved separately in heated, purified water, and the resultant solution is then filtered. Tobramycin sulphate powder is also dissolved in heated purified water using a Silverson mixer (3,800 rpm) to aid dissolution, and then the hydroxybenzoates filtrate solution is added very slowly to the tobramycin solution into the vortex created by the mixer. The mixer speed is increased to 6,000 rpm, orange syrup is added, followed by purified water to make up to volume. Finally, dilute hydrochloric acid 10% is added to adjust the pH to between 4.6 and 5.1 USP = United States Pharmacopoeia REG SPEC = Regional Specification BP = British Pharmacopoeia

incidence of necrotising enterocolitis (NEC) [40], it is therefore recommended that all three PTA ingredients be diluted in water.

Observers also suggest that PTA may delay gastric emptying/absorption of feeds, and the binding of colistin and tobramycin by food proteins is a factor known to reduce the lethal intestinal antibiotic levels required to eradicate AGNB [41]. This interference with food has been shown as the reason for SDD failure when oral contaminated feeds were given to a premature neonate [41]. In our PICU, we recommend that SDD doses be administered 30 min before feeds and not with feeds [30].

Although there are a limited number of commercially available products that could be used for SDD, problems with pack sizes, expiry dates and strengths of the commercial products mean that most ICUs prefer to use extemporaneously prepared products. For example, colistin syrup is available commercially at a strength of 250,000 units in 5 ml (Colomycin®, Forest). This means that to give a dose of 3,000,000 units ($\equiv$ 100 mg) for a patient >12 years of age, 60 ml would be required to be administered per dose, i.e., 240 ml/day. The same dose using an extemporaneously prepared colistin 100 mg/ml oral solution would equate to a volume of 1 ml, i.e., 4 ml/day. Recent discontinuations of some of the products that were available commercially (Fungilin® suspension and tablets) may have also hindered the application of the SDD concept to clinical practice.

Table 27.10 Costs of selective decontamination of the digestive tract (SDD) hospital preparations (June 2010)

Drug	Supplier	Pack size	Cost (£)	Total daily dose >12 years of age	Cost/day (£)
Amphotericin 100 mg/ml suspension	Western Infirmary, Glasgow	100 ml	80	2,000 mg	16
Colistin oral solution 100 mg/ml	Stockport Pharmaceuticals, Manchester	30 ml	42.37	400 mg	5.65
Tobramycin base oral solution 80 mg/ml	Stockport Pharmaceuticals, Manchester	60 ml	51	320 mg	3.4
SDD gel	Western Infirmary, Glasgow	5 g	9.50	A pea-sized application four times a day	1.9
SDD paste	Western Infirmary, Glasgow	5 g	14.70	A pea-sized application four times a day	2.94
SDD pastilles	Western Infirmary, Glasgow	28	45.15	1 pastille four times a day	6.45

27.7 Costs of Decontaminating Agents

Formal cost–benefit analyses of SDD in ICU patients have not been performed. In theory, successful prevention of infection may make ICU more cost effective in that reduced infection rates secondary to SDD may lead to a shorter patient ICU stay and lower ICU, parenterally administered antibiotic usage and microbiology laboratory costs. It has not been firmly established whether these potential savings offset the additional costs that the SDD regimen incurs through the use of non-absorbable antimicrobials, systemic antimicrobials and additional microbiological cultures [43].

The costs of drugs used in the PTA regimen using products prepared by hospital manufacturing units are listed in Table 27.10, and the costs of commercially available products are listed in Table 27.11 [44]. The cost of treating a patient >12 years of age using hospital or commercial products is also shown, although a complete daily cost comparison cannot be made due to the lack of commercial products.

It should be noted that the costs of hospital-made products have escalated dramatically over the past few years, perhaps because of further research and development costs in the production of more stable products, lack of competition from commercial products in driving prices down and problems affecting the

Table 27.11 Costs of commercially available preparations (British National Formulary March 2010) [44]

Drug	Supplier	Pack size	Cost (£)	Total daily dose >12 years of age	Cost/day (£)
Colomycin® syrup (colistin sulphate 250,000 units/5 ml)	Forest	80 ml	3.48	400 mg($\equiv$ 12,000,000 units)	10.44
Colomycin® tablets (colistin sulphate 1.5 million unit tablets)	Forest	50	58.28	400 mg($\equiv$ 12,000,000 units)	9.32
Fungilin® lozenges (amphotericin 10 mg lozenges)	Squibb	60	3.53	1 lozenge four times a day	0.24

Table 27.12 Possible sources of ingredients

Ingredient	Supplier
Sodium carboxymethylcellulose Ph. Eur; sodium benzoate Ph. Eur, tobramycin sulphate powder USP, amphotericin B powder Ph. Eur; glycerol Ph. Eur; citric acid monohydrate Ph. Eur; sodium citrate Ph. Eur; liquid paraffin Ph. Eur; peppermint concentrate BP	Fagron UK
	Tel/fax: +44-845-6522525
	www.fagron.co.uk
Colistin sulphate powder Ph. Eur.	Duchefa Farma
	Haarlem, The Netherlands.
	Tel: +31-235-319093
Nipasept®	Clariant UK Ltd
	Calverley Lane, Horsforth, Leeds, UK.
	LS18 4RP
	Tel: +44-113-2584646
Orange syrup BP	J.M. Loveridge Ltd
	Southbrook Rd, Southampton, UK.
	SO15 1BH
	Tel: +44-170-3228411
	Fax:+44-170-3639836

global economy. However, due to the commercial unavailability of tobramycin oral solution, an SDD gel and—more recently—amphotericin suspension and tablets (discontinued by the manufacturers), it would not be possible to follow the PTA regimen without the provision of hospital-made products.

One factor that may make it difficult for a hospital pharmacy to begin manufacturing preparations for SDD regimes is sourcing the raw ingredients necessary to make the products. Table 27.12 therefore provides useful information to overcome this problem.

27.8 Conclusion

Although application of the SDD concept to intensive care medicine has been proven to reduce ICU-related morbidity and mortality rates, and despite a publication validating SDD as an evidence-based medicine manoeuvre [25], the SDD approach is still not widely used in ICUs. Proposed reasons for this may be:
1. SDD is contrary to the traditional concept that prophylaxis creates resistance.
2. A primacy of opinion over evidence.
3. Opinion leaders control the medical media.
4. SDD formulations are not marketed by the pharmaceutical industry.
5. There is little physician–pharmaceutical industry interaction to stimulate industry interest in manufacturing SDD products.

In a climate with a lack of commercial products, the necessary extemporaneous production of SDD formulations must be undertaken by a pharmacy department that is able to commit to the additional workload that this entails. This means that, at present, the formulation and supply role of the hospital pharmacist is vital in order to facilitate application of the SDD concept to clinical practice.

References

1. Silvestri L, de la Cal MA, van Saene HKF (2009) Selective decontamination of the digestive tract [SDD]. Twenty five years of European experience. In: Gullo A, Besso J, Lumb PD, Williams GF (eds) Intensive care and critical care medicine. Springer, Milan, pp 273–283
2. Stoutenbeek CP, Van Saene HKF, Miranda DR, Zandstra DF (1984) The effect of selective decontamination of the digestive tract on colonization and infection rate in multiple trauma patients. Intensive Care Med 10:185–192
3. Silvestri L, Mannucci F, van Saene HK (2000) Selective decontamination of the digestive tract: a life saver. J Hosp Infect 45:185–190
4. Abdel-Razek SM, Abdel-Khalek AH, Allam AM et al (2000) Impact of selective gastrointestinal decontamination on mortality and morbidity in severely burned patients. Ann Burns Fire Disasters 13:213–216
5. Barret JP, Jeschke MG, Herndon DN (2001) Selective decontamination of the digestive tract in severely burned paediatric patients. Burns 27:439–445
6. Bergmans DC, Bonten MJ, Gaillard CA et al (2001) Prevention of ventilator-associated pneumonia by oral decontamination: a prospective, randomised, double- blind, placebo-controlled study. Am J Respir Crit Care Med 164:382–388
7. Bouter H, Schippers EF, Luelmo SA et al (2002) No effect of preoperative selective gut decontamination on endotoxemia and cytokine activation during cardiopulmonary bypass: a randomised, placebo-controlled study. Crit Care Med 30:38–43
8. Camus C, Bellissant E, Sebille V et al (2005) Prevention of acquired infections in intubated patients with the combination of two decontamination regimens. Crit Care Med 33:307–314

9. de Jonge E, Schultz MJ, Spanjaard L et al (2003) Effects of selective decontamination of the digestive tract on mortality and acquisition of resistant bacteria in intensive care: a randomised controlled trial. Lancet 362:1011–1016
10. de Smet AM, Kluytmans JA, Cooper BS et al (2009) Decontamination of the digestive tract and oropharynx in ICU patients. N Engl J Med 360:20–31
11. Farran L, Llop J, Sans M, Kriesler E et al (2008) Efficacy of enteral decontamination in the prevention of anastomotic dehiscence and pulmonary infection in esophagogastric surgery. Dis Esophagus 21:159–164
12. Hellinger WC, Yao JD, Alvarez S et al (2002) A randomised, prospective, double-blinded evaluation of selective bowel decontamination in liver transplantation. Transplantation 73: 1904–1909
13. Krueger WA, Lenhart FP, Neeser G et al (2002) Influence of combined intravenous and topical antibiotic prophylaxis on the incidence of infections, organ dysfunctions and mortality in critically ill surgical patients: a prospective, stratified, randomised, double-blind, placebo-controlled clinical trial. Am J Respir Crit Care Med 166:1029–1037
14. Pneumatikos I, Koulouras V, Nathanail C (2002) Selective decontamination of subglottic area in mechanically ventilated patients with multiple trauma. Intensive Care Med 28:432–437
15. Rayes N, Seehofer D, Hansen S et al (2002) Early enteral supply of Lactobacillus and fiber verses selective bowel decontamination: a controlled trial in liver transplant recipients. Transplantation 74:123–128
16. Stoutenbeek CP, van Saene HK, Little RA, Whitehead A, Working Group on Selective Decontamination of the Digestive Tract (2007) The effect of selective decontamination of the digestive tract on mortality in multiple trauma patients: a multicenter randomised controlled trial. Intensive Care Med 33:261–270
17. Zwaveling JH, Maring JK, Klompmaker IJ et al (2002) Selective decontamination of the digestive tract to prevent postoperative infection: a randomised placebo-controlled trial in liver transplant patients. Crit Care Med 30:1204–1209
18. Safdar N, Said A, Lucey MR (2004) The role of selective decontamination for reducing infection in patients undergoing liver transplantation: a systematic review and meta-analysis. Liver Transpl 10:817–827
19. Liberati A, D'Amico R Pifferi S et al (2004) Antibiotic prophylaxis to reduce respiratory tract infections and mortality in adults receiving intensive care (Cochrane Review). In: The Cochrane Library Issue 1, Chichester, UK: Wiley
20. Silvestri L, van Saene HKF, Milanese M, Gregori D (2005) Impact of selective decontamination of the digestive tract on fungal carriage and infection; systematic review of randomised controlled trials. Intensive Care Med 31:898–910
21. Silvestri L, van Saene HKF, Milanese M et al (2007) Selective decontamination of the digestive tract reduces bloodstream infections and mortality in critically ill patients: a systematic review of randomised controlled trials. J Hosp Infect 65:187–203
22. Silvestri L, van Saene HKF, Casarin AL et al (2008) Impact of selective decontamination of the digestive tract on carriage and infection due to gram-negative and gram-positive bacteria. Systematic review of randomised controlled trials. Anaesth Intensive Care 36:324–338
23. Silvestri L, van Saene HKF, Weir I, Gullo A (2009) Survival benefit of the full selective digestive decontamination regimen. J Crit Care 24:474.e7–14
24. Liberati A, D'Amico R, Pifferi S et al (2009) Antibiotic prophylaxis to reduce respiratory tract infections and mortality in adults receiving intensive care. Cochrane Database Syst Rev, CD000022
25. Masteron RG, Galloway A, French G et al (2008) Guidelines for the management of hospital-acquired pneumonia in the UK: report of the working party on hospital—acquired pneumonia of the British Society for antimicrobial chemotherapy. J Antimicrob Chemother 62:5–34
26. Rommes JH, Selby A, Zandstra DF (2005) Therapy of infection. In: van Saene HKF, Silvestri L, de la Cal MA (eds) Infection control in the intensive care unit, 2nd edn edn. Springer, Milan, pp 515–533

27. Sanchez M, Pizer BP, Alcock SR (2005) Enteral antimicrobials. In: van Saene HKF, Silvestri L, de la Cal MA (eds) Infection control in the intensive care unit, 2nd edn edn. Springer, Milan, pp 171–187
28. Silvestri L, Milanese M, Oblach L et al (2002) Enteral vancomycin to control methicillin-resistant *Staphylococcus aureus* outbreak in mechanically ventilated patients. Am J Infect Control 30:391–399
29. van Saene HKF, Petros AJ, Sarginson RE et al (2009) Is selective decontamination of the digestive tract a solution to the anti-microbial problem in the UK? JICS 10(2):86–89
30. Guidelines for the use of selective digestive decontamination (SDD) (1999, updated 2010). Alder Hey Children's NHS Foundation Trust, Liverpool, UK
31. Crome D (1989) Pharmaceutical technology in selective decontamination. In: van Saene HKF, Stoutenbeek CP, Lawin P, McA Ledingham I (eds) Infection control by selective decontamination. Springer, Berlin, pp 109–112
32. Data on file. Alder Hey Children's NHS Foundation Trust, Liverpool, UK
33. Data on file. Western Infirmary, Glasgow, UK
34. Symonds RP, Mcillroy P, Khorrami J et al (1996) The reduction of radiation mucositis by selective decontamination antibiotic pastilles: a placebo-controlled double-blind trial. Br J Cancer 74:312–317
35. Spijkervet FKL, van Saene HKF, van Saene JJM et al (1991) Effect of selective elimination of the oral flora on mucositis in irradiated head and neck cancer patients. J Surg Oncol 46:167–173
36. Data on file. Organon, Oss, The Netherlands
37. van Saene JJM (1990) Colonic delivery of polymyxin E and four quinolones for flora suppression. PhD thesis, University of Groningen. PAL, Amsterdam
38. van der Spoel JI, Schultz MJ, van der Voort PHJ, de Jonge E (2006) Influence of severity of illness, medication and selective decontamination on defecation. Intensive Care Med 32: 875–880
39. Smit MJ, van der Spoel JI, de Smet AMGA et al (2007) Accumulation of oral antibiotics as an adverse effect of selective decontamination of the digestive tract: a series of three cases. Intensive Care Med 33: 2025–2026
40. Jew RK, Owen D, Kaufman D, Balmer D (1997) Osmolality of commonly used medications and formulas in the neonatal intensive care unit. Nutr Clin Practice 12:158–163
41. van Saene HKF, Stoutenbeek CP, Faber-Nijholt R, van Saene JJM (1992) Selective decontamination of the digestive tract contributes to the control of disseminated intravascular coagulation in severe liver impairment. J Pediatr Gastroenterol Nutr 14(4):436–442
42. Personal Communication (2010) Stockport pharmaceuticals, Stepping Hill Hospital, Manchester, UK
43. Bonten MJ, Kullberg BJ, Van Dalen R et al (2000) Selective digestive decontamination in patients in intensive care. The Dutch Working Group on Antibiotic Policy. J Antimicrob Chemother 46(3):351–362
44. British National Formulary (BNF) No 59 (2010) British Medical Association and the Royal Pharmaceutical Society of Great Britain, March 2010

Antimicrobial Resistance

N. Taylor, I. Cortés Puch, L. Silvestri, D. F. Zandstra
and H. K. F. van Saene

28.1 Introduction

Resistance to antimicrobial drugs is a serious risk factor for infection-related morbidity and mortality in critically ill patients. Gut overgrowth by potentially pathogenic microorganisms (PPMs) is a major risk for de novo development of drug-resistant microorganisms. Selective decontamination of the digestive tract (SDD), in which enteral administration of antimicrobial agents is the essential element, significantly reduces the risk of gut overgrowth and the subsequent development of drug-resistant pathogens.

28.2 Definition

SDD is a prophylactic antimicrobial strategy aiming to reduce infection-related morbidity and mortality in the critically ill patient. It is a four-component protocol consisting of enteral, nonabsorbable antimicrobial administration (polymyxin E/tobramycin/amphotericin B (PTA)) and a short course of parenterally administered antibiotics (cefotaxime), together with a high standard of hygiene and surveillance cultures [1].

N. Taylor (✉)
Institute of Ageing and Chronic Disease, University of Liverpool,
Liverpool, Merseyside, UK
e-mail: nia.taylor@liv.ac.uk

28.3 Philosophy: Carriage

SDD is based on the observation that critical illness changes body flora by two methods: qualitatively and quantitatively. Carriage of normal flora is eroded and then replaced by abnormal flora [2], and the density of growth shifts from low to high grade (gut overgrowth) [3]

1. *Normal flora* consists of six potential pathogens that are commonly found in the oropharynx and/or gut of healthy people. *Streptococcus pneumoniae, Haemophilus influenzae, Moraxella catarrhalis*, which are found in the oropharynx only; *Escherichia coli* in the gut; and *Staphylococcus aureus* and *Candida albicans* in both the oropharynx and gut.
2. *Abnormal flora* consists of nine abnormal potential pathogens. Eight aerobic Gram-negative bacilli (AGNB) and methicillin-resistant *S. aureus* (MRSA), found in both the oropharynx and gut. The eight AGNB are *Klebsiella, Enterobacter, Citrobacter, Proteus, Morganella, Serratia, Acinetobacter,* and *Pseudomonas* spp.

Critical illness changes the normal carrier state into the abnormal carrier state, which is the persistent presence of abnormal flora in the patient's oropharynx and/or gut [2, 4].

28.3.1 Low- and High-Grade Carriage

Low-grade to high-grade carriage is the quantitative change brought about by critical illness. Low-grade carriage is defined as $<10^5$ potential pathogens per millilitre of saliva or gram of faeces (or $<2+$), whereas high-grade carriage is defined as $\geq 10^5$ potential pathogens per millilitre of saliva or gram of faeces (or $\geq 2+$) [5]. High-grade carriage is synonymous with gut overgrowth and is the crucial event that precedes endogenous infection [6].

28.4 Infection Types

Infection, when classified according to the carrier state, can be categorised into three different groups [7]: primary endogenous, secondary endogenous and exogenous. All require a different prophylactic manoeuvre (Table 28.1).

1. Primary endogenous infection is the most frequent type, causing approximately 55% of infections in the intensive care unit (ICU). It occurs when the causative microorganism is present in the patient's admission flora in overgrowth concentrations, generally within 1 week of admission. The component of SDD that prevents primary endogenous infections is the short course of parenterally administered antibiotics given when the patient is admitted and for the next 4 days.
2. Secondary endogenous infection occurs when the causative microorganism is not present in the patient's admission flora but the abnormal flora is acquired

Table 28.1 Carriage classification of severe infections of lower airways and bloodstream

Infection	PPM	Timing	Frequency (%)	Manoeuvre
1	6 normal 9 abnormal	<1 week	55	Parenteral antimicrobials
2	9 abnormal	>1 week	30	Hygiene and enteral antimicrobials
3	9 abnormal	Anytime during ICU treatment	15	Hygiene and topical antimicrobials

1 primary endogenous, *2* secondary endogenous, *3* exogenous, *PPM* potentially pathogenic microorganism, 6 normal PPM, *Streptococcus pneumoniae, Haemophilus influenzae, Moraxella catarrhalis, Candida albicans, Staphylococcus aureus, Escherichia coli,* 9 abnormal PPM, *Klebsiella, Enterobacter, Citrobacter, Proteus, Morganella, Serratia, Acinetobacter, Pseudomonas* spp. and methicillin-resistant *Staphylococcus aureus* (MRSA), *ICU* intensive care unit

during treatment in the ICU, and the patient subsequently develops the carrier state in overgrowth concentrations, which precedes the infection. Secondary endogenous infection occurs after a week of ICU treatment at a frequency of 30%. The manoeuvre to impact this type of infection is enterally administered nonabsorbable antimicrobials and high standards of hygiene.

3. Exogenous infection may occur at anytime during ICU treatment and develops when the abnormal flora is introduced directly into the patient, bypassing the carrier state. Approximately 15% of all ICU infections are exogenous. The manoeuvre designed to combat this infection is hygiene and topical application of antimicrobials. Enteral administration of antimicrobials also contributes to exogenous infection control by reducing the reservoir of potential pathogens in the unit that may be introduced into a patient

Surveillance cultures, the fourth component of SDD, are essential for three reasons:
1. They are required to distinguish primary endogenous from secondary endogenous and exogenous infections.
2. They allow ongoing monitoring of eradication of gut overgrowth during SDD.
3. They are the most sensitive sampling methods for detecting antimicrobial resistance.

28.5 Mechanisms of Action Explaining Efficacy: Control of High-Grade Carriage or Overgrowth

The reason for SDD efficacy requires the understanding of two points
1. Acknowledgement of carriage classification [8]: In order to accept the concept of SDD, it must be understood that carriage occurs. Primary carriage is when the patient is admitted to the ICU with flora in the digestive tract; secondary

Table 28.2 Four components of selective decontamination of the digestive tract (SDD)

Target PPM and antimicrobials	Total daily dose (4 times daily)		
	<5 years	5–12 years	>12 years
1. Parenteral antimicrobials: normal PPM cefotaxime (mg)	150/kg	200/kg	4,000
2. Hygiene with enteral antimicrobials: abnormal PPM A. Oropharynx			
• AGNB: polymyxin E with tobramycin	2 g of 2% paste or gel		
• MRSA: Vancomycin	2 g of 4% paste or gel		
• Yeasts: amphotericin B or nystatin	2 g of 2% paste or gel		
B. Gut			
• AGNB: polymyxin E (mg) with tobramycin (mg)	100 80	200 160	400 320
• MRSA: vancomycin (mg)	20–40/kg	20–40/kg	500–2,000
• Yeasts: amphotericin B (mg) or nystatin units	500 2×10^6	1,000 4×10^6	2,000 8×10^6
3. Hygiene with topical antimicrobials: abnormal PPM	2% PTA paste/4% vancomycin paste		
4. Surveillance swabs of throat and rectum on admission, Monday, Thursday			

PPM potentially pathogenic microorganisms, *AGNB* aerobic Gram-negative bacilli, *MRSA* methicillin-resistant *Staphylococcus aureus*, *PTA* polymyxin E/tobramycin/amphotericin B

carriage when the patient acquires flora in the digestive tract during treatment in the ICU.
2. The antimicrobials selected for SDD were selected for specific reasons and invariably clear high-grade carriage (Table 28.2):
   - parenteral cefotaxime clears carriage of normal bacteria; it is active against normal and against some abnormal pathogens and, moreover, has a good safety profile;
   - enterally administered polyenes clear normal fungal carriage;
   - enterally administered polymyxin/tobramycin with or without vancomycin clears carriage of abnormal bacteria AGNB and MRSA; these antimicrobials are nonabsorbable and manage to achieve high intraluminal concentrations.

SDD antimicrobials are required in high concentrations against prevailing microorganisms (Table 28.3). These concentrations are deemed more important than sparing the colonisation resistance [9]. Colonisation resistance is the mechanism whereby indigenous flora are a barrier against the abnormal flora acquired, e.g. from food, and then carried in the digestive tract.

Gut overgrowth [10] harms the critically ill in four main ways:
1. *Infection*. There is a quantitative relationship between surveillance and diagnostic samples. As soon as there is overgrowth in surveillance samples, the

Table 28.3 Effective concentrations against prevailing microorganisms are more important than sparing the colonisation-resistant flora

Antimicrobials selected for SDD	Concentrations (mg/L) in		
	Saliva	Bile	Faeces
Cefotaxime	6	20	
Polymyxin E			16–1,000
Tobramycin			100
Amphotericin B or Nystatin			60 <100
Vancomycin			3,000–24,000

SDD selective decontamination of the digestive tract

diagnostic samples become positive, which is the first stage in infection development [11].
2. *Immunosuppression.* Overgrowth of abnormal AGNB (and associated endotoxin) impairs systemic immunity due to generalised inflammation following absorption of AGNB and/or endotoxin [12].
3. *Inflammation.* Overgrowth of abnormal AGNB and/or endotoxin leads to cytokinaemia and inflammation of major organ systems [13].
4. *Resistance.* The abnormal carrier state in overgrowth concentrations guarantees increased spontaneous mutation, leading to polyclonality and antibiotic resistance [14].

SDD is a prophylactic measure using selected antimicrobials to control gut overgrowth, thereby reducing the four harmful overgrowth side effects, i.e. infection [6], immunosuppression [15], inflammation [16] and resistance [17].

28.6 Efficacy

SDD is one of the most investigated clinical interventions in critically ill patients. Its efficacy in preventing infection-related morbidity and mortality has been assessed in 11 meta-analyses [18–28] covering 65 randomised controlled trials (RCTs) [29–93] (Table 28.4). Of the 11 meta-analyses, lower airway infection was the endpoint in six [18–20, 24, 26, 28]. All meta-analyses invariably demonstrated a significant reduction in lower airway infections (odds ratio (OR) 0.28, 95% confidence interval (CI) 0.20–0.38). Bloodstream infection was the endpoint in three meta-analyses [22–24] and was significantly reduced (OR 0.63, 95% CI 0.46–0.87). When assessing bloodstream infection, AGNB septicaemias were significantly reduced, Gram-positive septicaemias were increased but not significantly and fungaemia was reduced but not significantly due to the low incidence in the control group (Table 28.4). Multiple organ dysfunction syndrome (MODS)

Table 28.4 Efficacy of selective decontamination of the digestive tract (SDD): 65 randomised controlled trials (RCTs) and 11 meta-analyses

Author	No. RCTs	Sample size	Lower airway infection OR (95% CI)	Bloodstream infection OR (95% CI)	Multiple organ dysfunction syndrome OR (95% CI)	Mortality rate OR (95% CI)
Vandenbroucke-Grauls [18]	6	491	0.12, 0.08–0.19	NR		0.92, 0.45–1.84
D'Amico [19]	33	5727	0.35, 0.29–0.41	NR		0.80, 0.69–0.93
Safdar [20]	4	259	NR	NR		0.82, 0.22–2.45
Liberati [21]	36	6922	0.35, 0.29–0.41	NR		0.78, 0.68–0.89
Silvestri [22] yeasts	42	6075	NR	0.89, 0.16–4.95		NR
Silvestri [23]	51	8065	NR	0.63, 0.46–0.87		0.74, 0.61–0.91
Silvestri [24] Gram− Gram+	54	9473	0.07, 0.04–0.13 0.52, 0.34–0.78	0.36, 0.22–0.60 1.03, 0.75–1.41		NR NR
Silvestri [25]	21	4902	NR	NR		0.71, 0.61–0.82
Liberati [26]	36	6914	0.28, 0.20–0.38	NR		0.75, 0.65–0.87
Silvestri [27]	7	1270	NR	NR	0.50, 0.34–0.74	0.82, 0.51–1.32
Silvestri [28]	12	2252	0.54, 0.42–0.69	NR		NR

OR odds ratio, *CI* confidence interval, *NR* not reported

was the endpoint in one meta-analysis [27]; the relative reduction of 50% was significant. Mortality was the endpoint in nine meta-analyses [18–21, 23, 25–28]. SDD consistently reduced mortality rates as long as the sample size was large enough; the sample size was too small in three meta-analyses [18, 20, 27].

28.7 Safety

SDD safety relies on the long-term level of resistance not emerging against the SDD antimicrobials [94]. The concept of exposing vast numbers of critically ill patients to broad-spectrum multiple drug cocktails runs counter to existing theoretical models (and dogma), as it is related to the genesis and promotion of antimicrobial resistance in pathogens acquired in the ICU [95]. The dynamics of resistance are driven by three mechanisms:
1. *Import.* The patient comes into the ICU with resistant microorganisms in overgrowth concentrations in the gut [3].
2. *Transmission.* 33% of patients admitted as normal carriers to a mixed ICU developed abnormal carriage of multi-drug-resistant *K. pneumoniae* and/or *A. baumannii*, the two abnormal AGNB endemic in the ICU at the time of the 1-year prospective observational study [96]. A higher Severity of Illness score on admission was a significant risk factor: the Simplified Acute Physiologically Score (SAPS) was 13 ± 4.6 in carriers versus 11.3 ± 5 in noncarriers ($p = 0.0006$).
3. *De novo development.* Gut overgrowth defined as $\geq 10^5$ potential pathogens per gram of faeces has been identified as a risk factor for de novo resistance development [14, 97]. The gut of the critically ill patient with microbial overgrowth is the ideal site for de novo development of new clones following increased spontaneous mutation, termed hypermutation. In hypermutation, microbial populations start mutating vigorously at random, presumably as an adaptive mechanism that may cause a mutant to arise that would enable them to overcome the unfavourable surroundings, resulting in polyclonality. A high proportion of patients who require long-term ICU treatment receive parenterally administered antimicrobials, which are invariably excreted via the bile into the gut. Although low and fluctuating, the antibiotic levels will kill the sensitive clones, promoting the emergence of clones resistant to the antibiotics.

Each mechanism is responsible for a third of antimicrobial resistance in the ICU. The common denominator of all three mechanisms is gut overgrowth.

There are four categories in which antimicrobial resistance is a problem in the ICU:
1. AGNB
    (a) *Sensitive to decontaminating agents polymyxin/tobramycin.* de Jonge et al. conducted a prospective open-label RCT in which 934 critically ill adult patients were randomly assigned on admission to either a medical/surgical ICU using routine SDD or a similar ICU in the same hospital that did not

use SDD [43]. Study participants were patients with expected duration of mechanical ventilation of at least 48 h and/or ICU stay >3 days. Surveillance cultures from the throat and rectum were obtained at ICU admission and at discharge, weekly during ICU treatment and for the first week postdischarge. The in-hospital mortality rate was significantly lower for SDD recipients than for control patients (24 vs. 31%; $p = 0.02$). Carriage of AGNB resistant to polymyxin E, tobramycin, ceftazidime, ciprofloxacin and imipenem was significantly reduced in SDD patients compared with controls (16 vs. 26%; $p = 0.001$). Similar results were observed by de Smet et al. in their cluster RCT [45]. Monthly point-prevalence surveys for carriage of multi-drug-resistant AGNB were obtained. The proportion of rectal swabs with resistant AGNB was lower for SDD compared with standard-care patients.

(b) Resistant to decontaminating agents polymyxin/tobramycin:
- there is only one potential pathogen intrinsically resistant to polymyxin/tobramycin—*Serratia* species. In case of *Serratia* endemicity, polymyxin/tobramycin must be replaced by paromomycin [98, 99].
- extended-spectrum beta-lactamase (ESBL) producing AGNB are often resistant to tobramycin but always sensitive to polymyxin [100]. In case of ESBL producing AGNB endemicity, tobramycin needs to be replaced by another aminoglycoside, e.g. neomycin, paromomycin [39, 93, 99].

2. MRSA
   (a) *Sensitive to glycopeptides.* Practically all MRSA strains are sensitive to glycopeptides such as vancomycin and teicoplanin. All RCTs [34, 52, 59, 60, 69, 80] and prospective studies [6, 101, 102] assessing the efficacy of enterally administered vancomycin on the abnormal MRSA carrier state demonstrated its efficacy. Therefore, it is recommended to add vancomycin to PTA in cases of MRSA endemicity.
   (b) *Resistant to glycopeptides.* MRSA is now endemic in many hospitals throughout the world. Several clusters of glycopeptide-resistant MRSA have been reported. A 39-case outbreak, defined as involving any patient carrying or infected by a strain of MRSA with reduced or intermediate susceptibility to glycopeptides, was recorded in a hospital in Paris, France, from October 1998 to March 1999 [103]. Another outbreak from Lyon, France, included 15 patients [104]. MRSA has been acknowledged as a gut rather than a nasal bacterium [6, 101, 102]. Patients requiring long-term ICU treatment invariably develop gut overgrowth of MRSA when it is endemic. MRSA gut overgrowth precedes endogenous MRSA infection, which—in general—is treated with glycopeptides. The combination of low antimicrobial concentrations in the faeces following biliary excretion and overgrowth leads to increased spontaneous mutation, polyclonality and antimicrobial resistance against glycopeptides [14].

3. Azole-resistant *Candida* spp.
   Practically all critically ill patients who require long-term ICU treatment have fungal overgrowth [105]. Parenteral azoles administered either prophylactically

or therapeutically fail to clear fungal overgrowth, because the faecal levels are not fungicidal and/or fluctuating following biliary excretion [106]. In contrast, fungal overgrowth promotes increased spontaneous mutation, polyclonality and antifungal resistance [107, 108].

4. Vancomycin-resistant enterococci (VRE)

   Enterococci are normal residents of the large bowel but not the oropharynx. Enterococci are organisms of low-level pathogenicity present in the gut of healthy people at concentrations between 10^{3-6} enterococci/gram of faeces. *Enterococcus faecalis* and *E. faecium* are the two most common enterococci associated with infection: *E. faecalis* is carried by 80% of healthy individuals at concentrations between 10^{5-7} CFU/g of faeces; *E. faecium* is carried by 30% of healthy individuals at lower concentrations. Enterococci are resistant to many antimicrobials but in general sensitive to glycopeptides (vancomycin, teicoplanin) and linezolid. A VRE is defined as an *Enterococcus* with a minimum inhibitory concentration (MIC) of ≥ 16 mg of vancomycin per litre [109].

   (a) *Linezolid sensitive VRE*. Carriage of VRE even sensitive to linezolid is abnormal [110]. As far as we are aware, there are no trials attempting to eradicate VRE carriage. Theoretically, it is not impossible to clear abnormal VRE carriage using vancomycin enterally: 2 g is associated with faecal vancomycin levels varying between 3,000 and 24,000 mg per litre, with an MIC around 16 mg/L [111].

28.8 No Resistance During SDD (Meta-Analysis)

Five RCTs of SDD involving 5,229 patients (2,631 SDD, 2,598 controls) reported data on resistance [39, 43, 45, 50, 61]. There were 74 (2.8%) patients with resistant microorganisms in the SDD group and 124 (4.8%) in controls, indicating a 44% reduction in the odds of resistance by SDD (OR 0.56, 95% CI 0.41–0.76; $p < 0.001$) (Fig. 28.1). Heterogeneity was not shown ($\chi^2 = 2.58888$, $p = 0.63$; $I^2 = 0$).

28.8.1 Subgroup Analysis

We investigated the impact of SDD on resistance among subgroups with different types of regimens (Fig. 28.1). Three studies using the full SDD protocol of parenterally and enterally administered antimicrobials [43, 45, 50] involved 5,076 patients (2,612 SDD, 2,566 control). Resistance was demonstrated in 76 (2.9%) patients in the SDD group and 118 (4.6%) in the control group, resulting in a significant 44% reduction in the odds of resistance. In contrast, in studies using only enterally administered antimicrobials [39, 61] and involving 153 patients (69 SDD, 84 controls), the number of patients with resistant microorganisms was two (2.9%) in the SDD and six (7.14%) in the control group. This reduction was not significant.

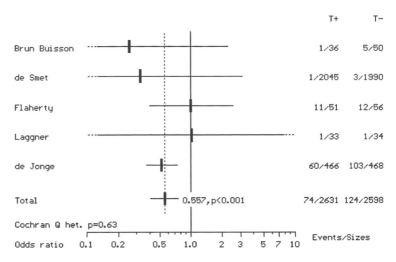

Fig. 28.1 Meta-analysis of five randomised controlled trials (RCTs) of selective decontamination of the digestive tract (SDD) with relevant data on resistance Odds ratio <1 favours SDD; >1 favours controls. Results presented with the fixed-effect model, as heterogeneity was not demonstrated T+, test; T–, control Brun-Buisson [39], de Smet [45], Flaherty [50], Laggner [61], de Jonge [43]

However, the sensitivity analysis showed that after excluding the de Jonge trial [43], the reduction in resistance was not significant (OR 0.75, 95% CI 0.35–1.61; $p = 0.46$; heterogeneity not significant).

28.9 SDD: Only EBM Manoeuvre with Grade 1A Recommendation

In recent years, RCTs have shown that five different manoeuvres reduce mortality rates:
- ventilation with low tidal volumes for acute lung injury and respiratory distress syndrome [112];
- recombinant human activated protein C for severe sepsis [113];
- intensive insulin therapy [114];
- low doses of steroids in patients with septic shock [115];
- SDD [43, 45, 60].

Table 28.5 reports the levels of evidence obtained using the Grading of Recommendations Assessment, Development and Evaluation (GRADE) system [116], which classifies the quality of evidence as high (A), moderate (B), low (C) or very low (D). RCTs may be downgraded due to limitations in implementation, inconsistency or imprecision of results, indirectness of the evidence and possible reporting bias [116]. An example of this is tight glucose control (A down to C): the

Table 28.5 Intensive care unit (ICU) interventions that reduce mortality rates

Intervention	Relative risk (95% CI)	AMR (%) (95% CI)	Number needed to treat	Grade of recommendation
1. Low tidal volume [112]	0.78 (0.65–0.93)	8.8 (2.4–15.3)	11	1B
2. Activated protein C [113]	0.80 (0.69–0.94)	6.1 (1.9–10.4)	16	2B
3. Intensive insulin [114]	0.44 (0.36–0.81)	3.7 (1.3–6.1)	27	2C
4. Steroids [115]	0.90 (0.74–1.09)	6.4 (-4.8–17.6)	16	2C
5. SDD [43, 45, 60]	0.65 (0.49–0.85)	8.1 (3.1–13.0)	12	1A

CI confidence interval, *AMR* absolute mortality reduction, *1* strong, *2* weak, *A* high, *B* moderate, *C* low

success of the original Belgian RCT [114] in reducing mortality rates has not to date been reproduced [117–121]. The GRADE system classifies recommendations as strong (1) or weak (2). The grade of strong or weak is considered of greater clinical importance than a difference in letter level of quality of evidence. A strong recommendation in favour of an intervention reflects that the desirable effects of adherence to a recommendation (beneficial health outcomes, less burden on staff and patients and cost savings) will clearly outweigh the undesirable effects (harms, more burdens, greater costs).

All RCTs and meta-analyses of SDD that assessed the full four-component protocol consistently demonstrated a significant survival benefit, providing the sample size was large enough. Mortality data show an intriguing observation that trial design determines the magnitude of the survival benefit [122]. The relative reduction in the OR for mortality was 41% when all patients received the full SDD protocol [43], 29% when half the patients received SDD [122] and 17% when one third of the population was treated with SDD [45, 123]. In the trial of the unit-wide application of SDD [43], SDD virtually eliminated transmission of potential pathogens via the hands of carers and hence exogenous infection in decontaminated patients. Survival benefit is diluted by mixing decontaminated and nondecontaminated patients in the same unit. This is the case in the RCT design, wherein patients receiving and not receiving SDD are treated within the same unit [45, 122]. Decontaminated patients protect control patients from transmission, acquisition, carriage, and subsequent infection, whereas patients receiving SDD remain at risk of acquiring potential pathogens and subsequent exogenous infections, resulting in a reduction in the true effect of SDD. The most recent multicentre RCT with a 17% relative reduction—albeit statistically significant—clearly emphasises the issue of diluting the SDD effect by increasing the number of nondecontaminated patients treated in the same unit with patients receiving SDD [45, 122].

28.10 Costs Implication for Using SDD

Although the cost-effectiveness of SDD has not yet been formally calculated, the daily costs of 6–12 euros [45, 70] can hardly be an issue for an ICU intervention that reduces pneumonia, septicaemia and mortality rates by 72, 37 and 29%, respectively (Table 28.4).

References

1. WFSICCM congress Firenze 2009 Gullo A (2009) Intensive and Critical Care Medicine. Springer, Milan, pp 273–283
2. Johanson WG, Pierce AK, Sanford JP (1969) Changing pharyngeal bacterial flora of hospitalized patients. Emergence of Gram-negative bacilli. N Engl J Med 281:1137–1140
3. Viviani M, van Saene HK, Pisa F et al (2010) The role of admission surveillance cultures in patients requiring prolonged mechanical ventilation in the intensive care unit. Anaesth Intensive Care 38:325–335
4. Mobbs KJ, van Saene HK, Sunderland D, Davies PD (1999) Oropharyngeal Gram-negative bacillary carriage: a survey of 120 healthy individuals. Chest 115:1570–1575
5. van Saene HKF, Damjanovic V, Murray AE, de la Cal MA (1996) How to classify infections in intensive care units—the carrier state, a criterion whose time has come? J Hosp Infect 33:1–12
6. de la Cal MA, Cerdá E, van Saene HKF et al (2004) Effectiveness and safety of enteral vancomycin to control endemicity of methicillin-resistant *Staphylococcus aureus* in a medical/surgical intensive care unit. J Hosp Infect 56:175–183
7. Stoutenbeek CP, van Saene HKF, Liberati A (1994) Prevention of respiratory tract infections in intensive care by selective decontamination of the digestive tract. In: Niederman MS, Sarosi GA, Glassroth J (eds) Respiratory infections, 1st edn. A scientific basis for management, Philiedelphia, pp 579–594
8. Silvestri L, van Saene HK, de la Cal MA, De Gaudio AR (2009) Carriage classification of pneumonia rather than time improves survival. Chest 136:1188–1189
9. Vollaard EJ (1991) The concept of colonization resistance. PhD thesis, Benda BV, Nijmegen, The Netherlands
10. Husebye E (1995) Gastrointestinal motility disorders and bacterial overgrowth. J Intern Med 237:419–427
11. Van Uffelen R, van Saene HK, Fidler V, Löwenberg A (1984) Oropharyngeal flora as a source of bacteria colonizing the lower airways in patients on artificial ventilation. Intensive Care Med 10:233–237
12. Deitch EA, Xu DZ, Qi L, Berg RD (1991) Bacterial translocation from the gut impairs systemic immunity. Surgery 104:269–276
13. Baue AE (1993) The role of the gut in the development of multiple organ dysfunction in cardiothoracic patients. Ann Thorac Surg 55:822–829
14. van Saene HKF, Taylor N, Damjanovic V, Sarginson RE (2008) Microbial gut overgrowth guarantees increased spontaneous mutation leading to polyclonality and antibiotic resistance in the critically ill. Curr Drug Targets 9:419–421
15. Horton JW, Maass DL, White J, Minei JP (2007) Reducing susceptibility to bacteremia after experimental burn injury: a role for selective decontamination of the digestive tract. J Appl Physiol 102:2207–2216
16. Conraads VM, Jorens PG, De Clerck LS (2004) Selective intestinal decontamination in advanced chronic heart failure: a pilot trial. Eur J Heart Fail 6:483–491
17. van Saene HKF, Stoutenbeek CP, Zandstra DF (1988) Cefotaxime combined with selective decontamination in long term intensive care patients. Virtual absence of emergence of rsistance. Drugs 35(Suppl 2):29–34

18. Vandenbroucke-Grauls CMJ, Vandenbroucke JP (1991) Effect of selective decontamination of the digestive tract on respiratory tract infections and mortality in the intensive care unit. Lancet 338:859–862
19. D'Amico R, Pifferi S, Leonetti C et al on behalf of the Study Investigators (1998) Effectiveness of antibiotic prophylaxis in critically ill adult patients: systematic review of randomised controlled trials. BMJ 316:1275–1285
20. Safdar N, Said A, Lucey MR (2004) The role of selective decontamination for reducing infection in patients undergoing liver transplantation: a systematic review and meta-analysis. Liver Transpl 10:817–827
21. Liberati A, D'Amico R, Pifferi S et al (2004) Antibiotic prophylaxis to reduce respiratory tract infections and mortality in adults receiving intensive care (Cochrane Review). In: The Cochrane Library Issue 1. Wiley, Chichester
22. Silvestri L, van Saene HKF, Milanese M, Gregori D (2005) Impact of selective decontamination of the digestive tract on fungal carriage and infection: systematic review of randomized controlled trials. Intensive Care Med 31:898–910
23. Silvestri L, van Saene HKF, Milanese M (2007) Selective decontamination of the digestive tract reduces bloodstream infections and mortality in critically ill patients: a systematic review of randomized controlled trials. J Hosp Infect 65:187–203
24. Silvestri L, van Saene HKF, Casarin AL et al (2008) Impact of selective decontamination of the digestive tract on carriage and infection due to Gram-negative and Gram-positive bacteria. Systematic review of randomized controlled trials. Anaesth Intensive Care 36:324–338
25. Silvestri L, van Saene HKF, Weir I, Gullo A (2009) Survival benefit of the full selective digestive decontamination regimen. J Crit Care 24(474):e7–e14
26. Liberati A, D'Amico R, Pifferi S et al. (2009) Antibiotic prophylaxis to reduce respiratory tract infections and mortality in adults receiving intensive care. Cochrane Database Syst Rev CD000022
27. Silvestri L, van Saene HKF, Zandstra DF et al (2010) Selective decontamination of the digestive tract reduces multiple organ failure and mortality in critically ill patients: systematic review of randomized controlled trials. Crit Care Med 38:1370–1376
28. Silvestri L, van Saene HKF, Zandstra DF (2010) Selective digestive decontamination reduces ventilator-associated tracheobronchitis. Respir Med 104(12):1953–1955
29. Abdel-Razek SM, Abdel-Khalek AH et al (2000) Impact of selective gastrointestinal decontamination on mortality and morbidity in severely burned patients. Ann Burns Fire Disasters 13:213–216
30. Abele-Horn M, Dauber A, Bauernfeind A et al (1997) Decrease in nosocomial pneumonia in ventilated patients by selective oropharyngeal decontamination (SOD). Intensive Care Med 23:187–195
31. Aerdts SJ, van Dalen R, Clasener HA et al (1991) Antibiotic prophylaxis of respiratory tract infection in mechanically ventilated patients. A prospective, blinded, randomized trial of the effect of a novel regimen. Chest 100:783–791
32. Arnow PM, Carandang GC, Zabner R, Irwin ME (1996) Randomized controlled trial of selective bowel decontamination for prevention of infections following liver transplantation. Clin Infect Dis 22:997–1003
33. Barret JP, Jeschke MG, Herndon DN (2001) Selective decontamination of the digestive tract in severely burned pediatric patients. Burns 27:439–445
34. Bergmans DC, Bonten MJ, Gaillard CA et al (2001) Prevention of ventilator-associated pneumonia by oral decontamination: a prospective, randomized, double-blind, placebo-controlled study. Am J Respir Crit Care Med 164:382–388
35. Bion JF, Badger I, Crosby HA et al (1994) Selective decontamination of the digestive tract reduces Gram-negative pulmonary colonization but not systemic endotoxemia in patients undergoing elective liver transplantation. Crit Care Med 22:40–49
36. Blair P, Rowlands BJ, Lowry K et al (1991) Selective decontamination of the digestive tract: a stratified, randomized, prospective study in a mixed intensive care unit. Surgery 110:303–310

37. Boland JP, Sadler DL, Stewart WA et al. (1991)Reduction of nosocomial respiratory tract infections in multiple trauma patient requiring mechanical ventilation by selective parenteral and enteral antisepsis regimen (SPEAR) in the intensive care unit. 17th International congress of chemotherapy, Berlin, Abstract 0465
38. Bouter H, Schippers EF, Luelmo SA et al (2002) No effect of preoperative selective gut decontamination on endotoxemia and cytokine activation during cardiopulmonary bypass: a randomized, placebo-controlled study. Crit Care Med 30:38–43
39. Brun-Buisson C, Legrand P, Rauss A et al (1989) Intestinal decontamination for control of nosocomial multiresistant Gram-negative bacilli. Study of an outbreak in an intensive care unit. Ann Intern Med 110:873–881
40. Camus C, Bellissant E, Sebille V et al (2005) Prevention of acquired infections in intubated patients with the combination of two decontamination regimens. Crit Care Med 33:307–314
41. Cerra FB, Maddaus MA, Dunn DL et al (1992) Selective gut decontamination reduces nosocomial infections and length of stay but not mortality or organ failure in surgical intensive care unit patients. Arch Surg 127:163–169
42. Cockerill FR 3rd, Muller SR, Anhalt JP et al (1992) Prevention of infection in critically ill patients by selective decontamination of the digestive tract. Ann Intern Med 117:545–553
43. de Jonge E, Schultz MJ, Spanjaard L et al (2003) Effects of selective decontamination of digestive tract on mortality and acquisition of resistant bacteria in intensive care: a randomised controlled trial. Lancet 362:1011–1016
44. de la Cal MA, Cerdá E, García-Hierro P et al (2005) Survival benefit in critically ill burned patients receiving selective decontamination of the digestive tract: a randomized, placebo-controlled, double-blind trial. Ann Surg 241:424–430
45. de Smet AM, Kluytmans JA, Cooper BS et al (2009) Decontamination of the digestive tract and oropharynx in ICU patients. N Engl J Med 360:20–31
46. Diepenhorst GM, van Ruter O, Besselink MG, van Santvoort HC, Wijnandts PR, Renooij W, Gouma DJ, Goosen HG, Boermeester MA (2011) Influence of prophylactic probiotics and selective decontamination on bacterial translocation in patients undergoing pancreatic surgery: a randomized controlled trial. Shock 35: 9–16
47. Farran L, Llop J, Sans M et al (2008) Efficacy of enteral decontamination in the prevention of anastomotic dehiscence and pulmonary infection in esophagogastric surgery. Dis Esophagus 21:159–164
48. Ferrer M, Torres A, González J et al (1994) Utility of selective digestive decontamination in mechanically ventilated patients. Ann Intern Med 120:389–395
49. Finch RG, Tomlinson P, Holiday M, Sole K, Stack C, Rocker G. (1991) Selective decontamination of the digestive tract (SDD) in the prevention of secondary sepsis in a medical/surgical intensive care unit. 17th International congress of chemotherapy, Berlin, Abstract 0474
50. Flaherty J, Nathan C, Kabins SA, Weinstein RA (1990) Pilot trial of selective decontamination for prevention of bacterial infection in an intensive care unit. J Infect Dis 162:1393–1397
51. Gastinne H, Wolff M, Delatour F, Faurisson F, Chevret S (1992) A controlled trial in intensive care units of selective decontamination of the digestive tract with nonabsorbable antibiotics. The French Study Group on Selective Decontamination of the Digestive Tract. N Eng J Med 326:594–599
52. Gaussorgues PH, Salord F, Sirodot M, Tigaud S, Cagin S, Gerard M, Robert D (1991) Efficacite de la decontamination digestive sur la survenue des bacteriemies nosocomiales chez les patients sous ventilation mecanique et recevant des betamimetiques. Rean Soins Intens Med Urg 7:169–174
53. Georges B, Mazerolles M, Decun JF, Rouge P, Pomies S, Cougot P, Andrieu P, Virenque CH (1994) Décontamination Digestive Sélective Résultats D'une Étude Chez Le Polytraumatisé. Rean Urg 3:621–627

54. Gosney M, Martin MV, Wright AE (2006) The role of selective decontamination of the digestive tract in acute stroke. Age Ageing 35:42–47
55. Hammond JM, Potgieter PD, Saunders GL, Forder AA (1992) Double-blind study of selective decontamination of the digestive tract in intensive care. Lancet 340:5–9
56. Hellinger WC, Yao JD, Alvarez S, Blair JE, Cawley JJ, Paya CV et al (2007) A randomized, prospective, double-blinded evaluation of selective bowel decontamination in liver transplantation. Transplantation 73:1904–1909
57. Jacobs S, Foweraker JE, Roberts SE (1992) Effectiveness of selective decontamination of the digestive tract (SDD) in an ICU with a policy encouraging a low gastric pH. Clin Intensive Care 3:52–58
58. Kerver AJ, Rommes JH, Mevissen-Verhage EA, Hulstaert PF, Vos A, Verhoef J et al (1988) Prevention of colonization and infection in critically ill patients: a prospective randomized study. Crit Care Med 16:1087–1093
59. Korinek AM, Laisne MJ, Nicolas MH, Raskine L, Deroin V, Sanson-Lepors MJ et al (1993) Selective decontamination of the digestive tract in neurosurgical intensive care unit patients: a double-blind, randomized, placebo-controlled study. Crit Care Med 21:1466–1473
60. Krueger WA, Lenhart FP, Neeser G, Ruckdeschel G, Schreckhase H, Eissner HJ et al (2002) Influence of combined intravenous and topical antibiotic prophylaxis on the incidence of infections, organ dysfunctions, and mortality in critically ill surgical patients: a prospective, stratified, randomized, double-blind, placebo-controlled clinical trial. Am J Respir Crit Care Med 166:1029–1037
61. Laggner AN, Tryba M, Georgopoulos A et al (1994) Oropharyngeal decontamination with gentamicin for long-term ventilated patients on stress ulcer prophylaxis with sucralfate? Wien Klin Wochenschr 106:15–19
62. Lingnau W, Berger J, Javorsky F, Lejeune P, Mutz N, Benzer H et al (1997) Selective intestinal decontamination in multiple trauma patients: prospective, controlled trial. J Trauma 42:687–694
63. Luiten EJ, Hop WC, Lange JF, Bruining HA (1995) Controlled clinical trial of selective decontamination for the treatment of severe acute pancreatitis. Ann Surg 222:57–65
64. Martinez-Pellús AE, Merino P, Bru M, Conejero R, Seller G, Muñoz C et al (1992) Can selective digestive decontamination avoid the endotoxemia and cytokine activation promoted by cardiopulmonary bypass? Crit Care Med 21:1684–1691
65. Martinez-Pellús AE, Merino P, Bru M, Canovas J, Seller G, Sapiña J et al (1997) Endogenous endotoxemia of intestinal origin during cardiopulmonary bypass. Role of type of flow and protective effect of selective digestive decontamination. Intensive Care Med 23:1251–1257
66. Oudhuis GJ, Bergmans DC, Dormans T, Zwaveling JH, Kessels A, Prins MH, Stobberingh EE, Verbon A (2011) Probiotics versus antibiotic decontamination of the digestive tract: infection and mortality. Intensive Care Med 37:110–117
67. Palomar M, Alvarez-Lerma F, Jorda R, Bermejo B (1997) Catalan study group of nosocomial pneumonia prevention. Prevention of nosocomial infection in mechanically ventilated patients: selective digestive decontamination versus sucralfate. Clin Intensive Care 8:228–235
68. Pneumatikos I, Koulouras V, Nathanail C, Geo D, Nakos G (2002) Selective decontamination of subglottic area in mechanically ventilated patients with multiple trauma. Intensive Care Med 28:432–437
69. Pugin J, Auckenthaler R, Lew DP, Suter PM (1991) Oropharyngeal decontamination decreases incidence of ventilator-associated pneumonia. A randomized, placebo-controlled, double-blind clinical trial. JAMA 265:2704–2710
70. Quinio B, Albanèse J, Bues-Charbit M, Viviand X, Martin C (1996) Selective decontamination of the digestive tract in multiple trauma patients. A prospective double-blind, randomized, placebo-controlled study. Chest 109:765–772

71. Rayes N, Seehofer D, Hansen S et al (2002) Early enteral supply of Lactobacillus and fiber versus selective bowel decontamination: a controlled trial in liver transplant recipients. Transplantation 74:123–128
72. Rios F, Maskin B, Saenex Valiente A, Galante A, Cazes Camarero P, Aguilar L et al (2005) Prevention of ventilator associated pneumonia (VAP) by oral decontamination (OD). Prospective, randomized, double-blind, placebo-controlled study. American Thoracic Society International Conference, San Diego, USA, C95; poster 608
73. Rocha LA, Martin MJ, Pita S, Paz J, Seco C, Margusina L et al (1992) Prevention of nosocomial infection in critically ill patients by selective decontamination of the digestive tract. A randomized, double blind, placebo-controlled study. Intensive Care Med 18:398–404
74. Rodríguez-Roldán JM, Altuna-Cuesta A, López A, Carrillo A, Garcia J, León J et al (1990) Prevention of nosocomial lung infection in ventilated patients: use of an antimicrobial pharyngeal nonabsorbable paste. Crit Care Med 18:1239–1242
75. Rolando N, Gimson A, Wade J, Philpott-Howard J, Casewell M, Williams R (1993) Prospective controlled trial of selective parenteral and enteral antimicrobial regimen in fulminant liver failure. Hepatology 17:196–201
76. Rolando N, Wade JJ, Stangou A, Gimson AE, Wendon J, Philpott-Howard J et al (1996) Prospective study comparing the efficacy of prophylactic parenteral antimicrobials, with or without enteral decontamination, in patients with acute liver failure. Liver Transpl Surg 2:8–13
77. Roos D, Dijksman LM, Oudemans-van Straaten HM, de Wit LT, Gouma DJ, Gerhards MF (2011) Randomized clinical trial of perioperative selective decontamination of the digestive tract versus placebo in elective gastrointestinal surgery. Br J Surg [Epub ahead of print]
78. Ruza F, Alvarado F, Herruzo R, Delagado MA, Garcia S, Dorao P et al (1998) Prevention of nosocomial infection in a pediatric intensive care unit (PICU) through the use of selective digestive decontamination. Eur J Epidemiol 14:719–727
79. Sánchez García M, Cambronero Galache JA, López Diaz J, Cerdá Cerdá E, Rubio Blasco J, Gómez Aguinaga MA et al (1998) Effectiveness and cost of selective decontamination of the digestive tract in critically ill intubated patients. A randomized, double-blind, placebo-controlled, multicenter trial. Am J Respir Crit Care Med 158:908–916
80. Schardey HM, Joosten U, Finke U Staubach KH, Schauer R, Heiss A et al (1997) The prevention of anastomotic leakage after total gastrectomy with local decontamination. A prospective, randomized, double-blind, placebo-controlled multicenter trial. Ann Surg 225:172–180
81. Smith SD, Jackson RJ, Hannakan CJ, Wadowsky RM, Tzakis AG, Rowe MI (1993) Selective decontamination in pediatric liver transplants. A randomized prospective study. Transplantation 55:1306–1309
82. Stoutenbeek CP, van Saene HKF, Zandstra DF (1996) Prevention of multiple organ system failure by selective decontamination of the digestive tract in multiple trauma patients. Faist E, Baue AE, Schildberg FW (Eds.) In: The immune Consequence of Trauma, Shock and Sepsis–Mechanisms and Therapeutic Approaches. Pabst Science, Lengerich, pp 1055–1066
83. Stoutenbeek CP, van Saene HK, Little RA, Whitehead A for the Working Group on Selective Decontamination of the Digestive Tract (2007) The effect of selective decontamination of the digestive tract on mortality in multiple trauma patients: a multicenter randomized controlled trial. Intensive Care Med 33:261–270
84. Tetteroo GW, Wagenvoort JH, Castelein A, Tilanus HW, Ince C, Bruining HA (1990) Selective decontamination to reduce Gram-negative colonisation and infections after oesophageal resection. Lancet 335:704–707
85. Ulrich C, Harinck-de Weerd JE, Bakker NC, Jacz K, Doornbos L, de Ridder VA (1989) Selective decontamination of the digestive tract with norfloxacin in the prevention of ICU-acquired infections: a prospective randomized study. Intensive Care Med 15:424–431

86. Unertl K, Ruckdeschel G, Selbmann HK, Jensen U, Forst H, Lenhart FP et al (1987) Prevention of colonization and respiratory infections in long-term ventilated patients by local antimicrobial prophylaxis. Intensive Care Med 13:106–113
87. Verwaest C, Verhaegen J, Ferdinande P, Schetz M, Van den Berghe G, Verbist L et al (1997) Randomized, controlled trial of selective digestive decontamination in 600 mechanically ventilated patients in a multidisciplinary intensive care unit. Crit Care Med 25:63–71
88. Wiener J, Itokazu G, Nathan C, Kabins SA, Weinstein RA (1995) A randomized, double-blind, placebo-controlled trial of selective digestive decontamination in a medical-surgical intensive care unit. Clin Infect Dis 20:861–867
89. Winter R, Humphreys H, Pick A, MacGowan AP, Willatts SM, Speller DCE (1992) A controlled trial of selective decontamination of the digestive tract in intensive care and its effect on nosocomial infection. J Antimicrob Chemother 30:73–87
90. Yilamazlar A, Ozyurt G, Kahveci F, Goral G (2009) Selective digestive decontamination can be an infection-prevention regimen for the intoxicated patients. J Pharmaco Toxicol 4:36–40
91. Yu J, Xiao YB, Wang XY (2007) Effects of preoperatively selected gut decontamination on cardiopulmonary bypass-induced endotoxemia. Chin Traumatol 10:131–137
92. Zobel G, Kuttnig M, Grubbauer HM, Semmelrock HJ, Thiel W (1991) Reduction of colonization and infection rate during pediatric intensive care by selective decontamination of the digestive tract. Crit Care Med 19:1242–1246
93. Zwaveling JH, Maring JK, Klompmaker IJ, Haagsma EB, Bottema JT, Laseur M et al (2002) Selective decontamination of the digestive tract to prevent postoperative infection: a randomized placebo-controlled trial in liver transplant patients. Crit Care Med 30:1204–1209
94. Baxby D, van Saene HKF, Stoutenbeek CP et al (1996) Selective decontamination of the digestive tract: 13 years on, what it is and what it is not. Intensive Care Med 22:699–706
95. Laupland KB, Fisman DN (2009) Selective digestive tract decontamination: A tough pill to swallow. Can J Infect Dis Med Microbiol 20:9–11
96. Garrouste-Orgeas M, Marie O, Rouveau M et al (1996) Secondary carriage with multi-resistant *Acinetobacter baumannii* and *Klebsiella pneumoniae* in an adult ICU population: relationship with nosocomial infections and mortality. J Hosp Infect 34:279–289
97. Verma N, Clarke RW, Bolton-Maggs PHB et al (2007) Gut overgrowth of vancomycin-resistant enterococci (VRE) results in linezolid-resistant mutation in a child with severe congenital neutropenia. J Pediatr Hematol Oncol 29:557–560
98. Abecasis F, Kerr S, Sarginson RE et al (2007) Comment on: emergence of multidrug-resistant Gram-negative bacteria during selective decontaminiation of the digestive tract on an intensive care unit. J Antimicrob Chemother 60:445
99. Bodey GP (1981) Antibiotic prophylaxis in cancer patients: regimens of oral non-absorbable antibiotics for prevention of infection during induction of admission. Rev Infect Dis 3(Suppl):S259–S268
100. Brun-Buisson C, Legrand P, Philippon A et al (1987) Transferable enzymatic resistance to third-generation cephalosporins during nosocomial outbreak of multi-resistant Klebsiella pneumoniae. Lancet ii:302–306
101. Viviani M, van Saene HKF, Dezzoni R et al (2005) Control of imported and acquired methicillin-resistant *Staphylococcus aureus* (MRSA) in mechanically ventilated patients: a dose-response study of enteral vancomycin to reduce absolute carriage and infection. Anaesth Intensive Care 33:361–372
102. Cerda E, Abella A, de la Cal MA et al (2007) Enteral vancomycin controls methicillin-resistant *Staphylococcus aureus* endemicity in an intensive care burn unit: a 9-year prospective study. Ann Surg 245:397–407

103. Guerin F, Buu-Hoi A, Mainardi JL (2000) Outbreak of methicillin-resistant *Staphylococcus aureus* with reduced susceptibility to glycopeptides in a Parisian hospital. J Clin Microbiol 38:2985–2988
104. Pina P, Marliene C, Vandenesch F et al (2000) An outbreak of *Staphylococcus aureus* strains with reduced susceptibility to glycopeptides in a French general hospital. Clin Infect Dis 31:1306–1308
105. van Saene HKF, Damjanovic V, Pizer B et al (1999) Fungal infections in ICU. J Hosp Infect 41:337–340
106. Bozzette SA, Gordon RL, Yen A et al (1992) Biliary concentrations of fluconazole in a patient with candidal cholecytitis: case report. Clin Infect Dis 15:701–703
107. Martins MD, Rex JH (1996) Resistance to antifungal agents in the critical care setting: problems and perspectives. New Horiz 4:338–344
108. Rex JH, Rinaldi MG, Pfaller MA (1995) Resistance of *Candida* species to fluconazole. Antimicrob Agents Chemother 39:1–8
109. Malathum K, Murray BE (1999) Vancomycin-resistant enterococci: recent advances in genetics, epidemiology and therapeutic options. Drug Resiste Updat 2:224–243
110. Coque TM, Tomayko JF, Ricke SC et al (1996) Vancomycin-resistant enterococci from nosocomial, community, and animal sources in the United States. Antimicrob Ag Chemother 40:2605–2609
111. Currie BP, Lemos-Filho L (2004) Evidence for biliary excretion of vancomycin into stool during intravenous therapy: potential implications for rectal colonization with vancomycin-resistant enterococci. Antimicrob Ag Chemother 48:4427–4429
112. The Acute Respiratory Distress Syndrome Network (2000) Ventilation with lower tidal volumes as compared with traditional tidal volumes for acute lung injury and the acute respiratory distress syndrome. N Engl J Med 342:1301–1308
113. Bernard GR, Vincent JL, Laterre PF et al (2001) Efficacy and safety of recombinant human activated protein C for severe sepsis. N Engl J Med 344:699–709
114. Van den Berghe G, Wouters P, Weekers F et al (2001) Intensive insulin therapy in the critically ill patients. N Engl J Med 345:1359–1367
115. Annane D, Bellissant E, Bollaert P et al (2009) Corticosteroids in the treatment of severe sepsis and septic shock in adults: a systematic review. JAMA 301:2362–2375
116. Atkins D, Best D, Briss PA et al (2004) Grading quality of evidence and strength of recommendations. BMJ 328:1490–1494
117. Van den Berghe G, Wilmer A et al (2006) Intensive insulin therapy in the medical ICU. N Engl J Med 354:449–461
118. Preiser J, Devos P, Ruiz-Santana S et al (2009) A prospective randomised multi-centre controlled trial on tight glucose control by intensive insulin therapy in adult intensive care units: the Glucontrol study. Intensive Care Med 35:1738–1748
119. Brunkhorst FM, Engel C, Bloos F et al (2008) Intensive insulin therapy and pentastarch resuscitation in severe sepsis. N Engl J Med 358:125–139
120. The NICE-SUGAR Study Investigators (2009) Intensive versus conventional glucose control in critically ill patients. N Engl J Med 360(13):1283–1297
121. Wiener RC, Wiener RC, Larson RJ (2008) Benefits and risks of tight glucose control in critically ill adults: a meta-analysis. JAMA 300(8):933–944
122. Silvestri L, van Saene HKF, Weir I et al (2009) Survival benefit of the full selective digestive decontamination regimen. J Crit Care 24:474.e7–474.e14
123. Oostdijk EA, De Smet AM, Blok HE et al (2010) Ecological effects of selective decontamination on resistant Gram-negative bacterial colonization. Am J Respir Crit Care Med 181(5):452–457

ICU-Acquired Infection: Mortality, Morbidity, and Costs

29

J. C. Marshall and K. A. M. Marshall

29.1 Introduction

Nosocomial infection is a common complication of critical illness [1]. Ambiguities in diagnostic criteria and variation in patient demographics render reliable estimates of its prevalence imprecise, but infection is generally reported to complicate the course of between a quarter and a half of all intensive care unit (ICU) admissions [2–4] and to be associated with increased morbidity and mortality rates and costs. ICU-acquired infection, however, is not a random complication but, rather, one that affects the sickest and most vulnerable of patients, and it has been considered by many to be not so much a cause of morbidity as a reflection of the state of being critically ill [5, 6].

Decisions about optimal strategies for preventing and managing ICU-acquired infection hinge on assumptions about the attributable morbidity and costs of such infections, assumptions that are only tenuously grounded in robust data. The adoption of strategies to prevent nosocomial infection presupposes that these infections produce excess morbidity or generate increased costs of care; the decision to treat nosocomial infections assumes that eradicating infection will improve the patient's clinical status and so reduce morbidity. These assumptions, self-evident on initial inspection, require closer scrutiny. This chapter reviews the concepts of attributable morbidity, mortality, and costs of nosocomial ICU-acquired infection, with the objective of providing an informed basis for clinical decision making.

J. C. Marshall (✉)
Department of Surgery and Interdepartmental Division of Critical Care,
General Hospital and University of Toronto, Toronto, Canada
e-mail: MarshallJ@smh.ca

29.2 Outcome Analyses: Methodological Considerations

Estimating the impact of nosocomial infection on an outcome—whether mortality, morbidity, or cost—is a complex process, the conclusions of which are critically dependent on assumptions made by the investigator, on the variables considered in constructing the analytic model, and, in the case of cost analyses, whose perspective is being considered—the patient, the hospital, or society.

29.2.1 Crude and Attributable Mortality

ICUs concentrate a variety of life-sustaining technologies with the explicit objective of intervening to avert patient death. The implication, therefore, appears to be that mortality is an unequivocal measure of the success or failure of ICU care. However, a moment's reflection reveals the limitations inherent in such an assumption. First, mortality as an outcome measure is time dependent: whereas 1 h survival might be an appropriate measure of the effectiveness of an intervention during cardiac arrest, successful treatment for cancer is generally measured as 5-year survival. The duration of survival that best defines success or failure in the ICU is unclear. Regulatory agencies have adopted the philosophy that 28-day mortality is the best measure of the effectiveness of novel mediator-directed therapies [7]. However, a patient who dies in the ICU after 47 days can hardly be considered a treatment success, whereas another patient who survives an acute illness to be discharged from hospital on the 13th day but who dies when struck by a car while heading home does not really represent a treatment failure.

Second, mortality is of variable importance to ICU patients and their families [8]. Critical illness is often a complication of other diseases developing in an already compromised host. For the elderly patient whose health has been failing, death may be less a concern than the prospect of institutionalization and loss of independence. Finally, for the patient with multiple comorbid conditions, it may be very difficult to ascribe mortality to a specific condition. Is pneumonia that develops in the patient admitted with congestive heart failure, diabetes, and advanced chronic obstructive pulmonary disease the cause of death, or simply a reflection of the further deterioration of a tenuous state of health? The concept of attributable mortality attempts to define the incremental increase in mortality that results from the disease process of interest or the decrement in mortality that occurs as the consequence of an intervention.

The most reliable method of defining attributable mortality of nosocomial ICU-acquired infection is by means of a randomized control trial (RCT) of an intervention that reduces the risk of infection or that attenuates its severity. The technique of randomization ensures that patient characteristics and health care interventions that might independently impact on outcome—both those that are known and those that are unknown—are roughly equally distributed between the two populations. As the only variable that differs systematically between the two populations is the experimental intervention, documentation of differential survival between the study populations implicates the intervention as the cause of that difference.

Clinical trials are costly and time consuming, and alternate approaches have been used to derive estimates of attributable morbidity from observational data. The technique of logistic regression analysis relates an outcome (survival or death) to a number of potential explanatory factors (infection, acute severity of illness, premorbid health status, etc.). A univariate analysis is generally performed first to identify those variables associated with the outcome of interest. Those that are found to be predictive of outcome (a p value of 0.10 is typically chosen for this analysis) are then entered into a stepwise analysis that identifies the independent determinants of outcome by adjusting for the strongest prognostic variable to determine the independent contribution of the next most potent predictor variable. The process is then repeated until none of the remaining variables is significantly related to the outcome of interest. The conclusions drawn from such an analysis depend on the potential explanatory variables chosen, which in turn reflect the assumptions and biases of the investigator. For example, although the adequacy (or lack of) of antibiotic therapy is commonly considered as a potential explanatory variable for adverse outcome in nosocomial infection, the corollary—the effect of administering unnecessary antibiotics—is not, thus potentially biasing the analysis toward the conclusion that use of broad-spectrum antibiotics is an important determinant of outcome.

Another approach to quantifying attributable mortality entails the use of a matched cohort study. Each patient with the risk factor of interest is matched to a contemporaneous control with similar baseline characteristics but lacking the risk factor. If we are interested in the attributable mortality of bacteremia, for example, we might match each patient with bacteremia with a control patient whose age, gender, and admission acute physiology and chronic health evaluation (APACHE) II score was the same as our case. Such an approach can only control for the variables used in matching and may overestimate the attributable outcome because of the unrecognized influence of variables that are not used in the matching process. In our example, we would not be matching for events that occurred following ICU admission that might modify mortality risk, such as the development of renal failure or the need for prolonged mechanical ventilation. The use of a sensitivity analysis—altering the assumptions associated with the use and weighting of discrete variables—can increase one's confidence in the conclusions reached [9].

A variation on this technique was employed by Connors et al. [10] to estimate the mortality attributable to the use of a Swan Ganz catheter. Recognizing that there was considerable variability in the use of the catheter from one unit to the next, the authors developed a propensity score that reflected the factors that predicted use of the catheter in those units where it was used frequently. Patients in low-use units were then matched by propensity score, and the mortality rates of the two groups were compared. The authors' conclusion was that use of the right heart catheter was associated with an attributable increase in mortality of 24%. Once again, however, the conclusion is potentially biased by those variables that are not included in the matching process.

The most reliable method of quantifying outcomes attributable to a particular risk factor, however, is by means of an RCT. In an adequately powered study, randomization controls for both known and unknown confounding factors by distributing them equally between the two groups. Other methods of estimating the impact of a factor such as infection on outcome must be interpreted with caution [11].

29.3 Cost Analyses

Some general comments on economic analysis are in order prior to a consideration of the differing approaches to estimating therapy costs. Costs are inherently difficult to calculate. The cost of an intervention includes both explicit costs—the costs expended to achieve the outcome desired—and implicit costs—the potential revenues that are not realized as a result of the decision that is made. For example, an intervention that increases survival for an individual patient may increase ICU costs by limiting the admission of a less seriously ill patient who might have consumed fewer resources and brought in greater revenues from a payer. Usually, such implicit costs are not incorporated into analyses of the costs of medical therapy, for their perspective is not that of the patient but of the payer. Implicit costs, however, have a potent impact on decisions regarding whether a particular patient or population of patients will be cared for at a given institution and so shape patterns of delivery of care within the health system. Explicit costs include fixed costs—those such as staffing or building maintenance—that are incurred regardless of the specific intervention, and variable costs—those such as the costs of drugs, operative procedures, and radiological investigations that depend on the specific decisions made for a particular patient.

Four types of economic analysis are typically employed to compare treatments (Table 29.1) [12].

1. Cost-minimization analysis: proceeds from the assumption that two interventions result in comparable outcomes, and seeks—by enumerating the spectrum of costs associated with each alternative—to identify the one that results in the lowest costs. The units of analysis are monetary units: dollars, euros, etc.
2. Cost–benefit analysis: considers both the costs and the outcome in monetary units and so must assign a specific dollar value to the outcome to be achieved—the cost of a life or other clinical outcome—to create meaningful comparisons.
3. Cost-effectiveness analysis: considers the costs generated per unit of clinical benefit, for example, the cost per life saved or episode of pneumonia prevented.
4. Cost-utility analysis: uses a weighted measure of outcome—quality adjusted life years—to express costs incurred for a comparable degree of clinical benefit. This strategy permits comparison of the costs of very divergent therapies; for example, liver transplantation with ventilator-associated pneumonia (VAP) prevention. Utilities reflect the value placed on an outcome by patients and are developed using techniques such as a standard gamble, time tradeoff, or through administration of a questionnaire.

Table 29.1 Types of economic analyses (adapted from Second American Thoracic Society Workshop on Outcomes Research [12])

Type of study	Numerator (costs)	Denominator (outcome)	Comments
Cost minimization	Dollars	None	Compares costs of two or more therapies without consideration of consequences
Cost benefit	Dollars	Dollars	Converts clinical effects into associated costs
Cost-effectiveness	Dollars	Measure of clinical efficacy	Expresses costs in terms of outcome of intervention (e.g., cost per case of pneumonia prevented)
Cost utility	Dollars	Quality-adjusted life years	Expresses costs relative to a standardized estimate of benefit and so allows comparisons of differing therapies

Each approach recognizes that patient-centered values represent a compromise between the outcome achieved and the adverse consequences of the interventions required to achieve that outcome. Whereas a cost-utility analysis provides the most relevant measure of costs related to patient-centered outcomes, utilities are difficult to measure and are dependent on a number of highly subjective assumptions.

29.4 Attributable Mortality of ICU-Acquired Infection

The most compelling evidence that nosocomial ICU-acquired infection is responsible for increased morbidity and mortality rates derives from RCTs of selective decontamination of the digestive tract (SDD). The most recent meta-analysis from 2009, that of 6,914 patients enrolled in randomized trials of SDD, documented a significant reduction in mortality rates from 30 to 24% in patients receiving the prophylactic regimen, in association with a reduced odds ratio (OR) for developing pneumonia to 0.28 [95% confidence interval (CI) 0.20–0.38] [13]. Whereas it is possible that the benefits of the intervention arose for reasons other than preventing subsequent nosocomial infection (for example, treating occult community-acquired infection or reducing the absorption of endotoxin from the gastrointestinal tract), the most plausible interpretation of these data is that nosocomial infection is responsible for a relative increase in the risk of ICU mortality rates of 22% (an absolute 5% increase from a baseline risk of 24%). For surgical patients, a population in which comorbid diseases are less prevalent, the relative risk reduction is even greater [14], consistent with the hypothesis that the attributable morbidity and mortality of infection is greatest in patients with minimal concomitant risk factors for an adverse outcome.

Table 29.2 Attributable mortality of nosocomial infection in the intensive care unit (ICU)

Type of infection	Attributable mortality (%)
Bloodstream infection	0–50
Primary bacteremia	20
Catheter-related bacteremia	12
Secondary to nosocomial infection	55
Ventilator-associated pneumonia	20–30
Urinary tract infection	5

Attributable mortality is highly population dependent: for patient populations with minimal comorbidity; the signal attributable to an acute event is relatively greater than it is for patient populations with significant comorbidities. Thus, prophylactic strategies such as SDD show their greatest benefit in patients with no significant premorbid illness and acute physiological derangement that is only mild to moderate. Available estimates of attributable mortality of common ICU-acquired infections are summarized in Table 29.2.

29.4.1 Bloodstream Infections

A cohort study of primary bloodstream infections in ICU patients found an overall incidence of 1%, increasing to 4%—or 4.0 infections per 1,000 catheter-days—in patients with central venous catheters [15]. Similar figures have been reported for pediatric patients. Gray et al. [16] found an incidence of nosocomial bloodstream infection of 25/1,000 ICU admissions, or 6.8/1,000 bed-days. Crude mortality rates for patients with bloodstream infection were higher (26.5 vs. 8.1%); however, 87% of patients with these infections had significant underlying disease [16]. The mortality associated with ICU-acquired bacteremia, however, is higher in adults, with rates ranging from 43 to 53% [15, 17–19]. Premorbid illness, reflected, for example, in a "do not resuscitate" order, is an important independent predictor of mortality. However, bacteremia was also an independent risk factor for death in a study of 1,052 patients with severe sepsis or septic shock [20].

A French study of >2,000 critically ill patients reported that bacteremia occurs in 5% of patients who remain in the ICU for >48 h. When the episode of bacteremia was judged to be primary (no obvious focus), the excess mortality attributable to the event was 20%, whereas catheter-related bacteremia led to an excess mortality of 11.5%. When it was judged as secondary nosocomial bloodstream infection, the excess mortality attributable to the bacteremia was estimated to be 55%, and patients remained in the ICU for a median of 9.5 days longer [21]. In contrast, a study of 2,076 episodes of infection in surgical patients, employing logistic regression analysis to control for the potentially confounding influences of comorbidities, concluded that although associated with critical illness and death, bacteremia is not independently predictive of outcome but is, rather, a surrogate measure of underlying severity of illness [22]. Digiovine et al. [23], in a study of primary bacteremia in ICU patients, reported that when stratified by illness severity, bacteremic patients did not experience a higher mortality risk, although the length of ICU stay was extended by a median of 5 days [23]. Our own work suggests that when patients are stratified by the clinical severity of the inflammatory response, bacteremia per se does not contribute to adverse outcome but may, paradoxically, be associated with a superior outcome [3].

Several studies have attempted to evaluate the impact of bacteremia with particular pathogens on ICU outcome. Harbarth et al. [24] evaluated 1,835 episodes of Gram-negative bacteremia in Swiss hospitals and found that bacteremia caused by *Klebsiella* spp. or by *Pseudomonas aeruginosa*, but not by multidrug-resistant organisms, was associated with an elevated risk of death. Blot et al. [25] matched 53 patients with *P. aeruginosa* bacteremia to 106 controls based on APACHE II score and diagnosis. Hospital mortality was higher for cases (62.3 vs. 47.2%), but APACHE proved to be the only predictor of survival in a multivariate analysis. These investigators performed a similar study of 73 critically ill patients with candidemia and found that although candidemia was associated with a prolonged ICU and hospital stay, it did not increase the mortality risk, which was determined primarily by age, acute illness severity, and preexisting underlying disease [26]. In contrast, the authors found that bacteremia with methicillin-resistant *Staphylococcus aureus* (MRSA) carried a significantly elevated attributable mortality rate of 23.4% [27].

29.4.2 Ventilator-Associated Pneumonia

Fagon et al. [28] evaluated the impact of VAP on ICU outcome. They demonstrated a crude mortality rate of 52.4% for 328 patients developing pneumonia, significantly higher than the 22.4% ICU mortality experienced by the 1,650 patients who did not develop pneumonia. The APACHE II score, number of failing organs, presence of pneumonia, development of nosocomial bacteremia, presence of significant underlying disease, and admission from another ICU were all independently associated with adverse outcome by logistic regression analysis. Similarly, a French case–control study suggested that VAP was responsible for a twofold increase in mortality and a 5-day prolongation of ICU stay [29]. A Canadian study found that pneumonia was associated with an increased length of stay and a trend toward an increased mortality rate [9]. In contrast, a Spanish study of 1,000 consecutive ICU admissions found that the development of VAP increased the length of stay, but not the mortality rate, of ventilated ICU patients [30]. This conclusion was also reached by a French matched case–control study, which showed rates of VAP to be comparable in patients who died while in the ICU compared with those who survived, when matched on the basis of a panel of risk factors for adverse outcome [31]. A study of pneumonia complicating the course of acute respiratory distress syndrome reported that the development of VAP increases the duration of mechanical ventilation but does not adversely impact on patient survival [32]. Pooled data from a systematic review suggest that the development of VAP results in an increased ICU length of stay of 4 days and an attributable mortality rate of 20–30% [33].

29.4.3 Other Nosocomial Infections

There is little available evidence regarding the attributable morbidity and mortality rates of other nosocomial infections in critically ill patients. Urinary tract infections, although relatively common, are generally thought to be of only modest clinical significance. For example, an Argentinian study reported that catheter-related infections, the most common ICU-acquired infection (comprising 32% of all infections), carry an attributable mortality of 25% and are associated with an excess length of stay of 11 days. VAP (25% of all nosocomial infections) was associated with a 35% attributable mortality and a prolongation of ICU stay of 10 days. In contrast, urinary tract infections (23% of infections) had a 5% attributable mortality and an increased length of ICU stay of 5 days [34].

29.4.4 Summary: Attributable Mortality of ICU Infections

Estimates of the attributable mortality of the two most common nosocomial ICU-acquired infections—bacteremia and VAP—are highly variable depending on study methodology, country of origin, and criteria used to define an optimal control population. The most commonly used techniques of analysis—matched cohort studies or population studies using multivariate techniques to control for potential confounders—yield estimates that likely overestimate the true attributable morbidity, for they are unable to completely eliminate the effects of unmeasured confounders. Moreover, inherent uncertainty in the diagnostic criteria used to define nosocomial infections introduces substantial uncertainty into the estimate of attributable outcome. Estimates of attributable morbidity are generally limited to estimates of prolongation of ICU stay. These, however, uniformly indicate an increased burden of illness resulting from the development of infection.

Because of the uncertainty and bias inherent in retrospective studies, the most reliable estimates of the attributable mortality are those deriving from prospective randomized trials of interventions to prevent infection. Pooled data from trials of SDD suggest a 5% absolute and a 22% relative attributable mortality associated with ICU-acquired infection [13]. Even this estimate, however, must be interpreted with caution, for it is not possible to determine whether the increased risk arises from the infection or from the additional interventions undertaken to treat that infection. The distinction is subtle but important. Two RCTs of antibiotic minimization strategies in the ICU both demonstrated that antimicrobial resistance is minimized [35] and mortality reduced [36] when explicit diagnostic and therapeutic approaches are used to minimize antibiotic exposure in the patient with suspected VAP.

29.5 Costs of Nosocomial Infection

Reliable estimates of the costs of an ICU complication such as nosocomial infection are difficult to determine for the same reasons that attributable outcomes are difficult to estimate. However, if we adopt the plausible assumption that there is at least some degree of mortality and morbidity attributable to the development of a nosocomial infection, it follows that interventions that can prevent infection can reduce that toll: whether they are worth the cost is the domain of cost-effectiveness analysis.

Cost-effectiveness analysis is predicated on the assumption that an intervention has an effect, and reflects the tradeoff that must be made between the cost of an intervention and the extent to which clinical benefit is achieved. In Fig. 29.1, the cost-effectiveness of a variety of ICU therapies is presented. Increasing cost is represented on the y axis, increasing benefit on the x axis. Obviously, the ideal therapy would be one that reduced costs while bringing increased benefit to the patient, the situation reflected in the lower right quadrant of the graph and exemplified by the use of a lower transfusion threshold in the anemic critically ill patient [37]. An intervention such as the use of activated protein C brings clinical benefit but at a substantial cost [38], whereas the use of growth hormone increases costs and morbidity [39] and so is clearly undesirable. It will be appreciated that ascertainment of the net costs and benefits is challenging and that the results are both qualitative and potentially controversial.

The perspective of the analysis also differs depending upon whether the primary effect of the intervention is to treat a disease or to prevent its occurrence. If we assume that measures taken to prevent a disease will have few or no consequences on long-term health-related quality of life but that the treatment of a disease will not necessarily restore a patient to his or her full premorbid state of health, then the tradeoff in prevention is the cost of the intervention against the percentage of patients who might develop the complication. The tradeoff for a therapeutic measure is the cost of the intervention against the predicted improvement in health-related quality of life. The former is a cost-effectiveness analysis, the latter a cost-utility analysis.

29.5.1 Costs of ICU-Acquired Infection

Several authors have attempted to generate estimates of the costs associated with infection in critically ill patients. Angus et al. [40] used administrative data to generate an estimate that there are approximately 750,000 new cases of severe sepsis (sepsis in association with organ dysfunction) in the United States each year and that the total costs attributable to these are US $16.7 billion annually. However, these estimates include cases of community-acquired sepsis and sepsis developing in patients who are not in an ICU, and they fail to include the costs of episodes of nosocomial ICU-acquired infection that do not meet the criteria for severe sepsis. Brun-Buisson et al. [41] found that the costs of sepsis in association with

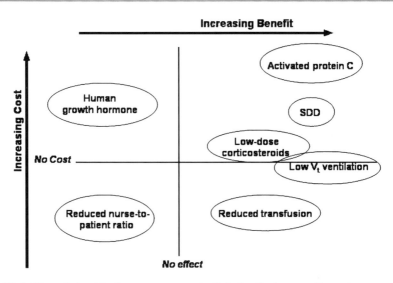

Fig. 29.1 The relationship between cost and clinical effectiveness. Increasing costs are represented on the y axis, with increasing clinical benefit on the x axis. Examples shown are approximations of the incremental cost associated with increased (or reduced) clinical benefit

ICU-acquired infection were three times higher than those incurred when sepsis was present at the time of ICU admission. The total costs were approximately 40,000 € for each patient developing sepsis in the ICU. Nosocomial infection complicating community-acquired sepsis increased costs by 2.5 times. These observations mirror those of a British study that found a fivefold increase in costs when patients developing sepsis after the second day of their ICU stay were compared with patients admitted with a diagnosis of sepsis [42]. Thus, preventing nosocomial infection in the ICU has the potential to significantly impact on the costs of ICU care.

29.5.2 Nosocomial Bacteremia

Pittet et al. [43] reported that nosocomial bloodstream infections complicate the course of 3% of patients admitted to an ICU and prolong both the ICU and hospital stay, generating costs of approximately US $40,000 per survivor. Similar estimates have been derived by others. Digiovine et al. [23], for example, found that although nosocomial bloodstream infection in the ICU did not increase mortality rates, it was associated with increased direct costs of US $34,508 per episode, whereas Dimick et al. (unpublished data) suggested that catheter-related bloodstream infection in the ICU results in increased total hospital costs of US $56,167 per case. Two analyses concluded that the use of antibiotic-coated catheters is cost effective in preventing nosocomial bloodstream infections [44, 45]. However, the conclusion is highly dependent on the estimate of the efficacy of such catheters, and intrinsic limitations in the design of the studies evaluating them limit the estimate of their benefits [46].

29.5.3 Ventilator-Associated Pneumonia

Warren et al. [47] estimated the attributable cost of an episode of VAP in the United States to be approximately US $12,000. Because a variety of prophylactic strategies have been shown to be effective in preventing VAP [48], and because these are generally relatively inexpensive to institute, VAP prevention is readily demonstrable to be cost effective. Zack et al. [49], for example, showed that instituting a comprehensive preventive program resulted in a 57.6% reduction in VAP rate and in cost savings of as much as US $4 million/year. Other strategies, such as minimizing intubation through the use of noninvasive positive-pressure ventilation [50] and reducing the frequency of ventilator circuit changes [51] are also cost effective.

29.5.4 Infection with Antibiotic-Resistant Organisms

Independent of infection site, nosocomial infection with resistant organisms is associated with increased costs [52]. Chaix et al. [53] undertook a case–control study of patients with MRSA and reported that the attributable costs of such infections were US $9,275 per episode. An infection control program that could lower transmission by 14% or more was calculated to be cost effective. Infection with Enterobacter spp. resistant to third-generation cephalosporins was associated with an attributable cost of US $29,379 per case [54]. Divergent conclusions have been drawn with respect to infection with vancomycin-resistant enterococci (VRE). Whereas one matched cohort study suggested an 11% increase in mortality rates and increased hospital costs of more than US $20,000 per case [55], a second study using stepwise logistic regression analysis failed to demonstrate that such infections were associated with either attributable morbidity or increased costs [56].

Because indiscriminate antibiotic use is a risk factor for the emergence of resistance, implementation of restrictive antimicrobial prescribing practices cannot only reduce costs but also limit the development of resistance in an ICU environment [35, 57].

29.6 Costs of Effective Treatment

Our focus has been on infectious complications that are amenable to prevention, in no small part because there are few proven effective therapies for infection in the ICU. Thus, although it is widely believed that specific antimicrobial therapy, adequate surgical source control, and the spectrum of supportive measures that comprise ICU care will improve clinical outcome, the attributable effect of any of

Table 29.3 Proven and promising strategies to reduce the morbidity and cost of ICU-acquired infection

Strategy	Examples
Prevent abnormal colonization	Selective digestive tract decontamination Minimize antibiotic exposure Enteral feeding
Reduce device-related infection	Antibiotic-coated catheters Noninvasive ventilation Coated endotracheal tubes or Foley catheters Reduced frequency of ventilator circuit changes
Prevent aspiration	Semi-recumbent positioning

these in the patient with infection is unknown, and therefore cost-utility analyses are impossible.

The approval of activated protein C for treating patients with severe sepsis has provided the first opportunity for cost-utility analyses in critically ill infected patients. Treatment with activated protein C has been shown in a cohort of patients with severe sepsis to reduce mortality rates by 6.1% but at a cost of approximately US $7,000 per course of therapy. Two independent analyses of the cost-effectiveness of activated protein C show a favorable profile when it is used in the sickest patients. Manns et al. [38] calculated the cost per life-year gained to be US $27,936 for all patients in the cohort, whereas Angus et al. [58] suggested that the cost-utility of activated protein C is US $48,800 per quality-adjusted life year.

29.7 Conclusions

The development of nosocomial infection in the critically ill patient results in increased morbidity and significantly increases the costs of care. Although the magnitude of both effects is difficult to know with certainty, it is clear that measures that can prevent nosocomial infection in the critically ill patient can both reduce costs and improve clinical outcomes (Table 29.3). More rigorous evaluation of the economic impact of these is needed.

References

1. National Nosocomial Infections Surveillance System (NNIS) (2002) System report, data summary from January 1992 to June 1992, issued August 2002. Am J Infect Control 30:458–475
2. Richards MJ, Edwards JR, Culver DH et al (1999) Nosocomial infections in medical intensive care units in the United States. National nosocomial infections surveillance system. Crit Care Med 27:887–892
3. Marshall JC, Sweeney D (1990) Microbial infection and the septic response in critical surgical illness. Sepsis, not infection, determines outcome. Arch Surg 125:17–23

4. Ponce de Leon-Rosales SP, Molinar-Ramos F, Dominguez-Cherit G et al (2000) Prevalence of infections in intensive care units in Mexico: a multicenter study. Crit Care Med 28:1316–1321
5. Fagon JY, Novara A, Stephan F et al (1994) Mortality attributable to nosocomial infections in the ICU. Infect Control Hosp Epidemiol 15:428–434
6. Nathens AB, Chu PTY, Marshall JC (1992) Nosocomial infection in the surgical intensive care unit. Infect Dis Clin North Am 6:657
7. Schwieterman W, Roberts R (1997) FDA perspective on study design for therapies for severe sepsis. Sepsis 1:69
8. Patrick DL, Pearlman RA, Starks HE et al (1997) Validation of preferences for life-sustaining treatment: implications for advance care planning. Ann Intern Med 127:509–517
9. Heyland DK, Cook DJ, Griffith L, Keenan SP, Brun-Buisson C (1999) The attributable morbidity and mortality of ventilator-associated pneumonia in the critically ill patient. Am J Respir Crit Care Med 159:1249–1256
10. Connors AF Jr, Speroff T, Dawson NV et al (1996) The effectiveness of right heart catheterization in the initial care of critically ill patients. JAMA 276:889–918
11. Asensio A, Torres J (1999) Quantifying excess length of postoperative stay attributable to infections: a comparison of methods. J Clin Epidemiol 52:1249–1256
12. Second American Thoracic Society Workshop on Outcomes Research (2002) Understanding costs and cost-effectiveness in critical care. Am J Respir Crit Care Med 165:540–550
13. Liberati A, D'Amico R, Pifferi S et al (2009) Antibiotic prophylaxis to reduce respiratory tract infections and mortality in adults receiving intensive care (Cochrane Review). In: The Cochrane library, issue 1. Wiley, Chichester
14. Nathens AB, Marshall JC (1999) Selective decontamination of the digestive tract in surgical patients. Arch Surg 134:170–176
15. Warren DK, Zack JE, Elward AM et al (2001) Nosocomial primary bloodstream infections in intensive care unit patients in a non-teaching community medical center: a 21-month prospective study. Clin Infect Dis 33:1329–1335
16. Gray J, Gossain S, Morris K (2001) Three-year survey of bacteremia and fungemia in a pediatric intensive care unit. Pediatr Infect Dis J 20:416–421
17. Jamal WY, El-Din K, Rotimi VO, Chugh TD (1999) An analysis of hospital-acquired bacteraemia in intensive care unit patients in a university hospital in Kuwait. J Hosp Infect 43:49–56
18. Crowe M, Ispahani P, Humphreys H et al (1998) Bacteraemia in the adult intensive care unit of a teaching hospital in Nottingham, UK, 1985–1996. Eur J Clin Microbiol Infect Dis 17:377–384
19. Pittet D, Thievent B, Wenzel RP et al (1996) Bedside prediction of mortality from bacteremic sepsis. A dynamic analysis of ICU patients. Am J Respir Crit Care Med 153:684–693
20. Brun-Buisson C, Doyon F, Carlet J et al (1995) Incidence, risk factors, and outcomes of severe sepsis and septic shock in adults. A multicenter prospective study in intensive care units. JAMA 274:968–974
21. Renaud B, Brun-Buisson C (2001) Outcomes of primary and catheter-related bacteremia. A cohort and case-control study in critically ill patients. Am J Respir Crit Care Med 163:1584–1590
22. Raymond DP, Pelletier SJ, Crabtree TD, Gleason TG, Pruett TL, Sawyer RG (2001) Impact of bloodstream infection on outcomes among infected surgical inpatients. Ann Surg 233:549–555
23. Digiovine B, Chenoweth C, Watts C, Higgins M (1999) The attributable mortality and costs of primary nosocomial bloodstream infections in the intensive care unit. Am J Respir Crit Care Med 160:976–981
24. Harbarth S, Rohner P, Auckenthaler R et al (1999) Impact and pattern of gram-negative bacteraemia during 6 y at a large university hospital. Scand J Infect Dis 31:163–168
25. Blot S, Vandewoude K, Hoste E, Colardyn F (2003) Reappraisal of attributable mortality in critically ill patients with nosocomial bacteraemia involving *Pseudomonas aeruginosa*. J Hosp Infect 53:18–24
26. Blot SI, Vandewoude KH, Hoste EA, Colardyn FA (2002) Effects of nosocomial candidemia on outcomes of critically ill patients. Am J Med 113:480–485

27. Blot SI, Vandewoude KH, Hoste EA, Colardyn FA (2002) Outcome and attributable mortality in critically ill patients with bacteremia involving methicillin-susceptible and methicillin-resistant *Staphylococcus aureus*. Arch Intern Med 162:2229–2235
28. Fagon J-Y, Chastre J, Vuagnat A et al (1996) Nosocomial pneumonia and mortality among patients in intensive care units. JAMA 275:866–869
29. Bercault N, Boulain T (2001) Mortality rate attributable to ventilator-associated nosocomial pneumonia in an adult intensive care unit: a prospective case-control study. Crit Care Med 29:2303–2309
30. Rello J, Quintana E, Ausina V et al (1991) Incidence, etiology, and outcome of nosocomial pneumonia in mechanically ventilated patients. Chest 100:439–444
31. Bregeon F, Ciais V, Carret V et al (2001) Is ventilator-associated pneumonia an independent risk factor for death? Anesthesiology 94:554–560
32. Markowicz P, Wolff M, Djedaini K et al (2000) Multicenter prospective study of ventilator-associated pneumonia during acute respiratory distress syndrome. Am J Respir Crit Care Med 161:1942–1948
33. Cook D (2000) Ventilator associated pneumonia: perspectives on the burden of illness. Intensive Care Med 26(1):S31–S37
34. Rosenthal VD, Guzman S, Orellano PW (2003) Nosocomial infections in medical-surgical intensive care units in Argentina: attributable mortality and length of stay. Am J Infect Control 31:291–295
35. Singh N, Rogers P, Atwood CW et al (2000) Short-course empiric antibiotic therapy for patients with pulmonary infiltrates in the intensive care unit. A proposed solution for indiscriminate antibiotic prescription. Am J Respir Crit Care Med 162:505–511
36. Fagon J-Y, Chastre J, Wolff M et al (2000) Invasive and noninvasive strategies for management of suspected ventilator-associated pneumonia. A randomized trial. Ann Intern Med 132:621–630
37. Hebert PC, Wells G, Blajchman MA et al (1999) A multicentre randomized controlled clinical trial of transfusion requirements in critical care. N Engl J Med 340:409–417
38. Manns BJ, Lee H, Doig CJ et al (2002) An economic evaluation of activated protein C treatment for severe sepsis. N Engl J Med 347:993–1000
39. Takala J, Ruokonen E, Webster NR et al (1999) Increased mortality associated with growth hormone treatment in critically ill adults. N Engl J Med 341:785–792
40. Angus DC, Linde-Zwirble WT, Lidicker J et al (2001) Epidemiology of severe sepsis in the United States: analysis of incidence, outcome, and associated costs of care. Crit Care Med 29:1303–1310
41. Brun-Buisson C, Roudot-Thoaval F, Girou E et al (2003) The costs of septic syndromes in the intensive care unit and influence of hospital-acquired sepsis. Intensive Care Med 29:1464–1471
42. Edbrooke DL, Hibbert CL, Kingsley JM et al (1999) The patient-related costs of care for sepsis patients in a United Kingdom adult general intensive care unit. Crit Care Med 27:1760–1767
43. Pittet D, Tarara D, Wenzel RP (1994) Nosocomial bloodstream infection in critically ill patients. Excess length of stay, extra costs, and attributable mortality. JAMA 271:1598–1601
44. Shorr AF, Humphreys CW, Helman DL (2003) New choices for central venous catheters: potential financial implications. Chest 124:275–284
45. Marciante KD, Veensra DL, Lipsky BA, Sainst S (2003) Which antimicrobial impregnated central venous catheter should we use? modeling the costs and outcomes of antimicrobial catheter use. Am J Infect Control 31:1–8
46. McConnell SA, Gubbins PO, Anaissie EJ (2003) Do antimicrobial-impregnated central venous catheters prevent catheter-related bloodstream infection? Clin Infect Dis 37:65–72

47. Warren DK, Shukla SJ, Olsen MA et al (2003) Outcome and attributable cost of ventilator-associated pneumonia among intensive care unit patients in a suburban medical center. Crit Care Med 31:1312–1317
48. Kollef MH (1999) The prevention of ventilator-associated pneumonia. N Engl J Med 340:627–634
49. Zack JE, Garrison T, Trovillion E et al (2002) Effect of an education program aimed at reducing the occurrence of ventilator-associated pneumonia. Crit Care Med 30:2407–2412
50. Sinuff T, Cook DJ (2003) Health technology assessment in the ICU: noninvasive positive pressure ventilation for acute respiratory failure. J Crit Care 18:59–67
51. Kotilainen HR, Keroack MA (1997) Cost analysis and clinical impact of weekly ventilator circuit changes in patients in intensive care unit. Am J Infect Control 25:117–120
52. Niederman MS (2001) Impact of antibiotic resistance on clinical outcomes and the cost of care. Crit Care Med 29(Suppl):N114–N120
53. Chaix C, Durand-Zaleski I, Alberti C, Brun-Buisson C (1999) Control of endemic methicillin-resistant *Staphylococcus aureus*: a cost-benefit analysis in an intensive care unit. JAMA 282:1745–1751
54. Cosgrove SE, Kaye KS, Eliopoulos GM, Carmeli Y (2002) Health and economic outcomes of the emergence of third-generation cephalosporin resistance in *Enterobacter species*. Arch Intern Med 162:185–190
55. Carmeli Y, Eliopoulos G, Mozaffari E, Samore M (2002) Health and economic outcomes of vancomycin-resistant enterococci. Arch Intern Med 162:2223–2228
56. Pelz RK, Lipsett PA, Swoboda SM et al (2002) Vancomycin-sensitive and vancomycin-resistant enterococcal infections in the ICU: attributable costs and outcomes. Intensive Care Med 28:692–697
57. Bantar C, Sartori B, Vesco E et al (2003) A hospital-wide intervention program to optimize the quality of antibiotic use: impact on prescribing practice, antibitoic consumption, cost savings, and bacterial resistance. Clin Infect Dis 37:180–186
58. Angus DC, Linde-Zwirble WT, Clermont G et al (2003) Cost-effectiveness of drotrecogin alfa (activated) in the treatment of severe sepsis. Crit Care Med 31:1–11

Evidence-Based Medicine in ICU 30

A. J. Petros, K. G. Lowry, H. K. F. van Saene and J. C. Marshall

30.1 Introduction

Evidence-based medicine (EBM) was extolled by David Sackett, who described two processes: one for assessing the quality of a therapy on a scale of 1–4, and a second for making recommendations for using that therapy on a scale of A–D. However, more recently, a newer method of grading the quality of evidence and strength of recommendation for a new therapy has been developed. The Grading of Recommendations Assessment, Development and Evaluation (GRADE) Working Group reported its suggestions in 2004, with further refinement in 2008 [1, 2]. The use of a structured approach to collect, analyse and summarise all the relevant evidence allows the production of grades of recommendations. GRADE is being increasingly used as the structure on which to develop guidelines [3] and is used widely by the World Health Organization, the American College of Physicians, the American Thoracic Society, the Cochrane Collaboration and many other organisations, with up to 25 groups demonstrating GRADE's success as a methodology [4].

GRADE guides assessment of the quality of evidence for a particular treatment or therapy in one of four levels—high (A), moderate (B), low (C) and very low (D). Study design, quality, consistency and directness are all assessed. The factors influencing the decision on quality are described in Table 30.1. Evidence from randomised controlled trials (RCTs) contributes to high-quality evidence, but confidence in that evidence may be decreased for several reasons: study limitations; inconsistent results; indirectness of evidence; imprecision; reporting bias [1] (Table 30.1). Observational studies, such as cohort and case-control studies, start with a low-quality rating; grading upwards may be possible if, for example,

A. J. Petros (✉)
PICU, Great Ormond Street Hospital, London, UK
e-mail: petroa@gosh.nhs.uk

Table 30.1 Descriptions of levels and quality used in the GRADE system

Quality, and confidence in the quality, of GRADE evidence		
Quality	Level	Description
High quality	A	Further research is very unlikely to change our confidence in the estimate of effect. Randomized control trials
Moderate quality	B	Further research is likely to have an important impact on our confidence in the estimate of effect and may change the estimate
Low quality	C	Further research is very likely to have an important impact on our confidence in the estimate of effect and is likely to change the estimate. Observational studies
Very low quality	D	Any estimate of effect is very uncertain. Any other evidence
Confidence in the quality of evidence used in GRADE		
Decreases if		
Serious (−1) or very serious (−2) limitation to study quality		
Important inconsistency (−1)		
Some (−1) or major (−2) uncertainty about directness		
Imprecise or sparse data (−1)		
High probability of reporting bias (−1)		
Increases grade if		
Strong evidence of association: significant relative risk of >2 (<0.5) based on consistent evidence from two or more observational studies, with no plausible confounders (+1)		
Very strong evidence of association: significant relative risk of >5 (<0.2) based on direct evidence, with no major threats to validity (+2)		
Evidence of a dose-response gradient (+1)		
All plausible confounders would have reduced the effect (+1)		

the size of the treatment effect is very large, or if there is a strong causal relationship. GRADE also makes recommendations from strong (1) to weak (2). The former is where the intervention clearly outweighs its undesirable effects and the latter where the trade-off between desirable and undesirable effects is less clear. Making recommendations for a specific therapy involves a balance between benefits and harms and inevitably involves placing a relative value on each outcome, though it is difficult to judge how much weight to give to different outcomes [1]. In making a recommendation, four main factors should be considered [1] (Table 30.2):
- trade-offs—these should consider the estimated size of the effect for the main outcomes, confidence limits around those estimates, and relative values placed on each outcome;
- quality of evidence;

Table 30.2 Recommendations by the GRADE system

Recommendations	
Net benefits	The intervention clearly does more good than harm
Trade-offs	There are important trade-offs between benefits and harms
Uncertain trade-offs	It is not clear whether the intervention does more good than harm
No net benefits	The intervention clearly does not do more good than harm

- translation of evidence into specific practice, allowing for factors that could qualify the expected effect, such as proximity to a hospital or availability of necessary expertise;
- uncertainty about the baseline risk for the population of interest.

The strong or weak grading is felt to be of greater clinical important than classifying the quality of the intervention.

Using GRADE provides a framework for structured assessment and can help ensure that appropriate judgments are made about a new therapy or manoeuvre. We screened intensive care unit (ICU) literature using these GRADE rules for manoeuvres that may impact on infectious morbidity and mortality rates and classified the most common manoeuvres according to levels of evidence and grades of recommendations (Table 30.3).

30.2 Infection-Control Manoeuvres: Nonantibiotic Interventions

30.2.1 Hand Washing, Isolation, Protective Clothing, Equipment Care and Environment

It has never been shown in a RCT that hand hygiene prevents pneumonia and reduces mortality rates in ventilated patients. The efficacy of hand hygiene on the incidence of infection was studied in eight nonrandomised studies [5–12] (Table 30.4); however, the incidence of pneumonia was not presented. The only study demonstrating an impact on mortality due to hand hygiene was the cohort study of Semmelweis in 1861 in postpartum women for reducing mortality due to puerperal sepsis, with a decrease from 11 to 3% [13]. There are no data available on the effect of isolation, protective clothing, equipment care and environment on pneumonia and mortality rates in ventilated patients.

These five traditional infection control measures target microorganism transmission via carriers' hands. Although they are important, the impact should not be overestimated. An optimal infection-control policy can only reduce infections due to microorganisms acquired in the ICU, i.e. secondary endogenous and exogenous infections. They fail to influence primary endogenous infections due to

Table 30.3 Analysis of the literature, grading of evidence and recommendations for controlling morbidity and mortality rates due to infection in ventilated patients in the intensive care unit

	Reduced infection		Reduced mortality	
	Level of evidence	Grade of recommendation	Level of evidence	Grade of recommendation
Nonantibiotic interventions				
Handwashing/isolation/protective clothing/care of equipment and environment	2	D	2	D
Positioning				
Rotation therapy	None	None	None	None
Semi-recumbent position	None	None	None	None
Subglottic secretion drainage	None	None	None	None
Oral antiseptic decontamination	None	None	None	None
Immunomodulation				
Steroids	1	A	None	None
Immunoglobulins	None	None	1	B
Activated protein-C	None	None	2	C
Anti-inflammatory modulators	None	None	1	B
	None	None	1	A
Antibiotic interventions				
Selective Decontamination of the Digestive Tract (SDD) (four-component)	1	A	1	A

Level: *1–4*; Grade: *A* high, *B* moderate, *C* low, *D* very low

microorganism present in admission flora. This type of infection is the major infection problem in the ICU, varying between 60 and 85%.

30.2.2 Positional Therapy

30.2.2.1 Rotational Therapy

Severely ill patients who require ventilation are traditionally treated in the supine position. This leads to collapse of the lower parts of the lung and reduced clearance of lower-airway secretions. These two factors increase the risk of pneumonia. Theoretically, treating a patient in a specialised rotating bed in which the patient is continuously rotated from -40 to $+40°$ around their longitudinal axis could help prevent pneumonia. One meta-analysis of six RCTs and two RCTs [14–16] indicated a significant reduction in pneumonia in patients who received rotational therapy. Of the six studies, five were performed in surgical or neurological patients. The sixth trial, in which no reduction in pneumonia was found, involved nonsurgical ICU patients; a more recent RCT in a mixed ICU population did not

Table 30.4 Studies into the effect of hand hygiene on the incidence of nosocomial infections, including pneumonia

Author	Year	Study design	No.	Outcome: infectious morbidity	Evidence
Casewell [5]	1977	Sequential	Not mentioned	Significant reduction in nosocomial infections during *Klebsiella* outbreak Effect on pneumonia not mentioned	2D
Massanari [6]	1984	Crossover	5,859	Significant reduction of nosocomial infection on some ICUs Effect on pneumonia not mentioned	2A
Maki [7]	1989	Crossover	Not mentioned	Significant reduction of nosocomial infection on some ICUs Effect on pneumonia not mentioned	2B
Simmons [8]	1990	Historically controlled	Not mentioned	No effect	2D
Doebbeling [9]	1992	Crossover	1,894	Significant reduction of nosocomial infection on some ICUs No effect on pneumonia	2A
Webster [10]	1994	Sequential	Not mentioned	Control of MRSA outbreak. Significant reduction of nosocomial infections	2D
Koss [11]	2001	Prospective, randomised	153	No effect on pneumonia	2A
Slota [12]	2001	Prospective, randomised	98	No effect on pneumonia	2A

MRSA methicillin-resistant *Staphylococcus aureus*

Table 30.5 Randomised controlled trials and meta-analyses into the effect of nonantibiotic interventions on pneumonia and mortality rates in ventilated patients

Manoeuvre	Author	Year	Study Design	No.	Pneumonia	Mortality	Evidence
Rotation therapy	Choi [14]	1992	MA 6 studies	419	RR 0.50 $P = 0.002$	No difference	2A
	Traver [16]	1995	RCT	103	RR 0.62 $P = 0.21$	RR 0.62 $P = 0.21$	2A
Semirecumbent position	Silvestri [21]	2010	MA 3 studies	337	OR, 0.59; 95% (0.15–2.35) ($P = 0.45$)	OR 0.86 (0.54–1.37) ($P = 0.53$)	1A
	Van Saene [54]	2009	MA 2 studies	311	OR 0.56 (0.06–5.54)	OR 0.81 (0.47–1.41)	1A
Subglottic suction drainage	Dezfoulian [32]	2005	MA 5 studies	896	RR 0.5 (0.35–0.71) ($P < 0.001$)	Not significant	1A
	Silvestri L [33]	2008	MA 9 studies	1953	OR 0.43 (0.32–0.58) ($P < 0.001$)	OR 0.93 (0.71–1.21) ($P = 0.57$)	1A
	Van Saene [54]	2009	MA 7 studies	1178	OR 0.40 (0.28–0.56)	OR 0.99 (0.71–1.38)	1A

(continued)

Table 30.5 (continued)

Manoeuvre	Author	Year	Study Design	No.	Pneumonia	Mortality	Evidence
Oropharyngeal decontamination using antiseptics	Pineda [50]	2006	MA 4 studies	1202	OR 0.42 (0.16–1.06)	OR 0.77 (0.28–2.11)	1A
	Chlebicki [51]	2007	MA 7 studies	1650	RR 0.70 (0.47–1.04) ($P = 0.83$)	RR 1.07 (0.76–1.51) ($P = 0.69$)	1A
	Chan [52]	2007	MA 7 studies	2144	RR 0.56 (0.39–0.81)	RR 0.96 (0.69–1.33)	1A
	Kola [53]	2007	MA 7 studies		RR 0.58 (0.45–0.74)	Not significnat	1A
	van Saene [54]	2009	MA 11 studies	2752	OR 0.49 (0.35–0.67)	OR 0.98 (0.64–1.50)	1A
	Carvajal [55]	2010	MA 10 studies		OR 0.56 (0.44–0.73)	Not significant	1A

RCT randomised controlled trial, *MA* meta-analysis, *SR* systematic review, *RR* relative risk (95% confidence intervals)

support the meta-analysis. Rotational therapy requires special beds, is associated with considerable costs and is unpleasant for the patient; a cost-effective analysis is not available.

30.2.2.2 Semirecumbent Position

Although in general the throat has been considered internal source of potential pathogenic microorganisms (PPMs) causing pneumonia, some believe that aspiration of PPMs carried in the stomach may play a role, the so called stomach–lung route [17]. Based on this concept, ventilating patients in a semirecumbent position is thought to have a beneficial effect on reducing the incidence of reflux and aspiration from the stomach, whereby pneumonia in ventilated patients could be prevented. This manoeuvre has been investigated in three RCTs [18–20] (Table 30.5). The first shows a significant reduction in pneumonia. Mortality rates however, were identical in both test and control group. Patients who underwent abdominal or neurosurgery, patients with refractory shock and patients who were readmitted to ICU within 1 month were excluded. The second RCT, published in abstract form, failed to confirm these results. There was no difference in pneumonia or mortality rates. Treating ventilated ICU patients in a semirecumbent position at an angle of 45° is difficult in practice and is often associated with frequent changes in patient position. Keeley [20] was unable to demonstrate any reduction in ventilator-associated pneumonia (VAP) in patients nursed at 45° ($P < 0.176$). Meta-analysis of these studies reveals no significant impact on VAP by this manoeuvre; cost was not reported [21].

30.2.3 Continuous Aspiration of Subglottic Secretions

Stasis of saliva contaminated with potential pathogens above the cuff on the endotracheal tube increase the risk of aspiration pneumonia. Removing and preventing this salivary stasis using continuous aspiration via a specially designed endotracheal tube is thought to prevent pneumonia. The intervention of subglottic secretion drainage (SSD) was evaluated in ten RCTs [22–31] performed in a mixed ICU population requiring ventilation for >72 h, and the fourth study in cardiac surgery patients. Results were not consistent. Two studies showed a significant reduction in pneumonia; the other two failed to show any impact on pneumonia during ventilation. There was no difference in mortality rates between test and control groups in any of these studies. Although the specially designed tubes and suction equipment are expensive, this technique has been suggested to be cost effective on theoretical grounds. There were no harmful side effects associated with this manoeuvre in any of the studies. Bo et al. found that the presence of subglottic secretion may be an origin of the pathogenetic organisms of VAP [27]. The morbidity rate of VAP in mechanically ventilated patients can be reduced by SSD. Liu et al. confirmed that migration of the dominant bacteria of the subglottic secretion was one of the important factors for ventilator-associated lower airway infection [28]. Concentration of bacteria in subglottic secretion was significantly reduced by subglottic secretion drainage when SSD was used, and SSD reduced the incidence of ventilator-associated airway infection and pneumonia in patients ventilated for <5 days. Zheng et al. supported these conclusions [30]. However, Lorente et al. found that the use of an endotracheal tube with polyurethane cuff and subglottic secretion drainage helps prevent early- and late-onset VAP [29]. Bouza et al. demonstrated that continuous aspiration of subglottic secretions reduces the incidence of VAP in at-risk patients [31].

There are two meta-analyses [32, 33]: Dezfulian et al. reported on five RCTs involving 896 patients [32]. They found that SSD reduced the incidence of VAP by nearly 50% (relative risk (RR) 0.51; 0.37–0.71) by reducing early-onset pneumonia (occurring within 5–7 days after intubation). SSD also shortened the duration of mechanical ventilation by 2 days and the length of ICU stay by 3 days; it also delayed the onset of pneumonia by 6.8 days. The authors concluded that SSD appears effective in preventing early-onset VAP among patients expected to require >72 h of mechanical ventilation. Silvestri et al. analysed ten RCTs of SSD [33] (Table 30.5), nine of which reported results on pneumonia rates. In 1,953 patients studied, there was a 57% reduction in VAP [odds ratio (OR) 0.43, 95% confidence interval (CI) 0.32–0.58; $P < 0.001$] in 1,846 patients in seven RCTs but no effect on mortality rates. Subglottic drainage seems to be effective in preventing VAP, though subgroup analysis revealed it was not effective in cardiac surgery patients.

30.2.4 Oropharyngeal Decontamination Using Antiseptics

There are 16 RCTs that report varying degrees of success with oropharyngeal decontamination using antiseptics [34–49]. However, the outcome of six meta-analyses revealed that antiseptic usage has no benefit in reducing pneumonia or mortality rates [50–55] (Table 30.5). In 1,202 patients, Pineda et al. [50] reported that use of oral decontamination with chlorhexidine did not result in significant reduction in the incidence of nosocomial pneumonia in patients who received mechanical ventilation, and it did not alter the mortality rate. Chlebicki and Safdar [51] demonstrated no mortality benefit with chlorhexidine, though in seven small RCTs there was a reduction in VAP, which was most marked in cardiac surgery patients. Neither antiseptic nor antibiotic oral decontamination reduced mortality, duration of mechanical ventilation or ICU stay in a meta-analysis of 11 studies by Chan et al. [52]. Kola and Gastmeier [53] found in seven RCTs a reduction in RR of lower respiratory tract infections in patients receiving chlorhexidine [RR (random): 0.58]. However, these results only applied to patients ventilated for up to 48 h. From 10 studies—but not all RCTs—Carvajal et al. [55] report a reduction in the risk of VAP with chlorhexidine (OR 0.56, 95% CI 0.44–0.73). However, no reduction in mortality rates, length of mechanical ventilation or ICU length of stay was seen.

Table 30.6 Randomised controlled trials into the effect of nonantibiotic interventions on the general infection and mortality rates in ventilated patients

Manoeuvre	Author	Year	Study Design	No.	Infection Rate	Mortality	Evidence
Immunonutrition	Beale [56]	1999	Meta-analysis of 12 studies	1,482	RR 0.67 (0.50–0.89) $P = 0.006$	RR 0.05 (0.78–1.41) $P = 0.76$	2A
	Heyland [57]	2001	Meta-analysis of 22 studies	2,419	RR 0.66 (0.54–0.80)	RR 1.1 (0.93–1.31)	2A
Steroids	Cronin [58]	1995	Meta-analysis of 9 RCTs	1,232	No difference	RR 1.13 (0.99–1.29)	2A
	Lefering [59]	1995	Meta-analysis of 10 RCTs	1,329	No difference	Difference in mortality −0.2% (−9.2 to 8.8)	2A
	Bollaert [60]	1998	RCT	41	No difference	Difference in mortality 31% (1–61)	2A
	Briegel [61]	1999	RCT	40	No difference	No difference	2A
	Annane [62]	2002	RCT	300	No difference	Significant reduction	2A

RCT randomised controlled trial, *RR* relative risk (95% confidence intervals)

30.2.5 Immunomodulation

30.2.5.1 Immunonutrition (Enteral Feeding)

Total parenteral nutrition (TPN) has been shown to be harmful in terms of infection rates and liver impairment. This prompted enteral feeding the ICU patient as soon as possible, because it is thought to be essential for the gut anatomy and physiology into prevent loss of mucosal integrity and subsequent translocation. In addition, several nutrients added to the enteral feed have been shown to influence immunologic and inflammatory responses in humans. There are two meta-analyses available on immunonutrition in the critically ill [56, 57] (Table 30.6). Both demonstrate a significant reduction in overall infection rate, although they do not specifically state pneumonia. There was no reduction in mortality rate in either meta-analysis. Surgical patients seemed to benefit more than medical patients. In two large RCTs, mortality rate was significantly higher in the subgroup who received immunonutrition. Some have speculated that adding arginine may have been detrimental to the immune system.

30.2.5.2 Steroids

High doses of steroids given to septic patients are thought to be beneficial for three reasons [58–62] (Table 30.6): steroids effectively suppress generalised inflammation due to microorganisms and their toxins; they have been shown to significantly reduce septic shock and early mortality within 72 h; they have been shown to significantly reduce mortality rates due to particularly severe invasive infection, including meningitis, typhoid and *Pneumocystis carinii* pneumonia (PCP). The major perceived side effects of high-dose steroids are the associated immune suppression and subsequent risk of superinfections. Indeed, the two meta-analyses show a trend towards increased mortality rates from secondary infection in patients receiving steroids. A systematic review by Annane et al. [63] examining the benefits and risks of steroids in sepsis reviewed 17 RCTs encompassing 2,138 patients, and three quasi-RCTs of 246 patients. Sub group analysis of prolonged low-dose corticosteroid therapy suggests a beneficial effect on short-term mortality rates [63]. The Corticosteroid Treatment and Intensive Insulin Therapy for Septic Shock in Adults (COIITSS) study [64] demonstrated that intensive insulin therapy together with hydrocortisone for septic shock did not improve in-hospital mortality rates. The addition of oral fludrocortisone did not result in a statistically significant improvement in in-hospital mortality [64].

The next logical step would be to combine steroids with SDD, whereby the perceived harmful effects of steroids could be abolished. In that way, the early survival benefit from steroids can be preserved, while keeping the patient free from secondary infections using SDD. The time has come to perform a randomised trial of SDD and steroids versus SDD only, with the endpoint as mortality rate.

30.2.5.3 Immunoglobulins

Polyclonal intravenously administered immunoglobulins significantly reduce mortality rates and can be used as an extra treatment option for sepsis and septic shock [65]. Overall mortality rates were reduced in patients who received polyclonal immunoglobulin i.v. (492; RR 0.64; 95% CI 0.51–0.80). For the two high-quality trials on polyclonal immunoglobulin i.v., the RR for overall mortality was 0.30, but the CI was wide (0.09–0.99; $n = 91$). However, all trials were small, and the totality of the evidence is insufficient to support a robust conclusion of benefit. Adjunctive therapy with monoclonal immunoglobulins i.v. remains experimental.

30.2.5.4 Activated Protein-C

Drotrecogin alfa (activated), or recombinant human activated protein C, is thought to have anti-inflammatory, antithrombotic and profibrinolytic properties. In a randomised trial of 1,690 patients, the mortally rate was 30.8% in the placebo group and 24.7% in the drotrecogin alfa group, which translates into an absolute reduction in risk of death of 6.2% ($P = 0.005$). The incidence of serious bleeding was higher in the drotrecogin alfa (activated) group than in the placebo group [66]. This is level 1 evidence and a grade B recommendation.

30.2.5.5 Anti-Inflammatory Mediators

Almost 60 randomised controlled clinical trials have tested the hypothesis that modulating the endogenous host inflammatory response can improve survival for patients with a clinical diagnosis of sepsis. The results have been frustrating, and no new agent has been introduced into clinical practice for this purpose [67].

Pooled data from studies using a monoclonal antibody to neutralise tumour necrosis factor (TNF) demonstrates a statistically significant 3.5% reduction in mortality rates. In aggregate, the three completed studies using recombinant interleukin-1 (IL-1) receptor antagonists to neutralise IL-1 also showed an absolute mortality rate reduction of 5%. Zeni et al. [68] showed that he combined results of all completed trials, independent of the therapeutic agents employed, demonstrate a statistically significant 3% overall reduction in 28-day all-cause mortality. It is debateable whether this small clinical benefit is sufficiently important to justify clinical use of these therapies, given the costs and potential toxicity of the agent involved.

30.2.5.6 Tight Glucose Control

Van den Berghe et al. [69] demonstrated that intensive insulin therapy reduces morbidity and mortality rates in cardiac surgical ICUs. However, intensive insulin therapy significantly reduced morbidity but not mortality rates among all patients in the medical ICU [70].

The American Diabetes Association and Surviving Sepsis Campaign recommend tight glucose control in critically ill patients based largely on one trial that shows decreased mortality rates in a surgical ICU. Because similar studies report

Table 30.7 Classification of microorganisms based upon their intrinsic pathogenicity

Intrinsic pathogenicity	Type	Site	Microorganism	Flora
Low level IPI = 0.01	Indigenous flora	Throat Gut Vagina Skin	*Peptostreptococcus, Veillonella* spp., *Streptococcus viridans* *Bacteroides* spp., *Clostridium* spp., enterococci, *E. coli* *Peptostreptococcus, Bacteroides* spp., *Lactobacillus* spp. *Propionibacterium acnes*, coagulase-negative staphylococci	Normal
Potential IPI = 0.3–0.6	Normal PPM Abnormal PPM	Throat Gut Throat and Gut	*Streptococcus pneumoniae, Haemophilus influenzae, Moraxella catarrhalis,* *Staphylococcus aureus, Candida* spp. *Escherichia coli, S. aureus, Candida* spp. *Klebsiella, Enterobacter, Citrobacter, Proteus, Morganella, Serratia, Pseudomonas, Acinetobacter* spp., MRSA	Normal Abnormal
High level IPI = 0.9–1.0	Epidemic Micro-organisms	Throat Gut	*Neisseria meningitidis* *Salmonella* spp.	Abnormal

The intrinsic pathogenicity index (IPI) is the ratio between the number of ICU patients with an infection due to a particular microorganism and the number of ICU patients who carry the same particular microorganism. Normal PPMs are carried by healthy individuals in throat and gut. Individuals with an underlying condition carry both normal and abnormal PPMs in throat and gut
IPI International Prognostic Index; *MRSA* methicillin-resistant *Staphylococcus aureus*

conflicting results and tight glucose control can cause dangerous hypoglycaemia, data underlying this recommendation should be critically evaluated [71].

An RCT by Vlasselaers et al. [72] of intensive insulin therapy to achieve age-adjusted normal fasting concentrations showed improved short-term outcome of patients in a paediatric ICU (PICU). However, the Neonatal Insulin Replacement Therapy in Europe (NIRTURE) study of tight glucose control in neonates and infants did not conclusively demonstrate the value of insulin therapy in preterm infants [73].

The practice of tight glucose control is accompanied by an increased incidence of hypoglycaemia. Hermanides et al. [74] demonstrated that hypoglycaemia increased the rate of death to 40:1,000 in those who experienced hypoglycaemia and 17:1,000 for those who were not hypoglycaemic.

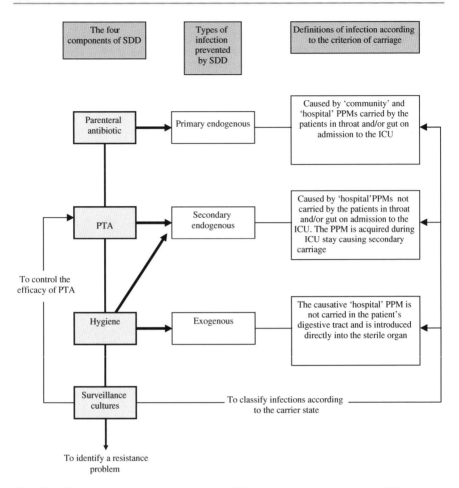

Fig. 30.1 The full four component protocol of SDD, that aims to control the three different types of infection that occur on ICU

30.3 Infection-Control Manoeuvres: Antibiotic Interventions

30.3.1 Selective Decontamination of the Digestive Tract

SDD is based on the observation that critical illness changes body flora, promoting a shift: (1) from normal (*Streptococcus pneumoniae* in the throat and *Escherichia coli* in the gut) towards abnormal [aerobic Gram-negative bacilli (AGNB) and methicillin-resistant *Staphylococcus aureus* (MRSA) in throat and gut] carriage (Table 30.7); (2) from low- to high-grade carriage (gut overgrowth) of both normal and abnormal flora. Parenterally administered cefotaxime controls gut overgrowth due to normal bacteria; enterally administered polyenes control gut overgrowth

Table 30.8 Carriage classification of severe infections of lower airways and blood

Infection	PPM	Timing	Frequency (%)	Manoeuvre
1	6 normal; 9 abnormal	>1 week	55	Parenteral antimicrobials
2	9 abnormal	>1 week	30	Hygiene and enteral antimicrobials
3	9 abnormal	Anytime during ICU treatment	15	Hygiene and topical antimicrobials

1 primary endogenous, *2* secondary endogenous, *3* exogenous *PPM* potentially pathogenic microorganism, *6 normal*: *Streptococcus pneumoniae, Haemophilus influenzae, Moraxella catarrhalis, Candida albicans, Staphylococcus aureus, Escherichia coli*, *9 abnormal*: *Klebsiella, Enterobacter, Citrobacter, Proteus, Morganella, Serratia, Acinetobacter, Pseudomonas* spp., methicillin-resistant *Staphylococcus aureus* (MRSA), *ICU* intensive care unit

due to normal *Candida* spp. Enterally administered polymyxin/tobramycin (without or with vancomycin) eradicates (if already present) and prevents overgrowth with abnormal bacteria.

Gut overgrowth is the crucial event preceding two classes of infections: primary and secondary endogenous infections (Table 30.8).

1. Primary endogenous infection is caused by normal or abnormal potential pathogens present in the patient's admission flora. This infection generally develops within 1 week and is the most frequent type of infection (55%).
2. Secondary endogenous infection is invariably caused by abnormal bacteria not present in the admission flora but acquired during treatment in the ICU. This infection generally occurs after 1 week in the ICU (30%).
3. Exogenous infection is caused by abnormal bacteria never carried in the patient's oropharynx and/or gut and may occur anytime during ICU treatment (15%).

Each of these three types of ICU infection requires different prophylaxis: primary endogenous can only be controlled by parenterally administered antimicrobials; secondary endogenous are prevented by enterally administered antimicrobials and high hygiene standards; exogenous are controlled by topically applied antimicrobials and hygiene. These three classes of intervention were first combined by Stoutenbeek et al., who expanded the prophylaxis to include surveillance cultures, thus creating the full four-component SDD protocol, the main mechanism of action being gut overgrowth control [75] (Fig. 30.1).

SDD has been assessed in 11 meta-analyses [76–86] covering 60 RCTs (Table 30.9), showing that SDD reduces pneumonia (72%), septicaemia (37%) and mortality rates (29%) without resistance emerging. Of the 11 meta-analyses, lower airway infection was the endpoint in six [76, 77, 79, 82, 84, 86]. All meta-analyses invariably demonstrate a significant reduction in lower airway

Table 30.9 Overview: efficacy of SDD: 60 RCTs and 11 meta-analyses

Author	No. of RCTs	Sample size	Lower airway infection OR (95% CI)	Bloodstream infection OR (95% CI)	Multiple organ dysfunction syndrome OR (95% CI)	Mortality OR (95% CI)
Vandenbroucke-Grauls [76]	6	491	0.12, 0.08–0.19	NR		0.92, 0.45–1.84
D'Amico [77]	33	5,727	0.35, 0.29–0.41	NR		0.80, 0.69–0.93
Safdar [78]	4	259	NR	NR		0.82, 0.22–2.45
Liberati [79]	36	6,922	0.35, 0.29–0.41	NR		0.78, 0.68–0.89
Silvestri [80] yeasts	42	6,075	NR	0.89, 0.16–4.95		NR
Silvestri [81]	51	8,065	NR	0.63, 0.46–0.87		0.74, 0.61–0.91
Silvestri [82] G– G+	54	9,473	0.07, 0.04–0.13 0.52, 0.34–0.78	0.36, 0.22–0.60 1.03, 0.75–1.41		NR NR
Silvestri [83]	21	4,902	NR	NR		0.71, 0.61–0.82
Liberati [84]	36	6,914	0.28, 0.20–0.38	NR		0.75, 0.65–0.87
Silvestri [85]	7	1,270	NR	NR	0.50, 0.34–0.74	0.82, 0.51–1.32
Silvestri [86]	12	2,252	0.54, 0.42–0.69	NR		NR

infection (OR 0.28, 95% CI 0.20–0.38). Bloodstream infection was the endpoint in three meta-analyses [80–82] and was significantly reduced (OR 0.63, 95% CI 0.46–0.87). When assessing bloodstream infection, AGNB septicaemias were significantly reduced; Gram-positive ones were increased but not significantly due to the low incidence in the control group (Table 30.9). Multiple organ dysfunction syndrome (MODS) was the endpoint in one of the most recent meta-analyses [85], in which the relative reduction of 50% was significant. Mortality was the endpoint in eight meta-analyses [76–79, 81, 83–85]. SDD consistently reduced mortality rates as long as the sample size was large enough; the sample size was too small in three meta-analyses [76, 78, 85].

References

1. Atkins D, Best D, Briss PA et al, for the GRADE working group (2004) Grading quality of evidence and strength of recommendations. BMJ 328:1490–1495
2. Schünemann HJ, Oxman AD, Brozek J et al, for the GRADE working group (2008) Grading quality of evidence and strength of recommendations for diagnostic tests and strategies. BMJ 336:1106–1110
3. Jaeschke R, Guyatt GH, Dellinger P et al, for the GRADE working group (2008) Use of GRADE grid to reach decisions on clinical practice guidelines when consensus is elusive. BMJ 337:a744
4. Guyatt GH, Oxman AD, Vist GE et al, for the GRADE working group (2008) GRADE: an emerging consensus on rating quality of evidence and strength of recommendations. 336:924–926
5. Casewell M, Philips I (1977) Hands as route of transmission for *Klebsiella* species. BMJ 2:1315–1317
6. Massanari RM, Hierholzer J (1984) A cross-over comparison of antiseptic soaps on nosocomial infection rates in the intensive care units. Am J Infect Control 12:247–248
7. Maki DG (1989) The use of antiseptics for handwashing by medical personnel. J Chemother 1(Suppl 1):3–11
8. Simmons B, Bryant J, Neiman K et al (1990) The role of handwashing in prevention of endemic intensive care unit infections. Infect Control Hosp Epidemiol 11:589–594
9. Doebbeling RN, Stanley G, Sheetz CT et al (1992) Comparative efficacy of alternative handwashing agents in reducing nosocomial infections in intensive care units. New Engl J Med 327:88–93
10. Webster J, Faogali JL, Cartwright D (1994) Elimination of methicillin-resistant *Staphylococcus aureus* from a neonatal intensive care unit after handwashing with tricloson. J Paediatr Child Health 30:59–64
11. Koss WG, Khalili TM, Lemus JF et al (2001) Nosocomial pneumonia is not prevented by protective contact isolation in the surgical intensive care unit. Am Surg 67:1140–1144
12. Slota M, Green M, Farley A et al (2001) The role of gown and glove isolation and strict handwashing in the reduction of nosocomial infection in children with solid organ transplantation. Crit Care Med 29:405–412
13. Silvestri L, Petros AJ, Sarginson RE et al (2005) Handwashing in the intensive care unit: a big measure with modest effects. J Hosp Infect 59:172–179
14. Choi SC, Nelson LD (1992) Kinetic therapy in critically ill patients: combined results based on meta-analysis. J Crit Care 7:57–62
15. Summer WR, Curry P, Haponik EF et al (1989) Continuous mechanical turning of intensive care unit patients shortens length of stay in some diagnostic-related groups. J Crit Care 4:45–53

16. Traver GA, Tyler ML, Hudson LD et al (1995) Continuous oscillation: outcome in critically ill patients. J Crit Care 10:97–103
17. Craven DE, Steger KA (1996) Nosocomial pneumonia in mechanically ventilated patients: epidemiology and prevention in 1996. Semin Respir Infect 11:32–53
18. Drakulovic MB, Torres A, Bauer TT et al (1999) Supine body position as a risk factor for nosocomial pneumonia in mechanically ventilated patients: a randomised trial. Lancet 354:1851–1858
19. van Nieuwenhoven CA, van Tiel FH, Vandenbroucke-Grauls C et al (2002) The effect of semi-recumbent position on development of ventilator-associated pneumonia (VAP). Intensive Care Med 27(Suppl 2):S285, Abstract 585
20. Keeley L (2007) Reducing the risk of ventilator-acquired pneumonia through head of bed elevation. Nurs Crit Care 12:287–294
21. Silvestri L, Gregori D, van Saene HKF, Belli R (2010) Semirecumbent position to prevent ventilator-associated pneumonia is not evidence based. J Critical Care 25:152–153
22. Mahul P, Auboyer C, Jaspe R et al (1992) Prevention of nosocomial pneumonia in intubated patients: respective role of mechanical subglottic secretions drainage and stress ulcer prophylaxis. Intensive Care Med 18:20–25
23. Valles J, Artigas A, Rello J et al (1995) Continuous aspiration of subglottic secretions in preventing ventilator-associated pneumonia. Ann Intern Med 122:179–186
24. Kollef MH, Skubas NJ, Sundt TM (1999) A randomised clinical trial of continuous aspiration of subglottic secretions in cardiac surgery patients. Chest 116:1339–1346
25. Smulders K, van der Hoeven H, Weers-Pothoff I et al (2002) A randomised clinical trial of intermittent subglottic secretion drainage in patients receiving mechanical ventilation. Chest 121:858–862
26. Metz C, Linde HJ, Gobel L et al (1998) Influence of intermittent subglottic lavage on subglottic colonization and ventilator associated pneumonia. Clin Intensive Care 9:20–24
27. Bo H, He L, Qu J et al (2000) Influence of the subglottic secretion drainage on the morbidity of ventilator associated pneumonia in mechanically ventilated patients. Zhonghua Jie He He Hu Xi Za Zhi 23:472–474
28. Liu SH, Yan XX, Cao SQ et al (2006) The effect of subglottic secretion drainage on prevention of ventilator-associated lower airway infection. Zhonghua Jie He He Hu Xi Za Zhi 29:19–22
29. Lorente L, Lecuona M, Jimenez A et al (2007) Influence of an endotracheal tube with polyurethane cuff and subglottic secretion drainage on pneumonia. Am J Respir Crit Care Med 176:1079–1083
30. Zheng RQ, Lin H, Shao J et al (2008) A clinical study of subglottic secretion drainage for prevention of ventilator associated pneumonia. Zhongguo Wie Zhong Bing Ji Jiu Yi Xue 20:338–340
31. Bouza E, Perez MJ, Munoz P et al (2008) Continuous aspiration of subglottic secretions (CASS) in the prevention of ventilator-associated pneumonia in the postoperative period of major heart surgery. Chest 134:938–946
32. Dezfulian C, Shojania K, Collard HR et al (2005) Subglottic secretion drainage for preventing ventilator associated pneumonia: a meta-analysis. Am J Med 118:11–18
33. Silvestri L, Milanese M, van Saene HKF et al (2008) Impact of subglottic secretion drainage on ventilator-associated pneumonia and mortality: systematic review of randomized controlled trials. In: Proceedings of the 21st anesthesia and ICU symposium Alpe Adria. Udine, 5–6 Sept 2008, pp 26–29
34. De Riso AJII, Ladowski JS, Dillon TA et al (1996) Chlorhexidine gluconate 0.12% oral rinse reduces the incidence of total nosocomial respiratory infection and nonprophylactic systemic antibiotic use in patients undergoing heart surgery. Chest 109:1556–1561
35. Fourrier F, Cau-Pottier E, Boutigny H et al (2000) Effects of dental plaque on antiseptic decontamination on bacterial colonisation and nosocomial infections in critically ill patients. Intensive Care Med 26:1239–1247

36. Houston S, Houghland P, Anderson JJ et al (2002) Effectiveness of 0.12% chlorhexidine gluconate oral rinse in reducing prevalence of nosocomial pneumonia in patients undergoing heart surgery. Am J Crit Care 11:567–570
37. MacNaughton PD, Bailey J, Donlin N et al (2004) A randomised controlled trial assessing the efficacy of oral chlorhexidine in ventilated patients. Intensive Care Med 30(Suppl 1):S12 Abstract 029
38. Grap MJ, Munro CL, Elswick RE et al (2004) Duration of action of a single early oral application of chlorhexidine on oral microbial flora in mechanically ventilated patients: a pilot study. Heart Lung 33:83–91
39. Fourrier F, Dubois D, P Pronnier et al (2005) Effect of gingival and dental plaque antiseptic decontamination on nosocomial infections acquired in the intensive care unit: a double-blind placebo-controlled multicenter study. Crit Care Med 33:1728–1735
40. Segers P, Speckenbrink RGH, Ubbink DT et al (2006) Prevention of nosocomial infection in cardiac surgery by decontamination of the nasopharynx and oropharynx with chlorhexidine gluconate. JAMA 296:2460–2466
41. Koeman M, van der Ven AJAM, Hak E et al (2006) Oral decontamination with chlorhexidine reduces the incidence of ventilator-associated pneumonia. Am J Respir Crit Care Med 173:1348–1355
42. Bopp M, Darby M, Loftin KC et al (2006) Effects of daily oral care with 0.12% chlorhexidine gluconate and a standard care protocol on the development of nosocomial pneumonia in intubated patients: a pilot study. J Dent Hyg 80:9
43. Tad YD (2007) Efficacy of Chlorhexidine oral decontamination in the prevention of VAP. Chest 51:498S
44. Tantipong H, Morkchareonpong C, Jaiyindee S et al (2008) Randomised controlled trial and meta-analysis of oral decontamination with 2% chlorhexidine solution for the prevention of ventilator-associated pneumonia. Infect Control Hosp Epidemiol 29:131–136
45. Panchabhai TS, Dangayach NS, Krishnan A et al (2009) Oropharyngeal cleansing with 0.2% chlorhexidine for prevention of nosocomial pneumonia in critically ill patients. Chest 135:1150–1156
46. Scannapieco FA, Yu J, Raghavendran K et al (2009) A randomised trial of chlorhexidine gluconate on oral bacterial pathogens in mechanically ventilated patients. Crit Care 13:R117
47. Munro CL, Grap MJ, Jones DJ et al (2009) Chlorhexidine, toothbrushing, and ventilator-associated pneumonia in critically ill adults. Am J Crit Care 18:428–438
48. Bellissimo-Rodrigues F, Bellissimo-Rodrigues WT et al (2009) Effectiveness of oral rinse with chlorhexidine in preventing nosocomial respiratory tract infections among intensive care unit patients. Infect Control Hosp Epidemiol 30:952–958
49. Cabov T, Macan D, Husedzinovic I et al (2010) The impact of oral health and 0.2% chlorhexidine oral gel on the prevalence of nosocomial infections in surgical intensive-care patients: a randomized placebo-controlled study. Wien Klin Wochenschr 122:397–404
50. Pineda LA, Saliba RG, El Solh AA (2006) Effects of oral decontamination with chlorhexidine on the incidence of nosocomial pneumonia: a meta-analysis. Crit Care 10:R35
51. Chlebicki MP, Safdar N (2007) Topical chlorhexidine for prevention of ventilator-associated pneumonia: a meta-analysis. Crit Care Med 35:595–602
52. Chan EY, Ruest A, O'Meade M et al (2007) Oral decontamination for prevention of pneumonia in mechanically ventilated adults: systematic review and meta-analysis. BMJ 334:889–893
53. Kola A, Gastmeier P (2007) Efficacy of oral chlorhexidine in preventing lower respiratory tract infections: meta-analysis of randomised controlled trials. J Hosp Infect 66:207–216
54. van Saene HKF, Silvestri L, de la Cal MA et al (2009) The emperor's new clothes: the fairy tale continues. J Crit Care 24:149–152
55. Carvajal C, Pobo A, Diaz E et al (2010) Oral hygiene with chlorhexidine on the prevention of ventilator-associated pneumonia in intubated patients: a systematic review of randomized clinical trials. Med Clin (Barc) 135:491–497

56. Beale RJ, Bryg DJ, Bihari DJ (1999) Immunonutrition in the critically ill: a systematic review of clinical outcome. Crit Care Med 27:2799–2805
57. Heyland DK, Novak F, Drover JW et al (2001) Should immunonutrition become routine in critically ill patients? a systematic review of the evidence. JAMA 286:944–953
58. Cronin L, Cook DJ, Carlet J et al (1995) Corticosteroid treatment for sepsis: a critical appraisal and meta-analysis of the literature. Crit Care Med 23:1430–1439
59. Lefering R, Neugebauer EAM (1995) Steroid controversy in sepsis and septic shock: a meta-analysis. Crit Care Med 23:1294–1303
60. Bollaert PE, Charpentier C, Levy B et al (1998) Reversal of late septic shock with supraphysiologic doses of hydrocortisone. Crit Care Med 26:645–650
61. Briegel J, Forst H, Haller M et al (1999) Stress doses of hydrocortisone reverse hyperdynamic septic shock: a prospective, randomised, double-blind, single-center study. Crit Care Med 27:723–732
62. Annane D, Sebille V, Charpentier C et al (2002) Effect of treatment with low doses of hydrocortisone and fludrocortisone on mortality in patients with septic shock. JAMA 288:862–871
63. Annane D, Bellissant E, Bollaert PE et al (2009) Corticosteroids in the treatment of severe sepsis and septic shock in adults: a systematic review. JAMA 301:2362–2375
64. Annane D, Cariou A, Maxime V et al, for the COIITSS study investigators (2010) Corticosteroid treatment and intensive insulin therapy for septic shock in adults: a randomized controlled trial. JAMA 303:341–348
65. Alejandria MM, Lansang MA, Dans LF, Mantaring JBV (2000) Intravenous immunoglobulin for treating sepsis and septic shock (Cochrane review). In: The Cochrane library, issue 3. Update Software, Oxford
66. Bernard GR, Vincent JL, Laterre PF et al (2001) Efficacy and safety of recombinant human activated protein C for severe sepsis. New Engl J Med 344:699–709
67. Marshall J (2000) Clinical trials of mediator-directed therapy in sepsis: what have we learned? Intensive Care Med 26:575–583
68. Zeni F, Freeman B, Natanson C (1997) Anti-inflammatory therapies to treat sepsis and septic shock: a reassessment. Crit Care Med 25:1095–1100
69. van den Berghe G, Wouters P, Weekers F et al (2001) Intensive insulin therapy in the critically ill patients. N Engl J Med 345:1359–1367
70. Van den Berghe G, Wilmer A, Hermans G (2006) Intensive insulin therapy in the medical ICU. N Engl J Med 354:449–461
71. Wiener RS, Wiener DC, Larson RJ (2008) Benefits and risks of tight glucose control in critically ill adults: a meta-analysis. JAMA 300:933–944
72. Vlasselaers D, Milants I, Desmet L et al (2009) Intensive insulin therapy for patients in paediatric intensive care: a prospective, randomised controlled study. Lancet 373:547–556
73. Beardsall K, Vanhaesebrouck S, Ogilvy-Stuart AL et al (2007) A randomised controlled trial of early insulin therapy in very low birth weight infants, NIRTURE (neonatal insulin replacement therapy in Europe). BMC Pediatr 7:29
74. Hermanides J, Bosman RJ, Vriesendorp TM (2010) Hypoglycemia is associated with intensive care unit mortality. Crit Care Med 38:1430–1434
75. Stoutenbeek CP, van Saene HKF, Miranda DR et al (1984) The effect of selective decontamination of the digestive tract on colonization and infection rate in multiple trauma patients. Intensive Care Med 10:185–192
76. Vandenbroucke-Grauls CMJ, Vandenbroucke JP (1991) Effect of selective decontamination of the digestive tract on respiratory tract infections and mortality in the intensive care unit. Lancet 338:859–862
77. D'Amico R, Pifferi S, Leonetti C et al, on behalf of the study investigators (1998) Effectiveness of antibiotic prophylaxis in critically ill adult patients: systematic review of randomised controlled trials. BMJ 316:1275–1285

78. Safdar N, Said A, Lucey MR (2004) The role of selective decontamination for reducing infection in patients undergoing liver transplantation: a systematic review and meta-analysis. Liver Transpl 10:817–827
79. Liberati A, D'Amico R, Pifferi S et al (2004) Antibiotic prophylaxis to reduce respiratory tract infections and mortality in adults receiving intensive care (Cochrane review). In: The Cochrane library, issue 1. Wiley, Chichester
80. Silvestri L, van Saene HKF, Milanese M, Gregori D (2005) Impact of selective decontamination of the digestive tract on fungal carriage and infection: systematic review of randomized controlled trials. Intensive Care Med 31:898–910
81. Silvestri L, van Saene HKF, Milanese M et al (2007) Selective decontamination of the digestive tract reduces bloodstream infections and mortality in critically ill patients: a systematic review of randomized controlled trials. J Hosp Infect 65:187–203
82. Silvestri L, van Saene HKF, Casarin AL et al (2008) Impact of selective decontamination of the digestive tract on carriage and infection due to Gram-negative and Gram-positive bacteria: systematic review of randomized controlled trials. Anaesths Intens Care 36:324–338
83. Silvestri L, van Saene HKF, Weir I, Gullo A (2009) Survival benefit of the full selective digestive decontamination regimen. J Crit Care 24:474.e7–474.e14
84. Liberati A, D'Amico R, Pifferi S (2009) Antibiotic prophylaxis to reduce respiratory tract infections and mortality in adults receiving intensive care. Cochrane Database Syst Rev 4:CD000022
85. Silvestri L, van Saene HKF, Zandstra DF et al (2010) Selective decontamination of the digestive tract reduces multiple organ failure and mortality in critically ill patients: systematic review of randomized controlled trials. Crit Care Med 38:1370–1376
86. Silvestri L, van Saene HKF, Zandstra DF (2010) Selective digestive decontamination reduces ventilator-associated tracheobronchitis. Respir Med 104:1953–1955

Index

A

Abnormal bacteria, 3, 18, 51, 55, 116–118, 172, 412, 431, 475
Abnormal colonization, 457
Acute pancreatitis, 25, 200, 242–244, 256, 268, 269, 379, 396, 442
AGNB, 3, 6, 18–21, 24, 31, 40, 42, 44, 50–57, 63, 67, 69, 70, 72–74, 77, 78, 80, 81, 83, 86, 116–125, 127, 128, 163, 165, 168, 170, 171, 178, 179, 181, 186, 187, 193, 197, 273, 274, 277, 279–281, 284, 305, 376, 412, 413, 416–418, 422, 429, 431, 432, 434, 435, 474, 477
AIDS, 22, 104, 321, 334–340, 342–344, 346–348, 350–353
Airway, 4, 5, 7, 9, 13, 15–19, 21–25, 28, 40–42, 41, 42, 48, 52, 56–59, 123, 145, 153, 160, 168, 169, 171, 173, 176, 193–195, 204–206, 208, 210–212, 214, 216, 250, 258, 274–277, 281, 285, 320, 356, 357, 358, 362–365, 367, 381, 383–386, 411, 412, 430, 432, 433, 439, 464, 468, 469, 475–478
Albumin, 64, 76, 81, 253, 254, 261, 337, 392, 393, 399
Amphotericin b, 9, 24, 42, 94–98, 100, 101, 102, 112–115, 119, 120, 122, 123, 125, 132, 165–167, 169, 171, 175, 185, 191, 193, 194, 198, 213, 251, 280, 283, 284, 292, 296, 298–300, 302, 310–312, 347, 348, 356, 358–360, 412, 413, 415, 417–420, 424, 428, 431, 432
Antacids, 209, 212, 213, 372, 401, 407, 412
Antibiotic therapy, 34, 37, 41, 69–71, 89, 99, 112, 115, 128, 145, 158, 171, 173, 176, 215, 234, 236, 240, 250, 259, 262, 265, 267, 287, 288, 289, 291, 293, 294, 295, 305, 341, 367, 448, 459
Antibiotics, 3–5, 18, 21, 25, 42, 43, 49, 59, 61–73, 75, 77, 79, 81, 83, 85–87, 89–91, 98, 119, 123, 128–130, 133, 134, 137, 155, 158, 163, 165, 166, 168, 169, 171–174, 176, 179, 183, 187, 191, 193, 197, 200, 205, 207, 209, 213–215, 220, 230, 231, 240, 241, 245, 251, 258, 259, 261, 265, 268, 270, 273, 277, 279, 281, 284, 285, 288–293, 295, 300, 307, 309, 342, 354–358, 362, 364, 367, 368, 370, 375, 376, 386, 398, 404, 405, 417, 421, 427–429, 434, 441, 444, 448
Antifungal therapy, 97, 99, 111, 113, 115, 185, 251, 364
Antimicrobial resistance, 8, 33, 35, 51, 61, 67, 89, 90, 123, 124, 133, 134, 147, 172–174, 193, 197, 290, 428, 430, 432–436, 438, 440, 442, 444, 453
Antimicrobials, 9, 24, 51, 56, 62, 116–128, 130, 132, 134, 136, 156, 162–166, 168–172, 186, 188, 191–194, 197, 198, 201, 279, 282, 284, 287–290, 292, 295, 313, 355, 356, 358, 359, 361, 363, 364, 367, 404, 406, 409, 411, 412, 414, 416, 418, 419, 423, 427, 430–432, 434, 436, 443, 475
Arginine, 251, 391, 396–398, 400, 471
Azole-resistant candida spp, 93, 104, 435

B

Bacteremia, 3, 10, 13, 25–27, 34, 36, 37, 47, 48, 72, 77, 81, 129, 190, 196–198, 202, 206, 215, 216, 222, 225, 228–230, 232–234, 238, 250, 289, 304, 308, 340, 342, 346, 352, 360, 369, 395, 439, 448, 451–453, 455, 458, 459
Bacterial colonization, 18, 24, 134, 148, 153, 203, 210–214, 285, 383, 385, 445
Bacterial pneumonia, 78, 89, 254, 340, 352
Bacterial translocation, 13, 23, 26, 58, 199, 259, 267, 268, 302, 307, 374–376, 378, 391, 399, 439, 441

B (*cont.*)
Bladder, 4, 11, 15–17, 21, 22, 28, 42, 52, 101, 157, 158, 166, 168, 262–264, 266, 276, 277, 279, 360, 361, 363, 364
Blood and body fluid, 315, 325, 328
Blood stream, 193, 274, 278
Bloodstream infection, 2, 3, 12, 14, 37, 99, 115, 124, 147, 149, 151, 155, 160, 194, 195, 202, 218–222, 224, 226, 228, 230, 232–234, 274, 277, 281, 285, 289, 299, 300, 342, 343, 362, 363, 367, 368, 377, 392, 399, 400, 426, 430, 432, 433, 440, 451, 455, 458, 459, 476, 477, 481
Bone marrow transplant, 110, 296, 302, 307, 309, 313, 332
Bundles, 209, 230, 231

C
Carriage, 2–5, 7, 9, 15–17, 19–21, 23–25, 28, 29, 31, 32, 35, 39, 41, 43–47, 49–59, 71, 116–122, 125–128, 132, 134, 135, 145, 148, 163, 169–173, 179, 182, 183, 186, 188–192, 194, 197, 198, 202, 273, 275, 281, 285, 299, 354–356, 360, 364, 365, 368, 370–372, 388, 411, 412, 416, 417, 426, 429–431, 434–436, 438–440, 444, 474, 475, 481
Carrier state, 3, 4, 9, 13, 16, 18, 24, 28, 36, 39, 41–44, 46, 47, 49–53, 55, 57–59, 116–118, 121, 134, 168, 169, 171, 172, 176, 191–193, 195, 275, 285, 412, 429, 430, 432, 435, 439, 474
Catheter, 2, 3, 11, 25, 28, 72, 111, 112, 136, 142–144, 149, 151, 155–161, 168, 180, 185, 205, 207, 214, 219, 220, 222–225, 233, 234, 239, 242, 246, 248, 264–266, 269, 271, 274, 279, 289, 296, 299, 304, 306, 308, 342, 356, 360–364, 366, 368, 382, 392, 395, 396, 398, 448, 451, 453, 455, 457–459
Cholangitis, 356
Classification, 12, 27, 29, 31–37, 39–49, 56, 57, 59, 78, 82, 83, 90, 121, 137, 138, 164, 166, 227, 232, 234–236, 243, 259, 262, 268, 270, 275, 388, 430, 439, 473, 475
Clinical experience, 93–95, 97, 129, 403
Cohorting, 142, 189, 316, 317, 319, 323
Colistin, 66, 67, 72, 74, 86, 91, 130, 132, 150, 152, 165, 292, 358, 413–415, 417–424
colonic ileus, 368, 372, 377, 409
Colonisation, 24, 25, 38, 56, 112, 115, 146, 147, 173, 174, 176, 180, 182–184, 189, 190, 201, 273, 277, 284, 312, 369, 412, 431, 432, 443, 478
Combination therapy, 81, 97, 98, 295, 355, 357–359, 361, 363
Community-acquired infection, 129, 232, 234, 297, 450
Compliance, 121, 123, 136, 140, 141, 143, 155, 193, 383, 418–420
Costs, 113, 144, 147, 172, 173, 206, 208, 213, 224, 233, 261, 271, 290, 291, 293, 300, 334, 380, 393, 394, 398, 423, 424, 438, 439, 446, 448–450, 452, 454–460, 468, 472
Critical illness, 13, 18, 23, 26, 49, 50, 51, 53, 63, 64, 66, 89, 176, 285, 292, 368, 370, 376, 377, 389–391, 396, 398–400, 405, 409, 429, 446, 447, 451, 474
Critically ill patient, 4, 8, 9, 12, 13, 15, 16, 19, 21, 23, 24, 39, 52, 55, 57–59, 61, 64, 65, 72, 90, 111, 117, 124, 129, 132, 159, 160, 168, 172, 175, 186, 190, 193, 200, 202–205, 212, 214, 217, 219, 221, 227, 230, 234, 237, 239, 250, 290, 291, 293–295, 355, 356, 362, 364, 367, 368, 371, 374, 375, 378, 384, 387, 389, 390, 392, 394–403, 405, 407–409, 426, 428, 432, 434, 435, 440, 442, 443, 445, 451–454, 457–459, 472, 477–481
Critically ill, 4, 8, 9, 12, 13, 15, 16, 19, 21, 23, 24, 26, 37, 39, 40, 51, 52, 55, 59, 61, 64, 65, 72, 89, 90, 111, 115–117, 119, 121, 123, 124, 129, 132–134, 159–161, 166, 168, 172, 175, 184, 186, 190, 193, 199–205, 212, 214, 217, 219, 221, 224, 227, 230–234, 237, 239, 249–251, 266, 267, 270, 281, 285, 286, 290, 291, 293–295, 333, 355, 356, 362, 364, 367, 368, 370–379, 384, 387, 389, 390, 400–410, 426, 428, 431, 432, 434, 435, 439–443, 445, 446, 451–454, 457–459, 471, 472, 477–481

D
De novo development, 428, 434
De-escalation, 71, 72, 90, 290, 293, 295
Definitions, 1–5, 7, 9, 11–15, 24, 28, 33, 41, 47, 48, 52, 192, 204, 216, 232, 233, 259, 266, 474

Diagnostic samples, 6, 16, 17, 43, 51–53, 57, 121, 186, 354, 357, 362, 366, 432
Drainage, 11, 157–159, 209, 220, 229, 236, 239, 241, 242, 246–248, 251, 266, 268–270, 310, 359–361, 364, 382, 384–387, 464, 466, 468, 469, 478

E

Echinocandins, 92, 94, 97, 99, 107–111, 114, 348
Efficacy, 9, 24, 64, 66–68, 81, 89, 94–96, 111, 121, 123, 126, 134, 137, 150, 151, 158, 162, 168–170, 172, 173, 186, 191–196, 199, 201, 209, 214, 215, 234, 245, 281, 284, 288, 292, 302, 312, 320, 355, 357, 381, 383, 387, 396, 406, 411, 414, 419, 426, 430, 432, 433, 435, 441, 443, 445, 450, 455, 463, 474, 476, 477, 479, 480
Empirical antibiotic treatment, 230, 288
Empirical, 4, 5, 65, 72, 81, 92, 94, 99, 108, 112, 113, 115, 172–174, 230, 240, 251, 283, 284, 288–291, 293, 294, 297, 306, 309, 354–356, 359, 361, 367, 368
Endogenous, 3, 5–7, 9, 11, 17, 21, 29, 39, 42–47, 51, 53, 55–57, 116, 118, 121, 123, 124, 127, 133, 168–170, 173, 179, 186, 191–193, 200, 205, 211, 275–277, 297, 300, 356, 362, 365, 370, 378, 385, 406, 408, 411–413, 429, 430, 435, 442, 463, 472, 474, 475
Endotracheal tube, 21, 23, 72, 136, 144, 150, 151, 153, 159, 160, 205, 210, 211, 214, 216, 277, 356, 364, 366, 381, 384, 385, 387, 388, 457, 468, 469, 478
Enteral feeding, 151, 208, 212, 270, 359, 386, 392, 394, 396, 399, 400, 402, 405–407, 457, 471
Enteral nutrition, 18, 19, 23, 26, 129, 151, 156, 209, 210, 217, 245, 268–270, 277, 285, 375, 381, 382, 385, 395–397, 399, 400, 409, 471
Eradication, 9, 24, 66, 117, 119, 121, 123, 171, 182, 184, 190, 197, 300, 324, 326, 359, 364, 365, 404, 418, 430
Evidence-based practice, 137
Exogenous infection, 5–7, 9, 42, 45–47, 53, 55–57, 123, 127, 173, 191, 193, 275, 277, 364, 385, 412, 430, 438, 463, 475

Exogenous, 3, 5–9, 11, 21, 23, 25, 29, 42, 43, 45–47, 53, 55–57, 59, 121, 123, 125, 127, 170, 173, 176, 179, 183, 186, 188, 191–193, 205, 211, 275, 277, 356, 363, 364, 367, 382, 385, 393, 394, 396, 411, 412, 429, 430, 438, 463, 474, 475
Extended infusion, 65

F

Faecal–oral transmission
Formulations, 113, 140, 302, 312, 397, 411, 415, 416, 418, 425
Four-quadrant method, 53, 54

G

Ganciclovir, 296, 298, 303, 309, 312, 313, 343, 344
Glutamine, 391, 396–398, 400
Grade, 50, 51, 55, 93, 94, 97, 111, 113, 180, 212, 236, 246, 312, 338, 367, 375, 429–431, 437, 438, 461–464, 472, 474, 477
Gut overgrowth, 8, 13, 23, 26, 50, 51, 53, 55, 58, 117, 124, 126, 129, 184, 187, 190, 285, 413, 428–431, 434, 435, 439, 444, 474, 475

H

Haart, 335, 336, 338, 340, 343, 346–351
Hand hygiene, 55, 126, 127, 137, 138, 140, 141, 146, 155, 158, 191, 319, 323, 324, 332, 366, 380, 463, 465
Hand washing, 6, 11, 111, 140, 225, 316, 317, 324, 325, 329, 365, 366, 463
Helicobacter pylori, 402, 404, 406, 409
High-level pathogen, 6, 191, 275
HIV infection, 327, 334, 335, 338–346, 348, 351–353
Hospital, 4, 6, 7, 13, 18, 19, 27, 29, 31–34, 36, 37, 39–42, 47, 48, 57, 58, 69, 72, 83, 90, 111, 115, 116, 125, 128, 129, 134, 136, 137, 139, 140, 143, 144, 146, 147, 149, 152, 154, 157, 164, 168, 172, 174, 176, 179–185, 188–190, 197, 198, 204, 206, 208, 215, 216, 218–220, 222–225, 227–229, 231–234, 236, 237, 258–260, 263, 265, 270–272, 276, 280, 287, 288, 290, 291, 294, 296, 297, 299, 303, 312,

317–324, 328, 331, 332, 335, 337, 342, 343, 352, 355, 361, 377, 380, 383, 387, 389–393, 395, 397, 398, 411, 414, 416, 418, 423–427, 434, 435, 439, 444–447, 452, 455, 456, 458–461, 463, 471, 474

I

IA abscess, 235, 253, 258
Immunonutrients, 390, 391
Immunonutrition, 391, 399, 406, 409, 470, 471, 480
Immunosuppression, 8, 18, 19, 33, 42, 44, 51, 55, 56, 129, 260, 289, 297, 299, 303, 306, 309, 310, 322, 338, 342, 343, 346, 364, 390, 432
Import, 1, 2, 4, 18, 20–22, 24, 25, 33, 37, 39, 42–45, 53, 55, 58, 63, 67–69, 71, 77, 85, 92, 98, 111, 116–119, 125, 126, 128, 135, 140, 155, 168, 172, 179, 181, 184, 186, 193, 197, 198, 204, 205, 208, 212, 215, 219, 221, 224–227, 231, 234, 238, 245, 251, 254, 258, 260, 261, 264, 266, 273, 274, 278, 285, 299, 310, 314, 319, 321, 323, 325, 330, 340, 342, 344, 354, 355, 364, 366, 370, 375, 376, 382–384, 386, 389–392, 395, 397, 398, 401–407, 413, 431, 432, 434, 438, 444, 447, 448, 451, 453, 462, 463, 468, 472
Indigenous flora, 7, 17, 20, 21, 31, 32, 34, 118, 119, 163, 164, 275, 366, 413, 431, 473
Infection control, 1, 7, 15, 24, 27, 39, 47, 48, 50, 57, 59, 61, 92, 113, 116, 128, 130, 135, 136, 138, 140, 142, 144, 146–149, 159, 161, 162, 177, 179, 180, 183, 187–189, 191, 204, 216, 218, 232, 235, 270, 272, 277, 284, 287, 296, 314, 316, 319, 320, 323, 327, 329, 331–334, 354, 356, 370, 380, 381, 383, 388, 389, 401, 405, 411, 426–428, 430, 446, 456, 461, 463
Infection, 1–29, 31, 33–53, 55–63, 65, 66, 69, 71, 72, 75–78, 80–83, 86, 89, 90–92, 94–101, 104, 108, 112–116, 118, 121–152, 154–163, 165, 166, 168–481
Inflammation, 2, 5, 6, 8, 12, 16–18, 24, 28, 42, 51, 52, 55, 129, 165, 166, 168, 169, 238, 241, 244, 256, 259, 277, 279, 339, 340, 344, 359, 362–364, 366, 367, 370, 371, 375, 392, 402, 403, 405, 413, 432
Inoculum effect, 62, 63
Intra-abdominal, 6, 89, 96, 97, 220, 222, 223, 225, 231, 235, 236, 238, 239, 241, 242, 253, 266–268, 270, 279, 355, 356, 359, 362, 368, 372, 393
Intrinsic pathogenicity index, 32, 48, 275, 285, 473
Isolation, 6, 11, 12, 17, 28, 30, 31, 54, 56, 57, 112, 137, 139, 141, 142, 146, 147, 184, 220, 221, 233, 279, 287, 316, 317, 319, 323–325, 328–330, 346, 348, 350, 362, 365, 463, 464, 477

K

Kaposi's sarcoma, 334, 335, 345, 348–350, 353

L

Leadership, 145
Lowest resistance potential, 163
Low-level pathogen, 44, 128, 191, 241, 275, 362, 436

M

Macconkey agar, 54
Mediastinitis, 248–251, 269, 270
Meningitis, 4, 63, 68, 101, 104, 278, 329, 347, 355, 356, 361, 471
MIC, 2, 13, 15, 18, 20–45, 47–73, 75–85, 87, 89–102, 104, 106–136, 138–142, 144–147, 151–158, 160, 162–176, 179, 180, 182–195, 197, 203, 205, 207, 211, 213–216, 218–226, 228–230, 232–238, 240, 241, 243–245, 249, 251–254, 256–267, 270, 272–295, 299–301, 303, 305, 307, 309, 311–323, 328–335, 337–342, 346, 348, 351, 352, 354–380, 383–387, 389, 391, 392, 394–396, 398, 401, 403–409, 411–419, 423, 426–436, 438–440, 442–445, 449–460, 463, 464, 468, 471, 473, 475–481
Morbidity, 7, 28, 72, 115, 118, 123, 128, 133, 147, 154, 172, 173, 179, 198, 208, 209, 218, 224, 242, 250, 252, 257, 258, 263, 270, 274, 281, 285, 288, 289, 293, 294, 314, 321, 330, 340, 342, 347, 367, 376, 380, 384, 389–391, 394–396, 398, 401, 405, 412, 425, 428, 432, 440, 446–448, 450, 454, 456–458, 460, 463–465, 468, 472, 478
Mortality, 7, 13, 18, 28, 33–35, 37, 40, 47, 53, 58, 60, 65, 72, 96, 99, 111, 112, 115,

118, 121, 123–125, 128, 129, 132, 133, 144, 147, 152, 154, 172, 173, 175, 179, 180, 184, 185, 187, 188, 195, 196, 198–203, 206, 208, 209, 213, 215–217, 224, 226, 229, 230, 232–235, 238, 240, 242–252, 257, 258, 263, 270, 273, 274, 276, 281, 282, 285, 286, 288–295, 297, 300–303, 305, 306, 308, 312, 314, 318, 320, 321, 329, 330, 334, 336–348, 351, 355, 357, 361, 366–369, 372–374, 376–378, 380, 383–392, 394–399, 401, 402, 405, 407, 408, 412, 425, 426, 428, 432–435, 437–444, 446–448, 450–460, 463, 464, 466–472, 475, 478, 480, 481
MRSA, 3, 6, 8, 18, 19, 21, 34, 42–44, 50–58, 65, 73, 74, 76–79, 82, 84, 86–88, 91, 116–122, 124–127, 132, 134, 135, 137, 142, 144–147, 163, 167–171, 178–180, 186–188, 193, 198, 205–208, 215, 222, 228–230, 250, 276, 277, 280, 289, 290, 299, 306, 307, 358, 364–366, 368, 412, 413, 429–431, 435, 444, 452, 456, 465, 473–475
Multiorgan dysfunction, 389, 390
Multiple organ dysfunction syndrome (MODS), 12, 131, 195, 196, 202, 215, 370, 379, 390, 401, 410, 432, 477, 433, 476
Mycobacterial infections, 350, 353

N
Neonatal intensive care unit, 36, 135, 175, 187, 190, 272, 283, 285, 286, 317, 332, 427, 477
Neostigmine, 357, 359, 368, 372, 377, 406, 409
Neuroendocrine system, 390
Nonabsorbable antimicrobials, 9, 24, 118, 123, 169, 364, 411, 412, 430
Nonantibiotic management, 381
Normal bacteria, 3, 18, 51, 55, 116–118, 128, 172, 412, 431, 475
Nosocomial infections, 36, 37, 40, 47, 59, 86, 135, 144, 147, 159, 174, 199, 206, 208, 216, 232, 259, 271, 285, 314, 324, 368, 390, 399, 441, 444, 446, 453, 457–459, 465, 477–479
Nutrition, 18, 19, 23, 26, 119, 129, 147, 151, 156, 205, 209, 210, 212, 217, 220, 241, 245, 260, 261, 268–270, 277, 285, 301, 340, 375, 381, 382, 385, 386, 389–400, 406, 409, 470, 471, 480

O
Open treatment, 240
Oral chlorhexidine, 387, 479
Oral decontamination, 132, 152, 159, 199, 201, 384, 387, 425, 440, 443, 469, 479
Outbreaks, 7, 35, 116, 118, 127, 142, 162, 177–190, 273, 284, 314, 315, 321–325, 334, 344
Overgrowth, 3, 8, 9, 13, 15–17, 19, 21, 23–26, 44, 47, 50–56, 58, 71, 116–118, 120–122, 124–129, 163, 169, 170, 184, 186, 187, 190, 193, 285, 360, 365, 366, 370, 372, 374, 376, 392, 400, 413, 428–432, 434–436, 439, 444, 474, 475

P
paediatric intensive care unit, 273, 284
Parenteral nutrition, 19, 23, 26, 129, 156, 245, 268, 269, 277, 285, 375, 396, 399, 400, 471
Peritoneal lavage, 239, 240, 267
Peritonitis, 6, 25, 81, 96, 108, 129, 235–242, 266, 267, 279, 304, 308, 358, 359, 367, 368, 395
Pharmacist, 162, 411, 412, 414, 425
Pharmacodynamics, 89, 114, 130, 288, 291, 295
Pharmacokinetics, 89, 91, 114, 129, 133, 291, 295
Pharmacological properties, 75, 76, 79, 80, 85, 93, 95, 97
PK/PD, 61, 89, 292, 293
Pneumocystis jiroveci pneumonia, 351
Pneumonia, 1, 3, 6–8, 12, 17, 18, 24–26, 28, 30, 32–34, 36, 37, 39–42, 44, 45, 47–49, 56, 59, 62, 69, 72, 76–83, 85, 86, 89, 90, 116, 117, 124, 130–132, 144, 147, 149–154, 159, 160, 167, 168, 171, 174, 176, 181, 185, 189, 194, 196–199, 201–218, 221, 225, 226, 228, 230, 231, 237, 252, 254, 256, 276–278, 281–285, 289–291, 294, 295, 298, 300, 301, 303–309, 318, 320–322, 334, 336–338, 340–343, 346, 347, 350–353, 355–357, 361, 362, 364, 367, 368, 372, 373, 379–384, 386–388, 393, 403–406, 408, 411, 412, 425, 426, 429, 430, 434, 439, 440, 442–444, 447, 449, 452, 456, 458–460, 463–469, 471, 473–475, 477–479
Polymyxin e, 9, 42, 86, 119, 122, 125, 130, 165, 167, 169, 170, 191, 193, 213, 280, 356, 358, 360, 412, 413, 415, 427, 431, 432, 435

P (*cont.*)
Posaconazole, 92–94, 103, 104–106, 113, 348
Postoperative complications, 261, 296, 389, 393, 399
Potential pathogen, 3, 7, 9, 11, 17, 23, 33, 50, 53, 55, 119, 126, 128, 165, 167–273, 275–277, 283, 284, 301, 355–357, 364, 429, 430, 434, 435, 438, 468
Pre-emptive, 92, 112, 320
Pregnancy, 68, 253, 256, 271, 322
Prevention, 12, 25, 36, 40, 47, 48, 58, 59, 104, 113, 117, 122, 129, 130, 132, 136, 137, 142, 145–147, 153, 155, 157–161, 175, 176, 179, 186, 199–201, 204, 206, 208, 209, 214, 219, 224, 233, 268, 270, 271, 279, 280, 284, 286, 296, 309, 310, 312, 331, 333, 350, 352, 354, 367, 368, 372, 376, 380, 381, 383, 386–388, 403–408, 423, 425, 426, 439, 440–444, 449, 454, 456, 460, 477, 478, 479
Probiotics, 90, 199, 200, 214, 217, 301, 375, 376, 379, 384, 387, 398, 441, 442
Prokinetics, 359, 376
Prolonged hospitalization, 389
Prophylaxis, 9, 24, 59, 60, 92, 93, 95, 96, 104, 108, 111–114, 127, 130, 132–134, 151, 156, 158, 161, 166, 168–171, 174, 175, 185, 191, 199–202, 208–210, 212, 213, 217, 259, 261, 262, 268, 270, 272, 279–281, 285, 286, 298–303, 309, 311, 312, 314, 320, 322, 325–327, 333, 334, 338, 346, 349, 351, 352, 368, 370, 372, 376, 377, 379, 381, 382, 387, 401, 402, 405–410, 425, 426, 440, 442, 444, 458, 475, 478, 480, 481

S
Secondary endogenous infection, 5, 29, 42, 43, 45, 169, 186, 193, 412, 429, 475
Selective decontamination of the digestive tract (sdd), 3, 134, 145, 168, 191, 280, 296, 403, 411, 415, 417–419, 422, 423, 431, 433, 437, 450, 464
Semirecumbent position, 159, 160, 210, 212, 381, 385, 386, 388, 466, 468, 478
Sepsis, 1, 2, 9, 10, 12–14, 23, 26, 37, 64, 69, 72, 89, 112, 115, 129, 138, 175, 179, 184, 199, 201, 223, 226, 229–234, 237, 238, 240, 241, 246–248, 250, 251, 258, 266, 267, 270, 274, 278, 285, 287–289, 291, 294, 295, 307, 322, 324, 332, 335, 336, 343, 355, 356, 359, 360, 362, 366, 367, 368, 370–372, 376–378, 391, 393, 397, 401–403, 406, 408, 409, 437, 441, 443, 445, 451, 454, 455, 457–460, 463, 471, 472, 480
Septic shock, 2, 9, 10, 12, 13, 64, 69, 89, 112, 223, 226, 229–232, 234, 250, 263, 267, 287–291, 294, 295, 337, 355, 359, 360, 362, 366, 367, 369, 371–374, 377, 378, 437, 445, 451, 458, 471, 480
Severe infections, 56, 72, 145, 362, 430, 475
Shock, 2, 9, 10, 12, 13, 26, 37, 64, 69, 70, 89, 112, 199, 201, 215, 223, 226, 229–232, 234, 241, 243, 244, 249–251, 263, 267, 287–291, 294, 295, 322, 328, 337, 341, 355, 359, 360, 362, 366, 367, 369, 371–374, 376–378, 383, 392, 401, 402, 408, 413, 437, 441, 443, 445, 451, 458, 468, 471, 472, 480
Silver-coated endotracheal tube, 150, 151, 160, 385
Solid organ transplant, 296, 298, 300, 301, 303, 307, 312, 313
Source control, 240, 267, 363, 456
Spectrum of activity, 75–77, 79, 80, 82, 83, 85–88, 93, 95, 96, 100, 103, 107, 166, 167, 261
Stress-ulcer prophylaxis, 208, 212, 213, 381, 382
Stress-ulcer-related bleeding (surb), 401, 406
Subglottic secretion drainage, 159, 209, 382, 384–387, 464, 469, 478
Surgical site, 125, 258, 260, 270
Surveillance cultures, 3, 9, 31, 43, 47, 52, 53, 55–58, 121, 126, 145, 147, 179, 184, 186–188, 190–192, 274, 275, 354, 360, 362, 364, 365, 367, 411, 428, 430, 439, 474, 475
Surveillance samples, 3, 8, 9, 15–17, 41, 50–53, 55–57, 59, 121, 123, 169, 172, 173, 193, 277, 300, 354, 365, 431
Surveillance, 2, 3, 8, 9, 12, 15–17, 29, 31, 33, 39, 41, 43, 47, 48, 50–59, 92, 98, 99, 115, 121, 123, 126, 134, 143–145, 147, 155, 169, 170, 172, 173, 176, 179, 180, 184–188, 190, 191–193, 208, 216, 219, 224, 232, 245, 274, 275, 277, 285, 297, 300, 328, 330, 333, 342, 354, 355, 360–362, 364, 365, 367, 380, 393, 411, 413, 419, 428, 430, 431, 439, 457, 474, 475
Systemic inflammatory response, 2, 9, 10, 13, 223, 237, 278, 366, 371, 389, 391

Systemic, 2, 8, 9, 10, 13, 18, 20, 21, 23, 25, 33, 41, 49, 51, 58, 59, 61, 63, 65, 67, 69, 71–73, 75, 77, 79, 81, 83, 85, 87, 89, 91, 92, 94, 96, 98, 100–102, 104, 106, 108, 110–119, 119, 124, 129, 131, 133, 156–158, 166, 168, 169, 175, 176, 193, 197, 199, 213, 223, 226, 229, 236–238, 241, 243–245, 251–253, 256–258, 263, 267, 278, 281, 284, 285, 299–301, 307, 309, 311, 352, 357–360, 362–364, 366–371, 373, 375, 389, 391, 392, 394, 395, 405, 406, 413, 423, 432, 439, 440, 478

T

Tobramycin, 9, 24, 42, 67, 69, 70, 74, 80, 81, 85, 119–124, 126, 130–132, 164, 165, 167, 169, 171, 191, 193, 197, 198, 213, 261, 280, 300, 356,
358, 360, 412, 413, 415, 417–419, 421–424, 428, 431, 432, 434, 435, 475

Toxicity, 65, 66, 78, 81, 85, 86, 95, 101, 102, 110, 130, 168, 169, 289, 292, 299, 310, 318–323, 355, 358, 472

Transmission, 8, 11, 35, 45, 47, 51, 53, 57, 59, 116, 125–128, 139, 142, 146, 147, 151, 179, 180, 182, 185, 186, 191, 193, 209, 272, 273, 315, 316, 318, 323, 325–327, 329–331, 364, 366, 383, 404, 434, 438, 456, 477

Treatment, 3, 8, 9, 13, 25, 31, 33–37, 41, 43, 51, 53, 55, 56, 59, 71, 72, 78, 89–91, 93–97, 108, 112–115, 122, 123, 126, 127, 129, 130, 132, 135, 149, 152, 154, 171, 172, 174, 175, 176, 182–187, 191, 200, 206, 208, 215, 216, 226, 229, 230, 232, 234–238, 240, 241, 246–248, 250, 251, 257–259, 261, 271, 282–284, 287–295, 297, 298, 301–303, 306, 307, 309, 310, 312, 314, 321, 322, 326–329, 332, 340, 341, 343–348, 351–355, 357–361, 363, 368, 370, 373, 376–378, 380, 386, 391, 405, 408, 411, 412, 414, 420, 430, 431, 434, 435, 442, 445, 447, 449, 454, 456–462, 471, 472, 475, 480

U

Urinary tract, 9, 11, 18, 22, 25, 28, 81, 82, 144, 149, 151, 157, 159, 161, 183, 219, 222, 225, 226, 229, 235, 237, 239, 241, 243, 245, 247, 249, 251, 253, 255, 257, 259, 261, 262, 263, 265, 267, 269, 271, 279, 299, 304, 308, 355, 360, 393, 451, 453

Urosepsis, 175, 356, 360

V

Vaccination, 298, 299, 309, 319

Vancomycin, 8, 13, 35, 37, 57–59, 62, 65, 74, 84–87, 91, 117–129, 131, 132, 134, 135, 144, 163, 165–167, 169–171, 173, 175, 178–180, 187–189, 193, 198, 203, 222, 250, 251, 261, 280, 292, 293, 301, 358, 360, 361, 364–366, 368, 413, 427, 431, 432, 435, 436, 439, 444–456, 460, 475

Vasodilators, 372, 376, 403, 405–407

Ventilator circuit, 209–211, 382, 384, 386, 456, 457

Ventilator-associated pneumonia, 1, 24, 33, 36, 37, 41, 48, 132, 144, 159, 160, 176, 201, 205, 208–210, 214, 216, 217, 294, 295, 298, 368, 380, 382, 384, 386–388, 403, 405, 411, 442, 449, 451, 452, 456, 458–460, 468, 478, 479

Viral, 8, 173, 177, 187, 253, 257, 274, 303, 304, 307, 312, 314, 318, 320, 321, 323, 324, 326, 328, 330–337, 342, 343, 345, 348, 351–353, 362, 363, 364

VRE, 8, 35, 48, 56, 86–88, 128, 135, 140, 143, 144, 163, 178–180, 186, 187, 198, 202, 222, 272, 279, 425, 429, 430, 436, 437, 441, 444, 456, 463, 466–468, 470, 474, 475

W

Wound, 7, 9, 12, 16, 17, 28, 41, 52, 138, 168, 170–172, 215, 219, 222, 227, 235, 237, 239, 241, 243, 245, 247, 249, 251–253, 255, 257–259, 261–263, 265, 267, 269–271, 276, 277, 279, 299, 300, 304, 308, 327, 330, 354, 356, 357, 360, 362–364, 393, 394, 412

Printed by Printforce, the Netherlands